Cerebral Palsy

Psiche Giannoni • Liliana Zerbino

Editors

Cerebral Palsy

A Practical Guide for Rehabilitation Professionals

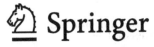

Editors
Psiche Giannoni
DIBRIS, University of Genoa
Genoa, Italy

Liliana Zerbino
DSS, University of Florence
Florence, Italy

Based on the Italian language edition "Fuori Schema" by Giannoni, Zerbino. Copyright © 2000 Springer-Verlag Italia. All rights reserved.

English translation of the original Italian edition published by Springer-Verlag Italia, Milan, 2000
ISBN 978-3-030-85621-2   ISBN 978-3-030-85619-9   (eBook)
https://doi.org/10.1007/978-3-030-85619-9

This Springer imprint is published by the registered company Springer Nature Switzerland AG
The registered company address is: Gewerbestrasse 11, 6330 Cham, Switzerland

Preface

This book has been written by therapists for therapists, with the intention of sharing a 50-year career in clinical and training experience in the field of cerebral palsy. It has been a 2-year challenge to prepare and is now an even greater responsibility to circulate, being fully aware from the beginning of two contrasting risks: that of seeming "rigid" by describing techniques on the one hand, and, at the same time, appearing too empirical, episodic, and fragmented on the other.

Today, rehabilitation treatments in cerebral palsy are based on both scientific evidence and clinical expertise, enhanced by those practical intervention strategies that therapists learn on-the-job every day, directly from the children, the parents, and caregivers. Formal education in this field has yet to be settled into an internationally agreed format and the numerous different "methods" and approaches that have emerged over the years continue to circulate and be applied separately or in casual, discordant combinations, mostly according to the professional's individual training opportunities.

As underlined throughout the text, techniques and technologies are necessary tools to be learned, understood, discussed, criticized, and applied in a rational, sensible, and flexible manner. However, techniques and technologies change over time, while the crucial requirement of addressing the global needs of the child and their family with open mindedness and appropriate clinical reasoning remains the same.

The leading authors are experienced and certified trainers in the neurodevelopmental treatment framework who are confident that the basic concepts advanced by their "trail-blazing" teacher, Berta Bobath, still remain extremely valid. For good reason, and as evident in this text, these principles have been further developed and enriched over the years by her "students," as it would have been impossible, and even unfair, to attempt to crystallize the Bobath approach in a rigid set of rules, frozen in time.

Berta herself invited her trainees to approach the child with special needs as a young person, caring for their rehabilitation with a holistic and individualized vision, not a treatment to be classified in a pre-arranged, standardized structure. This coincides with the key message that this text intends to transmit to its readers.

The book addresses the problems that involve the smaller child with cerebral palsy, together with certain aspects that follow through to adolescence. The child is always at the center of the proposed rehabilitation projects with the family fully integrated as proactive members of the team. On the basis of the authors' clinical experience and significant scientific references, each chapter of the book analyzes the different forms of the pathology, proposing the aims of treatment that can be used to guide the therapist's interventions, according to the functional potential and needs of each individual child and the specific phase of their development.

The text focuses particularly on the components related to the sensory-motor activities of the child, as well on those tasks related to the functional use of the upper limbs, all aimed at improving independence in daily life. Certain chapters share practical suggestions on feeding, communication, and visual problems which are frequently present in cerebral palsy. Attention is also given to the care of soft tissues, which is beneficial as the child moves from childhood towards adulthood. Last but not least, a chapter looks at the most recent technology, tools which are already assuming an essential and permanent role in pediatric rehabilitation.

Have we managed to meet the challenges and expectations that this publication represents? This has been the question on our minds from the beginning and it still remains. The answer can only come from the readers. In the meantime, we wished to have the opinion of distinguished colleagues who have kindly supported the text by reading the manuscript and expressed their views in the three commentaries following this Preface.

Genoa, Italy   Psiche Giannoni
Genoa, Italy   Liliana Zerbino

Commentary by Adrienne Davidson

The text *Cerebral Palsy: A Practical Guide for Rehabilitation Professionals*, prepared by Psiche Giannoni, Liliana Zerbino, and contributors is certainly a welcome addition to the publications available for therapists working with these very special young people and their great families. After working with children in Italy for 50 years, it is a particular pleasure to celebrate a book compiled by Italian physiotherapists, appreciating just how much good and hard work is done in this country by the teams of rehabilitation professionals.

The appraisal of the manuscript has been an occasion to reflect with an English friend and "sounding board" Tina Gericke, herself a pediatric occupational therapist who has shared parts of the Italian CP pioneering adventure. There is no doubt that our generations have been witness to, and participated in, a real revolution-evolution in rehabilitation for the pediatric age group. The field has certainly matured and expanded, particularly in the last 30 years, taking advantage of the teachings of many earlier "maestri." In fact, as "youngsters," all four of us were lucky enough to work closely with Professor Adriano Milani-Comparetti, who impressed us indelibly with many of the values that emerge in this book.

It is encouraging to know that the manual will be a source accessible to rehabilitation professionals working today, worldwide, in children's community and hospital services and in the different academic research and training contexts. The enthusiasm of younger professionals is rewarding to see, but also that of expert therapists, who take the trouble to publish in order to support the quality of the work done by others. The chapters of this text cover many areas of intervention in general, and of the early interventions for young infants, in preparation to enrich their activities and level of participation as they grow up.

Rehab in CP remains an intriguing and unexplainable challenge, still becoming a main field of interest for rehabilitation graduates moving into their pediatric specializations. They bring with them their energy and passion for the further development of the newer sectors of physical activity, recreation, sport, and technologies for the older children and adolescents.

All these realities will greet this publication because it represents a foundation stone for the treatment approach to these children. It can be considered a contribution to the state of the art. The distribution online will allow "nothing to be lost, nor forgotten," as it should be when colleagues select, write down, organize, and share their dedication and professional experiences with care, just like the authors have done in these pages.

Adrienne Davidson
Rehabilitation Department
Meyer Children's Hospital
Florence, Italy
University of Florence
Florence, Italy

Commentary by Daniela Morelli

It is with pleasure I write an introduction to this book, which is the result of the authors' expertise and their extensive experience in teaching many generations of therapists and doctors. I attended one of their courses in 2000, when I first became interested in pediatric rehabilitation, and this valuable experience greatly influenced my professional activity.

As a medical student of the 1970s and 1980s, I was trained on an approach to the doctor–patient relationship which was essentially "paternalistic," very different from the biopsychosocial model of the ICF.

The course I attended was, on the contrary, proposing a holistic approach to the child, where both the subject of observation first and the treatment later are seen as part of the environment where the child lives. The environment, in this case, refers not only to the physical environment around the child but also to a community that is caring, as defined by ICF. I am forever indebted to the authors for introducing me to this new approach to the child and their family.

It is no coincidence that one of the first pages of the handbook contains the following: "Taking the child on in therapy implies that the therapist is asking the family for 'permission' to enter a privileged relational context, and to accompany and support the child in their neurodevelopmental process. The therapist should never impose themselves intrusively on the parents–child relationship but should earn a 'mandate of trust' during the work together proposing a rehabilitation pathway characterized by sharing the aims to be achieved."

In this way, when the child is addressed directly at the beginning of the first visit, both child and parents are reassured, because they are recognized as "person" and it becomes clear that the examiner is interested in getting to know and establishing a relationship with the child, regardless of their abilities.

Many books today provide exhaustive and updated information on the state of the art of the research on normal motor development and on the main disorders of motor development. They address issues related to pathogenesis, new diagnostic tools based on the newest technologies with neuroimaging and neurophysiology, as well report on evidence-based therapeutic trends. Few books, however, deal with the topic in a practical way and make the reader reflect on the best observational practices and the best way to tackle the problems that may arise, and even fewer offer practical suggestions.

This handbook fills this gap in the literature and perfectly captures the rich experience and passion that have characterized the way the authors work. A book to read and consult whenever in doubt.

Daniela Morelli
Santa Lucia Foundation IRCCS
Rome, Italy

Commentary by Marjorie Woollacott and Anne Shumway-Cook

Cerebral Palsy: A Practical Guide for Rehabilitation Professionals is a highly readable text with extensive and up-to-date information on evaluating, creating, and carrying out rehabilitation plans for children with the different diagnoses of cerebral palsy.

We recommend its use in both academic setting in guiding the training of therapists in assessing and treating children with cerebral palsy and also as a reference tool for use in ongoing clinical practice.

Marjorie Woollacott
Department of Human Physiology
and Institute of Neuroscience
University of Oregon
Eugene, OR, USA

Anne Shumway-Cook
Department of Rehabilitation Medicine
University of Washington
Seattle, WA, USA

Acknowledgments

It is with gratitude that we dedicate this book to all children with impairment and their families that we have met during our professional life. These persons have contributed to making us understand their problems and to grow our experience.

We also acknowledge how important our *Maestri* were, who not only shared their know-how but taught us to be curious and urged to always update our minds, so as not to confine our work to a single technique or rehabilitation approach.

In particular, we wish to thank Pietro Morasso, who supported us in summarizing the state of the art about technological tools potentially useful in the field of rehabilitation.

We thank also the team of the Robert Hollman Foundation and Riccarda Barbieri for their collaboration.

Furthermore, we wish to express our gratitude to Adrienne Davidson who reviewed with extreme accuracy and competence this manuscript together with Tina Gericke and gave us excellent advice for the final draft.

Finally, we thank Gigi Degli Abbati and Serena Danieli, who with their creative hand drew the figures of this book with an intense expressive force that gave life to the drawn children, so much so that this book is now a small art gallery.

Contents

Child Evaluation Guide and Clinical Reasoning

Liliana Zerbino and Psiche Giannoni

Preliminary observation and treatment sessions are dedicated to knowing the child and their family, by observing the child's (approach to the environment, their ability to look around, move, listen, relate to an unfamiliar person, and adopt self-consoling strategies).

Taking the child on in therapy implies that the therapist is asking the family for "permission" to enter a privileged relational context and to accompany and support the child in their neuro-developmental process. The therapist should never impose themselves intrusively on the parent-child relationship but should earn a "mandate of trust" during the work together proposing a rehabilitation pathway characterized by sharing the aims to be achieved (Fig. 1.1).

The therapist, who meets face to face a child with neurodevelopmental problems for the first time, even if the child is a baby, cannot ignore the child's previous experiences. Association with the environment and with people has already impacted sometimes the experience in the short life of this baby and the family: for example, a preterm and/or problematic birth, followed by a long period of hospitalization in a neonatal intensive care unit, the time in an incubator, and diagnostic tests, may have created a challenging environment. The family itself emerges from the experience of a problematic birth and frequently manifests anxiety over the health of the child and their future, as well as a general sense of feeling at a loss (Negri 2014).

The therapist undertakes to think positively about the child's potential, trying to understand and enhance the child's uniqueness: their affectivity, emotions, perceptive style, ability to understand and express themselves, adaptive behavior, and motor problems. The theoretical reference model proposed here is specifically oriented to a holistic approach to clinical practice and underlines not only the need for

L. Zerbino
DSS, University of Florence, Florence, Italy

P. Giannoni (✉)
DIBRIS, University of Genoa, Genoa, Italy

© The Author(s), under exclusive license to Springer Nature Switzerland AG 2022   1
P. Giannoni, L. Zerbino (eds.), *Cerebral Palsy*,
https://doi.org/10.1007/978-3-030-85619-9_1

Fig. 1.1 Meeting with the child and their mother

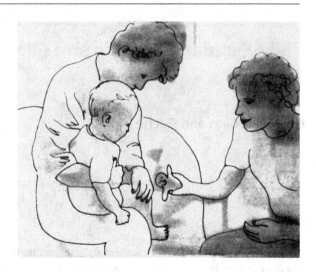

multidisciplinary intervention but also an interactive process between child and therapist (Bobath 1963; WHO 2007; Mayston 2016).

In all the rehabilitation phases, the assessment continually supports treatment, becoming a checking tool for what happens within the therapeutic setting. "[…]evaluation is a continuous process, it includes important variables that will emerge in the long term [...]. The therapist attempts to find out where the main problem lies and if anything can be changed" (Davies 2000).

The therapist begins to focus on some elements: initially, they observe the child in an overall context, with a gestaltic approach (Perls et al. 1951), and then they search for some particular element, linking situations and behaviors, asking themselves questions, in a sort of brainstorming, such as:

– What kind of relationship does the child establish with others? Do they have any referred references?
– What kind of "contacts" do they like and need? What ones do they not tolerate and make them annoyed?
– What communication strategies have they learned to use?
– What perceptive style does he do they adopt to get to know the environment?
– What functions have they already learned and use at the right time?
– What degree of independence have they already acquired?
– ………

Rehabilitation treatment is intended as the resolution of problems: the therapist must question all the "whys" that arise from careful observation of the child, using all their knowledge, experience, and creativity in search of possible solutions.

The questions posed by the therapist can address two research areas:

1. Interactive processes area
2. Area of spontaneous motor skills and functions

1.1   Interactive Process Area

From the very first moment that the therapist meets the child with the parents, they have the opportunity to detect and focus on the underlying elements in their relational exchange and the choice of posture/kinetics of both. They observe what the child can do, the communication strategies adopted when expressing primary needs or conveying moods, and the ways used to channel these messages.

The infant can draw the attention of the mother through how they look at her, how they cry, their vocal call, and the tonic/postural choice (e.g., the child stiffens in the mother's arms, to mean "no, I don't want"), while other children can communicate with verbal language, if present, with a mimic and gaze expression, the combined use of words and gestures, increased muscle stiffness, and more.

Inspired by the CARE-Index of Crittenden (2005), it is here suggested observation of the twosome caregiver/child, to avoid superficial interpretation by the therapist, of the quality of maternal care and any projections, addressed to the parental figure. The observation is directed toward both the twosome:

– Facial expression: Is the mother smiling? Are there any variations in expression? Does the child respond to a smile? Avoid eye contact? Does the child have a serious expression focused on the proposed activity?
– Vocal manifestations: Does the mother turn to her baby by speaking or humming, with sweetness and rhythm? Is the proposal appropriate for the age, state, and mood of the child? Does the child respond with vocalizations? Is the baby attentive?
– Position and body contact: How is the child held in her arms? Does the child turn their head toward the interlocutor, or is he/she held like a small baby in an all-encompassing embrace; is there a mutual body adaptation, or does the child demonstrate strongly increased stiffness or vice versa? Are they very hypotonic? Does the child's mother still manage to contain him/her?
– Affective expressions: Does the child's mother express pleasure in holding the child in her arms?
– Rhythm of role shifts: Does the mother give her baby time to organize an answer before making new proposals? Does she encourage them by alternating turns harmoniously? Does the child accept the adult's proposals? Does she touch them, whisper to them? Does the child participate in this joy prolonging eye, tactile, vocal contact, and are they able to initiate and interchange?
– Choice of activity: What activity or game does the mother propose to her child? Is it suitable for their age? Is it pleasant for the child? Does the child respond by accepting the game? Do they show interest?

It is always useful to ask the parents, at the time of the first meeting, to bring objects from home, toys that the child likes; in this way, the therapist will have further information on the child's skills and can better understand how they are perceived in the mind of the parents themselves.

The therapist should always approach the child, as "an interlocutor who, however compromised, is a person capable of weaving an interactive process, even by means of their own minimal signals." The therapist, at the time of the evaluation and during future treatments, must be aware of the interaction between parents and child, careful to grasp any communication cue, ready to facilitate not only the acquisition of skills but also the access to communication and expressive dialogue. "The therapist's action is not only a technical act but also, and simultaneously, a relational act" (Palazzoli Selvini 1987).

Also, the relationship modalities used by the therapist and the respect given to the child can become an indication for the family who, disoriented by the numerous problems, sometimes loses relationship spontaneity, often thinking that the child is unable to communicate.

> **The Family-Centered Care Model**
> In the rehabilitation process, the family-centered care model has the intention of improving the quality of life of the child, with neuro-developmental problems, together with that of the whole family, supporting parents considered as the experts of their child's needs and abilities. The participation of the family in the therapeutic program, from a partnership perspective, becomes of fundamental importance because it works together with professionals to make informed decisions about the services and interventions that the child and family receive (Law et al. 2003; King and Chiarello 2014). The aim of working with the family is therefore to promote the quality of life for all members, recognizing that each family is unique and a constant in the child's life and that the parents are the experts of their child.

The therapist analyzes verbal and non-verbal means of communication adopted by the child; discovers their interweaving, their evolution; and tries to understand them in light of the different cultural experiences of the families. The therapist is also careful to recognize all the information, as a noteworthy message that the child transmits, and tries to recognize its link with the environment (for further details, see Chap. 12).

1.1.1 Non-verbal Communication

Non-verbal communication is an important means for expressing emotions, attitudes, and conflicts.

This type of communication has the function of:

– Immediate control over the social environment (e.g., the therapist immediately understands if the child is bored or in disagreement with them, by observing their face, body position, sighs, etc.; in the same way, the child also tries to understand what is going on in the mind of the therapist)

– Support of oral communication, as further support to speech (e.g., the therapist who smiles and nods by moving their head communicates a non-verbal sign of approval)

– Replacement of oral communication which allows an alternative model to the verbal language

In non-verbal communication, the following signals are used:

- **Visual communication**
  This plays an important role in communicating interpersonal attitudes and in establishing relationships. It is closely linked to verbal oral and gestural communication. It is used in obtaining information on the other person's reactions, as a greeting to make contact and to show that the person understands what the other has expressed. The therapist should assess the child's use of visual communication observing the exchange of eye contact as a relational face-to-face dialogue, the recall, the escape, visual capture, co-orientation, harmony, etc. The visual system is the one most used in parent-child proto-communication, and it has a key role in promoting mutual attachment bonding (Fazzi et al. 2012). The child with CP impairment often has significant visual disturbances and, for example, could not look around giving an impression of refusal or indifference toward others.

  It is of fundamental importance that the therapist is aware of any visual system deficits in the children they are treating. They need to carefully investigate every child's visual function and have the opportunity to share their observations with visual rehabilitation professionals (for further information, see Chap. 11).

- **Facial mimicry**
  Facial expressions are manifestations of human emotions, and they convey all types of feelings like happiness with smiling and fear and apprehensive and "anxious face." The baby, as all young children, uses mimicry to capture the adult's immediate attention (for further details, see Chap. 12). Normally, a complex game of highly differentiated expressions is observed, made possible by the complex integrated activity of facial muscles, whereas, in the case of pathology, there can be a lack of facial mimicry or poorly modulated facial expressions, making it difficult to interpret the youngster's communication signals.

- **Hand gestures**
  Movements of hands can be highly expressive and useful for short communication tasks and can be considered a second language. They are embodied in specific cultural practices and so are learned and used very differently. Gestures are also connected to the emotional states of the mind and can have a particular meaning within oral communication. These signs can have a precise meaning (e.g., "hello," call someone with a nod), illustrate/accentuate words (e.g., tell the tale of *Pinocchio* describe the long nose with a gesture), and express mood (e.g., show a fist in a sign of anger). However, the person with an impairment—as the child with CP—often does not have the necessary dexterity.

- **Body language**

  As in adults, postures vary according to the emotional state of the child, and the therapist needs to be able to interpret the emotional and motor expression of the tonic modulations in the child with cerebral palsy (CP). Often these children have the limited repertoire of postural and movement choices which makes it hard to understand what they want to communicate through their body language. For example, a child in a wheelchair who extends with the identical excessive tonic movements can be communicating joy or pain or maybe acceptance or denial, making it extremely difficult for the interlocutor to decode the message.

- **Body space**

  The way a person occupies a space, and moves into the space of the other, has a meaning. For example, if there is no empathy/interest between the child and an adult (or other child), the two will "keep their distance." The orientation of the bodies of the persons in the interpersonal space can express the kind of relationships between them: collaboration, familiarity, intimacy, hierarchy, and so on. The movement and position of the body in space are a commonly used way of creating differentiated personal, peri-personal, and extrapersonal spatial relationships.

1.1.2 Verbal Communication

Language is a means of communication that carries out two important functions:

(a) Mutual communication, if those speaking and listening give the same meaning to the words
(b) Simplification of thought and behavior

Words have meanings. They are used to indicate different types of objects, to communicate an array of feelings and related ideas. In cerebral palsy, the children often use excessively words to escape from the required task or because words are the best way for the child to organize and control the environment around them.

Even the health professionals can use words to an excess to fill a silence or give commands, thus dominating the communication space.

All therapists are involved in the area of communication, working in close contact with the other rehabilitators including the specialized professionals like speech and language therapists and the augmentative and alternative communication team (see also Chap. 12). The common goal of the rehabilitation team regarding communication intervention in children with CP is to avoid that their communication impairments lead to a reduction in their social participation, adversely affecting cognitive and personality development.

1.2 Spontaneous Motor Skills and Functional Areas

1.2.1 The Newborn and Infant

Neurological and functional evaluation is based on the traditional neurological examination, through the exploration of evoked responses; the observation of spontaneous movements produced, endogenously, by the central nervous system; and various neurodevelopmental assessments. Over the past decades, numerous neurological examination protocols have been proposed, which are used during the first year of life, both for premature and term infants (André-Thomas and Saint-Anne Dargassies 1952; Amiel-Tison 1968; Prechtl and Beintema 1964; Touwen 1976; Milani Comparetti and Gidoni 1967; Milani Comparetti 1982; Prechtl 1990, 2001; Dubowitz and Dubowitz 1981; Dubowitz et al. 2005; Romeo et al. 2016; Picciolini et al. 2016).

Particular mention needs to be made of the work of Brazelton (1973) and Als (Als et al. 1982; Als 1986, 2009) who contributed greatly to the understanding of the newborn's responses to the outside world and to the assessment of their behavior, development, and neurological status.

Brazelton bases his approach on the concept that the newborn is a very capable individual who, at birth, already possesses their own complex behavioral repertoire. The author conceived the Neonatal Behavioral Assessment Scale (NBAS) as an interactive examiner-baby-parent assessment, which aims at bringing out the newborn's "best performances" in their behavioral organization with the support of the examiner. The use of this scale enhances the understanding of the behavioral characteristics of the newborn, focuses on their relationship with the environment, and facilitates the parents' understanding of the behavior of their child.

Als developed the synactive theory emphasizing the importance to observe the behavior of the premature infant and proposing individualized and evolutionary assistance programs respectful and adapted to the needs of the newborn and their family. After that she proposed the Neonatal Individualized Developmental Care and Assessment Program (NIDCAP) aiming to reduce the stress of the newborn and involve parents in the early care of them.

The protocol proposed by Prechtl is based on the observation of spontaneous movements of the preterm and term infant, from birth to 4 months of age. These movements are defined by Prechtl as "General Movements" (GM). If the examiner highlights elements of abnormality in GMs, a neurological motor pathology of the central nervous system is assumed (Ferrari et al. 2016).

1.2.2 The Toddler and Preschooler

The evaluation starts by observing a functional situation (e.g., the child eating a biscuit, taking off their sweater, putting on their shoes, etc.) or spontaneous play (e.g., the child sees a doll in the room, observes it, takes it, puts it to sleep, etc.). The therapist notes the quality and variability of the repertoire of movements that the child uses and the mental processes that seem to underlie their actions.

The physiotherapist must evaluate the child's behavior both through direct observation and through collecting indirect information (e.g., asking family and teachers, looking at video footages, etc.). The therapist must bear in mind not the chronological age of the child, but the repertoire of functional skills already learned, in progress or defect.

There are some privileged areas of observation, useful for a deeper knowledge and understanding of the child and for the reasoning of the treatment planning:

- **Dressing**
  The therapist observes which components of dressing and undressing skills have already been acquired by the child and how they are combined in the praxic-motor actuation (e.g., is the child able to get one or both arms out of the sleeves of their sweater? Do they need help to get it over their head? Are they able to take off their shoes? etc.). They need to keep in mind that independence in the dressing-undressing routine is neurodevelopmentally possible and more or less completed around the age of 4 or 5 years, even though these functional abilities are closely linked to the educational style in the home. Guided by the family member's attitude, the therapist can progressively suggest various praxic sequences and the best positions (e.g., the child can deal with their trousers either sitting, standing, or lying on their back, take off their shoes in sitting or standing, and so on).
- **Personal Hygiene and Toilet Use**
  (a) Self-care: the child learns to take care of their personal hygiene and the physiological rules and social expectations regarding cleanliness in their home environment and when they attend educational institutions like daycare centers, play groups, and preschool. The acquisition of complex tasks such as face washing, brushing teeth, bathing, and showering is a lengthy process which involves the gradual learning and practice of intermediate skills (e.g., the child initially learns to wash their hands and later their face and to clean their teeth) as they improve their dexterity and the use of the selective movements in the upper limbs.
  (b) Toilet training: the acquisition of sphincter control in infants is a delicate matter and, once again, a culturally and educational dependent issue where the therapist will need to know and respect the family's reference models. The admission of the child to preschool usually marks a time limit for these skills as children are usually toilet trained by around the age of 3 years.

In children with neurological impairment, the therapist needs to support not only the process of acquisition of sphincter control itself but also the best toileting positions and devices for the infant and then later the older child and adolescent.

- **Nutrition**

As for dressing, progressive learning is involved in self-feeding, beginning from weaning time at around 6 months of age. Normally children can be self-sufficient in feeding by around the age of 3 years, except for the ability to cut hard consistencies with a fork and knife.

Feeding and self-feeding are developmental milestones which need therapeutic support in cases of children with psychomotor impairment. In these cases, it is useful for both the physiotherapist and the speech therapist to observe the modalities chosen by parents to feed their child, to evaluate the child's level of postural control, their oro-motor function and eye-hand-mouth coordination, as well as the activities and rituals in use at the child's and the family's mealtimes in the home.

When the child is older, these assessments will be enriched by directly observing the mealtime routine at school or through video footage provided by parents. The therapists need to evaluate the child's position, their type of chair, the size of the table, how they hold the spoon, the motor control and coordination of their feeding actions, and the differentiated activity of the two hands.

It is also important to assess the different characteristics of the food proposed, including its tastes, smells, and presentation. Frequently, especially in cases of severe impairment, the children's main course is presented in a dish with all ingredients mixed together and thus with indefinable flavors, smells, and colors. The consistency of the food is other element to be evaluated. Foods which are too liquid can be a problem, while those that are too solid can make swallowing difficult (see also Chap. 10).

Intervention promoting self-feeding skills could include the guidance of the child's upper limb movements with tactile-kinesthetic information, as suggested by the Affolter-Modell (Affolter 1981, 2004) (see Chap. 6). Learning can be facilitated through the play feeding of an adult or older sibling and pretend play of feeding a doll.

- **Movement Within the Environment**

A child with traditional development gradually acquires the necessary skills to move independently. Through movement they receive sensory inputs that promote body awareness, and they understand the characteristics of the environment and the spatial-temporal relationships between themself and the outside world.

At birth, the baby has little ability to respond to the new gravitational forces, but, over a period of 12–18 months, they quickly learn to roll, creep, pivot, crawl on all fours, stand up, and finally walk in the erect position. Later on, they can go up and down stairs, run, jump, and skip.

In motor assessment of the child with CP, the therapist needs to observe not only the functional level reached but also the motor and cognitive strategies adopted to obtain a desired goal and to regulate their emotional and affective behavior in the process of separation from their primary adults. Sometimes the infant can improve their functional abilities with the use of an aid, which, at times, is the only way to reach the goal. Occasionally the temporary use of a piece of equipment can be the solution for a specific environmental context like using a wheelchair to go to the stadium when at home the youngster moves around walking.

The therapist takes into consideration:

(a)   The child's antigravity abilities, e.g., what transfers they can manage alone and which need assistance and how their tonic stiffness changes during tasks of different levels of complexity

(b)   The sensory-motor abilities of the child to adapt to their surroundings, e.g., to slow down, stop, change direction, overcome obstacles, and how they cope with large, noisy, and crowded spaces, different types of terrain, and climatic conditions like wind and rain

1.2.3   The School-Aged Child, the Adolescent, and Toward Adulthood

Starting school is very demanding for a child with CP and is a particular phase for the child themself, their family members, the teachers, and the entire rehabilitation team. The child's life will now be orientated not only on playing but also on learning to write and read and on becoming more independent in external environments.

The rehabilitation team needs to consider this new situation long before school starts and start dealing with the various challenges involved. They will need to focus on those functional needs that are emerging for the child and their family, considering that the child's most important, reachable neuromotor developmental milestones are more or less achieved in the first 5 years of life (Latash and Anson 1996). This does not mean that basic posturomotor requirements should be neglected, but, on the contrary, aspects like postural alignment to prevent soft tissue alterations and pain still require careful attention throughout middle childhood and adolescence.

Evaluation should involve the entire multidisciplinary team, which, according to ICF (WHO 2007), considers the following aspects:

- **Cognitive level**
  Identify the child's cognitive strengths and aspects that need to improve. It is not a question of labelling the child, but of understanding their potential and collaborating with teachers and pedagogists to overcome any learning difficulties. Cognitive assessment mainly includes verbal comprehension, perceptual reasoning, working memory, and speed of processing.
- **Motor abilities and needs**
  The therapist should verify the accesses and the architectural barriers to the school buildings and evaluate how the child can cope with them.

  It is necessary to verify if the child can move with or without aids, inside the classroom and in all other school environments. Are they able to transfer from the entrance to the classroom and then to their desk? Can they get from their classroom to the toilet and to the school canteen and recreation areas?

The team should assess the need for the postural care plan verifying if there are therapeutic indications to change the child's positions during school hours. For example, reduce sitting time to avoid muscle retraction at the hips and knees but, at the same time, allowing the child to continue their participation in class activities.

- **Vocal communication abilities**
  When the child does not have efficient vocal/verbal communication, an alternative strategy needs to be found to support the relationship between the child, the teachers, and companions, e.g., suggesting a communication board, speech-generating devices, etc. (for further details, see Chap. 12).
- **Writing/reading abilities**
  Verify if the school bench is suitable for the child's type of chair and if it facilitate their writing and reading activities

  Check if the child can efficiently use a writing tool, such as a pencil or an electronic device and whether a paper book or an electronic text is more appropriate for reading (see Chap. 12 and Sect. 13.1 of Chap. 13, for more details).
- **Leisure/recreational needs**
  Children and adolescents with CP, like all able-bodied people, need to participate and benefit from leisure activities, improving their health and well-being (Palisano et al. 2011; Shikako-Thomas et al. 2014).

  Fortunately, nowadays there are recreational and sporting initiatives available for young people with special needs. Therapists should be aware of these activities and help the youngsters and their families identify the most suitable, primarily to foster their social relationships and physical well-being. Many activities are comprehensive of both enjoyment and therapeutic benefits, such as horseback riding both for fun and to improve postural alignment and balance, as reported in several studies (Martín-Valero et al. 2018; Mutoh et al. 2019). Aquatic activities are also of great benefit to these young people, right though infancy, childhood, and adolescence, facilitating experiences of movement with less gravity and different sensory inputs (Gorter and Currie 2011; Ballaz et al. 2011).

Mobility and functional ability problems arise again when the adolescent with CP is introduced into employment. Such new events require updating the young person's functional and behavioral assessments considering the tasks involved, including overcoming architectural barriers and the use of work utensils and instruments. Technology will most likely help the older person adult with CP and the therapist to find adaptive solutions (see also Sect. 13.1).

Like all teenagers on the way to adulthood, the adolescent with CP will have many of the same psychological problems, some of which can be more challenging than others, like their different physical appearance and the sphere of their sexuality. For this, it may be wise to refer the adolescent to qualified counselling and/or psychological help.

Other problems arising in adults with CP include fatigue and pain due to increased immobility and worsening of musculoskeletal deformities (Sienko 2018; Pizzighello et al. 2019; Fosdahl et al. 2020). It is very important to maintain surveillance and assessment of their physical status over the years, providing all the necessary maintenance and preventive interventions to maintain an optimal quality of life (Bottos et al. 2001; Livingston et al. 2007; Opheim et al. 2009; Makris et al. 2019; Gjesdal et al. 2020; van der Slot et al. 2020) (see also Chap. 6, Sect. 6.2 and Chap. 7).

1.3   Clinical Reasoning

In health care, clinical reasoning (CR) is defined as a process of thinking and decision-making associated with clinical practice (Barrows and Tamblyn 1980). Clearly, there is not a single template to mechanically apply to all clinical situations, independently of the main focus of a specific application area: for example, diagnostic, prognostic, or rehabilitative.

In the field of rehabilitation, the main purpose of CR is to induce the therapist to first carry out a careful assessment of the person to be treated and their functional potential and then to develop an articulated plan which meets that person's individual, specific needs.

Furthermore, CR goes beyond the simple application of a single rehabilitation approach or method. It implies that the therapist uses a critical and analytical thought process in their decision-making procedure, without passively or automatically following any single therapeutic paradigm, applying current trends or intervention routines instead of solid, rational, evidence-supported guidelines (NICE 2017, 2019) and flexible interventions based on the problem-solving technique. CR is much more than a simple application of a theory even though the foundations offered by various theoretical models can undoubtedly enhance the professional's practical experience, but, alone, a single theory will never guarantee the *quality* of CR.

In fact, in the context of clinical practice, CR is a multifaceted process requiring multi-agent interactions. Particularly when treating children with CP, the therapist should establish not only a close relationship with the child, their parents, other family members, and caregivers but also with child's team of health professionals. According to the medical diagnosis, the team determines together the maximum functional prognosis and the goals of the rehabilitation project, establishing the necessary verification and measurements of the results of the various interventions. CR involves the therapists in a continuous problem-solving approach regarding the management of their specific interventions work, to guarantee that the therapeutic actions carried out have meaning and consistency with all that has previously been observed, evaluated, and reflected on.

CR leads the rehabilitation professional to formulate a set of fundamental actions that can be summarized as follows:

1. History-taking
2. Clinical and objective evaluation

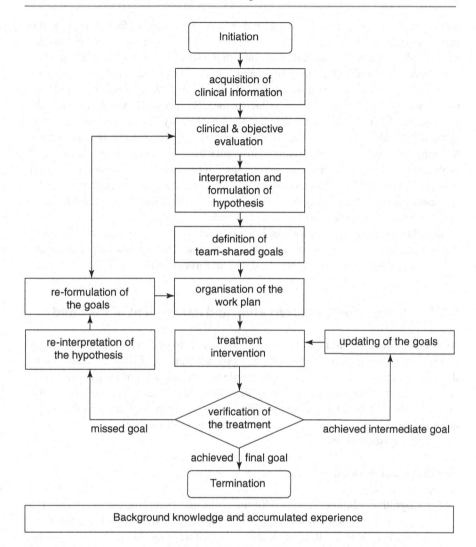

Fig. 1.2 Flowchart of the clinical reasoning process (courtesy of Pietro Morasso)

3. Analysis and definition of aims
4. Direct and indirect treatment intervention
5. Periodic reassessments and verification of results
6. Up-dating of needs and treatment plan
7. Discharge, when appropriate according to the pathology

Figure 1.2 shows the process more in detail:

The theoretical model of CR particularly useful in physical therapy practice is the hypothetical-deductive proposal (Jones 1995; Higgs and Jones 1995; Jones et al. 2000), to which many rehabilitation approaches refer. However, CR is also influenced by many external and internal factors. The external factors include the person to be treated and their family and person's needs, expectations, and fundamental values, while the internal ones concern the specific knowledge of the professional and their individual reasoning and clinical experience. CR also includes formulating and reflecting on hypotheses. Undoubtedly, the professional's individual knowledge and training greatly influence the CR process. However, it is not only the amount of knowledge that is decisive for good quality CR but also the ability to apply it profitably in the specific clinical situation. For this reason, an experienced therapist will have more professional substance and wisdom to draw on and will probably formulate more accurate and targeted intervention hypotheses, compared to a less experienced colleagues (Doody and McAteer 2002). Of course, this will be the result provided they apply their experience with open mindedness and flexibility, avoiding any dogmatic positions and attitudes.

Details on dealing with history-taking, observation, and evaluation are discussed in the next section, while other chapters address the characteristics, specific problems, and practical suggestions for the different forms of CP.

1.3.1 Outlines for the Observation and Assessment of the Child

After taking the medical history, the therapist begins to observe the child, focusing on and understanding their developmental potential and rehabilitation needs. First, they ask the child to carry out perform simple actions related to real-life, functional situations and previously agreed on with them or the parent. The context of the evaluation itself can suggest a function like undressing at the beginning of the evaluation session, activated with "Could you take off your sweater, please?"

The therapist observes:

- **What** the child does.
  Examples:
  (a) Cognitive relational ability: did the child understand verbal language? Do they need gestural, mimic-expressive emphasis? Did they associate the word "sweater" with the item of clothing they are wearing? Do they anticipate the gesture with their eyes? Do they need help? etc.
  (b) Adaptive skills: does the child find one or more solutions to solve the task? Can they simplify it? Do they choose an advantageous postural situation? Are they able to modify their strategy in the presence of environmental variables? etc.
- **How** does the child carry out the task, considering the type of environment, child-environment interactions, and the repertoire of movements used?
  Examples:
  (a) Postural choice: does the child sit down by themself? What characteristics does the sitting support base have? Is the child standing? What are the characteristics of the floor? Does the child need assistance? etc.
  (b) Interaction between the different parts of the body and the support base: does the child put their feet on the ground? Are the parts of the body aligned with

each other? Are there any balance reactions? Do they have selective pelvic movements? Do they have rotation of the girdles? etc.

(c) Use of sensory channels: does the child maintain postural control without visual feedback (e.g., when the sweater passes over their head)? Are they afraid of falling? Do they control their peri-personal space? etc.

(d) Use of upper limbs: does the child have sufficient proximal stability? How do they approach objects? Is there hand-eye coordination? Is bimanual exploration present? Do they have distal selective movements? Which ones? Is their praxic organization age-appropriate? etc.

With the specific characteristics of the pathology in mind, the therapist will pose certain questions:

- **Why** does the child make certain choices and exclude others?
  Example:
  (a) The child took off their sweater while remaining seated, with poor core sta-bility and balance reaction response, i.e., they straighten their trunk, move their center of gravity backward, and do not have efficient weight-bearing on their feet.
  Possible reasons:
  − Visual and/or vestibular disorders
  − Inadequate tonic recruitment
  − Poor selective pelvic movements
  − Proprioceptive disorders, e.g., in the feet
  − Contractures/retractions/alterations of the soft tissues
  − Presence of involuntary movements
  − Inadequate equipment
  − ...

1.3.2 Assessment Scales

Therapists should carefully evaluate the child with selected clinical scales that assess their functional potential and rehabilitation needs. These scales should be compiled after the initial meetings with the child and then again periodically throughout the intervention process to verify the results of the treatments.

The indications of ICF-CY may also be considered during assessment when using clinical scales. Its three classification domains of impairment, activities, and participation should reflect exactly the contents and the aims that lead a therapist to use one clinical scale rather than another.

In Table 1.1, clinical scales for the evaluation of the child or adolescent with CP are indicated. Some of them address assessment for impairment; other scales are more focused on functional activities and others (marked here with the sign *) con-sider both the domains. Other scales concerning specific forms or particular aspects of CP are reported in the chapters where the specific pathological forms are analyzed.

Table 1.1 Scales and instrumental evaluations in CP

Scales for the evaluation of the impairment

They aim to detect the impairment of the person, regarding:

- Range of movement (RoM) (instrumental):
  - PRoM (passive)
  - ARoM (active)
- Selective motor control
  - Selective Control Assessment of the Lower Extremity (SCALE) (Fowler et al. 2009)
  - Selective Control of the Upper Extremity Scale (SCUES) (Wagner et al. 2016)
- Muscle strength
  - Maximum Voluntary Isometric Contraction (MVIC)/Maximum Voluntary Contraction (MVC) (instrumental)
  - Maximum Voluntary Contraction (MVC) (instrumental)
  - Manual Muscle Test (MMT) (Manikowska et al. 2018)
- Muscle stiffness
  - Modified Tardieu Scale (MTS) (Haugh et al. 2006)
  - Modified Ashworth Scale (MAS) (Bohannon and Smith 1987)
  - Hypertonia Assessment Tool (HAT) (Jethwa et al. 2010)
- Sensation and perception
  - Sensory Integration and Praxis Test (SIPT) (Ayres 1989)
  - Revised Nottingham Sensation Assessment (rNSA), validated in adults (Lincoln et al. 1998)
  - Fugl-Meyer Assessment (FMA-UE, sect. H) (Fugl-Meyer et al. 1975)

Scales for the evaluation of the activity

These aim at defining the functioning level of the person, regarding:

- General functioning
  - Gross Motor Function Classification (GMFC)* (Russell et al. 2000)
  - Bayley Scales of Infant and Toddler Development™, Fourth Edition (Bayley™-4) (Bayley and Aylward 2019)
  - Goal Attainment Scaling (GAS) (Kiresuk and Sherman 1968; King et al. 2000)
  - Pediatric Evaluation of Disability Inventory (PEDI) (Haley et al. 1992)
  - Wee-Functional Independence Measure (WeeFIM) (Ottenbacher et al. 2000)
  - Neurosensory Motor Developmental Assessment (NSMDA) (Burns et al. 1989a, b)
  - Fugl-Meyer Assessment—Upper Extremities (FMA-UE)* (Fasoli et al. 2009)
  - Fugl-Meyer Assessment—Lower Extremities (FMA-LE)* (Balzer et al. 2016)
- Balance and reaching
  - Pediatric Reach Test (PRT) (Bartlett and Birmingham 2003)
  - Functional Reach Test (FRT) (Donohoe et al. 1994)
  - Segmental Assessment of Trunk Control (SATCo) (Butler et al. 2010)
  - Seated Postural and Reaching Control test (SP&R-co) (Santamaria et al. 2020)
  - Pediatric Balance Scale (PBS) (Franjoine et al. 2003)
  - Trunk Impairment Scale (TIS) (Sæther and Jørgensen 2011)
  - Trunk Control Measurement Scale (TCMS) (Heyrman et al. 2011)
- Walking
  - Timed Up and Go (TUG) (Williams et al. 2005) (instrumental)
  - 1-Minute Walk Test (1MWT) (McDowell et al. 2005) (instrumental)
  - Modified 6-Minute Walk Distance (6MVD) test (Geiger et al. 2007) (instrumental)
  - Edinburgh Visual Gait Score (EVGS) (Read et al. 2003)
  - Dynamic Gait Index (DGI) (Evkaya et al. 2020)
  - The Functional Assessment Questionnaire (FAQ) 22-item skill set (Gorton 3rd et al. 2011)

Table 1.1 (continued)

- Manual dexterity and perception
  - Manual Ability Classification System (MACS and Mini-MACS) (Eliasson et al. 2006, 2017)
  - Quality of Upper Extremity Skills Test (QUEST)* (DeMatteo et al. 1992)
  - ABILHAND-Kids (Arnould et al. 2004)
  - Box and Block Test (BBT) (Mathiowetz et al. 1985; Jongbloed-Pereboom et al. 2013)
  - Assisting Hand Assessment (AHA) (Krumlinde-Sundholm and Eliasson 2003)
  - Hand Assessment for Infants (HAI) (Krumlinde-Sundholm et al. 2017)
  - Melbourne Assessment of Unilateral Upper (Krumlinde-Sundholm and Eliasson 2003)
  - Limb Function (MUUL and MA2) (Randall et al. 1999, 2008)
  - In-Hand Manipulation Test (IMT) (Breslin and Exner 1999)
  - Tyneside Pegboard Test (TPT) (Basu et al. 2018)
  - Jebsen-Taylor Hand Function Test (JTHFT) (Tofani et al. 2020)
  - Test of Arm Selective Control (TASC) (Sukal-Moulton et al. 2018)
  - Bimanual Fine Motor Function (BFMF 2) (Elvrum et al. 2017)
  - Action Research Arm Test (ARAT): for individuals 13 years of age and older (Lyle 1981)
  - Besta Scale (Rosa-Rizzotto et al. 2014)
- Communication
  - Communication Function Classification System (CFCS) (Hidecker et al. 2011)

Scales for the evaluation of participation

Their aim is to define subjective implications, related to the person and their daily life in the community. Depending on the child's chronological age, their cognitive level, and the kind of investigation, the assessment requires the child's self-report or the parent proxi-report:

- Satisfaction and quality of life:
  - Pediatric Quality of Life Inventory (PedsQL™ 4.0) (Varni et al. 2001)
  - Child Health Questionnaire (CHQ) (Landgraf et al. 1998)
  - Quality of Life Questionnaire for Children (CP QOL-Child), Primary Caregiver Questionnaire (4–12 years) (https://www.ausacpdm.org.au/research/cpqol) (Gilson et al. 2014)
  - Quality of Life Questionnaire for Children (CP QOL-Child), Child Report Questionnaire (5–19 years)
  - Quality of Life Questionnaire for Adolescent (CP QOL-Teen), Primary Caregiver Questionnaire
  - Quality of Life Questionnaire for Adolescent (CP QOL-Teen) Adolescent Self-Report Questionnaire
- Self-evaluation:
  - Canadian Occupational Performance Measure (COPM) (Cusick et al. 2007)
  - Pediatric/Adolescent Shoulder Survey (PASS) (Edmonds et al. 2017)
  - Quick Disability of the Arm, Shoulder and Hand (*Quick*DASH); age, adolescents/adults (Gummesson et al. 2006)
  - Lower Limb Functional Index (LLFI); age, adolescents/adults (Gabel et al. 2012)
  - Upper Extremity Functional Index (UEFI); age, adolescents/adults (Stratford et al. 2001)
  - Craig Handicap Assessment and Reporting Technique (CHART); age, from 18 years (Whiteneck et al. 1992)
  - Community Integration Questionnaire; age, adolescents/adults (Willer et al. 1994)
- Pain:
  - Non-communicating Children's Pain Checklist—Revised (NCCPC-R) (Breau et al. 2002)
  - Brief Pain Inventory (BPI, short form) (Tyler et al. 2002)

1.3.2.1 Assessment Technology

Clinical scales are indispensable measurement tools for evaluating the potential of the child, and the therapist should undoubtedly use them. However, clinical scales can have necessarily some elements of subjective considerations, as well as their basic objective criteria and the final assessment score may be influenced by interpretative variables of the examiner. For this reason, where possible, it is worthwhile using assessment tools based on computational technologies as well, in order to obtain pure objective and repeatable measurements.

This specific topic is further elaborated in Chap. 13 "Rehabilitation Technologies for Sensory-Motor-Cognitive Impairments."

1.3.3 Aims of the Rehabilitation Project

In defining the intervention plan, the therapist should integrate functional, task-orientated aims and propose the appropriate activities that allow the child to achieve them immediately during the treatment sessions.

Of course, the rehabilitation project should be based on the close collaboration and integration of converging, common goals on the part of the three main participants (Fig. 1.3):

- The child
- The parents, family members, and caregivers
- The therapist and other professionals

Fig. 1.3 Sharing of common goals between child, parents, and therapist

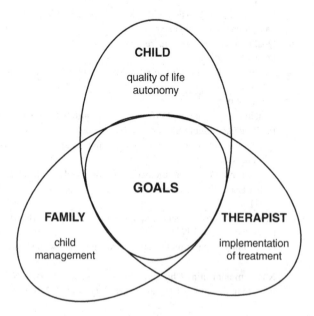

Figure 1.3 is a schematic representation illustrating how all the participants have specific roles:

- The *child* should be motivated to mature and to strive to overcome the difficulties related to their pathology.
- The *family* has the task of rearing, caring for, nurturing, and educating their child with special needs.
- The *therapist* is the facilitator who modifies the relationship between the child and the environment and promotes learning and new adaptations and skills.

The protagonists of the rehabilitation system, each contributing with their specific role and interacting constantly with each other, endeavor to achieve goals which are not immediate but are achieved after a journey extended over time. The overall goal is to acquire the highest possible level of autonomy and quality of life for each child.

The definition and sharing of aims imply good communication and the sharing of mutual expectations between the child, the family, and the therapists. These aspects should emerge in a well-documented, substantial, and precise therapeutic project which avoids generic and vague declarations of intent and wishful thinking with regard to the functional prognosis and the realistic outcomes of intervention.

The aims of rehabilitation treatment should indicate precise planning for the achievement of the results, and they need to be articulated in certain specific sub-goals, such as the following ones:

- *Short-term goals*: based on the main problem highlighted, the therapist immediately implements personalized treatment, to achieve a change in the child's adaptive behavior.
- *Medium-term goals*: based on planned functional goals agreed with the child, family and team, to be achieved within a short time.
- *Long-term goals*: based mainly on the prognostic functional evaluation, the interdisciplinary team elaborates a "personal profile" of the child, forecasting the most important milestones in their life, e.g., the access to education and recreation, orthopedic surgical interventions, future employment, etc.

Already in 1963 Berta Bobath indicated that the planned goals of a rehabilitation project should be:

- *Functional:* intending that the aims should be focused to resolve a child's real needs, within their daily life context. The skills acquired will therefore be essential for solving functional tasks at all times and in all different environments, with very significant impact on the quality of life of the child.
- *Realistic:* implying suitable and attainable in relation with the real potential of the child, therefore not too easy, but not too difficult, in such a way to challenge the child to reach the goal without frustrating them with the unattainable.

Frequently, it is when the goal is not tailored to the true potential of the child that it results to be a wrong goal of intervention.

- *Modifiable:* meaning the goal can be recalibrated by the therapist, based on the continual verification of the results obtained during treatment and updated according to the real functional situation of the child. This means that if the therapist does not observe any kind of improvement in the child's responses to treatment, the plan should be reset based on a new and deeper clinical reasoning. It may be that the earlier analysis account did not identify the most critical problems or, in the meantime, an unforeseen modification has occurred in the child's situation and development.

Following indications by Doran (1981) for the managerial field, currently, it is underlined that also the objectives to be pursued in a rehabilitation project should be "smart." This becomes the acronym meaning that a goal needs to be specific, measurable, achievable, relevant, and time-bound (SMART) (Bovend'Eerdt et al. 2009; Bexelius et al. 2018). Compared to those previously considered by Bobath, the two most significant SMART attributes are that one focusing on the need to quantify (measurable) with clinical scales or other objective assessment the potential of the child and to monitor their progress and the attribute (time-bound) relating to the time within which the results are supposed to be achieved.

Moreover, some authors added new items to the acronym, which now is often cited as SMARTER. According to the context, different meanings are given to the additions that in the rehabilitation context can be ecological and reviewed.

It is to remember that, when formulating the goals, the therapist should always bear in mind the child's background and their cognitive, emotional, and functional maturation and have an understanding of the educational styles of the parents and the teachers. Rosenbaum and Gorter (2012) underlined how all children are in a constant state of becoming. Therefore, the child is considered an *ever-evolving being* who shows rapid changes at various developmental stages through their activities and participation.

References

Affolter F (2004) Chapter 8: From action to interaction as primary root for development. In: Stockman IJ (ed) Movement and action in learning and development. Elsevier Academic Press, San Diego, pp 169–200. https://doi.org/10.1016/B978-012671860-7/50045-8

Affolter F (1981) Perceptual processes as prerequisites for complex human behaviour. Int Rehabil Med. 1981;3(1):3–10, https://doi.org/10.3109/03790798109167107

Als H (1986) A synactive model of neonatal behavioral organization. Phys Occup Ther Pediatr 6(3–4):3–53. https://doi.org/10.1080/J006v06n03_02

Als H (2009) Newborn individualized developmental care and assessment program (NIDCAP). New Frontier for Neonatal and Perinatal Medicine. J Neonatal-Perinatal Med 2(3):135–147. https://doi.org/10.3233/NPM-2009-0061

Als H, Lester BM, Tronick E, Brazelton TB (1982) Towards a systematic assessment of preterm infants' behavioral development. In: Fitzgerald HE, Lester BM, Yogman M (eds) Theory and research in behavioral pediatrics. Plenum Press, New York, pp 35–63

Amiel-Tison C (1968) Neurological Evaluation of the Maturity of Newborn Infants, Arch. Dis. Childh., 1968, 43(227):89–93, https://doi.org/10.1136/adc.43.227.89

André-Thomas, Saint-Anne Dargassies S (1952) Etudes neurologiques sur le nouveau-né et le jeune nourisson. Masson, Paris

Arnould C, Penta M, Renders A, Thonnard JL (2004) ABILHAND-Kids: a measure of manual ability in children with cerebral palsy. Neurology 63(6):1045–1052. https://doi.org/10.1212/01. wnl.0000138423.77640.37

Ayres AJ (1989) Sensory integration and praxis test. Western Psychological Services Publ, Los Angeles

Ballaz L, Plamondon S, Lemay M (2011) Group aquatic training improves gait efficiency in adolescents with cerebral palsy. Disabil Rehabil 33(17–18):1616–1624. https://doi.org/10.310 9/09638288.2010.541544

Balzer J, Marsico P, Mitteregger E, van der Linden ML, Mercer TH, van Hedel HJ (2016) Construct validity and reliability of the Selective Control Assessment of the Lower Extremity in children with cerebral palsy. Dev Med Child Neurol 58(2):167–172. https://doi.org/10.1111/ dmcn.12805

Barrows HS, Tamblyn R (1980) Problem-based learning: an approach to medical education. Springer Series on Med. Educ., Springer Publ. Co., New York

Bartlett D, Birmingham T (2003) Validity and reliability of a pediatric Reach Test. Pediatr Phys Ther 15(2):84–92. https://doi.org/10.1097/01.PEP.0000067885.63909.5C

Basu AP, Kirkpatrick EV, Wright B, Pearse JE, Best KE, Eyre JA (2018) The Tyneside Pegboard Test: development, validation, and observations in unilateral cerebral palsy. Dev Med Child Neurol 60(3):314–321. https://doi.org/10.1111/dmcn.13645

Bayley N, Aylward GP (2019) Bayley scales of infant and toddler development, 4th edn. Pearson, Bloomington

Bexelius A, Carlberg EB, Löwing K (2018) Quality of goal setting in pediatric rehabilitation-a SMART approach. Child: Care Health Dev 44(6):850–856. https://doi.org/10.1111/cch.12609

Bobath B (1963) Treatment principles and planning in cerebral palsy. Physiotherapy 49:122–124

Bohannon RW, Smith MB (1987) Interrater reliability of a modified Ashworth scale of muscle spasticity. Phys Ther 67(2):206–207. https://doi.org/10.1093/ptj/67.2.206

Bottos M, Feliciangeli A, Sciuto L, Gericke C, Vianello A (2001) Functional status of adults with cerebral palsy and implications for treatment of children. Dev Med Child Neurol 43(8):516–528. https://doi.org/10.1017/s0012162201000950

Bovend'Eerdt TJH, Botell RE, Wade DT (2009) Writing SMART rehabilitation goals and achieving goal attainment scaling: a practical guide. Clin Rehabil 23(4):352–361. https://doi. org/10.1177/0269215508101741

Brazelton TB (1973) Neonatal behavioural assessment scale. Clinics in developmental medicine, vol 50. Spastics International Medical Publication/W. Heinemann Med. Books, London

Breau LM, McGrath PJ, Camfield CS, Finley GA (2002) Psychometric properties of the non-communicating children's Pain Checklist-Revised. Pain 99:349–357. https://doi.org/10.1016/ s0304-3959(02)00179-3

Breslin DM, Exner CE (1999) Construct validity of the In-Hand Manipulation Test: a discriminant analysis with children without disability and children with spastic diplegia. Am J Occup Ther 53(4):381–386. https://doi.org/10.5014/ajot.53.4.381

Burns YR, Ensbey RM, Norrie MA (1989a) The Neuro-Sensory Motor Developmental Assessment Part I: development and administration of the Test. Aust J Physiother 35(3):141–149. https://doi.org/10.1016/S0004-9514(14)60503-1

Burns YR, Ensbey RM, Norrie MA (1989b) The Neuro-Sensory Motor Developmental Assessment Part II: predictive and concurrent validity. Aust J Physiother 35(3):151–157. https://doi.org/10.1016/S0004-9514(14)60504-3

Butler PB, Saavedra S, Sofranac M, Jarvis SE, Woollacott MH (2010) Refinement, reliability, and validity of the segmental assessment of trunk control. Pediatr Phys Ther 22(3):246–257. https://doi.org/10.1097/PEP.0b013e3181e69490

Crittenden PM (2005) Der CARE-Index als Hilfsmittel für Früherkennung, Intervention und Forschung. Frühförderung interdisziplinär (early interdisciplinary intervention). Special issue: Bindungs orientierte Ansätze in der Praxis der Frühförderung 24:S.99–S106

Cusick A, Lannin NA, Lowe K (2007) Adapting the Canadian Occupational Performance Measure for use in a paediatric clinical trial. Disabil Rehabil 29(10):761–766. https://doi.org/10.1080/09638280600929201

Davies PM (2000) Step to follow: the comprehensive treatment of patients with hemiplegia, 2nd edn. Springer, Berlin

DeMatteo C, Law M, Russell D, Pollock N, Rosenbaum P, Walter S (1992) Quest: quality of upper extremity skills test. https://slpemad.files.wordpress.com/2015/06/1992_quest_manual.pdf

Donohoe B, Turner D, Worrell T (1994) The use of functional reach as a measurement of balance in boys and girls without disabilities ages 5 to 15 years. Pediatr Phys Ther 6:189–193

Doody C, McAteer M (2002) Clinical reasoning of expert and novice physiotherapists in an outpatient orthopaedic setting. Physiotherapy 88(5):258–268. https://doi.org/10.1016/S0031-9406(05)61417-4

Doran GT (1981) There's a S.M.A.R.T. way to write management's goals and objectives. Manag Rev 70(11):35–36

Dubowitz LMS, Dubowitz V (1981) The neurological assessment of the preterm and full term newborn infant, Clinics in Developmental Med. 79, London, Spastic Int Med Publications/Heinemann Medical Books

Dubowitz L, Ricci D, Mercuri E (2005) The Dubowitz neurological examination of full-term newborn. Ment Retard Dev Disabil Res Rev 11:52–60. https://doi.org/10.1002/mrdd.20048

Edmonds EW, Bastrom TP, Roocroft JH, Calandra-Young VA, Pennock AT (2017) The Pediatric/Adolescent Shoulder Survey (PASS): a reliable youth questionnaire with discriminant validity and responsiveness to change. Orthop J Sports Med 5(3):2325967117698466. https://doi.org/10.1177/2325967117698466

Eliasson A, Krumlinde-Sundholm L, Rösblad B, Beckung E, Arner M, Öhrvall A, Rosenbaum P (2006) The Manual Ability Classification System (MACS) for children with cerebral palsy: scale development and evidence of validity and reliability. Dev Med Child Neurol 48(7):549–554. https://doi.org/10.1017/S0012162206001162

Eliasson AC, Ullenhag A, Wahlström U, Krumlinde-Sundholm L (2017) Mini-MACS: development of the Manual Ability Classification System for children younger than 4 years of age with signs of cerebral palsy. Dev Med Child Neurol 59(1):72–78. https://doi.org/10.1111/dmcn.13162

Elvrum AG, Beckung E, Sæther R, Lydersen S, Vik T, Himmelmann K (2017) Bimanual capacity of children with cerebral palsy: intra- and interrater reliability of a revised edition of the Bimanual Fine Motor Function Classification. Phys Occup Ther Pediatr 37(3):239–251. https://doi.org/10.1080/01942638.2016.1185507

Evkaya A, Karadag-Saygi E, Karali Bingul D, Giray E (2020) Validity and reliability of the Dynamic Gait Index in children with hemiplegic cerebral palsy. Gait Posture 75:28–33. https://doi.org/10.1016/j.gaitpost.2019.09.024

Fasoli S, Fragala-Pinkham M, Haley S (2009) Fugl-Meyer assessment: reliability for children with hemiplegia. Abstract: Arch Phys Med Rehabil 90(10):E4–E5. https://doi.org/10.1016/j.apmr.2009.08.010

Fazzi E, Galli J, Micheletti S (2012) Visual impairment: a common sequela of preterm birth. Neo Rev 13(9):e542–e550. https://doi.org/10.1542/neo.13-9-e542

Ferrari F, Frassoldati R, Berardi A, Di Palma F, Ori L, Lucaccioni L, Bertoncelli N, Einspieler C (2016) The ontogeny of fidgety movements from 4 to 20 weeks post-term age in healthy full-term infants. Early Hum Dev 103:219–224. https://doi.org/10.1016/j.earlhumdev.2016.10.004

Fosdahl MA, Jahnsen R, Pripp AH, Holm I (2020) Change in popliteal angle and hamstrings spasticity during childhood in ambulant children with spastic bilateral cerebral palsy. A register-based cohort study. BMC Pediatr 20:11. https://doi.org/10.1186/s12887-019-1891-y

Fowler EG, Staudt LA, Greenberg MB, Oppenheim WL (2009) Selective Control Assessment of the Lower Extremity (SCALE): development, validation, and interrater reliability of a clinical tool for patients with cerebral palsy. Dev Med Child Neurol 51(8):607–614. https://doi.org/10.1111/j.1469-8749.2008.03186.x

Franjoine MR, Gunther JS, Taylor MJ (2003) Pediatric Balance Scale: a modified version of the Berg Balance Scale for the school-age child with mild to moderate motor impairment. Pediatr Phys Ther 15(2):114–128. https://doi.org/10.1097/01.PEP.0000068117.48023.18

Fugl-Meyer AR, Jääskö L, Leyman I, Olsson S, Steglind S (1975) The post-stroke hemiplegic patient. 1. A method for evaluation of physical performance. Scand J Rehabil Med 7(1):13–31

Gabel CP, Melloh M, Burkett B, Michener LA (2012) Lower Limb Functional Index: development and clinimetric properties. Phys Ther 92(1):98–110. https://doi.org/10.2522/ptj.20100199

Geiger R, Strasak A, Treml B, Gasser K, Kleinsasser A, Fischer V, Geiger H, Loeckinger A, Stein JI (2007) Six-minute walk test in children and adolescents. J Pediatr 150(4):395–399, 399. e1–399.e2. https://doi.org/10.1016/j.jpeds.2006.12.052

Gilson KM, Davis E, Reddihough D, Graham K, Waters E (2014) Quality of life in children with cerebral palsy: implications for practice. J Child Neurol 29(8):1134–1140. https://doi.org/10.1177/0883073814535502

Gjesdal BE, Jahnsen R, Morgan P, Opheim A, Mæland S (2020) Walking through life with cerebral palsy: reflections on daily walking by adults with cerebral palsy. Int J Qual Stud Health Wellbeing 15(1):1746577. https://doi.org/10.1080/17482631.2020.1746577

Gorter JW, Currie SJ (2011) Aquatic exercise programs for children and adolescents with cerebral palsy: what do we know and where do we go? Int J Pediatr 2011:712165. https://doi.org/10.1155/2011/712165

Gorton GE 3rd, Stout JL, Bagley AM, Bevans K, Novacheck TF, Tucker CA (2011) Gillette Functional Assessment Questionnaire 22-item skill set: factor and Rasch analyses. Dev Med Child Neurol 53(3):250–255. https://doi.org/10.1111/j.1469-8749.2010.03832.x

Gummesson C, Ward MM, Atroshi I (2006) The shortened disabilities of the arm, shoulder and hand questionnaire (QuickDASH): validity and reliability based on responses within the full-length DASH. BMC Musculoskelet Disord 7:44. https://doi.org/10.1186/1471-2474-7-44

Haley S, Coster W, Ludlow L, Haltiwanger J, Andrellos P (1992) Pediatric Evaluation of Disability Inventory (PEDI): development, standardization and administration manual. New England Medical Center Hospitals, Inc. and PEDI Research Group, Boston

Haugh AB, Pandyan AD, Johnson GR (2006) A systematic review of the Tardieu Scale for the measurement of spasticity. Disabil Rehabil 28(15):899–907. https://doi.org/10.1080/09638280500404305

Heyrman L, Molenaers G, Desloovere K, Verheyden G, De Cat J, Monbaliu E, Feys H (2011) A clinical tool to measure trunk control in children with cerebral palsy: the Trunk Control Measurement Scale. Res Dev Disabil 32(6):2624–2635. https://doi.org/10.1016/j.ridd.2011.06.012

Hidecker MJ, Paneth N, Rosenbaum PL, Kent RD, Lillie J, Eulenberg JB, Chester K Jr, Johnson B, Michalsen L, Evatt M, Taylor K (2011) Developing and validating the Communication Function Classification System for individuals with cerebral palsy. Dev Med Child Neurol 53(8):704–710. https://doi.org/10.1111/j.1469-8749.2011.03996.x

Higgs J, Jones M (1995) Clinical reasoning in the health Professions. Butterworth-Heinemann, London

Jethwa A, Mink J, Macarthur C, Knights S, Fehlings T, Fehlings D (2010) Development of the Hypertonia Assessment Tool (HAT): a discriminative tool for hypertonia in children. Dev Med Child Neurol 52:e83–e87. https://doi.org/10.1111/j.1469-8749.2009.03483.x

Jones M (1995) Clinical reasoning and pain. Man Ther 1(1):17–24. https://doi.org/10.1054/math.1995.0245

Jones M, Jensen G, Edwards I (2000) Clinical reasoning in physiotherapy. In: Higgs J, Jones N (eds) Clinical reasoning in the health professions. Butterworth/Heinemann, Oxford, pp 115–127

Jongbloed-Pereboom M, Nijhuis-van der Sanden MW, Steenbergen B (2013) Norm scores of the Box and Block Test for children ages 3-10 years. Am J Occup Ther 67(3):312–318. https://doi.org/10.5014/ajot.2013.006643

King G, Chiarello L (2014) Family-centered care for children with cerebral palsy: conceptual and practical considerations to advance care and practice. J Child Neurol 29(8):1046–1054. https://doi.org/10.1177/0883073814533009

King GA, McDougall J, Palisano R, Gritzan J, Tucker MA (2000) Goal Attainment Scaling. Its use in evaluating pediatric therapy programs. Phys Occup Ther Pediatr 19(2):31–52. https://doi.org/10.1080/J006v19n02_03

Kiresuk TJ, Sherman RE (1968) Goal Attainment Scaling: a general method for evaluating comprehensive community mental health programs. Community Ment Health J 4(6):443–453. https://doi.org/10.1007/BF01530764

Krumlinde-Sundholm L, Eliasson AC (2003) Development of the Assisting Hand Assessment, a Rasch-built measure intended for children with unilateral upper limb impairments. Scand J Occup Ther 10:16–26. https://doi.org/10.1080/11038120310004529

Krumlinde-Sundholm L, Ek L, Sicola E, Sjöstrand L, Guzzetta A, Sgandurra G, Cioni G, Eliasson AC (2017) Development of the hand assessment for infants: evidence of internal scale validity. Dev Med Child Neurol 59(12):1276–1283. https://doi.org/10.1111/dmcn.13585

Landgraf JM, Maunsell E, Nixon Speechley K, Bullinger M, Campbell S, Abetz L, Ware JE (1998) Canadian-French, German and UK versions of the Child Health Questionnaire: methodology and preliminary item scaling results. Qual Life Res 7:433–445

Latash ML, Anson JG (1996) What are "normal movements" in atypical populations? Behav Brain Sci 19(1):55–106. https://doi.org/10.1017/S0140525X00041467

Law M, Hanna S, King G, Hurley P, King S, Kertoy M, Rosenbaum P (2003) Factors affecting family-centred service delivery for children with disabilities. Child: Care Health Dev 29(5):357–366. https://doi.org/10.1046/j.1365-2214.2003.00351.x

Lincoln NB, Jackson JM, Adams SA (1998) Reliability and revision of the Nottingham Sensory Assessment for stroke patients. Physiotherapy 84:358–365. https://doi.org/10.1016/S0031-9406(05)61454-X

Livingston M, Rosenbaum PL, Russell DJ, Palisano RJ (2007) Quality of life among adolescents with cerebral palsy: what does the literature tell us? Dev Med Child Neurol 49(3):225–231. https://doi.org/10.1111/j.1469-8749.2007.00225.x

Lyle RC (1981) A performance test for assessment of upper limb function in physical rehabilitation treatment and research. Int J Rehabil Res 4(4):483–492. https://doi.org/10.1097/00004356-198112000-00001

Makris T, Dorstyn D, Crettenden A (2019) Quality of life in children and adolescents with cerebral palsy: a systematic review with meta-analysis. Disabil Rehabil 10:1–10. https://doi.org/10.1080/09638288.2019.1623852

Manikowska F, Chen BP, Jóźwiak M, Lebiedowska MK (2018) Validation of Manual Muscle Testing (MMT) in children and adolescents with cerebral palsy. NeuroRehabilitation 42(1):1–7. https://doi.org/10.3233/NRE-172179

Martín-Valero R, Vega-Ballón J, Perez-Cabezas V (2018) Benefits of hippotherapy in children with cerebral palsy: a narrative review. Eur J Paediatr Neurol 22(6):1150–1160. https://doi.org/10.1016/j.ejpn.2018.07.002

Mathiowetz V, Federman SM, Wiemer DM (1985) Box and Block test of manual dexterity: norms for 6-19 year olds. Can J Occup Ther 52(5):241–245. https://doi.org/10.1177/000841748505200505

Mayston M (2016) Bobath and NeuroDevelopmental Therapy: what is the future? Dev Med Child Neurol 58:994–994. https://doi.org/10.1111/dmcn.13221

McDowell BC, Kerr C, Parkes J, Cosgrove A (2005) Validity of a 1 minute walk test for children with cerebral palsy. Dev Med Child Neurol. 2005 Nov;47(11):744–8. https://doi.org/10.1017/S0012162205001568

Milani Comparetti A (1982) Semeitotica Neuroevolutiva Prospettive in Pediatria 48;305–14:1982

Milani Comparetti A, Gidoni EA (1967) Pattern analysis of motor development and its disorders. Dev Med Child Neurol 9;625–30:1967

Mutoh T, Mutoh T, Tsubone H, Takada M, Doumura M, Ihara M, Shimomura H, Taki Y, Ihara M (2019) Impact of long-term hippotherapy on the walking ability of children with cerebral palsy and quality of life of their caregivers. Front Neurol 10:834. https://doi.org/10.3389/fneur.2019.00834

Negri R (2014) The newborn in the Intensive Care Unit: a neuropsychoanalytic prevention model, ed. Karnac Books

NICE (Nat. Inst. for Health and Care Excellence) (2017) Cerebral palsy in under 25s: assessment and management. https://www.nice.org.uk/guidance/ng62

NICE (Nat. Inst. for Health and Care Excellence) (2019) Cerebral palsy in adults. https://www.nice.org.uk/guidance/ng119

Opheim A, Jahnsen R, Olsson E, Stanghelle JK (2009) Walking function, pain, and fatigue in adults with cerebral palsy: a 7-year follow-up study. Dev Med Child Neurol 51(5):381–388. https://doi.org/10.1111/j.1469-8749.2008.03250.x

Ottenbacher KJ, Msall M, Lyon N, Duffy LC et al (2000) The WeeFIM instrument: its utility in detecting change in children with developmental disabilities. Arch Phys Med Rehabil 81(10):1317–1326. https://doi.org/10.1053/apmr.2000.9387

Palazzoli Selvini M (1987) Una bussola relazionale per gli operatori della riabilitazione, Atti XV del Congresso Naz. S.I.M.F.E.R., La riabilitazione nell'età infantile pag. 533–535, ed. CLUP, Milano

Palisano RJ, Orlin M, Chiarello L, Oeffinger D, Polansky M, Maggs J et al (2011) Determinants of intensity of participation in leisure and recreational activities by youth with cerebral palsy. Arch Phys Med Rehabil 92(9):1468–1476. https://doi.org/10.1016/j.apmr.2011.04.007

Perls FS, Hefferline R, Goodman P (1951) Gestalt therapy: excitement and growth in the human personality. Julian Press, New York

Picciolini O, Montirosso R, Porro M, Giannì ML, Mosca F (2016) Neurofunctional assessment at term equivalent age can predict 3 year neurodevelopmental outcomes in very low birth weight infants. Acta Paediatr 105(2):e47–e53. https://doi.org/10.1111/apa.13248

Pizzighello S, Pellegri A, Vestri A, Sala M, Piccoli S, Flego L, Martinuzzi A (2019) Becoming a young adult with cerebral palsy. Res Dev Disabil 92:103450. https://doi.org/10.1016/j.ridd.2019.103450

Prechtl HFR (1990) Qualitative changes of spontaneous movements in preterm infants are a marker of neurological dysfunction. Early Hum Dev 23(3):151–158. https://doi.org/10.1016/0378-3782(90)90011-7

Prechtl HFR (2001) General Movements assessment as a method of developmental neurology: new paradigms and their consequences. Dev Med Child Neurol 43(12):836–842. https://doi.org/10.1017/s0012162201001529

Prechtl HFR, Beintema D (1964) The neurological examination of the full-term newborn infant. Little Club Clinics Develop. Med. No 12

Randall M, Johnson L, Reddihough D (1999) The Melbourne Assessment of Unilateral Upper Limb Function: test administration manual. Royal Children's Hospital, Melbourne, Melbourne

Randall M, Imms C, Carey L (2008) Establishing validity of a modified Melbourne Assessment for children ages 2 to 4 years. Am J Occup Ther 62(4):373–383. https://doi.org/10.5014/ajot.62.4.373

Read HS, Hazlewood ME, Hillman SJ, Prescott RJ, Robb JE (2003) Edinburgh visual gait score for use in cerebral palsy. J Pediatr Orthop 23(3):296–301

Romeo DM, Ricci D, Brogna C, Mercuri E (2016) Use of the Hammersmith Infant Neurological Examination in infants with cerebral palsy: a critical review of the literature. Dev Med Child Neurol 58(3):240–245. https://doi.org/10.1111/dmcn.12876

Rosa-Rizzotto M, Visonà Dalla Pozza L, Corlatti A, Luparia A, Marchi A, Molteni F, Facchin P, Pagliano E, Fedrizzi E, GIPCI Study Group (2014) A new scale for the assessment of performance and capacity of hand function in children with hemiplegic cerebral palsy: reliability and validity studies. Eur J Phys Rehabil Med 50(5):543–556

Rosenbaum P, Gorter J (2012) The "F-words" in childhood disability: I swear this is how we should think! Child: Care Health Dev 38(4):457–463. https://doi.org/10.1111/j.1365-2214.2011.01338.x

Russell DJ, Avery LM, Rosenbaum PL, Raina PS, Walter SD, Palisano RJ (2000) Improved scaling of the gross motor function measure for children with cerebral palsy: evidence of reliability and validity. Phys Ther 80(9):873–885

Sæther R, Jørgensen L (2011) Intra- and inter-observer reliability of the Trunk Impairment Scale for children with cerebral palsy. Res Dev Disabil 32(2):727–739. https://doi.org/10.1016/j.ridd.2010.11.007

Santamaria V, Rachwani J, Saussez G, Bleyenheuft Y, Dutkowsky J, Gordon AM, Woollacott MH (2020) The Seated Postural & Reaching Control Test in cerebral palsy: a validation study. Phys Occup Ther Pediatr 40(4):441–469. https://doi.org/10.1080/01942638.2019.1705456

Shikako-Thomas K, Kolehmainen N, Ketelaar M, Bult M, Law M (2014) Promoting leisure participation as part of health and well-being in children and youth with cerebral palsy. J Child Neurol 29(8):1125–1133. https://doi.org/10.1177/0883073814533422

Sienko SE (2018) An exploratory study investigating the multidimensional factors impacting the health and well-being of young adults with cerebral palsy. Disabil Rehabil 40(6):660–666. https://doi.org/10.1080/09638288.2016.1274340

Stratford PW, Binkley JM, Stratford DM (2001) Development and initial validation of the upper extremity functional index. Physiother Can 53:259–267. https://doi.org/10.2174/1874325001408010316

Sukal-Moulton T, Gaebler-Spira D, Krosschell KJ (2018) The validity and reliability of the Test of Arm Selective Control for children with cerebral palsy: a prospective cross-sectional study. Dev Med Child Neurol 60(4):374–381. https://doi.org/10.1111/dmcn.13671

Tofani M, Castelli E, Sabbadini M, Berardi A, Murgia M, Servadio A, Galeoto G (2020) Examining reliability and validity of the Jebsen-Taylor Hand Function Test among children with cerebral palsy. Percept Mot Skills 127(4):684–697. https://doi.org/10.1177/0031512520920087

Touwen B (1976) Neurological development in infancy. Clin. Dev. Med. 58, SIMP, London Heinemann Medical Books, pp 109–122

Tyler EJ, Jensen MP, Engel JM, Schwartz L (2002) The reliability and validity of pain interference measures in persons with cerebral palsy. Arch Phys Med Rehabil 83:236–239

van der Slot WMA, Benner JL, Brunton L, Engel JM, Gallien P, Hilberink SR, Månum G, Morgan P, Opheim A, Riquelme I, Rodby-Bousquet E, Şimşek TT, Thorpe DE, van den Berg-Emons RGB, Vogtle LK, Grigorios Papageorgiou G, Roebroeck ME (2020) Pain in adults with cerebral palsy: a systematic review and meta-analysis of individual participant data. Ann Phys Rehabil Med 64(3):101359. https://doi.org/10.1016/j.rehab.2019.12.011

Varni JW, Seid M, Kurtin PS (2001) PedsQL 4.0: reliability and validity of the Pediatric Quality of Life Inventory version 4.0 generic core scales in healthy and patient populations. Med Care 39(8):800–812. https://doi.org/10.1097/00005650-200108000-00006

Wagner LV, Davids JR, Hardin JW (2016) Selective control of the Upper Extremity Scale: validation of a clinical assessment tool for children with hemiplegic cerebral palsy. Dev Med Child Neurol 58(6):612–617. https://doi.org/10.1111/dmcn.12949

Whiteneck GG, Charlifue SW, Gerhart KA, Overholser JD, Richardson GN (1992) Quantifying handicap: a new measure of long-term rehabilitation outcomes. Arch Phys Med Rehabil 73(6):519–526

Willer B, Ottenbacher KJ, Coad ML (1994) The community integration questionnaire. A comparative examination. Am J Phys Med Rehabil 73(2):103–111. https://doi.org/10.1097/00002060-199404000-00006

Williams EN, Carroll SG, Reddihough DS, Phillips BA, Galea MP (2005) Investigation of the Timed 'Up & Go' test in children. Dev Med Child Neurol 47(8):518–524. https://doi.org/10.1017/s0012162205001027

WHO - World Health Organization (2007) International classification of functioning, disability and health: children and youth version: ICF-CY. World Health Organization

The Child with Bilateral Spastic Cerebral Palsy

Psiche Giannoni and Liliana Zerbino

According to the Surveillance of Cerebral Palsy in Europe (SCPE) (Krägeloh-Mann et al. 1994; Cans et al. 2007, 2008; Rosenbaum et al. 2007; Günel et al. 2014), a child with a bilateral spastic cerebral palsy (BSCP) presents an impairment that displays an increase in muscular tone and involves all the parts of the body. The impairment does not occur to the same extent in all the body, but one side can be more severely involved than the other, as well as the lower parts compared with the upper ones.

It is important to point out that in day-to-day practice, several practitioners use the general term spasticity to refer to the summary of the many features of the upper motor neuron syndrome (UMNS). However, many studies on UMNS report how muscle weakness, meaning the reduced ability for the muscle to generate force, coexists together with other features such as an altered muscle tone and decreased speed, accuracy, dexterity and endurance of the motor performance (Ivanhoe and Reistetter 2004; Segal 2018).

On this basis, it is necessary to have a more general and broader view of the problem relating to the features observed in CP. When a single able body segment plans to move, all the other parts move simultaneously and adapt by cooperating to successfully achieve the proposed goal. Anticipatory postural adjustments are activated before the forthcoming movement in order to sustain it without losing the balance, together with compensatory adjustments often supported by the contralateral part of the body (Santos et al. 2010; Xie and Wang 2019). In CP there is not such an efficient interplay (Liu et al. 2007; Girolami et al. 2011), and the motor patterns are performed in an ineffective, less functional, and laborious way.

P. Giannoni (✉)
DIBRIS, University of Genoa, Genoa, Italy

L. Zerbino
DSS, University of Florence, Florence, Italy

The limitation of motor functioning due to the different signs of the UMNS requires the nervous system to organize new strategies to overcome this lack of ability (Levin et al. 2009). These compensatory strategies are in themselves positive strategies when the severely impaired child nevertheless needs to carry out a function, but they can also cause considerable limitations and become significant negative learning, the so-called "bad use" (Alaverdashvili et al. 2008; Raghavan 2015) for a young nervous system with still so much to learn (Nudo and Milliken 1996; Nudo et al. 1996, 2001; Eyre et al. 2001; Martin et al. 2007; Eyre 2007; Johnston 2009).

Therefore, well-focused training with the child needs to pay attention first of all to their postural reactions against gravity and their alignment. Then, immediately afterwards, the therapist proposes reliable functional tasks for the child to organize, applying an individualized problem-solving approach, instead of offering the child pre-conceived solutions, and then encourages the repetition of many varied but similar tasks. As Bernstein (1967) wrote, and according to Schmidt's schema theory (Schmidt 1975, 1988), "repetition without repetition" can influence the nervous system not only to acquire more economic and functional skills but also to improve the generalization process. In this way, the child avoids learning and exploiting the use of "bad" movement patterns, which tend to increase misalignment, reduce range of movement and increase distal muscle stiffness.

2.1   The Child with Severe Bilateral Spastic Cerebral Palsy

The form of bilateral spastic cerebral palsy (BSCP) involves all the parts of the body and differs from the other forms not only because of very limited movement but also for the inability of the child to acquire antigravity competences and functionally maintain different postures. These children could be classified at level IV–V on the GMFCS (Palisano et al. 1997).

The severity of the neural damage causes constant and excessive recruitment of muscle tone, and the child has difficulty interacting with the surrounding environment. The altered and increased tone, as well as the many other associated problems which often characterize this form, does not allow the child to correctly receive and process information and to respond adequately.

The child's poor abilities induce them to interact with the environment only with a limited and stereotyped repertoire of movements. Feeling overwhelmed by an imponent quantity of sensory inputs, they gradually shut a lot out and relate to the environment through a reduced amount of sensory information creating a closed and stereotyped circuit. Due to poor head control and untrained eye-head coordination, the child often relies on the auditory sensory channel at the expense of the visual one, and they neglect the tactile inputs because they are unable to explore with their hands. The youngster also misses out on the first simple rhythmic movements of kicking, important for the recruitment of abdominal muscles; therefore, the already poor motor repertoire and interaction with the environment are gradually even more reduced.

On the other hand, considering these very limited resources, it would be a big mistake and misunderstanding to bombard the child therapeutically, overloading them with too many inputs, since the youngster with severe BPCP is unable to perceive and select them adequately.

These difficulties of interaction with the environment are common not only in this form of CP but in all the other forms characterized by poor motor repertoire, for example, in the very hypotonic floppy child (see also Chap. 4, Sect. 4.1).

Characteristics of BSCP Child with Severe Impairment
Movement:

– Difficulty in acquiring antigravity abilities (balance)
– Very limited and stereotyped motor repertoire

Muscle stiffness:

– Spasticity or increased muscle tone

Involvement of body parts:

– With different degrees of impairment

Hypertonia vs. Spasticity
When assessing, handling and treating a child with CP, therapist needs to consider the differences between tone, hypertonia and spasticity.

- Tone is the level of activity of a muscle, whose mechanical characteristics are expressed and/or measured in N/m by the muscular stiffness. Tone is considered "normal" when it allows a person to manage the effects of gravity, maintain a posture to move freely at the same time.
- Hypertonia is a condition in which muscle tone is too high, determining an exaggerated muscle stiffness associated with a high degree of coactivation around the joints. It is detected in the presence of resistance to passive movement; it is not velocity-dependent and can be present with or without spasticity.
- Spasticity is still defined as "a motor disorder characterized by an increase in the tonic-stretch reflexes due to hyper-excitability tensions, resulting from the hyper-excitability of the stretch reflex, as a component of the upper motor neuron syndrome" (Lance 1980). It remains the most accepted and recognized definition. A therapist can recognize spasticity as an increase in resistance to a sudden and passive movement because it is velocity-dependent, whereas hypertonia is not. Furthermore, spasticity always has the characteristics of hypertonicity, but hypertonia does not necessarily result from spasticity.

Many times, when the child with poor postural stability tries to maintain a posture or move a limb, there is an increase in distal stiffness due to a lack of "cooperative interaction" in the other parts of the body.

Additionally, the therapist can influence the child's tone recruitment by working towards a suitable body alignment creating the basis for more appropriate uprighting against gravity and by coaching them in functional activities. At the same time, nowadays it is possible to intervene on spasticity with pharmacological or surgical interventions, among which the most common are botulinum toxin injections, baclofen pump and selective dorsal rhizotomy.

2.1.1   Natural Clinical Development in Severe Bilateral Spastic Cerebral Palsy

The etiopathogenesis in BSCP refers most frequently to an alteration of the white matter at the periventricular and subcortical level during the prenatal period. This leads to a condition characterized not only by important impairment of motor function but also by the presence of other associated problems, such as microcephaly, seizure disorders and visual and cognitive deficits.

A clinical diagnosis of severe BSCP can be made early soon after birth, even in the preterm newborn, since the presence of a poor and stereotyped motor repertoire can be observed immediately (Prechtl et al. 1993; Ferrari et al. 2002). The General Movement Assessment of Prechtl describes the movements in these babies as "not fluid", "not elegant" and "lacking in harmony" that sometimes the untrained examiner's eye can capture almost instinctively in these more severe cerebral lesions.

The prognosis for functional autonomy in these children is very poor because, even when treatment is started early, the impairments and secondary complications such as nutritional and respiratory problems and muscular-skeletal deformities will likely increase over time (Sato 2020). For these reasons, medical and rehabilitation care needs to continue throughout childhood and into adulthood.

The limitation of soft tissue contractures and joint deformities is of great importance and needs to be considered since the early intervention. These limitations are caused by the permanent presence of spasticity or hypertonia in all parts of the body which increases when the child is moved and positioned without appropriate support (Fig. 2.1) and in highly emotional situations. Every attempt of the child to move is interfered with not only by stiffness but also by the presence of stereotyped reactions, such as the tonic-labyrinthine and tonic-symmetrical responses (related to the movements of the head), the startle reaction (which hinders antigravity organization) and the asymmetric tonic neck reflex (ATNR), which can cause postural misalignments and future deformities in children with dystonia, such as the hip dysplasia or subluxation (Shrader et al. 2019).

Children with severe BSCP have very static postural behaviour, with global motor synergies and few variable patterns (Bobath and Bobath 1975; Ferrari et al.

Fig. 2.1 Child with increased muscular stiffness

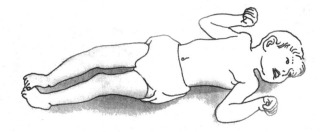

Fig. 2.2 Child with extensor synergy

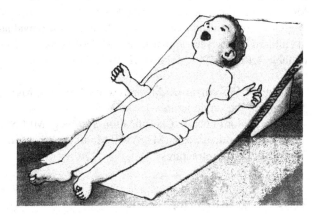

2019). The synergy in extension is accentuated when the child is supine, and the flexor synergy when in prone, but the lower limbs can be extended if a tonic labyrinthine reflex is still strongly present.

- Dominant *extensor synergy* motor behaviour, mainly in supine (Fig. 2.2):
  - *Extensor hypertonus, lungs often in forced inspiration*
  - *Lack of head control, mouth open*
  - *Retraction of shoulders, abnormal finger position*
  - *Extended lower limbs with plantarflexed feet and/or in everted ankles*

The child's attempt to respond to gravity occurs with extension, sometimes of a great degree, of all parts of the body, even in prone (propulsive reaction). Motor behaviour is often conditioned by reflex responses such as ATNR.

- Dominant *flexor synergy* motor behaviour, mainly in the prone position (Fig. 2.3)
  - *Flexed head and spine*
  - *Shoulders pulled forwards and down, arms in flexion under the body*
  - *Flexed hips and knees, but maybe in extension in the presence of strong tonic labyrinthine reflex*

Fig. 2.3 Child with flexor
synergy

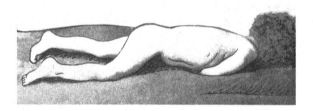

This child appears very still, as if wrapped up in paper envelope, showing very few attempts to move out of this position and interact with the environment. Movement is very poor. There is little initiative to move.

Below are the used assessment tools and clinical evaluations that are most used in children with severe impairment, and further specific clinical scales are reported in Table 1.1 of Chap. 1, Sect. 1.3.2:

– Range of Movement (RoM) and Active Range of Movement (ARoM) measurements of the single joints
– Gross Motor Function Classification System (GMFCS)
– Modified Tardieu Scale (MTS) and Modified Ashworth Scale (MAS) to evaluate stiffness and contractures

2.1.2 Practical Suggestions

The goals for the management and treatment of this severe type of CP are, above all, directed to achieve physical and psychological well-being through the care of the child, their parents and their caregivers. There is no doubt that the main aim is to improve the quality of life of the child as much as possible, not the acquisition of antigravity skills.

First of all, it will be necessary to work with the parents to organize the activities related to the daily care of the child: feeding, sleeping, washing and dressing, handling, carrying, positioning (particularly sitting) and chronic constipation (Bormley 2014; Rivi et al. 2014).

The aims of rehabilitation plan need to be achievable, and they should be related to solving practical functional problems, as well as achieving feasible and useful motor skills, however small.

Different aims of intervention of the therapist:
- *For the child (autonomy and quality of life)*
  – Improve breathing function.
  – Support control of oral functions (swallowing, chewing, closing of the lips, etc.).
  – Promote nutrition: acceptance of foods of different consistency and taste, etc.

- Encourage initiatives and interactions with the environment.
- Propose different postural settings, not only supine.
- Introduce the use of verbal/non-verbal communication strategies.
- *For the parents and caregivers (child management)*
  - Provide advice and support for parents to allow them to improve the daily handling of their child (e.g. hygiene, dressing, transfers from one position to another, etc.).
  - Suggest aids for the appropriate positioning of the child, at home and outside.
  - Promote appropriate ergonomic behaviours when caring for the child, e.g. to avoid parental back pain.
  - Advise and verify the facilitations for feeding the child to improve basic abilities, e.g. chewing/swallowing.
  - Suggest strategies to facilitate non-verbal dual communication: e.g. use of gaze, facial mimic, voice, touch, etc.
- *For the treatment session*
  - Encourage the child's initiative.
  - Select and request simple and meaningful motor behaviours.
  - Implement appropriate and diversified positioning.
  - Maintain the intrinsic characteristics of muscles, joints and connective tissues as long as possible (see Chap. 7 on body tissues care).
  - Provide care to the nasal and oral cavity to improve breathing and feeding functions (see Chap. 10 on feeding and swallowing problems).
  - Select suitable functional aids and orthoses.
  - Select strategies to improve verbal and non-verbal communication (see Chap. 12 on "augmentative and alternative communication").

2.1.2.1 Supine

For this severely affected child, the functional prognosis is not favourable. Treatment occurs most of the time in supine, and its aims are mainly to prevent both internal (e.g. respiratory illness) and external (e.g. retractions or rib cage deformities) complications.

Suggestion
- Organize a setting with environmental conditions that fit the needs of the child:
  - *Optimize the sensory input in the environment (regulate sounds, background noise, light sources, "atmosphere") to facilitate the child to feel at ease, to pay attention, to listen and to interact.*
  - *Lie the child on a stable, medium soft supporting surface of neither too hard nor too soft so the child feels comfortable but also perceives the sensory input from the support.*
  - *Provide a pillow, a wedge, or a U-pillow, to control and facilitate the movements and the alignment (avoid excessive extension or flexion) of the head.*

Fig. 2.4 Release of the tissues of the posterior muscle chain

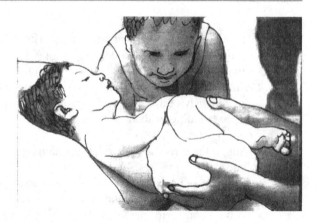

Fig. 2.5 Inducing rhythmic breathing

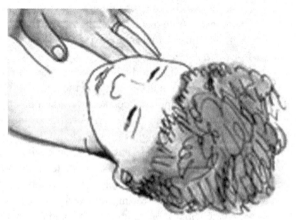

- Introduce some alternative components to control the extensor synergy:
  1. *Handle the child to release the tissues of the posterior muscle chain, to counteract the extension at the spine and to improve the alignment between the two girdles.*
  2. *Gradually bring the lower limbs into flexion, giving the child time to feel at ease and adapt to the postural change (Fig. 2.4).*
- Enhance a paced breath, emphasizing expiration versus inspiration:
  1. *Gently place hands on the child's ribs, and, with a light pressure, induce rhythmic breathing movements, moving the hands from the lower ribs towards the navel.*
  2. *With quiet rhythmic breathing (Fig. 2.5), induce the release of the muscular stiffness at the level of the upper trunk, which will allow the child's head to move more easily towards the midline and facilitate some distal movements (e.g. hands to the mouth, on the face, some visual coupling, etc.).*
  3. *Encourage the child to combine expiration with vocal emission (e.g. in a relationship game that includes the alternation of expressive initiatives and pauses).*

Note
- Children with severe BSCP often have respiratory problems, which need specific specialized medical interventions and respiratory physiotherapy with indications to parents for daily management (Ersöz et al. 2006; Marpole et al. 2020; Gibson et al. 2021).

2.1.2.2 Supine, with Extension Synergy

For a very immobile child with many difficulties to move from one posture to another, it is important to offer everyday experiences which allow them to perceive a wider quantity and variety of sensorial information.

Suggestion
- Let the child perceive other types of inputs, different from the usual:
  1. *First, align their head in midline, and check if the pelvis is available to be moved into posterior tilt.*
  2. *Work to release the muscle posterior chain, to reduce the stiffness not only at the lower trunk but also at the neck and shoulder girdle, which must be engaged as a stable reference point.*
  3. *First lift the pelvis of the child, and transfer their weight on the upper trunk, and then gradually rotate the pelvis towards a shoulder. Always wait and feel the reaction of the body and availability of the child to be moved, that they are ready to go back to the previous position.*
  4. *The weight-bearing felt on the upper trunk can create the conditions to free the child's arms, switch to a visual coupling, and have some hand-mouth movements (Fig. 2.6).*
  5. *After this, a slight tilt sidewards of the pelvis and an interesting input from the side (the parent's face, a toy, etc.) can induce the child to transfer their interest in it and attempt to move in that direction.*

Note
- The therapist should facilitate and encourage the initiative of the child, not move their body on their behalf.

Fig. 2.6 Weight-bearing on the shoulders

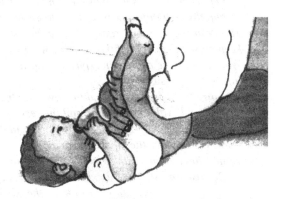

- To enhance the relationship with the adult of reference, it is important to propose play activities that involve:
  - (a) Visual function (visual coupling on person/object, pursuit and exploration of the environment)
  - (b) Knowledge of the body (exploring parts of their own body and of another person, e.g. the face of the parent)
  - (c) Communication (play by imitating sounds, vocalizations with sounds and coded pauses, etc.)
  - (d) Movement (playing with their own body, enjoying the pleasure of moving, etc.)

2.1.2.3 Supine, with Flexion Synergy

Here again, it is very important for this child with a posture fixed in flexion, to feel the different parts of their body and the different RoMs at the joints.

Suggestion
- Gradually mobilize the parts of the body with limited RoM joints, to increase the range and to modify the global postural alignment of the child:
  1. *Lie the child in the supine position, using a wedge instead of a pillow in case the child has many joints fixed in flexion.*
  2. *Mobilize the shoulder girdle first:*
     - *Feel and gently evaluate the RoM and the resistance to movement at the gleno-humeral joint, then the elbow and other distal parts.*
     - *Start to release, and gently stretch the pectoral muscles, to obtain some abduction and outward rotation of the arm.*
  3. *Mobilize the head with regard to the shoulder girdle:*
     - *Check if freer neck movements are now possible that allow the alignment of the head.*
     - *Release and gently stretch the superior* trapezius, scaleni *and* sternocleidomastoideus *muscles.*
     - *Hold the occiput of the child and make a light passive distraction of the cervical vertebrae.*
     - *Let the child feel some new movements, such a lateral rotation of the head, and through this new experience to explore the close environment.*
  4. *Maintain the previous situation, and solicit the child to actively close and keep closed their lips (if the nasal airways are free).*
  5. *Work to achieve a greater expansion of the rib cage, emphasizing this time* inspiration *versus* expiration.
  6. *Mobilize the pelvic girdle and the lower limbs.*
     - *Feel and evaluate the RoM and the resistance to passive movement of the* hamstrings, adductors, rectus femoris *and* iliopsoas.
     - *Work to reduce the hip flexion and obtain more RoM in extension, and then introduce some abduction and outward rotation of the femoris.*
     - *Release and stretch the posterior muscles of the leg and those of the sole of the foot, and then help to keep the leg in extension by working for a concentric activation of the* quadriceps femoris *as a knee extensor.*

Fig. 2.7 Transfer and weight shifts on the side with extended hip

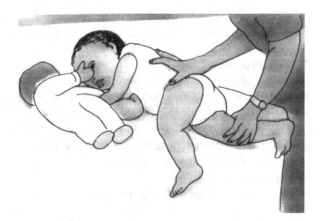

- Facilitate a transfer to side lying asking the child to collaborate actively as much as possible:
  1. *Mobilize the shoulder girdle to enhance their availability to move/be moved.*
     - *Feel and evaluate the RoM and the resistance at the gleno-humeral joint, at the elbow and other distal parts.*
     - *Prepare the joints to be more mobile, and then facilitate the child's hand to experience some touching or proprioceptive movements, avoiding over-recruitment that could cause the shoulder joint to return to fixation.*
  2. *Prepare and maintain in extension the hip joint of the lower side, while favouring the upper leg to be freer to move (Fig. 2.7).*
  3. *Invite the child to move the upper leg further forwards, e.g. as for attempting to reach the prone position, always maintaining a good extension of the hip of the lower side.*

Note
- A mobilization, even if passive, is appropriate and benefits severe children, but it must be followed by facilitation of some simple active and/or active-assisted movements, rather than limited to mere passive mobilization (Fragala et al. 2003; Pin et al. 2006).

  To reach these aims:

- Give the child time to feel and adapt to other possible transfers, e.g. towards the prone position.
- Work to maintain the visco-elastic properties of the muscles as long as possible.
- Work to prevent and delay the onset of retractions.

Furthermore, children who have blood circulation problems due to their limited movements benefit greatly from soft tissue mobilization. During movement, ask the child to adapt to the physical and sensory contact and to increase the level of tolerance to tactile input that their nervous system could otherwise perceive as nociceptive.

Mobilization is also a task that can also be entrusted to parents at home, encouraging the relationship and communication with their child.

2.1.2.4 Prone

It is very important to move a severe BSCP and vary their posture during the day. Particularly, it is very useful to have daily periods of tummy time (except for sleeping which is not safe) because it:

- Prevents/delays retractions at the joint, mainly at the hips
- Provides different sensory information
- Improves lung ventilation
- Invokes some antigravity response

The prone position is very useful for the child with an important flexor synergy because it induces the child to organize some antigravity responses and reduce the exaggerated flexion at the head, girdles and spine.

With greater attention than with a flexed child, it is useful to propose the prone position also to a child with extensor synergy, if adequately positioned on a wedge cushion that allows them to simultaneously maintain different joints in flexion and extension (e.g. shoulder girdle in flexion and hip in extension together with the abduction and some degrees of external rotation of the lower limbs).

Suggestion
- Create a suitable support where the child can maintain the prone position:
  1. *Lie the child prone on a wedge cushion (the height of the cushion must correspond to the distance between the armpit and the elbow of the child)* (Fig. 2.8).
  2. *Flex their shoulders, place the arms in front of the wedge, and induce the child to feel the upper trunk weight on the forearms.*
  3. *Enhance the feeling of weight-bearing by exerting light manual pressure on the child's shoulder girdle and along the* humerus, *and verify by feeling the real weight on forearms and open hands on the surface.*
  4. *Verify the extension of the hip joints.*

Fig. 2.8 Child in prone with support on forearms

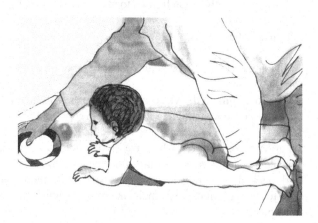

5. *Slightly abduct and externally rotate the lower limbs of the child, using, for example, a pad or rolled towel, to counteract the possible increase of tone in the lower limbs, probably induced by the extension of the hips.*
6. *Facilitate to maintain the head righting involving the child's interest towards someone/something important in the surroundings, like looking at parent's face or a loved toy.*
7. *Consider the distance and height of the object/person to look at, thus avoiding an unwanted hyperextension of the head.*
8. *Help the child to shift the weight-bearing from one side to the other involving one of their upper limbs in different tasks (moving to reach, touch, explore), while the other side manages the main weight-bearing task.*

Note
- Play situations proposed by the caregiver to engage the child's attention should not be too monotonous and never meaningless, such as repeatedly playing with a rattle. The proposals should involve the child in simple motor-cognitive-communication tasks. Moreover, the games should be selected, avoiding both too many toys at the same time and toys that are too chaotic which will make it difficult for the child to concentrate and focus their attention.

2.1.2.5 On a Prone-Standing Frame

Children with severe CP can benefit greatly from using a prone-standing system (Fig. 2.9). The different posture provides the child with new tactile-proprioceptive, visual and vestibular inputs, induces some head righting and can promote the involvement of the upper limbs for simple activities. The appropriate use of a prone-standing frame encourages the child's participation and interaction with the

Fig. 2.9 Prone-standing frame

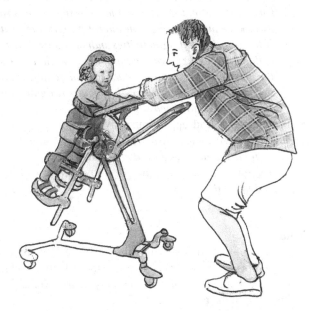

environment (people, family activities, toys and games, educational interventions, etc.) and helps maintain better body alignment and prevents/delays the onset of retractions of muscles (Pin 2007; Paleg et al. 2013).

Suggestion
- First of all, prepare the child for the use of the prone-standing frame:
    1. *Mobilize the child in supine or preferably in the prone position (on therapist's lap for a toddler) to obtain more range at the more comprised joints.*
    2. *Slowly bring the child close to the frame, and help them understand what will be happening together. This anticipation will reassure the child and give them time to adapt to the changes ahead.*
    3. *During the transfer, handle the child in such a way as to maintain the extension of the joints gained previously in point 1.*
    4. *The wide range of tilting possibilities of the frame must not trigger undesired synergies but contain them as much as possible, allowing a small amount of movement at the upper body. The child may have difficulty dealing with a greatly tilted frame which can provoke them to remain flexed. On the other hand, minimal tilting requires a considerable antigravity response that most likely this child will not have.*
    5. *Place a belt or other support at the level of the pelvis to counteract hip flexion and maintain the extension obtained. Assure that the child is comfortable, and, according to the amount of impairment, keep the various supports to a minimum, since excessive support will not allow the activation of the child's active antigravity postural reactions.*
    6. *Verify that the table in front is at a level no higher than the child's sternum, to allow the head, shoulder girdle and glenohumeral joint to move freely.*
    7. *Position the lower limbs with slight abduction and external, trying to extend the knees but without exceeding the extension. The position can be maintained using knee support pads, some lateral-posterior rests at the feet and ankle straps.*
    8. *If the prone-standing activities induce exaggerated tonic recruitment in the child's upper trunk, work again on all the shoulder girdle area to counteract the muscle stiffness around the neck, the scapula and the shoulder joints, trying to facilitate righting of the head, straightening of the spine and some simple active movements of the arms.*
- Facilitate eye-head-upper limb activity:
    1. *Place a recessed table in front of the frame, so that the child can support there on their forearms and lift their head.*
    2. *The presence of a caregiver or a toy in front will motivate the child to reach and move their arms.*

Note
- If the young child is very impaired, the use of a prone-standing frame could be inappropriate and will need to be postponed. To introduce a more extended position, the therapist can treat the child lying transversely on their lap or while leaving them in the parent's arms (Fig. 2.10).

Fig. 2.10 Child in prone lying in the parent's arms

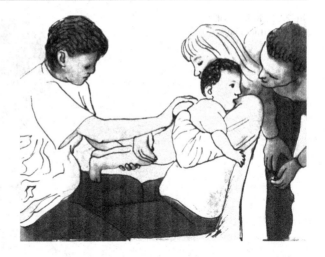

2.1.2.6 Rolling to Side

In BSCP, the transfer and maintenance of the side-lying position represent a conflicting experience requiring the child to remain between supine and prone, which means they need to control the synergies in extension and flexion with their own body. The therapist needs to create the environmental conditions to allow the child to actively achieve the goal and maintain the position with the least possible effort.

After careful evaluation of the alignment and the movement available between the shoulder and pelvic girdles, it is important to facilitate the transfer supine-to-side in both directions, so that the child can experience the variety of sensations arriving from the different sensory inputs. When moving onto the side, the body weight is shifted along the lower side of the body in contact with the support, which then becomes engaged in maintaining the body stable, while the upper side is free to organize some active movements. This transfer could be functional for the child and the parents if, for example, the child learns to use this movement in the night to change position in bed by themselves.

The return from side lying to supine is also important and requires a lot of attention, as described further on.

Note
- It is easy for the therapist to just roll the child onto the side with a passive flexion manoeuvre at the hip and knee with a quick side-to-side transfer. However, this way does not give the child time to understand and feel the task and to try to actively participate, even minimally. In all transfer tasks, it is essential to give the child time to collaborate. The caregiver needs always to assume the role of the "helper", not the "doer", facilitating for best way possible for the child to carry out the functional task.

Suggestion
- Prepare the transfer supine → side lying.
  1. *First of all, verify the muscle stiffness at the shoulder girdle and upper trunk of the child (see preparation in supine)* (Fig. 2.11).

Fig. 2.11 Release of the
muscle stiffness in the
upper trunk

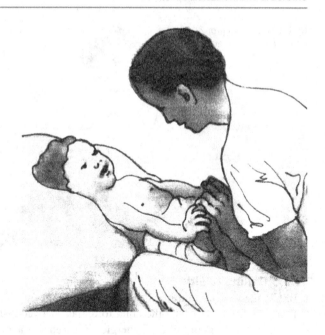

2. *Work to release the stiffness at the hemi-trunk that will act as the base during rolling to side, and introduce extension of the hip that will remain in contact with the mat, in order to avoid interference with the ensuing rolling.*
3. *Place one hand on the child's scapula, and with the other hand apply light pressure on the sternum to allow the child to feel more comfortable to rotate towards the side.*
4. *Give the child time to adapt to the new proprioceptive inputs.*
5. *Motivate the child to actively move towards a target (e.g. reach and touch parent, a toy, etc.), and wait for their attempt to rotate the head and shoulder girdle.*
6. *Facilitate the pelvic girdle to follow the rotation of the upper trunk, verifying the appropriate weight shifting on the hip on the mat and the advancement of the upper hip.*

Note
- A very flexed child may use synergy in flexion in an attempt to move the trunk and limbs. In this case, the therapist must not facilitate the flexion at the shoulder girdle, as suggested above, but to widen the RoM of the shoulder of the pivoting side, so that the body can move more freely forwards (Fig. 2.12).

2.1.2.7 Rolling from Side Lying to Supine
An able-bodied child is continually moving and experimenting with play in a variety of ways. The therapist give needs to provide the same chances to a child with poor motor repertoire, always keeping in mind the level of the functional potential of the child.

Fig. 2.12 Rolling prone without flexor synergy

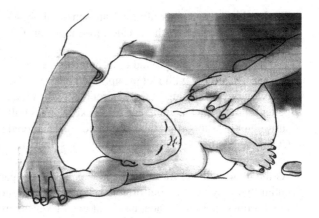

Fig. 2.13 Rolling back to supine with extension synergy

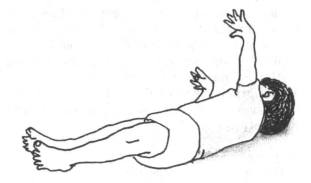

Suggestion
- Prepare the child to go back supine from side lying:
    1. *Before starting the transfer to supine, help the child to feel that their trunk is stable so that they can attempt to involve the pelvis and hip for the movement backwards. High tonic recruitment might not allow the lower limbs to start the movement backwards, and the body could just rotate all in one piece.*
    2. *Facilitate the child to start the movement backwards with the lower limbs as prime movers, while the rest of the body will follow immediately afterwards.*
    3. *If necessary, guide and facilitate the transfer sequence, which should preferably take place with abduction of the lower limb and extension of the hip.*

Note
- The movement from side lying to supine is crucial because the child could return to the supine position using first a strong extension of the head, which often causes the startle reaction (Fig. 2.13).

2.1.2.8 Sitting in a Chair: Child with Extensor Synergy
Most likely a child with severe BSCP will only be able to maintain the sitting posture but cannot move into sitting independently. However, it is essential to let them experience this antigravity position for several reasons:

- The head is the container of important sensorial organs, including the visual and vestibular systems, which provide information to regulate complex antigravity positions.
- The feet resting on the ground or a footrest receive tactile and weight inputs not present when lying with feet unsupported on.
- The wider eye-scanning of the environment when the child is sitting promotes a better relationship and more enriching experiences with people and objects in the surroundings, supporting their cognitive and relational maturation.
- Changing positions during the day improves the child's autonomic functions.

As the child with severe impairment spends a great part of the day sitting, it is essential that they have a comfortable seating system tailored to their basic needs and that allows them to be adequately aligned (Angsupaisal 2015). Therefore, the therapist needs to be extremely careful in choosing a chair of the right size (height, width and depth of the seat, the height of the backrest, etc.) considering the child's size and the characteristics related to their kind of impairment.

In addition to the positioning, it is also worth bearing in mind which activities the child will do when seated: socialization, eating, watching television, etc.

Also, the "right" chair is beneficial to the caregivers, as it facilities the management of the child. However, the child should not sit for long periods of time during the day, and the caregiver has to periodically move the child to alternative positions.

Suggestion
- Main characteristics of the chair:
  - *Measurements (to be taken in the seated position):*
    - (a) *Seat depth: distance from back of hip along posterior side of thigh to knee—minus approximately 5 cm. (2 in.)*
    - (b) *Seat width: the widest distance from hip to hip—plus approximately 5 cm. (2 in.) to consider garments*
  - *A seat of the right size gives the child feelings of "safe border". It is better not to use provisional cushions to fill empty spaces, to avoid unreliable stability inputs.*
  - *If planning simple activities with the upper arms, the backrest should be vertical or at most tilted slightly backwards. If it slopes too far back, it could force the child to continually bring the head and trunk forwards. The centre of gravity line should fall through the pelvis and not behind it.*
  - *For good pelvic positioning a chair with a moulded seat or a three-point belt could be useful that allows a certain abduction of the thighs and avoids the use of transverse belts or uncomfortable dividers.*
  - *The child's feet need to be in contact with the footrest, and the back of the chair must not be tilted too far back as this does not favour weight-bearing on them.*
  - *It is better to have a backrest that does not exceed the height of the shoulders because very often the constant tactile stimulus on the back of the head of a backrest surface stimulates the child to push back in extension. If severe*

impairment requires support to align the head, it is best to use a headrest that controls the upper back of the head instead of the nape of the neck.
– *A front table or recessed tray helps the child to maintain a better alignment and serves as an arm rest.*
– *This positioning helps the child to see their hands, to feel the contact on the table and perhaps to organize simple active movements.*
– *The child's hands can be guided for experiences of touching with open hands and for simple reaching.*
– *The arms on the tray shift the child's CoM a little forwards, allowing the child to maintain a better and more active posture.*

Note
• The above advice refers to an optimal positioning plan, but often severe impairment does not allow this. In children with an important extensor synergy, the main aim is limited to counteract this synergy, and therefore it is necessary to adopt a more reclined chair that induces flexion of the hip and knee joints. Consequently, the therapist should bear in mind that in this case it is necessary to work on the soft tissues to delay future muscle retractions.

2.1.2.9 Sitting in a Chair: Child with Flexor Synergy
The child with a prevalent flexor synergy has difficulty in keeping the trunk upright against gravity caused also by the increased muscular stiffness around the two girdles. The hips can neither extend nor flex adequately, and the protracted shoulders cannot sustain any reaching.

The child needs to be positioned in such a way as to keep their hips tilted further forwards and so facilitate some righting of the spine and active control of the head and trunk. With a straighter spine, the child is also more likely to feel some weight through their legs onto their feet.

• Different characteristics of the chair, compared with the extended child's chair:
– *First of all, work to obtain an anterior tilt of the child's pelvis and flexion of the hips.*
– *If necessary, use strips of adhesive tape to fasten a wedge a few inches high and inclined with the highest side towards the back of the seat, to introduce a physiological curve at the level of the lumbar spine. Alternatively, a shaped lumbar cushion may be useful to keep the back straight.*
– *As for the child with extensor synergy, the height of the recessed table should allow the "flexed" child to keep their forearms and hands in contact with the support surface, to enhance postural control.*
– *The table should not be too close to the child, to avoid a backward inclination of the trunk, contradictory to the previous work to activate an upright trunk control.*
– *If the child has a very precarious antigravity head and trunk control, a commercial or handmade harness can be used.*

2.1.2.10   Assisted Standing
With a severe BSCP child, the goal of the upright posture is not to achieve a functional antigravity competence but to provide the child with various environmental

inputs and to solicit some new upright responses compared to their spontaneous repertoire.

To achieve these results, the therapist needs to carefully set up a facilitating environment in order to obtain positive responses from the child.

Before proposing the upright position, it is essential to work on the soft tissues to prepare the various parts of the body to actively maintain such an antigravity position. This preparation will include release of the shortened muscles and activation of the stretched ones.

Suggestion
- Prepare the child for the postural change:
  1. *Assess the RoM at the main joints, to identify which muscles are too short and which are too stretched over lengthened. Both of these situations limit the range of movement of the joints.*
  2. *Release the contracted muscles (any "technique" can be used if applied after a careful specific, not generic, assessment, remembering to prepare soon after the postural muscles to maintain the upright position). These muscles will need to work to sustain the body weight and to provide some active antigravity responses.*
- Transfer the child towards the vertical position:
  1. *Pay close attention not to lose the advantages achieved with the soft tissue treatment. For this, transfer the child directly from the previous position to the upright one, and then give them time to adapt and organize some active reactions. The transfer from a horizontal to a standing position is quite drastic: so avoid doing it quickly because that could provoke exaggerated perceptive reactions in the child, in the same way as when the child is positioned on a prone-standing frame.*
  2. *Hold the child from behind, place their feet on the ground, and verify that extension is still present at the hip and trunk.*
  3. *Avoid just passively sustaining the child, but facilitate weight-bearing on the feet and propose some interesting activities, such as playing with parent or sibling (Fig. 2.14).*
  4. *Transfer the child on a prone-standing frame: a support table placed in front of the child can help them to cope with simple activities, as pointing on a communication board.*

Note
- The height of the table is of fundamental importance: for a very flexed child, the table should be slightly higher than the height usually indicated, with the aim of facilitating the active upright reaction in the head and trunk. On the other hand, for a child with extensor synergy, it is appropriate to have the table at a slightly lower height than usual, in such a way as to contrast the extension of the body backwards.

Fig. 2.14 The child with
severe BSCP in assisted
standing in front of parent

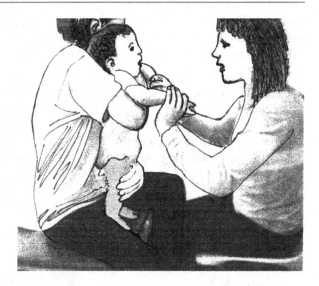

2.2 Child with Tetraparesis and Moderate Motor Impairment

Compared to the child with a very high muscle tone, the child with moderately increased stiffness can adapt more easily and organize their behaviour to solve functional environmental problems. Most of these children are classified in the GMFCS at the level II–III.

Although the therapist must work to promote functional activity in these children by limiting the recruitment of excessive stiffness, they need to consider that one of the signs of damage to the first motor neuron is muscle weakness, which will primarily affect the involvement of postural muscles. Due to this weakness, many children with BSCP have poor core stability (Hodges 1999) with difficulty sustaining postural muscles of the lower trunk, often conditioned also by perceptive impairments. These youngsters are very motivated to move and can transfer from one postural situation to another adopting compensatory strategies. However, the effort of performing in conditions of muscle weakness of the core can favour an increase in stiffness in the distal parts of their body.

It is more difficult for these children to solve a functional motor problem in a more upright posture, such as playing in the sitting position, where they have a smaller base of support (BoS) that requires more trunk stability, or in standing position, with an even more reduced base and a higher CoM compared with supine and prone.

The transfer from one position to another is conditioned by the child's ability not only to move stably against gravity but also to integrate information coming from the visual, vestibular and tactile-proprioceptive systems. Through the feedforward learning process, the child creates and preserves their "baggage" of sensory experiences, varies their attempts to solve problems and so increases their repertoire of functional strategies. On this basis, the therapist needs to pay attention to the problem-solving proposals addressed to the child, proposals that need to be tailored to their effective potential, be interesting and of functional value.

Characteristics of the Child with Moderate BSCP Impairment
Movement:

- Poor motor repertoire compared to the task
- Difficulty in acquiring antigravity abilities (balance) → lack of movement

Muscle stiffness:

- Weakness of postural muscles
- Increased muscle stiffness, mainly in distal parts of the body
- Mixed types of CP display also dystonia

Parts of the body:

- All segments of the body are involved, but with different severity

---

2.2.1 Natural Clinical Development in Tetraparesis and Moderate Motor Impairment

2.2.1.1 Supine

The child has a reduction in postural muscle recruitment at the level of the lower trunk. They will have difficulty building a valid core stability and consequently perceiving their body in contact with the supporting surface. When the central part of the body is unstable, the quality of movement of the limbs is limited by this lack of cooperation from the core.

Unlike the able-bodied child who takes advantage of the joy of kicking to strengthen their abdominal muscles, the child with poor core stability finds it difficult to kick with a good rhythmic sequence. As a result, any attempt to move requires a greater effort and increases the stiffness at the distal parts of the child's body.

The less able child has also a limited variety in motor patterns and more stereotyped synergies in extension or flexion. This behaviour, together with the misalignment of the pelvis, may cause future displacement of the hip joints (Shrader et al. 2019). The child has difficulties varying their motor behaviour, remains mainly with an extended spine, also conditioned by a still-present ATNR (Fig. 2.15). This position accentuates the misalignment of the body and alters the perception of the body schema.

During the first stage, the shoulder girdle is retracted with internal rotation at the shoulder joints and the elbows in flexion. The attempt of functional reaching occurs with parabolic movements from extension towards flexion, with raking movements of the whole arm instead of simply extending the arm towards the object.

Fig. 2.15 Typical posture
in supine

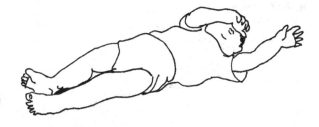

Fig. 2.16 Child with
flexion-extension patterns

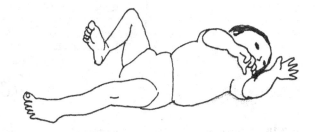

2.2.1.2 Side Lying

Compared to situations of severe impairment, this child has more motor initiative, but attempts to move actively increase stiffness (due to the initial misalignment) and the effort to accomplish a task.

When transferring to side lying, it is difficult for them to rotate the two girdles independently, move the shoulders forwards and stretch the arms towards the midline. Even their lower limbs have difficulty changing the repetitive flexion-extension patterns (Fig. 2.16). Often the young child tries to move to their side, but unfortunately the head and lower limbs do not easily move away from the supporting surface. The older child, on the other hand, uses a more economical strategy by pushing themselves en bloc onto their side (Fig. 2.17) using a massive head-induced flexion.

2.2.1.3 Prone

This position, compared to the supine one, does not appeal to the child because it requires more effort to resolve the upward control. When the child tries to lift their head, they have difficulty extending the shoulder girdle, and the upper limbs cannot move forwards efficiently to support the body weight (Fig. 2.18). The great effort to perform the task can cause an increase in stiffness in all the other parts of the body and hinder the initiative and the fluidity of movement.

The shoulder girdle, tightened by this situation, has a reduced RoM between scapula and arm, the rotator muscles are ineffective, and the Codman's scapulohumeral rhythm is limited. When the head is not straight and the shoulders do not extend adequately, the spine and pelvic girdle cannot be activated, and the lower limbs are not able to abduct and externally rotate to bear weight efficiently and transfer weight from one side to the other. Therefore, balance is very poor.

Fig. 2.17 Transfer en bloc
onto the side

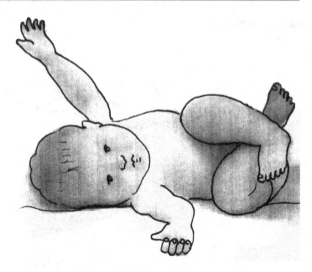

Fig. 2.18 Prone position
with poor support on
the arms

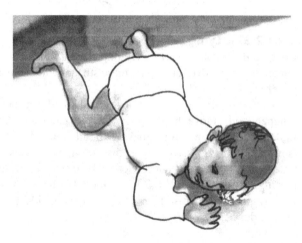

2.2.1.4 Sitting Position

Supported sitting begins early both for practical needs (e.g. to be fed) and to promote interaction with the environment. Children with less impairment adapt quite easily to the antigravity position, while others have greater difficulties. All of them need to organize themselves differently to maintain the CoM over the BoS of the pelvis. Compensatory strategies are useful, such as using hands for support or inclining the upper trunk further forwards, with protraction of head and shoulders, internal rotation and adduction of the lower limbs (Fig. 2.19).

This strategy is useful in one way because it stops the child from falling, but it also blocks them in a precarious, rigid, semi-flexed posture with no anterior tilt of the pelvis where the head and trunk righting reactions and movement initiatives are impossible. In the long run, it becomes a consolidated compensation strategy which prevents any further maturation of antigravity abilities in sitting.

Fig. 2.19 Sitting position with posterior tilt of the pelvis

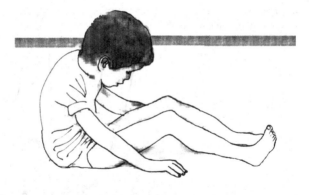

Fig. 2.20 Difficulty in the bimanual manipulation in semi-flexed sitting

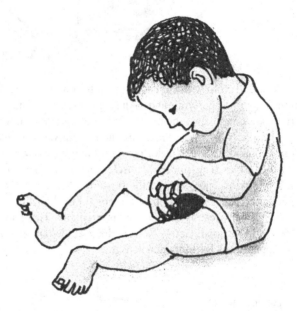

Immobilized in this semi-flexed posture, the child is also unable to move their head to visually explore and interact with the surrounding environment, two primary functional advantages of sitting. Any attempt to move their head or the arms to reach for a toy causes a shift of the CoM to which the child is unable to react with an adequate and immediate balance reaction. The child quickly learns that it is better to not even try and they remain as still as possible. Even raising their head just to look, focus or watch a person moving around the room is very demanding for them.

The upper limbs become tools not to reach and grasp, but rather to maintain the CoM within the pelvis. Another compromise to avoid falling is to grasp a stable support with one hand (the edge of the chair or sometimes their pants!), while the other hand grabs an object. Bimanual manipulation is severely limited as is the development of praxic skills (Fig. 2.20).

Fig. 2.21 Ileo-psoas
recruitment to maintain the
sitting position

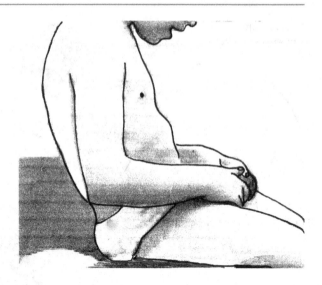

A skilled child with CP has more motor initiative which sometimes diverts attention from an underlying and enduring muscle weakness, particularly in the lower trunk, which prevents the maturation of antigravity trunk control.

The posterior postural muscles and the *transversus abdominis* do not work properly to create a good anterior pelvic tilt and the activation and strengthening of the spinal muscles. The *iliopsoas* muscles remain permanently contracted to fix the hips in semiflexion and stabilize the posture (Fig. 2.21). The stability of the trunk is maintained by a kyphotic posture which is exhausting for the child who will flop against a back rest as soon as one is available. This sitting compensation causes a gradual reduction in active RoM at the shoulder and pelvic girdles and in the use of the upper limbs for bimanual activities.

Advantages of sitting
  – Experience of an upright position
  – Better participation and interaction with the environment
Disadvantages of sitting
  – Consolidation of compensation strategies
  – Increased recruitment of muscle tone, to sustain the antigravity position
  – Gradual reduction in joint range

2.2.1.5 Kneeling

The child with moderate BSCP can achieve a functional kneeling position, but with few variable patterns. The transition from sitting is done using compensatory strategies and with poor alignment and righting of the trunk. Once in kneeling, this child

Fig. 2.22 Child sitting between feet with no trunk rotation

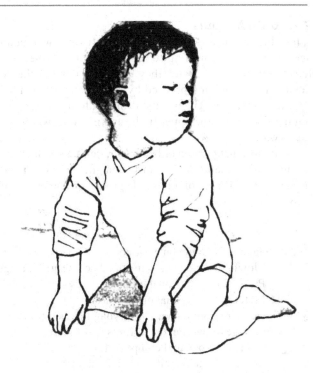

will sit between their heels, often asymmetrically, to maintain the CoM inside a BoS as wide as possible. This allows to stay balanced and to use the hands for playing and other praxic activities even though it blocks the lower spine in extension (Fig. 2.22). The hips and knees are fixed in flexion as are the feet in equinus, all of which contribute to future muscle retractions. The child with moderate BSCP usually does not pass through half-kneeling to stand up.

Advantages of kneeling
- Improvement of the visual range for scanning environment
- Facilitation of bimanual activities
- Improvement of praxic abilities
- Interaction with the surrounding activities

Disadvantages of kneeling
- Static position with legs stuck in flexion
- Bad use of functional but disadvantageous position compensation
- Increased muscle stiffness, mainly at the pelvic girdle and lower limbs
- Further reduction of RoM, mainly at the pelvic girdle and lower limb joints

2.2.1.6 On All Fours

If the child can lean forwards and support some weight on their arms, they manage to pass from kneeling to all fours, but with very flexed hips and inactive legs. To move on all fours, they take advantage of the flexion-extension movements of the head and proceed by moving their legs forwards together with no alternating pattern. The most skilful children manage to move without supporting themselves on the upper limbs and move forwards with a type of "kangaroo crawl walk".

With this repetitive motor behaviour, flexion will increase in hips and knees, and the feet will remain blocked in plantar flexion. The poor variability of patterns increases the stiffness of all muscle groups of the lower limb, in particular, the *triceps surae* muscle.

Advantages of moving on all fours
  - Moving independently in the adjacent surroundings
  - Promotion of personal initiative
  - Maturation of spatial organization
  - Greater participation in everyday interactive activities
Disadvantage of moving on all fours
  - Overuse of postural compensations
  - Increased muscle stiffness and risk of contractures/retractions
  - Further reduction of RoM at the main joints

2.2.1.7 Standing

The child must use alternative strategies to stand up since adequate balance skills and complete foot support and perception of the ground are lacking (Fig. 2.23).

Fig. 2.23 Reduced BoS, with support on the forefeet

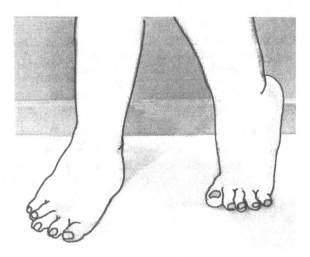

They pull themselves up with their arms to reach the erect position and then stay upright supporting with hands and trunk.

The child gains the upright position without any valid antigravity competences or adjustment at the ankle joints (ankle strategy). Postural instability leads the child to employ alternative strategies for standing, at the expense of good support on feet and extended hips, a well upright response of the trunk and variability of motor patterns. Instead, they use a flexion-adduction posture in the lower limbs to steady the body and to lower the CoM.

In presence of a fixed plantarflexed foot due to retraction of the *triceps surae*, the child will hyperextend at the knees in order to have the feet in contact with the ground to obtain more weight-bearing surface.

In standing, the child with mild tetraparesis has many of the same features as the child with diplegia but shows more head and shoulder compensations and misalignment of the girdles.

> Disadvantages of standing
> – Increased muscle stiffness and possible contraction/retraction of muscles of the lower limb (*triceps surae*, *iliopsoas*, hamstring and adductor muscles)

2.2.1.8 Walking

Few of these children can walk efficiently because the poor distal motor repertoire in the lower limbs does not allow sufficient balance reactions at the ankles and feet. There is substantial reduction in the BoS, and weight-bearing is only possible on the front of the feet.

The limited active movements of the pelvis on the three spatial planes and the lack of rotation between the two girdles further worsen the walking sequence: while one lower limb supports the weight, the other quickly transfers forwards en bloc without rotation at the hip joint but only with pelvis rotation (Fig. 2.24). The child walks forwards emphasizing side-to-side transfers of the whole body, pausing briefly in the weight loading phase.

> Advantages of walking
> – Experiences of independent movement in the environment
> Disadvantages of walking
> – Reduction of degrees of freedom (DoF) at different main joints
> – Difficulty in modulating walking speed
> – Learning of unvaried and inaccurate walking patterns

Fig. 2.24 Walk with
flexed hips and no rotation

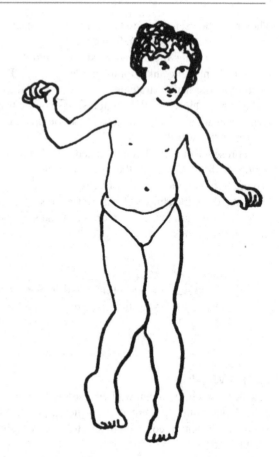

2.2.2 Practical Suggestions

The child with moderate tetraparesis can reach a functional level that includes
a satisfactory functional antigravity postural control. Each child will have
their own potential and the functional prognosis will be different. Therefore,
the therapeutic plan needs to be carefully personalized.

It is important that the child, also when quite young, experiences different
antigravity positions, including standing, even when they do not have all the
requirements to deal with them independently. From the first year of life, they
need to have occasions to process visual and vestibular sensory information,
with their head in an upright position as well as to experience tactile and proprioceptive weight-bearing through the legs onto the feet (Takakusaki
et al. 2016).

The functional rehabilitation plan need not follow a stereotyped path towards
independence but instead should be self-paced and versatile, e.g. walking
independently in easy and/or well-known surroundings and then using a stick
or a wheelchair in more difficult environments.

Different aims of the therapist:
- *For the child (autonomy and quality of life)*
  - Acquisition of adaptive skills diversified according to environmental demands, at different levels
  - Improvement of perceptual attention and processing of sensory information
  - Autonomy in daily functioning
  - Autonomy in interpersonal interactions (e.g. communication strategies, school participation, etc.)
- *For the parents and caregivers (everyday management)*
  - Understanding child's potential, difficulties and current problems
  - Learning and adapting the most appropriate everyday care to the needs of the child
  - Support in the promotion of independence and partnership in therapy choices such as surgery, medication, hands-on therapy sessions, use of orthoses and specific equipment
- *For the treatment session*
  - Postural adaptation of the child to different antigravity levels (based on the functional prognosis), with particular emphasis on the acquisition of movement skills
  - Recruitment of motor units for strengthening weak muscles
  - Integration of motor, sensory and perceptual systems
  - Soft tissue care to prevent or delay negative changes to joints and fasciae
  - Organization of gnosis-praxic skills
  - Prevention/reduction of deformities through team planning of interventions: orthoses, equipment, medications, surgery
  - Functional evaluation of the upper limbs to foster written communication
  - Identification of strategies to facilitate daily functioning

2.2.2.1 Holding and Carrying of Infant in Parent's Arms

Holding and carrying baby in the parent's arms is a simple and natural daily activity with wonderful benefits for both, especially for all newborns and infants with CP:

- Provides a state of well-being in all involved through reciprocal touch and physical contact
- Facilitates the adoption of consoling modalities
- Facilitates body postural adaptations of baby and parent
- Promotes baby's sensory, motor, communication and social development
- Facilitates eye-to-eye contact with the baby
- Facilitates the contacts with the external environments

Suggestion
- Suggest different ways for parents to hold and carry their baby/infant and help them understand the best ways to do this:
  - *Vertical chest to chest carry with the infant well supported at trunk and pelvis and shoulders and hips flexed* (Fig. 2.25)
  - *Hip carry with infant carried in the "koala" position, with legs astride parent's hip* (Fig. 2.25b)
  - *Front carry* (Fig. 2.26) *of infant with hips flexed and abducted and shoulder girdle slightly forwards*
  - *Lap sitting with parent seated and supporting infant's trunk stability as they look outwards*
  - *Back carry with the infant in a backpack or piggybacked on the parent's body*

Note
- "Babywearing" using a baby carrier (sling, wrap or pouch) an alternative functional way to facilitate the parent-child body contact, contributing to the adult's comfort (Fig. 2.27). The therapist can encourage the parents and caregivers to be babywearers and guide them in the choice of the best type to use for their particular baby and according to family preferences.
- It is advisable to start the treatment session with baby in parent's arms, the most comfortable and protected situation for both. The therapist gently enters into this privileged parent-child relationship making contact with the child, looking for eye contact, a head-trunk straightening and orientation of the upper limbs towards the midline, hand-hand contact, etc.

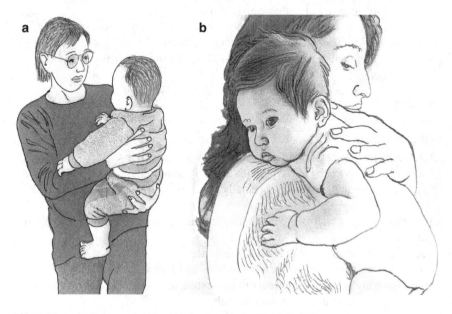

Fig. 2.25 (**a**, **b**) Baby carried chest to chest and in the "koala" position

Fig. 2.26 Front carry of
baby with legs apart

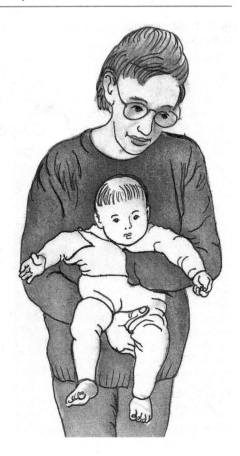

2.2.2.2 Supine
Although the supine posture is the child's usual position when sleeping, or lying in
a stroller for a walk, or during nappy changes, treatment can be started in any position based on the goals of the activity proposed.

The infant can be moved from the parent's arms to sitting on the therapist's lap
to introduce different motor, sensory and interacting therapeutic activities.

Suggestion
- Align the segments of the child's body to let them feel positions other than in
  extension:
  1. *Gently elongate the baby's neck and align their head in midline.*
  2. *Flex the lower limbs and hips and tilt the pelvis backwards.*
  3. *Elongate their back muscles, to let them feel the weight of the body on their
     shoulders, first on one side and then on the other. In this way, the muscle stiff-
     ness at the level of the shoulder girdle decreases, and the child can bring their
     arms forwards more easily.*

Fig. 2.27 Babywearing
using a kangaroo wrap

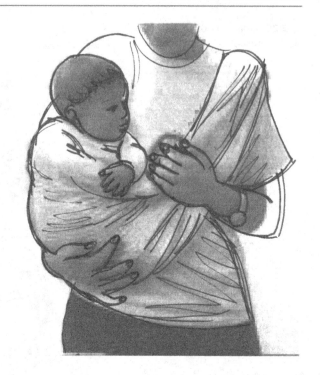

Fig. 2.28 Move sideways
to touch mom

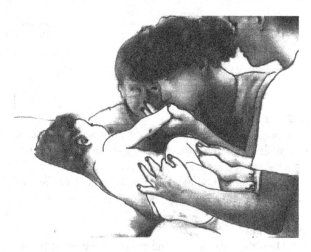

- Propose different transitions to move to/from supine:
  1. *Emphasize sensory information involving the child's upper limbs and intro-
     duce eye-hand-mouth-foot coordination.*
     Depending on the age of the child:
     - *Suggest the child touch the parent's or someone else's face in front*
       (Fig. 2.28).

Fig. 2.29 Touch and play
with bare feet

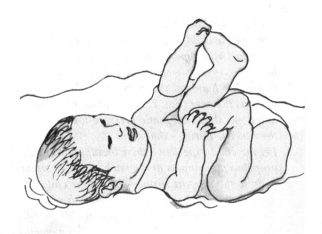

- *Facilitate the child's hands to touch and explore their mouth, face and tummy.*
- *Facilitate hand-object activity: reach for, grasp, hold, shake and play with toy.*
- *Facilitate bimanual play: touch, manipulate, explore toys with both hands.*
- *Facilitate hand-feet activity; find and play with bare feet, bring to mouth* (Fig. 2.29).
2. Facilitate active movement in the lower legs like kicking:
   - *Verify the alignment of parts of the body to increase RoM at the main joints.*
   - *Encourage active global and segmental rhythmic movements in flexion-extension-rotation in the lower limbs.*

2.2.2.3 Kicking

An active kicking is a milestone for the future ability to move against gravity because it involves the *transverse* and *rectus abdominis* muscles allowing the child to organize basic core stability. Moreover, the regular movements of the legs in flexion-extension bring to mind the rhythmic motor patterns produced by the central pattern generators (CPG) and which are a prerequisite for future walking. Also, regular movement of the lower limbs supports good growth and alignment in the coxo-femoral joints.

A child with poor antigravity postural control prefers more horizontal positions to bypass the problem of gravity and to have more ease of movement to play, for example. However, even in these positions, a child can acquire significant skills for future antigravity competences, recruiting more motor units through rhythmic kicking patterns, forearm support in prone lying, side sitting and later sitting.

The movement of the limbs requires the activation of the proximal parts of the body, and consequently, with a circular progression, the reinforced stability core allows the manifestation of the distal motor repertoire.

Suggestion

- Solicit valid and strong kicking:
    1. *Observe the child's chest wall and the movement of the diaphragm. If the ribs are wide with superficial breathing, give manual guidance to improve the breathing rhythm, emphasizing exhalation.*
    2. *Place one hand on the sternum of the child and apply a gentle pressure towards the core* (Fig. 2.30), *or place both hands laterally on the lower ribs and apply the same gentle pressure towards the core, to reduce the width of the rib cage during exhalation.*
    3. *Let the child experience their breathing through this manual guidance. The proprioceptive inputs at the back of trunk can facilitate the anchoring of the body to the support surface so that the child can have a better kicking and move the distal parts of the body more freely.*
    4. *To further strengthen the core, slightly lift the infant's pelvis when kicking, as this will improve diaphragmatic breathing and the function of the* transversus abdominis *muscle.*
    5. *Ask the infant to lift their head, to look at a toy on their tummy, for example, to engage the* rectus abdominis *muscles.*

Note

- Kicking can also be a pleasant game and activate the child's desire to move. It is possible that, shortly after working specifically on the activity, the child themself masters the movement, using it as an expression of joy, a way of attracting attention and to communicate with loved ones.

2.2.2.4 Turning Sideways and Prone

In neuro-motor development, rolling onto the side is the baby's first independent change of position. The first times it occurs is by chance: when the baby moves their legs in the air, they end up falling spontaneously to one side with gravity, rotating the pelvis, and they find themself in side lying. Later the child will be able to actively rotate the two girdles and arrive in the prone position with a complete roll. Although these sequences occur relatively easily on a wide and stable support, they can be a

Fig. 2.30 A gentle manual pressure on the chest enhances proprioception

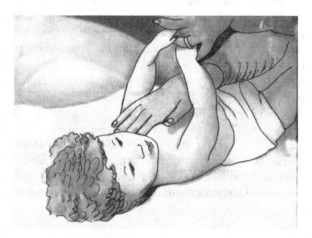

complex task for the child with motor impairment, because they require selective movements of the head, shoulder and pelvic girdles and limbs.

Suggestion
- Set up the biomechanical conditions that facilitate the child to move all parts of their body as best as possible:
  1. *Verify that there are no elements that hinder the freedom of movement, such as too much extension of the head or a tight posterior muscle chain.*
  2. *Verify that the child is ready to use their body axis as an active base on which to rotate: the hip joint on the side of the body that will weight bear during rolling should be extended so that the child does not just passively fall flexed in prone by gravity.*
  3. *The upper hip needs to be free to move. If necessary, manually increase the extension-abduction, to facilitate the transfer.*
- Motivate the child to turn by animating a toy or another attractive proposal on the side, and then wait, giving them time to initiate the roll. The adult helps by facilitating the movement avoiding passively turning the child.
  1. *Verify that the sequence begins with the rotation of the head and the child's eyes are looking at the endpoint.*
  2. *Encourage the upper arm to cross the midline. If necessary, help the body to turn by introducing slight trunk flexion at the level of the sternum to facilitate the forward movement of the shoulder.*
  3. *Verify that the upper leg and hip joint are also free to move and not stuck in adduction. For that, it is necessary to actively engage the* obliquus abdominis muscles, *the* gluteus medius *and* maximus *and* tensor fasciae latae.
  4. *Give the child time to enjoy the intermediate position on their side, and "play" with the flexion-extension movements of the leg and then maybe roll back actively to supine (Fig. 2.31).*
  5. *According to the child's task while in side lying and prone, be ready to facilitate the appropriate orientation of the arm and involvement of the hand. The arm and hand move differently if the task is to reach for a toy or lean on the forearm. However, to perform both tasks, the external rotator muscles of the shoulder must be engaged first and then the arm muscles such as the* triceps *and supinators of the forearm.*

Fig. 2.31 Facilitations to roll from side to prone

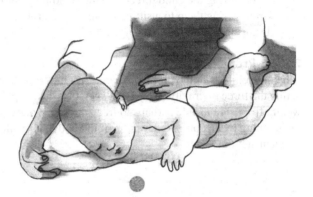

Note

- The therapist needs to be constantly attuned to the intentions of the child regarding their aspirations of interacting with the environment so that they can facilitate the achievement of their goals, modifying the environmental conditions, for example.
- They facilitate in such a way as to allow the child to try by themself, find adaptive strategies to complete the task, repeat the action and learn.

2.2.2.5 Moving the Child in Adult's Arm into Prone Lying on Lap

The way in which the small child with CP is moved by adults from one position to another (the so-called "handling") is extremely important. The therapist needs to educate the parents and other caregivers on the appropriate modalities to always use when moving their child.

Suggestion

- Below is an example of how to transfer the infant into the prone position on the adult's lap:
  1. *Place one arm transversely under the infant's shoulder girdle and the other under the pelvis.*
  2. *Verify that the hips are extended, and slowly turn the child onto one side, and rest them transversely on the adult's lap.*
  3. *Holding the joint of the external shoulder, complete the rotation towards the prone position. One of adult's legs should be at the level of the child's sternum, while the other at the level of the hip joints which should be positioned in extension.*
  4. *Once in the prone position, facilitate activities involving the upper limbs (e.g. reaching for a toy, look at and touch parent, etc.) which will activate trunk extension, with a straight spine and extended hips.*

Note

- The prone position on the adult's lap is a very useful starting point for transferring the child to other positions without introducing unwanted hip flexion.
- Some examples are:
  - Transferring the child directly to the standing position
  - Transferring them to a sitting position, with rotation between the two girdles
  - Dressing and undressing (Fig. 2.32)

2.2.2.6 Prone

When the child is in the prone position, they have to solve the problem of counteracting the force of gravity. They must keep their head up, lean on forearms and shift weight from side to side perhaps to free an arm for play. This position also requires maintaining extension in other parts of the body, particularly the hips, essential for efficient standing later on.

Fig. 2.32 Child undressed on adult's lap

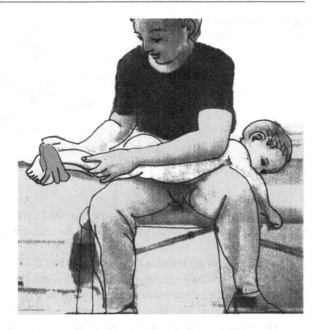

Suggestion
- Prepare the child to support on forearms, so that they can keep their head and trunk extended:
  1. *Verify the freedom of movement in the shoulder girdle, particularly the movement of the scapula. If limited, pectoralis muscles can be manually released to improve the gliding of the scapula on the ribcage.*
  2. *Verify the presence of a satisfactory Codman's rhythm between the scapula and the humerus, and, consequently, work to release the intra-rotator muscles (e.g. subscapularis) and to activate the extra-rotators.*

Note
- As with all manual therapy, the therapist's work on specific muscles requires visual and tactile information on ROM and muscle tension, and so the child should be undressed.

- Propose activities that require alternate weight-bearing shifts, pivoting on the tummy and rotation between the two girdles:
  1. *Verify that the shoulder girdle is not in flexion, the spine and pelvis are extended and the lower limbs abducted and slightly outwards rotated so that the child feels stable.*
  2. *Exert a slight pressure from the shoulder of the child on the axis of the humerus, to emphasize the weight-bearing perception on the forearm.*
  3. *Verify—and facilitate if necessary—that the child arrives in the prone position with open hands. Hands are a fundamental source to receive sensory information and tool for stabilizing the body (see also Chap. 6).*

Fig. 2.33 Support on one forearm and reaching a toy

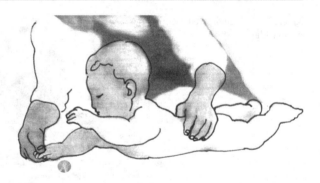

4. *Exert gentle manual pressure at the extended hips.*
- Propose functional tasks that require the activation of stability/mobility responses:
  - *Stretch one arm forwards to reach a toy* (Fig. 2.33).
  - *Pivot on the tummy and so move to reach something on the side.*
  - *Move into the sitting position transferring the weight first backwards and then pivoting on one hip, pushing on the arm and extending the trunk. If appropriate, propose returning to the prone lying position using the upper limbs for support.*

Note
- When the therapist gives light manual pressure to a part of the child's body, they draw perceptual attention to "that" part, which becomes the child's stability reference point. This allows them to be more confident in experimenting new activities with other parts of the body. This type of manual approach is different from the technique of pressure tapping, which instead aims to facilitate the contraction of postural muscles in hypotonic children (for further details, see Chap. 4, Sect. 4.2).

2.2.2.7 Transferring to the Sitting Position
The transfer from the supine to the sitting position requires the activity of the *obliquus externus* and *internus abdominis* muscles, generally less active in children with CP.

Suggestion
- To active transfer from supine to sitting:
  1. *Stabilize one hip joint with light manual pressure, to use that hip as the pivot base to rotate and extend the trunk.*
  2. *With the other hand behind the contralateral scapula, facilitate the child's shoulder to move forwards and cross the midline.*
  3. *Before the child rotates sidewards, verify that they are ready and motivated to move into sitting with full open hand contact on the surface; facilitate the hand for efficient support, as necessary.*

Fig. 2.34 Transfer to sitting position with hand support

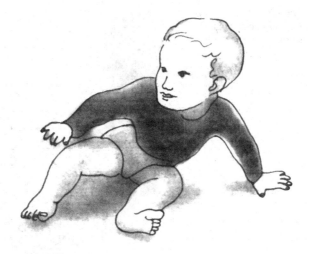

4. *Encourage the contralateral shoulder and upper arm to cross the midline, first with forearm support, then with the arm extended and righting of the trunk at the same time.*
5. *Let the child pause in intermediate positions of the transfer sequence, if they are interested in some activity, spontaneous or suggested by the adult.*
6. *Take into account that this transfer also involves the lower limbs, which have a very important role in balancing (Fig. 2.34).*
7. *Verify the final alignment of the body, at the end of transfer.*

Note

- The therapist should always keep their manual facilitation to a minimum according to the child's active involvement. The intention should be to influence and guide the child towards more functional motor behaviour, not act on the child's behalf.
- Excessive hands-on guidance can be a perceptual disturbance to the child. The therapist needs to select their input to the child's initiatives and not vice versa.

2.2.2.8 Sitting

In the sitting position, the CoM is higher than in the supine position and the BoS is smaller.

In severe forms of CP, sitting with appropriate postural support is a functional aim of treatment. It is also the most useful position for ADLs and for the training of fine movements at the upper limbs. Where possible, it is important for the child to learn to transfer to and from the sitting position independently, since it means that they are able to transit from a higher or lower position with selective movements of the trunk, pelvis and arms.

When promoting sitting, the aims for the child are not only to be able to sit independently but also to move and function in this position.

Fig. 2.35 The sideways transfer into and out of sitting

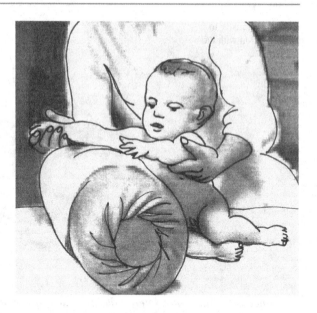

In the future, the child will spend much time seated, with the risk of developing contractions/retractions in the *iliopsoas* and *long rectus femoris*. It is important to encourage the child to be active because movement increases muscle contractility, extensibility and strength.

For the child with moderate impairment, interventions in sitting should be varied with the use of stools and benches rather than chairs with backs or arm-rests. These activities will promote reaching and bimanual activities and strengthen the muscles of the upper limbs, trunk and the lower limbs, as preparation for standing.

Sitting can be achieved through various postural transfers. Depending on their age and ability, the child will learn to move in and out of sitting, and the therapist should be guided by the child's choice in discovering the most suitable strategy.

The transfers to and in sitting include the following:

- From the supine position → rotation and righting of the trunk, using one arm for support
- From the prone position → extension and rotation of the trunk, pushing up on two arms
- From all fours → rotation of the trunk, transferring through side sitting (Fig. 2.35)
- From kneeling → transfer through half-kneeling then half-way and half standing with trunk rotation

Fig. 2.36 Sitting position
with facilitated upright
trunk

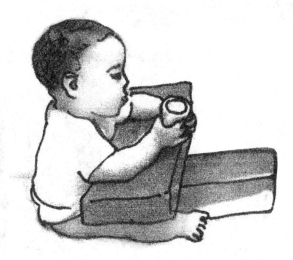

- From standing → with or without trunk rotation, according to the position and height of the seat
- From standing → sit on the corner of a bench, sit astride, or transfer to another seat
- ....

Suggestion
- Prepare the most suitable setting for the child to sit and move on a sitting surface:
  (a) Seat with a wide, non-slippery and moderately rigid surface.
  (b) Bench or stool of a height distance knee to heel, where the child's feet are supported on the floor.
    1. *Verify that the CoM projection is over the BoS and that head and trunk are upright* (Fig. 2.36). *This is possible with a minimal anterior tilt of the pelvis.*
    2. *Verify the freedom of movement in the lower limbs. In particular, if the child is long-sitting, release the adductor and hamstring muscles to obtain a wider base and more RoM at the hip joints.*
    3. *If the child is sitting on a stool or bench, emphasize the perception of the feet on the floor with a gentle manual pressure through the lower legs.*
    4. *Facilitate weight-bearing through the lower legs, to prepare the child for an efficient transfer into standing.*
    5. *When the child is in a comfortable situation, enrich play with distal haptic sensorial experiences to the feet, experimenting with surfaces of different textures (smooth/rough, wet/dry, hot/cold, soft/hard, with/without edges, etc.)* (Fig. 2.37).
- Propose different experiences in the sitting position.

Fig. 2.37 Sensorial inputs
for feet and hands

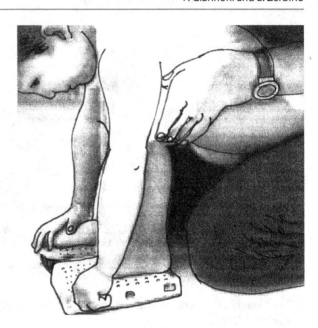

Fig. 2.38 Sitting inside a
box. Modified from
European Bobath Tutors
Assoc., with permission

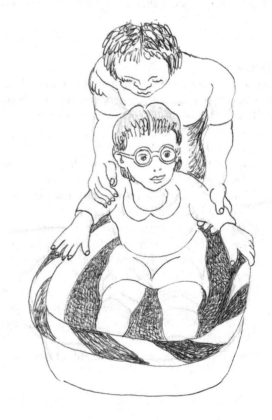

Note

- Certain conditions are essential for the child to maintain the sitting position independently and participate in activities such as looking around and playing with objects:
  - It is important that the child's feet are supported on a stable floor surface, with bare feet or shoes, rather than in socks only.
  - The presence of available anterior and posterior tilting of the pelvis, adequate head and trunk alignment and upright control.
- Haptic experiences are multisensorial, and they need to be appropriate with the functional task proposed to avoid confusing to the child. For example, the main goal could be to give sensory input to the feet to reinforce the perception of the body, or precise weight-bearing input to the feet at the right time during movement to allow the child to engage in more active and efficient transfers.
- For many functional tasks, the child needs to stay longer in a sitting position for specific ADL involving the upper limbs (e.g. during feeding time, at school) which require a stability of the trunk. Children with BSCP will have different levels of trunk impairment and therefore different abilities to maintain postural control that allows efficient use of the upper limbs. As reported by Butler et al. (2010), it is useful to assess the level of support that the individual child needs at the shoulder/axilla/inferior scapula/lower ribs to maintain valid righting of the trunk and the need to apply any support straps, stabilizing cushions or provide a personalized seating system.
- If the child has any vestibular disorder, the therapist must take into account this specific disturbance and propose adequate interventions not triggering this pathology. For example, the therapist can sit the child astride a roll and evoke balance responses or can solicit the child to do small side to side weight transfers, to practise vestibular adaptation to movement (Fig. 2.39).

2.2.2.9 Sitting: Link Between Core Stability and Upper Functioning

A child with good antigravity balance in sitting can maintain a stability even when moving and using the distal parts of the body. On the other hand, in a child with precarious core stability and so poor trunk control, even the head cannot be completely steady causing imprecise visual fixation and consequent difficulty in fine motor skills.

To improve the child's antigravity competences, it is essential to check and facilitate an adequate position of the pelvis on the sagittal and coronal planes, the straightening of the trunk and good foot support all to promote more efficient functional movement in the upper part of the body.

Suggestion

- Work for the linear acceleration of the child's trunk:
  - *Sit the child on a stable surface without back support, of a height that allows the child's feet to support on the ground.*

Fig. 2.39 Child seated on unstable roll surface. Modified from European Bobath Tutors Assoc., with permission

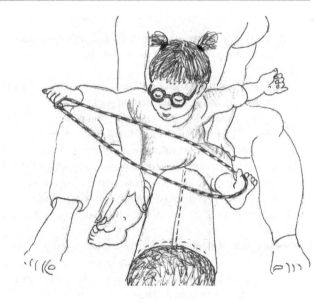

Fig. 2.40 Stability at the lower trunk with a wide elastic lumbar belt

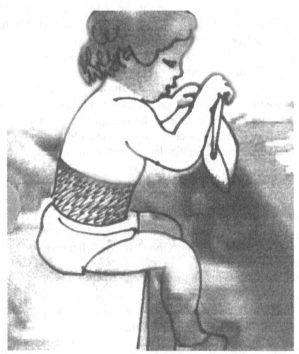

- *It can be useful to have the child wear a wide elastic belt around the lumbar spine area to enhance for a short time the perception of stability of their lower trunk (Fig. 2.40).*
- *Place a small wedge (high on one side no more than 6 cm.) under the child's buttocks, to facilitate the anterior tilting of the pelvis.*

- Facilitate more selective movements of the pelvis:
  - (a) *With an infant in long-sitting on a surface or the therapist's lap:*
    1. *Apply one steady proprioceptive manual reference point at the level of their anterior chest and the other on their back at the level of the lumbar spine, to induce the trunk righting reaction (Fig. 2.41).*
    2. *Propose appropriate, individualized activities that require weight shifts, so that the child can use one hip as a pivot and rotate the trunk, allowing the contralateral limbs (leg and/or arm) to move more freely.*
  - (b) *With a child sitting on a stool:*
    1. *Verify that the child's feet are in good contact with the ground; effective weight-bearing can be enhanced by exerting manual pressure on the knee through the axis of tibia to the feet.*
    2. *Allow the child to experience tilting movements of the pelvis on the sagittal plane and to weight shift from side to side (Fig. 2.42).*
    3. *Propose activities involving the upper limbs while the trunk remains straight and the two girdles rotate (Fig. 2.43).*
- Involve the child in activities that require visual-manual coordination:
  1. *Propose bi-/unimanual activities while the child keeps the trunk straight with no support (Fig. 2.36).*   (a)   *Undressing, dressing, combing a doll*
     - (b) *Hanging the doll's laundry*
     - (c) *Drawing in the air*
     - (d) *Playing games of gesture imitation*
     - (e) ......
  2. *Request visual exploration combined with gestural indications:*
     - (a) *Search for a hidden object in the room and indicate it.*
     - (b) *Play kids' bingo games, with figured tables hanging on the wall.*
     - (c) *Propose praxic sequences that require vision and gestures;*
     - (d) ......

Fig. 2.41 Proprioceptive input to straight up the trunk

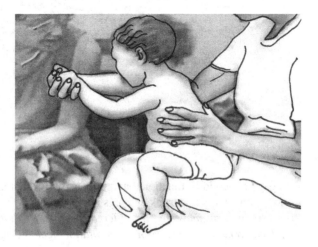

Fig. 2.42 Pelvic tilting in sitting

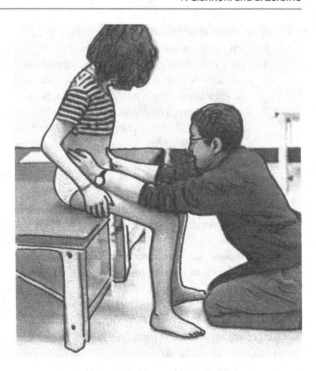

Fig. 2.43 Activities for rotation with straight trunk

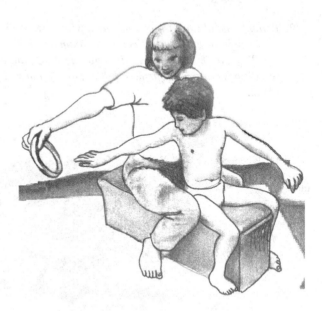

- Engage the child in functional and play activities that involve many upper limb movements while the trunk and legs remain stable:
    1. *Activate arm movement at different heights, so that the CoM rises and the trunk remains steady, even when rotation occurs* (Fig. 2.44).

Fig. 2.44 Combination of upper limb movement and trunk stability

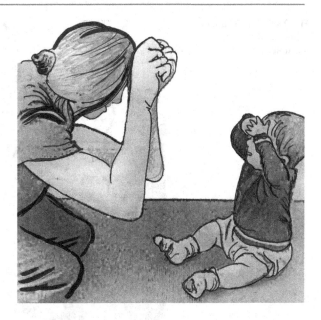

Note

- The need to maintain a constantly erect trunk is completely different if the child is sitting with a support in front. For a child with muscle weakness and poor antigravity postural control, leaning the trunk and/or forearms on an anterior support is certainly the easiest solution to maintain the upright position and use their hands at the same time. However, this is done without involving the postural muscles and with no real weight-bearing on the lower limbs.

Suggestions for a functional sitting position:

(a) To facilitate the anterior tilting of the pelvis:
    - Stool, bench or chair without back support
    - Seat surface with different degrees of inclination or a small wedge, to transfer the CoM forwards
    - Anti-slip mat on the seat surface
(b) To facilitate the maintenance of the upright reaction of the trunk:
    - Table positioned in front of the child, with an adjustable tilting top
    - Anti-slip mat under the child's feet

2.2.2.10   Sitting Without Foot Support

From a postural control point of view, it is very different to sit with or without foot support. With an average distance between the feet, foot support significantly increases the body's weight-bearing base. It provides a distal point of stability that improves the upright reaction of the head and trunk and enhances the child's core stability and their ability to perform selective distal movements. The sitting position without foot support requires different skills and is more tiring because the BoS is smaller and less defined, and more muscle work is required to maintain balance.

Fig. 2.45 Small base of
support and balance
reactions

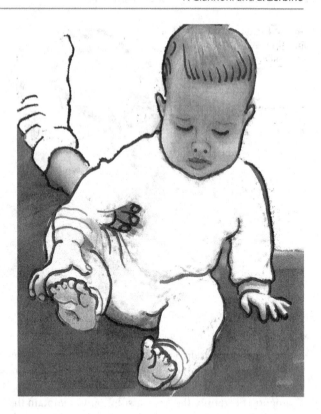

All activities in sitting without foot support require more balance skills and
involvement of core stability.

Suggestion
- Allow the child to practise balance reactions in the sitting position by proposing
  various dynamic activities while on both stable and unstable surfaces with varied
  conditions of foot support:
  - *Verify the availability of the child's pelvis to tilt on the sagittal and frontal
    planes during an activity with weight shifting, and allow them time to per-
    ceive and adapt to the new postural information.*
  - *Propose activities that require moving some distal parts of the body while
    maintaining a steady-state balance:*
    - *Turn the head to observe the surrounding environment.*
    - *Lean forwards or sideways to take a toy and then manipulate it.*
    - *Lift one foot while the other leg stabilizes the body, e.g. to take off a sock
      (Fig. 2.45).*
    - *........*

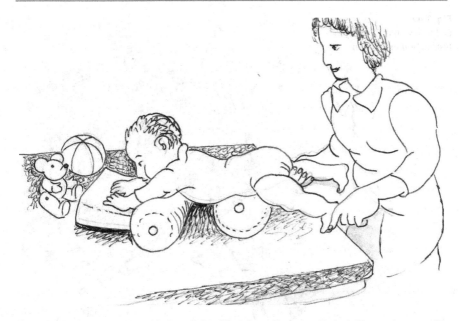

Fig. 2.46 Infant on ball and baby-roll Modified from European Bobath Tutors Assoc., with permission

2.2.2.11 On a Small Gym Ball

To facilitate dynamic righting reactions, the therapist can lie the infant on their tummy over a small ball and create a mobile situation to strengthen their posterior muscle chain, increase hip extension, and even experiment forefoot contact on the floor (Fig. 2.46).

Suggestion
- Prepare a safe and suitable setting:
  - *Place a ball on a non-slippery surface, so that it can be moved safely.*
  - *Create a limited environment around the child to support their perceptual spatial awareness.*
  - *Before transferring the toddler onto the ball, arrange for someone to be in front of them (e.g. parent) for reassurance.*
- Transfer the toddler from prone to an upright position:
  1. *Transfer the child prone onto the ball, in such a way to favour extension in the upper trunk and moving forward of the arms.*
  2. *Propose activities that induce active righting of head and trunk and extension of the hips.*
  3. *While holding the child's thighs, facilitate further extension of the hips introducing slight abduction and outward rotation of the lower limbs.*

Fig. 2.47 Facilitating leg
and foot weight-bearing in
preparation of standing

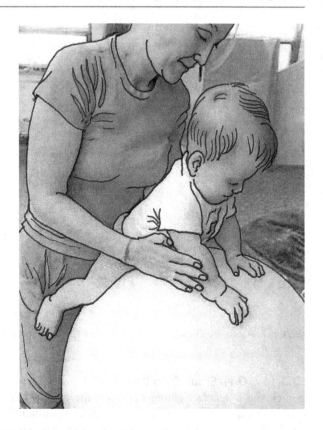

4. *Gently roll the ball backwards to slowly bring the child's feet (better if supported on the therapist's thighs, during the transition) down to the floor.
   Pause occasionally along the way to allow the child to perceive the gradual
   increase in weight-bearing (Fig. 2.47).*
5. *Let both feet, or one foot first, make contact with the floor, preparing them for
   complete support on the ground.*
6. *Encourage the child to fully stand up, with the protection of the ball in front.*

2.2.2.12   On a Big Gym Ball

In some daring children, a bigger ball can be proposed to facilitate the transfer in the
standing position, because it can engage them in dynamic and playful experiences
that improve balance.

This could be considered only a therapeutic technique, not related to the functional needs of the child. However, a capable therapist can easily combine fun for
the child and specific targeted activities to improve postural reactions and muscle
recruitment.

The therapist needs to take into account the great mobility of the ball and know
that the child may initially fear interacting with it. To gain the child's confidence,
the therapist needs to always let the child play with it first, touching it, pushing and

Fig. 2.48 Facilitation of hip extension and balance reactions on the gym ball

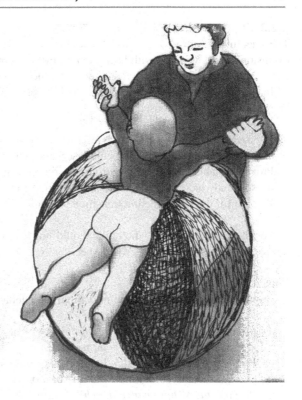

throwing it, etc., to make them feel safe. Activity on the ball should not be proposed if the child remains fearful.

Although activity on a gym ball can facilitate different experiences and several transfers from one position to another, the child's training on it has two main goals: to improve basic righting and balance reactions in the head and trunk (for this the ball should be moved slowly) and enhance more dynamic balance reactions (here the ball will be moved faster).

Suggestion

- Transferring the child onto the ball:
  - *Handle the young child in the same way as the transfer from the adult's arms to the prone position (see above): shoulder girdle and hip joint should be extended, and lower limbs abducted and slightly outwardly rotated.*
  - *Some children can start to interact with the ball positioned firmly in front of them, when they are standing.*
- Work to achieve active upright head control, engagement of the posterior muscle chain and balance reactions:
  1. *Move the ball in such a way as to open the kinetic chain in the child's lower limbs and then roll it very carefully in various directions to induce the desired balance responses in the child (Fig. 2.48).*

2.2.2.13　Kneeling

The kneeling position is not easy for a child with BSCP because it requires hip extension simultaneously with knee flexion. Furthermore, in this position a person cannot adopt any ankle strategy, and therefore they can use only a hip strategy.

In children with both the tetraparetic and diplegic forms of moderate BSCP, the kneeling position is proposed to:

- Improve the stability of the pelvic girdle through strengthening of the *gluteus maximus* and abdominals, particularly necessary in this position
- Provide a stable base to enhance trunk control while maintaining hip extension and consequently increase RoM at the shoulder joint and improve upper limb activities
- Prepare for the half-kneeling transition to stand up

For these specific goals, the child should not lean on a support surface (e.g. a table) with their trunk or arms when kneeling.

Suggestion
- Promote activities that require maximum engagement of *gluteus maximus* and active trunk righting reactions:
  1. *Assure that the child's feet are off the mat or other support surface, in order to involve some tibiotarsal joint movements.*
  2. *Verify that the pelvis is tilted backwards through a strong* gluteus maximus *and* transversus abdominis *muscle, to obtain an adequate postural alignment.*
  3. *Propose tasks that involve the child's upper limbs while maintaining steady trunk balance even when rotating or shifting on the frontal plane:* e.g. *take and manipulate a toy with two hands, hit a balloon, grab a scarf that moves in the air,* etc. (Fig. 2.49).

Note
- Often these children are uncomfortable maintaining the kneeling position for a long time because they present with "patella alta" caused by *quadriceps* and patellar tendon forces that are increased by standing and walking with semi-flexed knees (Lenhart et al. 2017).
- To overcome the lack of stability at the pelvic girdle, the child will try to stabilize in kneeling by blocking the hips in semi-flexion and intrarotation and so widen the base of support, lower the CoM and reduce the sway of the body axis. It is therefore wise to work hard on pelvic girdle stability and hip extension to avoid the need for this compensatory strategy which will compromise the quality of future walking.

2.2.2.14　Sitting to Standing

The ability to move independently from sitting and squatting to a standing position is essential for everyday functional motor activities. Sit to stand (STS) is very demanding for the child with CP because they need to control the destabilizing forces caused by the movements of the various parts of the body, both on the horizontal and sagittal planes. During this transfer, (1) the ankles dorsiflex, and the feet

Fig. 2.49 Stability of the
pelvic girdle when moving
the upper limbs

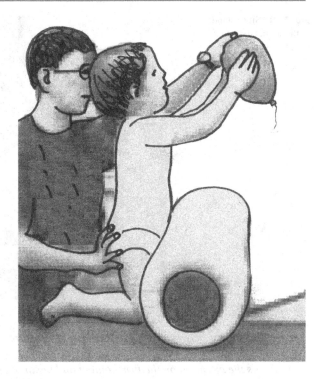

move backwards and push on the floor; (2) the hips flex, and the straight trunk moves forwards over the feet with the contribution of the *anterior tibialis* muscles; (3) an upright movement of the trunk brings the child to standing due to the coordinated activity of the extensor muscles of all three joints (ankle, knee and hip). The active preparation of feet and ankles is very important as well.

The therapist needs to work hard on training this basic STS sequence using repetition to improve balance and strengthen weak muscles through concentric and eccentric exercise (Shepherd 2014). Moreover, they should ask the child to carry out this task introducing different functional variables: stand up from seats of different heights, with foot placement in different positions; transfer from squatting and through half-kneeling, while holding an object, in quiet and noisy environments, with more or less visual control; etc. (Khemlani et al. 1999; Medeiros et al. 2015; Jeon et al. 2019). Scientific literature reports how the ability to perform STS strongly influences the functional level of the child with CP impairment (Pavão et al. 2014) and underlines that the transfer is very demanding for them mainly due to disturbed proprioception at the lower extremities (Gaul-Aláčová et al. 2003).

Suggestion
- Prepare the starting conditions for the transfer:
  1. *Verify the correct height and width of the seat: the child's feet need to be in full contact with the floor.*
  2. *If not yet planned to stand and walk, the child should have bare feet, never be only in socks.*

Fig. 2.50 Sit to standing
with the transfer of CoM
over the feet

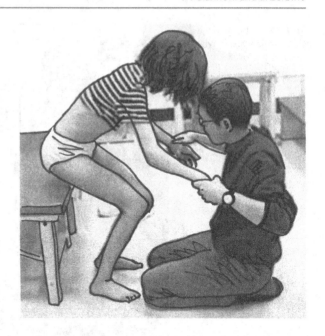

3. *The distance between the two feet should be more or less the width of the child's pelvis.*
4. *Focus the attention on the firm contact and position of the feet of the child, in order to provide a stable pushing up.*
5. *Assess, and facilitate if necessary, the postural adjustments of the upper body, which provide upright extension of the trunk and anterior tilting of the pelvis.*
6. *Facilitate the ankle mobility in moving the feet backwards and the alignment of the talocrural joints, the eccentric activation of the* soleus *and concentric activation of the* anterior tibialis. *Before starting the STS transfer, RoM in the ankle joint should be less than 90°.*
7. *Before moving the trunk forwards, verify the availability of the pelvis to adapt when slightly shifted to the sagittal and frontal plane.*
- Facilitate the forward transfer and the final extension of the three joints:
   1. *Enhance the activity of the ankle dorsiflexors to move the CoM over the feet, applying slight traction forwards and vertical pressure downwards* (Fig. 2.50).
   2. *Influence the uprighting phase facilitating first hip extension with righting of the trunk and immediately after the smooth continuum with extension of the knee.*
   3. *Stabilize the knee by engaging the* vasti *muscles.*

Note
- During STS the therapist should keep in mind the exact timing sequence of the muscle activation and facilitate them during treatment. On the other hand, they also need to enhance the child's sensory perception of this transfer, occasionally asking

Fig. 2.51 Moving in intermediate sit-to-standing positions

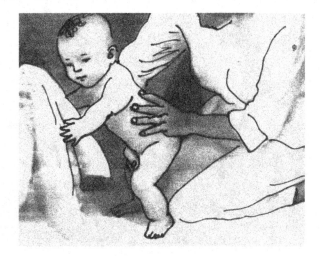

the child to pause, adapt and maintain intermediate positions. Competence in this transfer allows the child to cope with many functional problems: transferring from one seat to another, reaching for something at different heights, un/dressing and, in general, having a vaster functional repertoire at the upper limbs (Fig. 2.51).

- Sometimes the adult's leg is mistakenly put in front of the child's knee without leaving them the possibility to move their knees forwards and transfer the CoM over the feet. The result of this impediment is excessive extension of the body upwards, with a CoM outside the BoS. It is important to show parents and care-givers how to properly help the child in this transfer!

2.2.2.15   Back to Sitting

From a perceptive and muscle point of view, the back-to-sit (BTS) transfer is not the reversal of the STS sequence. There is a motor control perceptual problem here, because the child does not have visual guidance of the final target (the seat) during descent and they may fear falling. Similarly the postural sway during STS in children with CP is greater when performing the sequence with closed eyes (Pavão et al. 2018).

Compared to STS, there is a more eccentric muscle activity in the BTS, for example, in the *quadriceps* and *triceps surae,* and the need to maintain postural stability makes the movement slower, with less forward displacement of the trunk (Papaxanthis et al. 2003).

Suggestion

- Prepare the starting conditions for sitting down:
  1. *If the transfer is new, prepare the child by showing them what is expected: the seat, where to place their buttocks and so on.*
  2. *Verify the anticipatory adjustment of the trunk necessary to efficiently control the descending phase.*
  3. *Verify the availability of the pelvis to tilt in the sagittal plane to allow the knees to flex.*

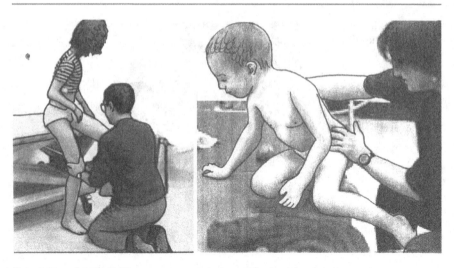

Figs. 2.52 and 2.53 Different ways to reach the standing position

- Start the BTS sequence:
  1. *During the first attempts, reassure the child with explicit manual facilitation at the pelvis, to flex the knees and lower the CoM to emphasize the vertical pressure on the feet.*
  2. *In competent children, reduce the hands-on facilitation, and only apply pressure along the axis of the femur to flex the knees and lower the CoM.*
  3. *In the meantime, monitor the eccentric work of the* erector spinae *which allows the trunk to move forwards.*
  4. *Guide the child in lowering themselves slowly, controlling the eccentric activity of* quadriceps *and* triceps surae *and maintaining good contact of the feet on the floor.*
  5. *The child moves their buttocks backwards and sits down.*

2.2.2.16 Transfer to the Standing Position
There are many different ways to stand up, including from lower and higher positions. It is wise for the child to experience a variety of them and so learn to adapt to their variables.

The therapist should not impose pre-packaged motor behaviours but support the child's initiative, since every experience offers a good opportunity to experiment and learn how to solve functional problems.

Suggestion
- Support the child's initiative to stand up in different ways:
  - *Standing up from seats of different heights, widths and consistencies.*
  - *Standing up from a sitting position on a roller, ball and other mobile supports.*
  - *Get off a table or other high surface with/without rotation of the trunk and then stand up (Figs. 2.52 and 2.53).*

> – *Standing up from a squatting or half-kneeling position (see Chap. 2, Sect. 2.3.2, and Chap. 3, Sect. 3.2).*
> – *............*

Note

- The use of aids (standing frame, sticks, elbow crutches, etc.) to help the child maintain an upright position should be carefully evaluated and proposed only with very specific aims in mind, because they limit the variability of the sensory-motor experiences offered in standing and the need for active adaptive responses. However, these aids are useful for preventing or counteracting probable muscle retractions and reduction of RoM at joints in the lower limbs in children with sustained stiffness. In these cases, the therapist needs to counterbalance the limited involvement of the lower limbs with active demands to the upper body.

2.2.2.17 Standing

An efficient upright position requires a good contact of the feet on the floor to control the body sway with the ankle strategy, core stability through the involvement of the postural muscles to maintain the extension of the main joints and balance reactions to move against gravity and improve the sensory-motor experience.

All this does not happen in the child with CP because muscle weakness does not allow proper recruitment of muscle activity which results in poor antigravity control. A strategy to solve this impasse from the biomechanical point of view is to "stand still" to reduce the body sway and stabilize the posture by fixing the hips and legs in flexion.

Suggestion

- Prepare the conditions for a good standing position by working for greater RoM at the shoulder girdle and better hip extension:
  - *Verify the linear acceleration of the trunk and the extension of the shoulders.*
  - *If necessary, modify with hands-on guidance the protraction of the shoulder blades, to facilitate a lateral or posterior support for the upper limbs, with outward rotation, extended elbows and open hands. The Light Touch Contact can be of help (see Chap. 6, Sect. 6.4.4).*
  - *Verify the effective weight-bearing on the feet, which facilitates sensory input to the midbrain from the soles and organizes the antigravity response.*
  - *Engage the* transverse *muscle and all the core stability muscles—including the diaphragm—to achieve greater extension of the hip joints. Facilitate strong recruitment of the* gluteus maximus *to emphasize weight-bearing on the feet and allow the upright reaction.*
  - *Remember that the straightening of the knees is closely related to the hips (hip extension → knee extension). Then stabilize the knees by recruiting the* vasti *muscles.*
- If the child initially has difficulty maintaining upright antigravity control independently, introduce some facilitation, and let them feel small weight shifting movements with extended hips:

Fig. 2.54 Standing position with extension facilitations

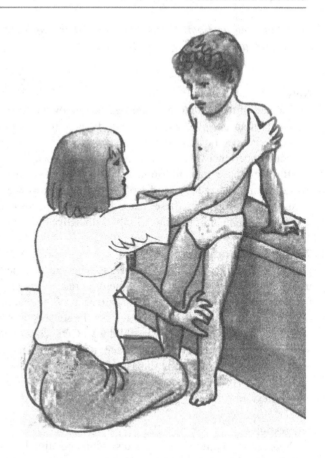

- *To practise independent standing, get the child to stand in the angle of the room, using the wall as perceptual reference points for the shoulders and hips. The child may also receive some perceptual input through the back of their hands and arms externally rotated along the body.*
- *Lean the child's pelvis against the edge of a table whose height corresponds to that of their buttocks and propose tasks that require pelvic shifting on the frontal plane, maintaining the buttocks in contact with the table (Fig. 2.54). Posterior support on externally rotated arms, extended elbows and open hands will help the child carry out the task.*
- *Repeat the exercise as before but with the child moving the pelvis forwards on the sagittal plane and so losing and regaining contact with the edge of the table.*
- *If the child has perceptual problems, place additional boundaries close to their body, e.g. standing between two tables, where the child can move supporting themself on open hands.*
- *Get the child to stand in front of a table of the height of their sternum, and ask them to put their arms on it at 90°. Since the child's trunk does not lean against the table, guide them in performing posterior tilting movements of the pelvis to engage the abdominal muscles, extend the hips and improve the core stability.*

Fig. 2.55 Dynamic upper
limb activity in standing

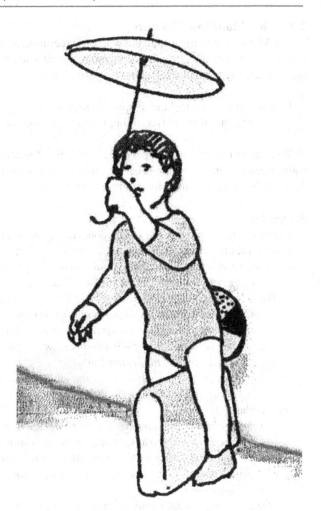

- Work for steady balance in standing:
  - *Propose play and functional activities that require weight shifting on the frontal plane, with or without mobile support at the pelvis (e.g. a soft overball).*
  - *Challenge the child with dynamic activities of the upper limbs (e.g. catching soap bubbles, keeping a small umbrella open, etc.) while maintaining steady balance in the standing position (Fig. 2.55).*
  - *Propose activities that require bimanual involvement of the upper limbs and some rotations between the two girdles.*

Note
- The therapist should avoid any front support because leaning forwards on it eliminates active uprighting and balance reactions, due to the wide, stable BoS. In the case that anterior support for the arms is provided, the height of its surface should be at the level of the child's sternum.

2.2.2.18   Standing: The Core

The child with mild impairment but with poor recruitment of motor units of the core muscles by-passes the difficulty of maintaining antigravity trunk control for a long time, by finding particular compensatory solutions:

- Fixation of the thoracolumbar spine in hyperlordosis
- Anterior tilting of the pelvis, fixing the hips and legs in flexion

With these restrictions, the pelvis is very limited in its movements on the three anthropometric planes, as are necessary for efficient walking. The same compensations as above are also used by children with diplegia.

Suggestion
- Evaluate the position of the pelvis concerning the three anthropometric planes and the relative muscle activation at the pelvic girdle:
    - *In the position considered most suitable (e.g. supine or standing), release the posterior muscles of the thoracolumbar tract and the hip flexor muscles.*
    - *While gaining some posterior tilt of the pelvis, engage the activity of the child's abdominal muscles, in particular the* transversus *and* rectus abdominis *muscles, using tactile-proprioceptive stimulation* (Fig. 2.56).
    - *In the same way, facilitate the recruitment of the* glutæi maximi *and* medii *to stabilize the hip with valid extension.*
- Based on the age and participation of the child, educate them through specific activities to feel and actively perform pelvic movements on the three anthropometric planes:
    - *On the sagittal plane, emphasize the posterior tilting of the pelvis through the engagement of the* transversus, rectus abdominis *and* glutæi *muscles to obtain more extension of the hips. Also, verify the concentric activity of the* vasti *muscles to obtain better extension and alignment in the lower limbs.*
    - *Regarding the frontal plane, propose activities that require lateral shifts of the CoM and different weight-bearings on the lower limbs. Also, include one-leg standing activities to strengthen the* gluteus medius.
    - *Solicit the movements of the pelvis on the horizontal plane with activities that require small rotations of the trunk as during walking.*

2.2.2.19   Basics for Walking

Functional and independent walking is a goal that children with an adequate motor repertoire can achieve because they are able to acquire sufficient balance reactions. However, the therapist needs to help the child to feel and adapt to the sensory-motor inputs that occur during each of the specific, different gait phases, before introducing them to functional walking. Even if later on the child will wear shoes with/without orthoses, at this stage of training, it is better that the child is barefoot during these proprioceptive experiences. Shoes will be worn normally at other times and for long transfers with the therapist.

Note on Walking

(a) On the horizontal plane: the rotation between the two girdles is particularly emphasized during fast walking. In the case of CP motor impairment, the child has limited degrees of freedom at the joints of lower trunk and limbs, and therefore the rotation of the pelvis on the horizontal plane is performed moving the body as a whole, without rotations between the two girdles.

(b) In the frontal plane: during the swing phase, a hemipelvis lowers towards gravity (4°–6°), and the contralateral pelvis "holds" the body weight by engaging the *gluteus medius* muscle. In cases of CP impairment, the child adopts the strategy of lifting the pelvis of the swinging limb due to the lack of stability on the contralateral supporting leg.

(c) In the sagittal plane: the tilting of the pelvis is minimal (3°–6°) and not very significant. In cases of CP impairment, it is necessary to counteract an excessive anterior tilt of the pelvis and engage the abdominal muscles, in order to have a better core stability before starting walking.

Fig. 2.56 Tactile-proprioceptive input to improve core stability

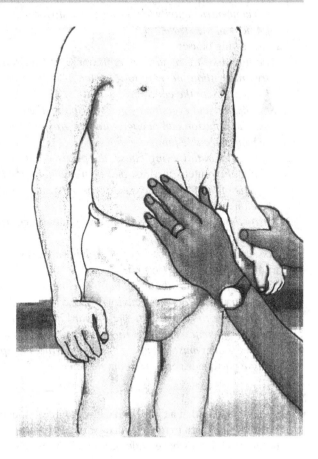

Suggestion
- Verify that the following components of efficient walking are present:
  - *Functional alignment of the different parts of the body.*
  - *Upright extension of the trunk and correct posterior tilting of the pelvis to obtain adequate core stability.*
  - *The child's feet provide effective support for the body weight, also during small shifts in the sagittal and frontal planes.*
  - *Steady-state balance.*
- Prepare the child for the stride sequence:
  1. *First of all, get the child to move the support leg forwards, and so have the contralateral one in hip extension and ready to start the swing phase.*
  2. *Apply extra manual input to the supporting leg to increase hip extension through activation of the hip extensor muscles.*
  3. *Assess and realign the joints of the foot of the contralateral limb, particularly at the heel, talus and cuboid bone. At the metatarsal-phalangeal level, verify the stability of the contact of the big toe on the ground and the presence of some abduction of the fifth toe.*
  4. *Verify the availability of the* triceps suræ *to work first in elongation and then with concentric activity to rock the foot onto the big toe, ready for the pushing-off phase of the stride.*
- Start the swing phase:
  1. *The initial swing requires dorsiflexion of the ankle to lift and move the foot forwards without needing to raise the ipsilateral pelvis. If necessary, manually accentuate the concentric activity of the* tibialis anterior *or facilitate the dorsiflexion and eversion by gently gripping the external part of the foot. The same dorsiflexion can be facilitated by grasping the child's fifth toe or guiding from the ankle joint.*
  2. *During the initial swing phase, the pelvis should not lift; to avoid this, first engage the* gluteus medius, *and then manually apply gentle pressure along the axis of the femur. The* quadriceps *must shorten as an elastic response to the elongation.*
  3. *Verify the activity of the contralateral* gluteus medius *to avoid the collapse of the pelvis on that side.*
  4. *Assist the forward rotation of the pelvis on the swing side, if necessary.*
- Start the contact and support phase:
  1. *Good contact with the heel requires continuous dorsiflexion of the foot; if necessary, facilitate this activity* (Fig. 2.57).
  2. *At the same time, facilitate the forward movement of the pelvis, in order to achieve efficient weight-bearing and extension at the hip on the support leg; the two* glutæi *must be engaged for supporting the upright trunk response, as well as the* quadriceps *to sustain the knee.*

Note
- It is very unlikely that a child with CP will achieve independent walking without aids if they first learn to move with quadripods or a trolley with low handles. This is because these aids have wide bases and are extremely stable. Relying on the

Fig. 2.57 The heel
contact phase in gait

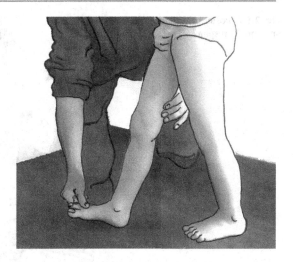

fact that these aids do not fall over, the child consequently can lean on them for support towards gravity eliminating the need for a vertical upright reaction of the trunk. Whereas a completely different result is achieved by using one-point sticks or forearm crutches, perhaps with an enlarged base, or otherwise a posterior walking frame.

- Today the posterior walker is more frequently proposed rather than the anterior type. It offers many advantages because it induces a greater anti-gravity righting and therefore more hip extension (Fig. 2.58). However, if the therapist introduces this walker too early when the child is still unable to regularly sustain a valid upright response, the use of the aid may trigger a general increase in stiffness. Furthermore, poor balance could induce the child to support themselves mainly with their upper limbs, accentuating the forward rounded position of the shoulders and the possibility of future muscular contractures that are difficult to deal with.

2.2.2.20   Walking

The decision of whether the therapist should guide the child in walking from behind or from the front depends on many factors and evaluations:

- Typically a child with CP presents with significant flexion in most joints and reduced RoM at hips, knees, ankles, shoulders and upper limbs. If the main problem is poor movements in the three planes at the pelvis and lower limbs, the therapist needs to guide the pelvic girdle, and therefore their position is irrelevant and will depend on the activities in progress with the child.
- On the other hand, a child with flexed shoulder girdle and a poor righting of the trunk will benefit from receiving manual guidance from behind to perceive and learn upper body extension.
- If there are some perceptual problems, such as spatial and/or vestibular difficulties, the child may be afraid to move forwards towards an empty space and feel safer when the therapist stays in front. However, the therapist should always be

Fig. 2.58 Posterior walker
and upright response

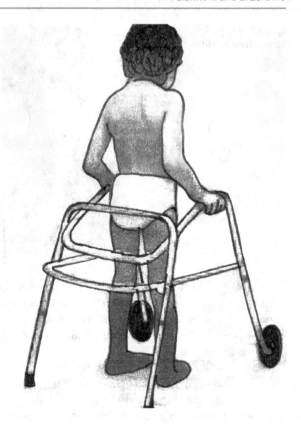

aware of these perceptual disorders of the child and create an appropriate spatial working environment (not too large nor too empty) in front of them. Even the child's mom, dad or sibling in front could be an interesting and pleasant target to reach.

Suggestion
- Engage the child in motor activities in standing that activate upright antigravity stability and extensive muscle work:
  - *First verify that there is an appropriate alignment of trunk, pelvis and lower limbs.*
  - *Guide the child from behind to obtain extension in the upper trunk and external rotation at the shoulders. Then get the child to hold a large object with both hands (e.g. a tray with something on it or a large ball or doll), and ask them to walk and take the object to a destination for a purpose (Fig. 2.59).*
- Create a setting which helps the child feel more confident despite any perceptual problems:
  - *Position the child between two tables parallel to each other, with distance slightly larger than their hip width.*

Fig. 2.59 Facilitated
walking carrying
something with two hands

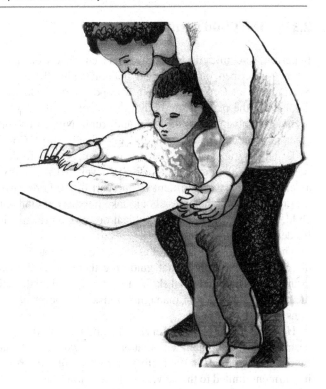

- *Encourage them to touch the table surface with both hands in light way while moving the legs forwards: this will provide an intermitted tactile feedback both on the hands and hips. The child should feel safer, and it will be easier for them to maintain the extended upright posture.*
- *In the same situation as above, propose to walk backwards (see also the Suggestions for the child with diplegia).*
- *Propose walking in other environments with different variables, e.g. in long and narrow paths created with chairs, inside long boxes or other containers with edges, up surfaces that are slightly inclined.*
- *Get the child to practise walking using various types of support that facilitate hip extension and steady balance, such as long sticks with vertical handles.*

Note
- There is the question: "During treatment sessions, should the child walk in shoes or barefoot?" This depends on the child's potential and therefore on the aim of therapy at each particular phase. If the child needs more localized sensory information to acquire more selective movement skills and to improve their step, it makes sense that they are barefooted.

  If, on the other hand, the goal of the treatment is to carry out more global functional tasks in walking, like reaching a distant destination, or the even more demanding activities of going up and down steps, walking over small obstacles, etc., it is more logical and facilitating for the child to wear shoes.

2.3   The Child with Diplegia

In current scientific literature, the motor characteristics of the diplegic form in CP are not described uniformly and unequivocally. To overcome this problem, the Surveillance of Cerebral Palsy in Europe (SCPE 2000) suggests describing topographically the parts of the body most involved, the evident asymmetries and the eventual involvement of the head and trunk. Numerous authors are more oriented towards abandoning the term diplegia (SCPE 2000; Colver and Sethumadhavan 2003; Hurvitz and Brown 2010), while others are still decidedly opposed to that (Cioni et al. 2008; Ferrari et al. 2008; Shevell 2010). However, if one considers that a definite primary impairment in one part of the body also affects function in the rest, rehabilitation therapies should take into account the holistic functioning of the child, and therefore the topographical description of impairment is not significant for deciding on the treatment plan.

The therapist should always assess the child's potential, regardless of the official diagnosis. The elements that guide the therapist's clinical reasoning include the evaluation of the functional skills already acquired by the child, the identification of their strategic choices in managing a task and the identification of essential functions still to be acquired.

However, by carefully observing the infant with a diagnosis of diplegia and comparing their development with that of a child with tetraplegia, it is obvious that their functional evolution is distinctive and clear-cut. At first, shows mainly a motor impairment limited to the pelvis and lower limbs, but the lack of muscle recruitment in the core and consequently the difficult interplay between the lower and upper parts of the body gradually require more functional adaptations also on the part of the latter. These compensations make the child perform functionally as if affected with mild tetraparesis (Giannoni and Zerbino 2000), and most of the time they are classified in the GMFCS at the level I–II.

Some authors (Ferrari and Cioni 2010; Ferrari et al. 2014; Damiano et al. 2013; Alboresi et al. 2020) underline the possible presence of perceptive impairment in children with diplegia basing this diagnostic orientation on the presence of certain characteristics:

- Exaggerated and low threshold startle reaction
- Upper limbs in startle position
- Avoidance of eye contact
- Frequent blinking and closing of eyes
- Facial grimaces
- Freezing of posture

Other studies indicate that, compared to a child with tetraparesis, the child with diplegia also has sensory-perceptual impairment (Ferrari and Cioni 2010) concerning vision (Pagliano et al. 2007; Ego et al. 2015), attention and executive functions (Di Lieto et al. 2017), due largely to periventricular leukomalacia.

Main Characteristics of the Child with Diplegia
Movement:

- Poor selective functional movements, initially limited to the pelvic girdle and lower limbs
- Subsequent motor involvement of all parts of the body parts, although with more impairment remaining in the lower trunk and limbs

Muscle stiffness:

- Initially moderate recruitment of stiffness and limited to the lower limbs
- Progressive worsening of stiffness, due to the antigravity functional demands

2.3.1   Natural Clinical Development of the Diplegic Form

2.3.1.1 Supine
When supine, this child easily relates to their parents, with visual contact and active participation within everyday interactions. The child does have kicking patterns, but they lack the physiological fluidity and variability. The reduction in the spontaneous motor repertoire in the lower limbs does not allow the strengthening of the abdominal muscles essential to build a valid core stability.

In the infant, kicking of the legs is characterized by two basic patterns, one with global flexion at the level of the three joints and the other with global extension. Some studies point out that in these children there is no combined pattern with hip flexion and knee extension in leg elevation, or isolated movements of the knee and tibiotarsal joint, the absence of which may be a specific diagnostic sign of CP impairment (Yokochi et al. 1991; Jeng et al. 2004; Fetters et al. 2010).

The kicking in these children is not coordinated and is often asymmetrical due to different levels of motor impairment between the two sides of the body. One limb moves with more flexion and abduction, while the other stabilizes by activating the internal rotator, adductor and ankle extensor muscles (Bobath and Bobath 1975; Shepherd 2014). This asymmetry causes misalignment of the pelvis on the horizontal and frontal plane. Early on, head movements and the functional use of the upper limbs do not seem to present any problems, as they are not yet significantly involved in more antigravity positions. In fact, the head is free to move, and the upper limbs can move to midline, although possibly one arm less than the other, due to the altered relationship between the girdles.

2.3.1.2 Side Lying
From supine the infant will fall or roll spontaneously onto their side with misaligned girdles, using the head, arms and shoulders as prime movers, as they have a fuller and more variable motor repertoire compared to the lower part of the body. The upper leg will follow the movement, but with little selectivity and an increase in

stiffness, due to the effort and limited fluidity of the transfer. The side position facilitates movement initiatives with the pelvis and kicking with the upper part of the leg, which reinforce the abdominal, hip, knee and foot muscles, useful for future locomotor abilities. The child with diplegia is unlikely to remain in side lying and will probably move into prone.

2.3.1.3 Prone

If the child is put in the prone position, or arrives by themself, they need to learn to push and support on their forearms, lift and move their head in all directions, shift their weight from side to side, stabilize on one forearm and extend the other to reach an object, activating the outward rotator muscles of the shoulder. It will be difficult for them to push up onto extended arms with open hands and to straighten the trunk properly, due to insufficient hip extension.

The lower limbs will tend to lie asymmetrically, due mainly to the misalignment of the pelvic girdle. Pivoting on the tummy will not be possible due to the lack of abduction-extension in the hips. Instead, it will be easier for this child to move forwards pushing on their forearms using a global, propulsive flexion pattern. This propulsive effort will increase the stiffness in the legs and in other parts of the body (Fig. 2.60).

Advantages of supine to side lying and prone
- First transfers and change of position
- Different relationships with the environment
- Reaching for objects
- Gratification for the child and family
- Maturation of motor and sensory abilities

Disadvantages of supine to side lying and prone
- Consolidation of simplified strategies
- Postural misalignments
- Progressive increase in muscle stiffness with decrease in RoM
- Scarce visual control and exploration of the environment
- Limited functional position for ADL or interpersonal experiences for the older infant

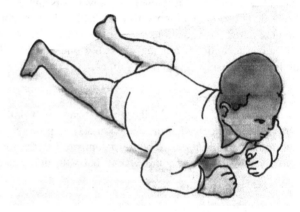

Fig. 2.60 Moving forwards in prone, pulling in global flexion on forearms

2.3.1.4 Sitting on the Floor

The child sits up without apparent difficulties and therefore can easily interact with the environment. However, without adequate pelvic postural control, they have difficulty performing selective anterior/posterior tilting of the pelvis at the lumbosacral joint and the flexion-extension of the hips. Limited experience in prone lying with the extensor muscle activity of the trunk does not favour a good sitting position.

The scarce anterior pelvic tilt limits adequate hip flexion and so the proper sitting position, and the chid begins to overuse the *iliopsoas* muscle and the long head of the *rectus femoris* (Fig. 2.21).

In this situation, the lower limbs do not abduct, and the body cannot move forwards, so the child should flex their head and shoulder girdle forwards, keeping the hip constantly semi-flexed to avoid falling backwards. All these compensations provoke an increase in general stiffness. The child then uses one hand, generally the most skilled, to reach and manipulate, while the other rests on the sitting surface to widen the BoS and to stabilize the position. A more able child can use both hands but increasing the use of the compensatory strategies described above.

2.3.1.5 Sitting on the Floor in W Position

As motor activities increase in the upper body, the young child who passes time on the floor will start sitting between their heels in the "W position" to create a wider BoS and stabilize the trunk. This leaves the upper limbs and hands free to be used for manual tasks. The upper trunk is now facilitated to move but rotation is limited; this makes it difficult for the arms to cross the midline, and so the child's field of action for manual experiences is restricted mainly to the anterior space.

Furthermore, overuse of the W sitting position stresses the coxo-femoral and knee joints, which can become painful. The misalignment of the pelvis makes the child sit with one lower limb inwards rotated and the other outwards, increasing the generalized muscle imbalance. Another way is sitting with both femurs inwards rotated. Both positions increase the risk of hip subluxation/dislocation and can contribute to future toe walking (Fig. 2.61).

Advantages of sitting on floor
  – Contact with the environment, with head and trunk upright
  – Better participation in social interactions
Disadvantages of sitting on floor
  – Increase of postural misalignment and compensation strategies
  – Progressive increase in muscle stiffness, including shoulder girdle
  – Progressive reduction of RoM in all areas, including upper body
  – Possible joint pain and modification of the intrinsic quality of soft tissues
  – Perceptive problems concerning peripersonal space

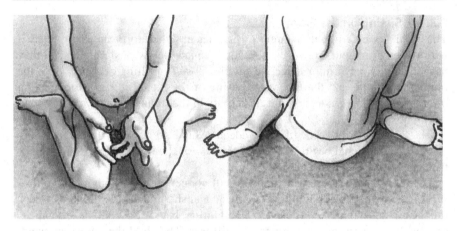

Fig. 2.61 Child in W sitting

2.3.1.6 Seated on Chair

When the child is seated on a chair, they have difficulty shifting the CoM forwards because of the poor core stability and the fixed position of the pelvis in semi-flexion. Therefore, they lean back against the backrest, missing out on the advantages of weight-bearing on the feet (Fig. 2.62). The misalignment of the pelvis directly affects the position of the legs: on the side of the pelvis rotated backwards, the hip is more externally rotated, and on the other side, it is internally rotated. The feet seem to be in contact with the floor, but in reality there is no valid weight support. Leaving the child to sit in this way gradually limits the functional abilities of the child.

> Advantages of sitting on a chair
> – Sharing activities and games with other mates
> – Carry out specific activities of daily life, such as undressing/dressing when seated
>
> Disadvantages of self-organized sitting on a chair
> – Inefficient weight-bearing on the feet
> – Overuse of the *iliopsoas* muscle and the long head of the *rectus femoris* to maintain the sitting position
> – Postural misalignment with progressive increase in muscular stiffness, including in the shoulder girdle
> – Progressive reduction of RoM of the joints and modification of the intrinsic quality of soft tissues

2.3.1.7 Kneeling

The lack of hip extension does not allow the child to stay in kneeling with the trunk properly uprighted, and the misalignment of the pelvis causes asymmetrical weight-bearing. The fixed semi-flexion of the hips and the need to maintain upper trunk

Fig. 2.62 Seated child without weight-bearing on feet

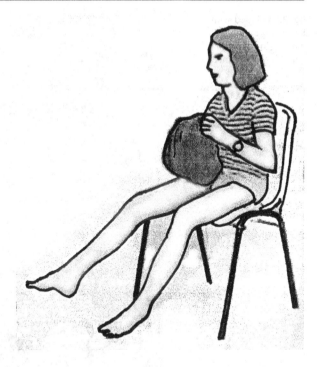

extension to use the upper limbs cause the child to compensate in hyperlordosis, with further loss of RoM at that level (Fig. 2.63).

Furthermore, the child cannot move on their knees with rhythmic alternated leg movements but instead adopts the strategy of bunny-hopping on all fours (Fig. 2.64).

Advantages of kneeling
  – Possibility of manipulation
  – Position of transition for transfers
  – Exploration of the environment through the transfers
Disadvantages of kneeling
  – Further loss of selective movements of the pelvic girdle and lower limbs
  – Increase in the lumbar lordotic curve
  – Increase in stiffness and reduction of RoM at the joints

2.3.1.8 Standing Up from Half-Kneeling

Spontaneously the child with diplegia has difficulty getting into proper half-kneeling, and therefore they cannot really use it to transfer to standing. Instead, to stand, they lean completely on their forearms and pull themself up, dragging the lower limbs up together (Fig. 2.65).

Another strategy for getting up from the floor can be the plantigrade transit. Here, the child places their hands on the floor and comes to their feet with a small

Fig. 2.63 Fixed semi-flexed hips and hyperlordosis compensation in kneeling

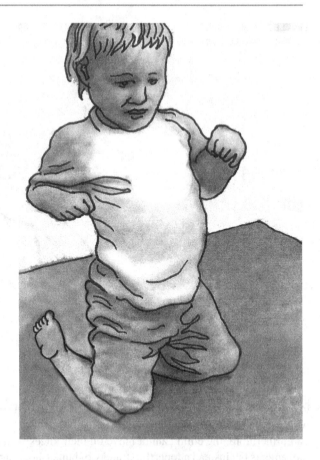

Fig. 2.64 Bunny-hopping

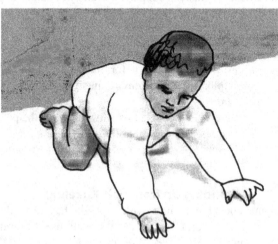

Fig. 2.65 Transfer
through half-kneeling
leaning on forearms

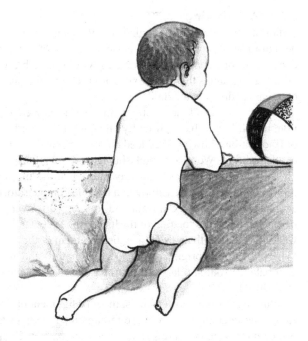

jump, then moving quickly supporting on furniture. The whole sequence takes place
very swiftly, and in the future it will be speed that becomes a strategic habit to
bypass accuracy during position transfers.

2.3.1.9 Standing

The child with diplegia can independently reach the standing position either from
squatting or with an STS transfer (see Chap. 2, Sect. 2.2.2). Once the child is standing, the weight on the lower limbs is asymmetrical. The limb on the side of the
pelvis which is rotated more posteriorly will have the predominant role of support,
with greater flexion of the hip and greater ankle RoM and foot contact. The other leg
will be even more flexed, with only the forefoot touching the floor. Therefore, the
child finds themself in only partial functional weight-bearing, which will require the
hands to be used for support or hanging on.

Advantages of standing
 – The gain of the erect position for functioning with upper limbs
 – Some small, independent steps on the spot, around the body axis
 – New perceptual inputs from the surrounding environment
Disadvantages of standing
 – Increase in misalignment of the pelvis and lower limbs
 – Compensatory strategies to maintain balance on a reduced BoS
 – Increase in muscle stiffness, including in the upper part of the body
 – Perceptive problems mainly regarding the posterior body space

2.3.1.10 Walking

Children with a form of diplegia usually manage to walk independently or with the help of orthoses and/or aids. The acquisition of this skill within 3–5 years of age is considered an excellent outcome and will be possible when the child has a good GMFS score and if there are no major problems of visual acuity and/or intelligence quotient (Fedrizzi et al. 2000).

With the posture-kinetic attitude that has developed to arrive in the standing position, the child will have difficulty engaging in a coordinated and smooth sequence of locomotion, showing a reduced ability to recover balance without adequate therapeutic training (Woollacott and Shumway-Cook 2005).

The retraction probably already present in the iliopsoas and adductor muscles limits complete hip extension, but a notable compensatory hyper-lordosis will be in action to keep the trunk upright and to proceed forwards (Romkes et al. 2007). In particular, adequate rotation of the hip on the horizontal plane is lacking, so forward walking occurs with an excessive displacement of the trunk on the frontal plane and to keep the trunk upright and to proceed forwards and an overuse of the upper limbs as a balance rod, similar to the strategy used by newly walking toddlers (Meyns et al. 2011).

With regard to the lower limbs, the misalignment of the pelvis on all three planes causes the internal rotation of the femurs, the flexion of the knees (in particular the one with less weight-bearing) and equinus at the feet (Ganjwala and Shah 2019). The heel-to-toe movement of the feet, necessary to have effective heel contact and push-off on the front foot, is missing which results in hasty, imprecise and tiring walking.

Furthermore, proprioceptive disturbances will have negative influences on locomotion.

Rodda and Graham (2001), continuing the studies of Sutherland and Davids (1993) on the typical features of CP gait, specifically analysed the characteristics of walking in children with diplegia, identifying the following four forms on the sagittal plane:

1. True equinus: ankle in plantar flexion and calf spasticity, knee and hip extended.
2. Jump gait: more proximal involvement with knee and hip flexion, and further spasticity of hamstrings and hip flexors; the activity of rectus femoris often causes stiff knee.
3. Apparent equinus: increased flexion of the hip and knee and more evident dorsiflexion of the ankle joint during the stance phase.
4. Crouch gait: excessive ankle dorsiflexion in combination with flexion at the hip and knee.

Few children maintain the typical pattern of the first form in childhood. The jump gait pattern is more common, with involvement of the pelvic girdle and the lower limbs in flexion. Moreover, the crouch gait is often observed in children who have had isolated heel cord lengthening when younger.

Over time, the adolescent and adult with diplegia may present torsional deformities at the long bones, the most common being the medial torsion of the femur and the lateral torsion of tibia. Associated with these are muscle-tendon contractures and/or retractions and flat-valgus-pronation deformities in the feet. For these reasons older persons frequently have to undergo both muscle and bone surgery (Simon et al. 2015; Putz et al. 2016; Gatamov et al. 2019).

2.3.2   Practical Suggestions

As explained above, from a postural-kinetic point of view, the child with diplegic has many aspects in common with a youngster with mild tetraparesis. However, the therapist always needs to pay particular attention to the pelvis and the ankle joints as well as any perceptual disturbances, which can negatively affect rehabilitation outcomes.

Different aims of the therapist:

- *For the child (functional independence and quality of life)*
  - Acquisition of various abilities (including good antigravity balance) in accordance with the needs in the everyday environments
  - Improvement of perceptual attention and elaboration of sensory information
  - Functional autonomy in daily activities, with specific aids, as necessary
- *For parents and caregivers (child management)*
  - Support to acknowledging the child's potential and offering guidance towards acquiring new functions
  - Support to acknowledging the current difficulties and problems of the child and understanding how to limit undesired compensatory strategies
  - Advice and education on childcare procedures
  - Sharing appropriate rehabilitation choices (orthesis, specific aids, surgical operations, etc.)
- *For the treatment session*
  - Postural adaptation of the child in the various levels of anti-gravity activities, including walking
  - Work on improving core stability through the strengthening of the weak muscles
  - Sensory problem-solving to help the child learn to cope with their perceptual problems
  - Organization of praxic and gnosic competencies
  - Training of functional strategies for daily independence
  - Maintenance of the intrinsic characteristics of body tissues as much as possible
  - Verifying and updating of the rehabilitation plan, with multidisciplinary teamwork for assessments for orthoses, aids, surgery, botox treatment, etc.

2.3.2.1 Infant with Their Parents

The parents of an infant with a possible history of prematurity or disorders in the autonomic sphere will have to face commitments of care.

Today, all parents of infants with a diagnosis of CP have the advantage of having specialized rehabilitation therapists to guide them in the best daily care for their babies: holding and carrying the child in their arms, feeding, changing, consoling, etc. The therapists will help them to understand their child and to learn ways to support the child's relationships and psychomotor development. This will include some simple natural interactive activities with mother and father, touching their baby, transmitting fine contact experience and tonic-body dialogue, privileging eye contact and facilitating different types of mutual sensory communication (Provenzi et al. 2020).

Suggestion
- Propose various and comfortable postural situations that also have stable perceptual reference points for a better understanding of the surrounding.
  - *Holding the infant in parent's arms, as indicated also for the child with tetraparesis*
  - *Supine, using a U-shaped cushion* (Fig. 2.66)
  - *Prone on a changing table, play mat or wedge*
  - *Seated in a postural system, with adequate cushions, if necessary*
- Guide parents in gently moving and playing with the various parts of the body of their baby, as a "small gymnastic interactions" (see also Chap. 7, Sect. 7.1):
  1. *Child supine, move the pelvis, looking for a better alignment.*
  2. *Playing, flex, extend and abduct the baby's hips, flex and extend the lower limbs, and mobilize ankles and feet.*
- Take care of sensorial information:
  1. *Gently massage the infant with a light baby oil* (McClure 2017), *in particular their abdomen and lower limbs.*

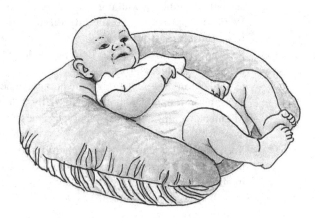

Fig. 2.66 Infant on a U-shaped cushion

Fig. 2.67 Toddler prone, on parent's chest

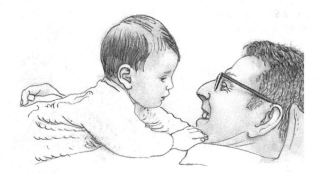

Note
- It is beneficial for the child to pass some time everyday in the prone position, to receive proprioceptive inputs on the extended hips, to enable the child to engage the muscles of the rear muscle chain and to mature the use of the upper limbs for support, for example, lying on mother's and father's chest (Fig. 2.67).
- However, the prone posture is contraindicated for sleep because it is proven to increase the risk of "cot death", the sudden infant death syndrome—SIDS (Hockenberry and Wilson 2019).

2.3.2.2 Moving While Supine/Prone

At first, the young child with diplegia seems to have good motor initiative, but in later childhood and adolescence, they present acquired functional abilities carried out using more or less consolidated compensatory strategies. The therapist can apply this practical knowledge to guide the child in the use of motor patterns with variable strategies and so expand their future functional abilities.

Suggestion
- Propose activities and postural transfers that solicit the activation of weaker muscles (i.e. *transversus abdominis*, *obliquus externus* and *internus abdominis*, *gluteus maximus* and *medius*, *extensor spinae*) and the involvement of the lower trunk, pelvis and lower limbs, reinforcing the core.
  - In supine touch and play with feet
  - Kicking
  - Rolling onto one side or remaining halfway, emphasizing the involvement of the pelvic girdle
  - Rolling prone and return (involving the pelvic girdle, as above)
  - Lying prone or supine
  - Pivoting on the abdomen in prone soliciting abduction of the hips
  - Sitting on a roller, climb over it, sit astride
  - Transfer into long-sitting and side-sitting
  - Transfer into kneeling and half-kneeling
- .....

Fig. 2.68 Activities in prone on a roller

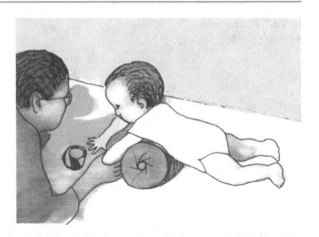

- Use practice in the prone position to recruit the posterior muscle chain and to maintain the extension of the pelvis:
  1. *With the baby prone on a rug/mat and on a wedge/roller, propose enjoyable activities that motivate them to pass some time in this position.*
  2. *Propose reaching or other activities with the upper limbs, to reinforce the trunk righting reaction (Fig. 2.68).*

2.3.2.3 Bridging

The child can be involved in motor activities similar to traditional gymnastics, which require performing more selective and precise movements, to reinforce the weak muscles listed previously.

The activity of bridging requires focusing the child's attention specifically on the pelvis and lower limbs, but the trunk and upper limbs also cooperate in this activity to increase the body's stability.

There are many alternatives to bridging that may be proposed to the child, according to their potential and age.

Suggestion
- Prepare the child in an appropriate starting position:
  1. *Position the child in supine lying with a small cushion under their head.*
  2. *Flex their knees and place their feet (without socks!) on the mat, slightly forwards with respect to the vertical line from the knee to the ground.*
  3. *Assure that the feet are in good contact with of the support surface: if necessary, release the stiffened muscles (*i.e. triceps suræ, tibialis posterior, medial gastrocnemius, flexor hallucis brevis *and* longus*), and/or activate others (*i.e. tibialis anterior, peronæi, abductor digiti quinti*).*
  4. *If necessary, apply a light pressure along the axis of the lower legs, to emphasize the perception of weight-bearing on the feet.*
- Verify and release the posterior muscle chain, reduce the hyperlordosis of the lumbar spine to get the pelvis tilted backwards:

Fig. 2.69 Preparation to bridging

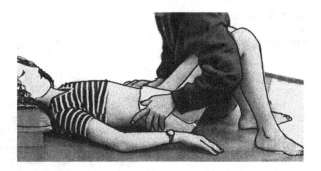

1. *Ask the child to tilt their pelvis backwards, guiding them manually only if necessary.*
2. *Emphasize the expiration phase of the diaphragmatic breathing, and, at the same time, guide the child to lower their ribs and maintain the lengthening of the spine, which is in contact with the mat surface.*
3. *Verify the lengthening of the cervical spine, and release the muscles around the shoulder girdle (pectoralis major and minor muscles in particular) to improve the involvement of the upper limbs during bridging.*
4. *Verify that the forearms and hands are properly in contact with the mat because they will help the child to maintain their balance during bridging.*
5. *Guide the child in carrying out active posterior tilting movements of the pelvis, and then return to the starting position without actively overusing anterior tilting (Fig. 2.69).*

- Monitor the correct execution of bridging:
  1. *Verify that the pelvis is actively mobile for backward tilting.*
  2. *Verify that forearms and hands have effective contact with the surface.*
  3. *Ask the child to actively tilt the pelvis backwards and then raise it from the support surface, facilitating the pubic symphysis to lift first, while the rest follows.*
  4. *During lifting, guide the upper legs to move forwards, to help the child transfer effectively weight onto their feet (Fig. 2.70).*
  5. *Assure that, at the end of the transfer, the two legs are perpendicular to the ground; otherwise the whole body will push backwards, causing global extension and loss of weight-bearing on the feet.*
  6. *Ask the child to return to the starting position by first lowering the lumbar spine and finally the pelvis on the mat while breathing out at the same time.*

Note
- The therapist should not block the child's feet before they lift the pelvis, because this does not facilitate the bridging, but causes a wrong movement pushing back of the body.
- Propose alternatives to bridging, according to the child's potential and to age.

Fig. 2.70 Manual facilitation to the lower limbs during bridging

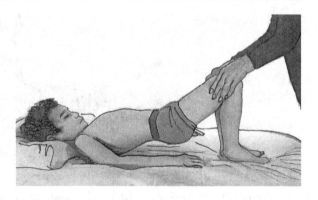

Suggestion

- *With the pelvis raised and the hips in extension, propose alternate movements of weight-bearing on the lower limbs, similar to the rhythmic movements evoked by the CPGs, aided by verbal or musical facilitations.*
- *Propose unilateral bridging exercises, maintaining one leg with knee flexed and the other in open kinetic chain with hip and knee extended.*
- *Combine the bridging exercises with anterior shoulder flexion and arm raising to 90°, e.g. holding a ball with both hands, in such a way as to further involve the abdominal muscles.*
- *If the child is managing well, during bridging ask them to carry out selective rotations of the pelvis on a horizontal plane, without losing the hip extension.*
- *......*

2.3.2.4 Prone

As in the tetraparetic form, also in the case of diplegia, attention needs to be given to preventing/limiting the possible future misalignment of the pelvis on the three planes and the exaggerated anterior tilting, caused by the prolonged and excessive action of the *iliopsoas*. It is, therefore, necessary to act on this problem early on and, beyond the treatment sessions, integrate play into the everyday activities in which the child is regularly positioned with their hips in extension, as in the prone position (see also suggestions for the child with tetraparesis).

Suggestion

- Organize the environment in such a way as to enable the child to play in the prone position:
  - *Verify the RoM of the hip joints, and, if necessary, manually release the long head of the* biceps femoris, *to obtain more extension and slight abduction in the hips.*
  - *Place a roller or a small wedge under the child's chest, so that they can stabilize and support themself on their forearms.*
  - *Place toys in front of them to attract their visual attention, so that they raise their head which activates the extensor muscles of the trunk and the* gluteus

maximus. *The toy needs to remain a little higher than the child's eye level but not too much so as not to lose the weight-bearing on the upper limbs.*
- Introduce head and trunk rotation activities:
  - *Move the target of interest, ensuring that it remains in the child's field of vision, to induce weight shifts to one side, and rotations of the trunk mainly at the lumbar level.*
  - *Verify that while carrying out these rotations, the child does not go backwards with their pelvis, but remains with their hips extended and abducted.*

2.3.2.5 Sitting

The sitting posture gives the therapist a lot of information related to the child's pelvis and its relationship with the spine and lower limbs.

When this type of child is sitting on a surface without a backrest, e.g. on a bench, it will be observed that the pelvis does not move on the three planes, the projection of the CoM is at the rear limit of the BoS and there is little support on the feet. The body weight is not equally distributed on both sides, and that affects the lower limbs, which are obliged into two different postures: one limb passively bears the weight, while the forefoot of the other limb points at the ground, widening in this way the BoS and coping with the postural instability. If maintained for a long time, this situation increases muscle and joint stiffness.

When required, the child does not have adequate pelvic tilting nor the active hip flexion necessary to straight the trunk properly. If movement on the frontal plane is required, e.g. for lifting one leg, the child accentuates the movement of the trunk backwards, and the upper body is forced to counterbalance with forwarding flexion. For all these reasons, it is necessary to train the child to perform very selective movements of the pelvis on the three planes.

Suggestion
- Verify the ability of the child to selectively move their pelvis on the sagittal plane:
  1. *Before directly addressing the mobility of the pelvis, verify the righting of the trunk and the appropriate weight-bearing on the pelvic girdle and lower limbs.*
  2. *Prepare the lower limbs to manage and maintain weight-bearing, with particular attention to the soles of the feet* (see also Chap. 6, Sect. 6.4.3, and Chap. 7, Sect. 7.2.1) (Fig. 2.71).
  3. *Facilitate anterior/posterior tilting of the pelvis by acting on the lumbosacral joint* (Fig. 2.42).
  4. *If necessary, give a manual stable reference point on the rib cage, more or less at the level of the sternum, so that the trunk is kept still, thus facilitating active and selective movements of the pelvis without involving the other parts of the body.*
  5. *Propose dynamic situations that require forward and backward tilting of the pelvis, so that the uprighting of the trunk is active and the feet perceive the different weight-bearing* (Fig. 2.72).

Fig. 2.71 Enhancing
proprioception to the foot

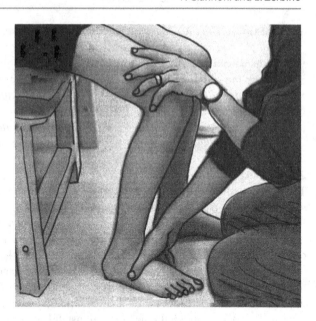

Fig. 2.72 Dynamic
adaptation to movement of
the pelvis

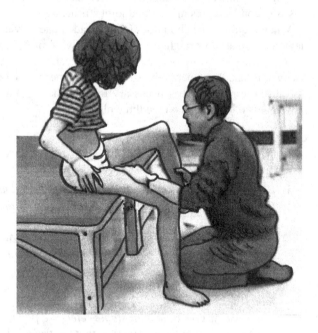

- Verify the active movements of the pelvis on the frontal plane:
    1. *Observe how the pelvis adapts to the movement, verifying that the child does not lose the uprighting of the trunk* (Fig. 2.73).
    2. *Induce transfer of the weight to one side, without the support of the upper limbs* (Fig. 2.74).

Fig. 2.73 Pelvis movements in the frontal plane without feet support

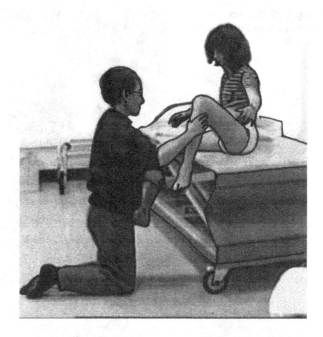

Fig. 2.74 Weight shifting with uprighting of the trunk

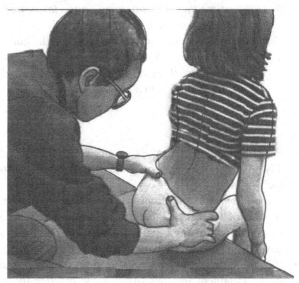

3. *Here too, verify the uprighting of head and trunk, and, if necessary, activate the abdominal oblique and transverse muscles to make one hip become an active pivot and reduce the weight to the other side.*
4. *Introduce even more selective motor activities, e.g. crossing one leg over the other: the child should first shift the weight on one hip, rotate the contralateral hemipelvis forwards, and then cross that leg over the other.*

Fig. 2.75 Sensory
perception of hands
and feet

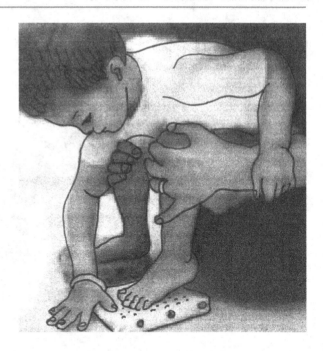

5. *Differentiate the weight-bearing on the lower limbs, raising alternately and rhythmically first one leg and then the other.*
- Verify the active movements of the pelvis on the horizontal plane:
  1. *To strengthen the obliqui muscles, sit the child on a wide surface without foot support, and ask them to shift their bottom forwards and backwards, rotating the pelvis alternately in a rhythmic way.*

Note
- Better perception of the foot's contact with the ground helps the child to gradually raise their tolerance threshold to the different sensory inputs arriving through the bottom of the feet. Copying the natural everyday environment that provides numerous tactile and proprioceptive inputs (e.g. when walking on the sand or pebbles of a beach, on the grass or in the water, etc.), the therapist can enrich treatment with many sensory inputs to the feet, e.g. with a wet sponge, a container with pebbles, sand, tree bark, etc. (Fig. 2.75).
- It is not sufficient to perform specific pelvic mobilization exercises repetitively in the treatment sessions. After some practice these new-learned movements need to be integrated into a series of more dynamic, complex activities, such as postural transfers and everyday functional experiences: e.g. take off/put on socks and shoes when sitting or adjust the skirt under the buttocks.
- The rehabilitation treatment for the child with diplegia needs to be focused above all on the extension of the hip joints and the selective movements of the pelvis. Hard work on the pelvic and hip components is priorities in the rehabilitation

treatment for the acquisition of functional motor abilities, particularly in efficient walking. For this, the therapist needs to promote regular everyday activities that include the standing and kneeling positions.

2.3.2.6 Standing Up from Half-Kneeling

Transit from sitting on the ground to standing is undoubtedly the most common transfer towards an upright position in young children, the one that the child performs frequently during the day. To facilitate this transfer, the therapist can follow the guidelines suggested for the tetraparetic form, with the advantage of now working with a child who is more able from a kinetic point of view.

Half-kneeling is often very difficult for the child with diplegic impairment, as in USCP. It requires selective control of the hips, each of which has to manage different tasks: after a shift of the pelvis on the frontal plane, a lower limb should take on the load function with hip in extension and knee in flexion. Meanwhile, the other leg has a more dynamic task which requires good flexion of all the joints, the forward movement of the limb and the stability of the hip while standing. During the whole sequence, the trunk should remain upright.

Suggestion
- Prepare the child in an appropriate starting position:
  1. *Control that the child is kneeling with extended hips and active contraction of the* gluteus maximus *muscle.*
  2. *Verify that there is enough freedom of movement to allow the child to shift their weight on a frontal plane, maintaining the hips in extension with the engagement of the* gluteus medius.
- Facilitate a lower limb to come forwards:
  1. *Before the child starts spontaneously with the sudden forward flexion of one leg, propose small shifts on the frontal plane to reinforce efficient weight-bearing of the contralateral limb with the hip extended.*
  2. *Guide the child to bring the limb forwards properly and place it with the tibia perpendicular to the ground: involve the* gluteus medius *and the internal rotators of the hip first and then the external hip rotators at the end of the transfer to align the thigh.*
  3. *Propose activities that involve the child's upper limbs in an open chain, to reinforce core stability and balance.*
  4. *Through these latter activities, prepare the child to move their weight forwards as a prerequisite for future standing.*
- Facilitate the final transfer into standing:
  1. *Emphasize the weight-bearing of the flexed limb forwards, guiding the thigh to move forwards if necessary.*
  2. *Furthermore, manually help the child to activate the* quadriceps *and arrive in the standing position with hip and knee extended.*
  3. *Contemporarily, control the sway of the contralateral leg, to enable completion of the sequence with a mainly inertial action of the* iliopsoas *and* rectus femoris *muscles to finally stand with the hip extended.*

Fig. 2.76 Elongation of
the posterior muscle chain
in prone trunk standing

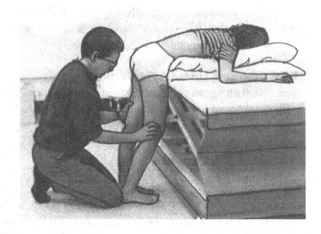

Note
- When a child with diplegia wants to stand up despite their poor balance, they usually try to hold on to something. To avoid this during therapy sessions, the therapist can propose activities that involve the child's upper limbs, e.g. holding a large, light toy with both hands or reaching for something higher, etc.

2.3.2.7 Prone Trunk Support in Standing

The main goal of the sequence "from standing to prone trunk support and back to standing" (Fig. 2.76) in the older child/adolescent is to strengthen the extensor muscles of the posterior muscle chain and improve the uprighting of the trunk. To make the sequence as active as possible, it is best to actively involve the upper limbs during the uprighting phase. Being a gymnastic type of exercise, it is suitable for interested and collaborative youngsters.

Suggestion
- Preparation of the setting:
  - *The treatment table should be of a height that will allow the young person's hips to be flexed to 90°.*
  - *Get the youngster to stand in front of the table in bare feet.*
- Verify that the starting position is appropriate:
  - *Control the alignment of the body and the effective contact of the feet on the floor, working for the elongation of tight muscles, if necessary.*
  - *Position the youth's hands open on the table with their arms straight and slightly abducted.*
  - *Guide the posterior tilt of the pelvic through the activation of the abdominal muscles.*
  - *Using a manual hold at the height of the armpits, guide the youngster into elongating and extending their trunk.*
- Begin the sequence:
  - *Maintaining the hold on the upper part of the trunk, act in unison with the youth as they lower themself slowly towards the table surface, keeping the trunk very straight.*

- *During the descent, the trunk performs small alternate rotations, and the open hands slide on the support while the arms abduct slightly.*
- *Check that the youngster turns their head to one side, and, if useful, add a small pillow or a wedge under the trunk for comfort.*
- *Since the posterior muscles of the trunk may be too tight and/or too weak, release the tightness first, and then work on activating and strengthening all the extensors, to improve the uprighting performance.*
- *Verify that the lower limbs remain straight throughout and with active foot contact in order to elongate the entire muscular posterior chain. Then ask the youngster to practise alternating knee bending (Fig. 2.76) while continuing to keep the feet in full contact with the floor, to prepare them to be active while returning to the upright position.*
- Preparing the return to upright standing:
  - *Guide the youngster with a manual hold on the upper trunk so that they align their head, and then slowly and actively upright their upper trunk, again with small alternated rotations and sliding of the hands.*
  - *During the movement ask the child to involve the upper limbs with an active hand contact for valid support.*
  - *Complete the sequence verifying the alignment and the uprighting of all the body.*

Note
- The sequence from standing to prone trunk support is not proposed, if the youngster has difficulty breathing.

2.3.2.8 Standing
Children with both tetraparesis and diplegia usually transfer to standing from sitting on a support (chair, stool, bench, etc.). In diplegic motor impairment, there is neither sufficient hip flexion for good functional sitting nor sufficient hip extension for good functional standing and walking. A lot of work needs to be done on the lower body, particularly to improve selective movements involving the lower trunk, the pelvic girdle and the hips.

Valid standing with efficient balance requires active ankle adjustments, sufficient foot support and core stability that activates the extensor muscles of the pelvis and lower limbs. On the contrary, the child with diplegia has multiple limitations at the ankle and hip joints, with tight muscles involving the *iliopsoas, adductor, quadriceps, triceps suræ* and *tibialis anterior.* The child is obliged to adopt compensation strategies to stabilize in standing.

The most typical are:

- The lowering of CoM through flexion and adduction-intrarotation of the hips, a compensation described later in crouch gait (Woollacott et al. 1998).
- Limitation of RoM in the main joints, to allow the use of the lower limbs as single segments "en bloc" and moving only the joints at a proximal level. These postural adjustments will be adopted in preparation of coping with dynamic functional motor tasks.

Fig. 2.77 Step exercise

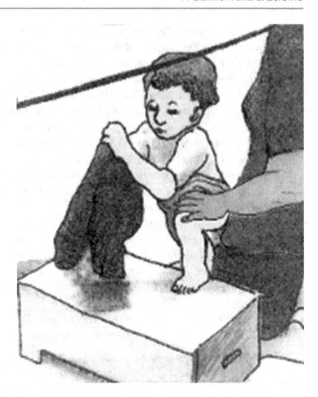

As in the sitting position, the misalignment of the pelvis also causes asymmetrical weight-bearing through the lower limbs in standing.

Suggestion
- Work for a standing position with hip extension, and *Induce an active and dynamic weight-bearing on the lower limbs, involving the hips in extension:*
  - *From sitting on a high table, the child lowers themself down into standing, sliding their pelvis forwards and arriving with hips extended.*
  - *As above, but arriving in standing first with one foot and then the other (and then returning to the high sitting position).*
  - *Standing in front of a low step support, the child shifts their weight onto one leg and then steps up onto the low support with the other (Fig. 2.77). This activity reinforces the* gluteus medius *and* quadriceps femoris *of the supporting leg and* tibialis anterior, peronei *and* extensor digitorum *muscles in the other.*
  - *Stand the child on the step block. Then ask them to put one foot on the floor as far back as possible so the hip moves into maximum extension, while the other limb remaining on the step sustains the body weight. This task is quite demanding and will need manual guidance and/or surveillance because the child does not have visual control of the space behind them (Fig. 3.25 Chap. 3).*

Fig. 2.78 Activity with manual guidance in standing

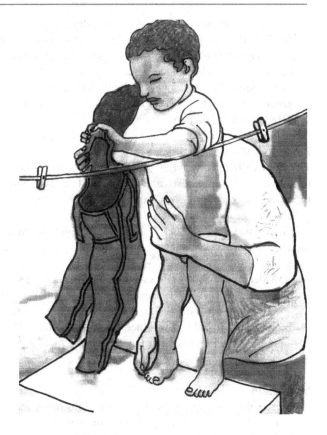

- *To improve balance in the standing position, get the child to play games with light objects, e.g. tapping balloons in the air, catching soap bubbles, pretending to hang out washing, etc. (Fig. 2.78).*
- *Play rocking the feet forwards and backwards, engaging the* triceps suræ *in a mobile sequence while maintaining the hips extended and the uprighting of the trunk.*
- ....

Notes
- Precarious balance in standing induces the child to search for some kind of support, e.g. a high or low table, a chair, etc. This allows them to support with the arms and/or abdomen which requires much less antigravity balance. At the same time, this causes not only an increase in trunk flexion but also a loss of the uprighting reaction.
- If the child needs to free up their hands for play or functional activities, they support more on the forearms compromising the open kinetic chain movements of the upper limbs and fine manual skills.
- To reduce these negative effects, the therapist should check that the child uses active hand contact on the surface without leaning on it and that they engage the core in appropriate alignment and uprighting of the trunk.

- If posterior support is proposed for standing (e.g. a table or a ball), the therapist should verify that the outermost edge of the support is in the middle of the child's *glutæi maximi*(Fig. 2.54); otherwise ischial support becomes appealing to sit on.
- Many authors underline the benefits of AFO orthoses or DAFO types, to prevent early plantar flexion retraction in the foot and to improve foot contact during stance (Abel et al. 1998; Radtka et al. 2004; Hassani et al. 2004; Lintanf et al. 2018) (see also Chap. 6, Sect. 6.4.3).

2.3.2.9 Walking

The child with diplegia has a more favourable prognosis about walking, compared to children with tetraparesis, and the therapist needs to build the foundations for this function from early on, when the child is very young.

It is necessary to train the different gait components first (see suggestions in "Basic for walking" in Sect. 2.2.2) and then get the child to carry out the whole sequence within functional tasks immediately with a cadence and speed close to the usual one.

Considering the sensorial-perceptual problems of this type of child, they should have bare feet for these therapeutic activities, to enhance the tactile and proprioceptive inputs on the soles of the feet and their adaptation to the different characteristics of the ground. Outside of the therapy sessions, the kids will wear shoes and/or orthoses for daily life, to contain the tibiotarsal joint at 90° and correct the flat, valgus foot, if necessary.

Suggestion
- Prepare the child for a valid uprighting of the trunk and extension of the hips, and propose functional activities that require walking:
  1. *Verify the child's posture and balance control in standing: functional body alignment, hips in extension and efficient foot contact on the ground.*
  2. *Provide tactile-proprioceptive input to the child's trunk to solicit its uprighting, and allow freer movements at the pelvic girdle. For this, apply stable manual reference points to the upper trunk, with one hand on the front and the other on the back.*
  3. *Verify that the child is ready to shift the weight on the frontal plane, necessary for initiating the first step.*
  4. *Facilitate the first step and walking forwards by proposing an interesting functional activity and/or destination point.*
  5. *The perceptive manual reference of the therapist's hands (sometimes two fingers are enough) can reduce swinging movement of the trunk and enhance the rotation of the pelvis on the horizontal plane (Fig. 2.79).*
- Propose walking experiences with a speed, cadence and mean stance time close to normal:
  - *Facilitate the step cadence by proposing activities with upper limbs while walking, e.g. clapping hands.*
  - *Facilitate speed with vocal rhythm, e.g. encouraging the child to sing together.*
  - *Propose walking games of "stop and go", changes of direction and overcoming obstacles.*

Fig. 2.79 Active walking
with reference upper trunk

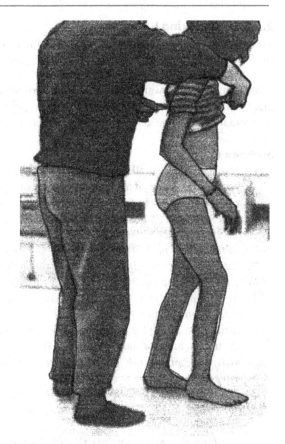

Suggestion

- Encourage the child to cope with walking in different environmental situations (surface consistency, with greater or lesser inertia, width, slope, presence of background noise, etc.), so that they learn to use different and appropriate strategies to adapt to everyday contexts.
  - *Let the child practise walking on smaller surface areas, where they have to move sideways, cross step and walk with legs closer together or one leg in front of the other.*
  - *Propose walking while holding onto safe mobile handrails, e.g. a semi-mobile piece of rope.*
  - *Introduce various walking experiences like moving forwards and backwards, along a narrow path, up and down stairs and walking up and down slopes*

Note

- If the child is capable enough, the therapist can propose fun motor activities with playmates, such as jumping and running games and riding a bicycle or kick scooter.

2.3.2.10 Walking Backwards

Training backward walking is very useful for the child with diplegia and others with moderate motor impairment because it requires good core stability, rotation between the two girdles and, above all, alternating extension of the hips. It should be remembered that the task of walking backwards is particularly demanding because it takes place without visual control of the destination point, so it enhances the use of the perceptual information arriving through the feet on the ground.

Suggestion
- Prepare the child to walk backwards:
  1. *Verify the position of the hips and pelvis, and reduce any excessive hip flexion and anterior pelvic tilt. Assure the validity of abdominal muscles for good core stability.*
  2. *Assure that the child is able to shift their weight forwards and backwards, and on the frontal plane.*
  3. *Verify that the two girdles can rotate on the horizontal plane.*
- With the child plan out the walking backwards practice and the destination point:
  1. *Guide the child from the front, at least initially, with two hands on the pelvis to facilitate rotation.*
  2. *Verify that, as the leg begins the swing phase and the foot leaves the ground, the* tibialis anterior muscle activates the *dorsiflexion of the ankle; contemporarily the ipsilateral hip should rotate backwards and internally, contrary to what happens for anterior walking.*
  3. *At the same time, pay attention that the contralateral hip activity guarantees full weight-bearing on the supporting limb, recruiting the* gluteus maximus and medius *muscles.*
  4. *The limb moving backwards should touch the ground first with the big toe. Therefore, before the foot touches the ground, verify, and facilitate if necessary, the dorxiflection of the metatarsophalangeal joints and the recruitment of the* triceps surae *muscle, together with elongation of the* tibialis anterior.

Note
- Nowadays, the treadmill is frequently used as an adjunct to physiotherapy treatment for the training of more active and independent walking in children with BSCP. Undoubtedly it is a challenging activity for the child, in particular because it requires them to exercise dorsiflexion of the ankle, extension of the hip and push-off of the foot in the various phases of walking, in an environmental context that forces the child to make various adaptations, especially with regard to the rhythm and speed of walking (Sheperd 2014). Many studies have highlighted how this type of training promotes the increase of muscle strength in the lower limbs, motor learning and control of the locomotion (Maltais et al. 2014) as well as balance (Ameer et al. 2019), endurance and gait speed (Yong-Gu and Chang-Kyo 2020) and lung ventilation capacity (Lauglo et al. 2016).

In all cases, after evaluating the characteristics, potential and motivation of the child, the therapist needs to share the aims of the proposed treadmill training, with the rehab team and the parents.

For further information on treadmill training, see Chap. 13, Sects. 13.3.1 and 13.2.2.

References

Abel MF, Juhl GA, Vaughan CL, Damiano DL (1998) Gait assessment of fixed ankle-foot orthoses in children with spastic diplegia. Arch Phys Med Rehabil 79:126–133. https://doi.org/10.1016/s0003-9993(98)90288-x

Alaverdashvili M, Foroud A, Lim DH, Whishaw IQ (2008) "Learned bad use" limits recovery of skilled reaching for food after forelimb motor cortex stroke in rats: a new analysis of the effect of gestures on success. Behav Brain Res 188(2):281–290. https://doi.org/10.1016/j.bbr.2007.11.007

Alboresi S, Sghedoni A, Borelli G, Costi S, Beccani L, Neviani R, Ferrari A (2020) Are perceptual disorder signs in diplegic cerebral palsied children stable over time? A retrospective cohort analysis. Mine Pediatr 72(2):79–84. https://doi.org/10.23736/S0026-4946.18.05237-4

Angsupaisal M, Maathuis CG, Hadders-Algra M. Adaptive seating systems in children with severe cerebral palsy across International Classification of Functioning, Disability and Health for Children and Youth version domains: a systematic review (2015) Dev Med Child Neurol. 2015 Oct;57(10):919–30. https://doi.org/10.1111/dmcn.12762.

Ameer MA, Fayez ES, Elkholy HH (2019) Improving spatiotemporal gait parameters in spastic diplegic children using treadmill gait training. J Bodyw Mov Ther 23(4):937–942. https://doi.org/10.1016/j.jbmt.2019.02.003

Bernstein NA (1967) The coordination and regulation of movements. Pergamon Press, Oxford

Bobath B, Bobath K (1975) Motor development in the different types of cerebral palsy. William Heinemann Medical Books, London

Bormley D (2014) Abdominal massage in the management of chronic constipation for children with disability. Community Pract 87(12):25–29

Butler PB, Saavedra S, Sofranac M, Jarvis SE, Woollacott MH (2010) Refinement, reliability, and validity of the segmental assessment of trunk control. Pediatr Phys Ther 22(3):246–257. https://doi.org/10.1097/PEP.0b013e3181e69490

Cans C, Dolk H, Platt MJ, Colver A, Prasauskiene A, Krägeloh-Mann, SCPE Collaborative Group (2007) Recommendations from the SCPE collaborative group for defining and classifying cerebral palsy. Dev Med Child Neurol Suppl 109:35–38. https://doi.org/10.1111/j.1469-8749.2007.tb12626.x

Cans C, De-la-Cruz J, Mermet MA (2008) Epidemiology of cerebral palsy. Paediatr Child Health 18(9):393–398. https://doi.org/10.1016/j.paed.2008.05.015

Cioni G, Lodesani M, Pascale R, Coluccini M, Sassi S, Paolicelli P, Perazza S, Ferrari A (2008) The term diplegia should be enhanced. Part II: contribution to validation of the new rehabilitation oriented classification. Eur J Phys Rehabil Med 44(2):203–211

Colver A, Sethumadhavan T (2003) The term diplegia should be abandoned. Arch Dis Child 88(4):286–290. https://doi.org/10.1136/adc.88.4.286

Damiano DL, Wingert JR, Stanley JC, Curatalo L (2013) Contribution of hip joint proprioception to static and dynamic balance in cerebral palsy: a case control study. J Neuroeng Rehabil 10:57. https://doi.org/10.1186/1743-0003-10-57

Di Lieto MC, Brovedani P, Pecini C, Chilosi AM, Belmonti V, Fabbro F, Urgesi C, Fiori S, Guzzetta A, Perazza S, Sicola E, Cioni G (2017) Spastic diplegia in preterm-born children: executive function impairment and neuro anatomical correlates. Res Dev Disabil 61:116–126. https://doi.org/10.1016/j.ridd.2016.12.006

Ego A, Lidzba K, Brovedani P, Belmonti V, Gonzalez-Monge S, Boudia B, Ritz A, Cans C (2015) Visual-perceptual impairment in children with cerebral palsy: a systematic review. Dev Med Child Neurol 57(Suppl 2):46–51. https://doi.org/10.1111/dmcn.12687

Ersöz M, Selçuk B, Gündüz R, Kurtaran A, Akyüz M (2006) Decreased chest mobility in children with spastic cerebral palsy. Turk J Pediatr 48(4):344–350

Eyre JA (2007) Corticospinal tract development and its plasticity after perinatal injury. Neurosci Biobehav Rev 31(8):1136–1149. https://doi.org/10.1016/j.neubiorev.2007.05.011

Eyre JA, Taylor JP, Villagra F, Smith M, Miller S (2001) Evidence of activity-dependent withdrawal of corticospinal projections during human development. Neurology 57(9):1543–1554. https://doi.org/10.1212/wnl.57.9.1543

Fedrizzi E, Facchin P, Marzaroli M, Pagliano E, Botteon G, Percivalle, Fazzi E (2000) Predictors of independent walking in children with spastic diplegia. J Child Neurol 15:228–234. https://doi.org/10.1177/088307380001500405

Ferrari A, Cioni G (2010) The spastic forms of cerebral palsy. Springer

Ferrari F, Cioni G, Einspieler C (2002) Cramped Synchronized General Movements in preterm infants as an early marker for cerebral palsy. Arch Pediatr Adolesc Med 156(5):460–467. https://doi.org/10.1001/archpedi.156.5.460

Ferrari A, Alboresi S, Muzzini S, Pascale R, Perazza S, Cioni G (2008) The term diplegia should be enhanced. Part I: a new rehabilitation oriented classification of cerebral palsy. Eur J Phys Rehabil Med 44(2):195–201

Ferrari A, Sghedoni A, Alboresi S, Pedroni E, Lombardi F (2014) New definitions of 6 clinical signs of perceptual disorder in children with cerebral palsy: an observational study through reliability measures. Eur J Phys Rehabil Med 50(6):709–716

Ferrari F, Plessi C, Lucaccioni L, Bertoncelli N, Bedetti L, Ori L, Berardi A, Della Casa E, Iughetti L, D'Amico R (2019) Motor and postural patterns concomitant with General Movements are associated with cerebral palsy at term and fidgety age in preterm infants. J Clin Med 8(8):1189. https://doi.org/10.3390/jcm8081189

Fetters L, Sapir I, Chen YP, Kubo M, Tronick E (2010) Spontaneous kicking in full-term and preterm infants with and without white matter disorder. Dev Psychobiol 52(6):524–536. https://doi.org/10.1002/dev.20455

Fragala MA, Goodgold S, Dumas HM (2003) Effects of lower extremity passive stretching: pilot study of children and youth with severe limitations in self-mobility. Pediatr Phys Ther 15(3):167–175. https://doi.org/10.1097/01.PEP.0000083045

Ganjwala D, Shah H (2019) Management of the Knee Problems in Spastic Cerebral Palsy. Indian J Orthop. 2019;53(1):53-62. https://doi.org/10.4103/ortho.IJOrtho_339_17

Gatamov OI, Chibirov GM, Borzunov DY, Dolganova TI, Dolganov DV, Popkov DA (2019) Correction of torsion deformities in adolescents and adults with cerebral palsy, impact on gait parameters. Genij Ortopedii 25(4):510–516. https://doi.org/10.18019/1028-4427-2019-25-4-510-516

Gaul-Aláčová P, Opavský J, Janura M, Elfmark M, Stehlíková J (2003) Analysis of the sitting-to-standing movement in variously demanding postural situations. Acta Univ Palacki Olomuc Gymn 33(1)

Giannoni P, Zerbino L (2000) Fuori Schema, ed. Springer, Italia, Milano

Gibson N, Blackmore AM, Chang AB, Cooper MS, Jaffe A, Kong WR, Langdon K, Moshovis L, Pavleski K, Wilson AC (2021) Prevention and management of respiratory disease in young people with cerebral palsy: consensus statement. Dev Med Child Neurol 63(2):172–182. https://doi.org/10.1111/dmcn.14640

Girolami GL, Shiratori T, Aruin AS (2011) Anticipatory postural adjustments in children with hemiplegia and diplegia. J Electromyogr Kinesiol 21(6):988–997. https://doi.org/10.1016/j.jelekin.2011.08.013

Günel MK, Türker D, Ozal C, Kara OK (2014) Physical management of children with cerebral palsy. In: Cerebral palsy—challenges for the future, cap. 2

Hagberg B, Hagberg G, Olow I, von Wendt L (1996) The changing panorama of cerebral palsy in Sweden. VII. Prevalence and origin in the birth year period 1987–90. Acta Paediatr 85:954–960

Hassani S, Roh J, Ferdjallah M, Reiners K, Kuo K, Smith P, Harris G (2004) Rehabilitative orthotics evaluation in children with diplegic cerebral palsy: kinematics and kinetics. In: Conf Proc IEEE Eng Med Biol Soc, pp 4874–4876. https://doi.org/10.1109/IEMBS.2004.1404348

Hockenberry MJ, Wilson D (2019) Wong's nursing care of infants and children, 11th edn. Elsevier

Hodges PW (1999) Is there a role for transversus abdominis in lumbo-pelvic stability? Man Ther. 1999 May;4(2):74–86. https://doi.org/10.1054/math.1999.0169

Hurvitz EA, Brown SH (2010) The terms diplegia, quadriplegia, and hemiplegia should be phased out. Dev Med Child Neurol 52:1070–1070. https://doi.org/10.1111/j.1469-8749.2010.03782.x

Ivanhoe CB, Reistetter TA (2004) Spasticity: the misunderstood part of the upper motor neuron syndrome. Am J Phys Med Rehabil 83(10 Suppl):S3–S9. https://doi.org/10.1097/01.phm.0000141125.28611.3e

Jeng SF, Chen LC, Tsou KI, Chen WJ, Luo HJ (2004) Relationship between spontaneous kicking and age of walking attainment in preterm infants with Very Low Birth Weight and Full-Term Infants. Phys Ther 84(2):159–172. https://doi.org/10.1093/ptj/84.2.159

Jeon W, Jensen JL, Griffin L (2019) Muscle activity and balance control during sit-to-stand across symmetric and asymmetric initial foot positions in healthy adults. Gait Posture 71:138–144. https://doi.org/10.1016/j.gaitpost.2019.04.030

Johnston MV (2009) Plasticity in the developing brain: implications for rehabilitation. Dev Disabil Res Rev 15:94–101. https://doi.org/10.1002/ddrr.64

Khemlani MM, Carr JH, Crosbie WJ (1999) Muscle synergies and joint linkages in sit-to-stand under two initial foot positions. Clin Biomech (Bristol, Avon) 14(4):236–246

Krägeloh-Mann I, Hagberg G, Meisner C, Schelp B, Haas G, Edebol Eeg-Olofsson K, Konrad Selbmann H, Hagberg B, Michaelis R (1994) Bilateral Spastic Cerebral Palsy—a comparative study between Germany and Western Sweden. II: epidemiology. Dev Med Child Neurol 36(6)

Lance JW (1980) Symposium synopsis. In: Feldman RG, Young RR, Koella KP (eds) Spasticity: disorder of motor control. Year Book, Chicago, pp 17–24

Lauglo R, Vik T, Lamvik T, Moholdt T (2016) High-intensity interval training to improve fitness in children with cerebral palsy. BMJ Open Sport Exerc Med 2(1):e000111. https://doi.org/10.1136/bmjsem-2016-000111

Lenhart RL, Brandon SC, Smith CR, Novacheck TF, Schwartz MH, Thelen DG (2017) Influence of patellar position on the knee extensor mechanism in normal and crouched walking. J Biomech 25(51):1–7. https://doi.org/10.1016/j.jbiomech.2016.11.052

Levin MF, Kleim JA, Wolf SL (2009) What do motor "recovery" and "compensation" mean in patients following stroke? Neurorehabil Neural Repair 23(4):313–319. https://doi.org/10.1177/1545968308328727

Lintanf M, Bourseul JS, Houx L, Lempereur M, Brochard S, Pons C (2018) Effect of ankle-foot orthoses on gait, balance and gross motor function in children with cerebral palsy: a systematic review and meta-analysis. Clin Rehabil 32(9):1175–1188. https://doi.org/10.1177/0269215518771824

Liu WY, Zaino CA, McCoy SW (2007) Anticipatory postural adjustments in children with cerebral palsy and children with typical development. Pediatr Phys Ther 19(3):188–195. https://doi.org/10.1097/PEP.0b013e31812574a9

Maltais DB, Wiart L, Fowler E, Verschuren O, Damiano DL (2014) Health-related physical fitness for children with cerebral palsy. J Child Neurol 29(8):1091–1100. https://doi.org/10.1177/0883073814533152

Marpole R, Blackmore AM, Gibson N, Cooper MS, Langdon K, Wilson AC (2020) Evaluation and management of respiratory illness in children with cerebral palsy. Front Pediatr 8:333. https://doi.org/10.3389/fped.2020.00333

Martin JH, Friel KM, Salimi I, Chakrabarty S (2007) Activity- and use-dependent plasticity of the developing corticospinal system. Neurosci Biobehav Rev 31(8):1125–1135. https://doi.org/10.1016/j.neubiorev.2007.04.017

McClure V (2017) Infant Massage: a handbook for loving parents, 4th edn. Bantam

Medeiros DL, Conceição JS, Graciosa MD, Koch DB, Santos MJ, Ries LG (2015) The influence of seat heights and foot placement positions on postural control in children with cerebral palsy during a sit-to-stand task. Res Dev Disabil 43–44:1–10. https://doi.org/10.1016/j.ridd.2015.05.004

Meyns P, Desloovere K, Gestel L, Massaad F, Smits-Engelsman B, Duysens J (2011) Altered arm posture in children with cerebral palsy is related to instability during walking. Eur J Paediatr Neurol 16:528–535. https://doi.org/10.1016/j.ejpn.2012.01.011

Nudo RJ, Milliken GW (1996) Reorganization of movement representations in primary motor cortex following focal ischemic infarcts in adult squirrel monkeys. J Neurophysiol 75(5):2144–2149. https://doi.org/10.1152/jn.1996.75.5.2144

Nudo RJ, Wise BM, SiFuentes F, Milliken GW (1996) Neural substrates for the effects of rehabilitative training on motor recovery after ischemic infarct. Science 272(5269):1791–1794. https://doi.org/10.1126/science.272.5269.1791

Nudo RJ, Plautz EJ, Frost SB (2001) Role of the adaptive plasticity in recovery of function after damage to motor cortex. Muscle Nerve 24(8):1000–1019. https://doi.org/10.1002/mus.1104

Pagliano E, Fedrizzi E, Erbetta A, Bulgheroni S, Solari A, Bono R, Fazzi E, Andreucci E, Riva D (2007) Cognitive profiles and visuoperceptual abilities in preterm and term spastic diplegic children with periventricular leukomalacia. J Child Neurol 22(3):282–288. https://doi.org/10.1177/0883073807300529

Paleg GS, Smith BA, Glickman LB (2013) Systematic review and evidence-based clinical recommendations for dosing of pediatric supported standing programs. Pediatr Phys Ther 25(3):232–247. https://doi.org/10.1097/PEP.0b013e318299d5e7

Palisano R, Rosenbaum P, Walter S, Russell D, Wood E, Galuppi B (1997) Gross Motor Function classification system for cerebral palsy. Dev Med Child Neurol 39:214–223. https://doi.org/10.1111/j.1469-8749.1997.tb07414.x

Papaxanthis C, Dubost V, Pozzo T (2003) Similar planning strategies for whole-body and arm movements performed in the sagittal plane. Neuroscience 117(4):779–783. https://doi.org/10.1016/s0306-4522(02)00964-8

Pavão SL, Dos Santos AN, de Oliveira AB, Rocha NA (2014) Functionality level and its relation to postural control during sitting-to-stand movement in children with cerebral palsy. Res Dev Disabil 35(2):506–511. https://doi.org/10.1016/j.ridd.2013.11.028

Pavão SL, Arnoni JLB, Rocha NACF (2018) Effects of visual manipulation in Sit-to-Stand movement in children with cerebral palsy. J Mot Behav 50(5):486–491. https://doi.org/10.1080/00222895.2017.1367641

Pin TW (2007) Effectiveness of static weight-bearing exercises in children with cerebral palsy. Pediatr Phys Ther 19:62–73. https://doi.org/10.1097/PEP.0b013e3180302111

Pin T, Dyke P, Chan M (2006) Effectiveness of passive stretching in children with cerebral palsy. Dev Med Child Neurol 48(10):855–862. https://doi.org/10.1017/S0012162206001836

Prechtl HFR, Ferrari F, Cioni G (1993) Predictive value of general movements in asphyxiated fullterm infants. Early Hum Dev 23:151–158. Elsevier Scientific Publ. Ireland Ltd. https://doi.org/10.1016/0378-3782(93)90096-d

Provenzi L, Rosa E, Visintina E, Mascheronia E, Guida E, Cavallini A, Montirosso R (2020) Understanding the role and function of maternal touch in children with neurodevelopmental disabilities. Infant Behav Dev 58. https://doi.org/10.1016/j.infbeh.2020.101420

Putz C, Wolf SI, Geisbüsch A, Niklasch M, Döderlein L, Dreher T (2016) Femoral derotation osteotomy in adults with cerebral palsy. Gait Posture 49:290–296. https://doi.org/10.1016/j.gaitpost.2016.06.034

Radtka SA, Skinner SR, Johanson ME (2004) A comparison of gait with solid and hinged ankle-foot orthoses in children with spastic diplegic cerebral palsy. Gait Posture 21(3):303–310. https://doi.org/10.1016/j.gaitpost.2004.03.004

Raghavan P (2015) Upper limb motor impairment after stroke. Phys Med Rehabil Clin N Am 26(4):599–610. https://doi.org/10.1016/j.pmr.2015.06.008

Rivi E, Filippi M, Fornasari E, Mascia MT, Ferrari A, Costi S (2014) Effectiveness of standing frame on constipation in children with cerebral palsy: a single-subject study. Occup Ther Int 21(3):115–123. https://doi.org/10.1002/oti.1370

Rodda JM, Graham HK (2001) Classification of gait patterns in spastic hemiplegia and diplegia: a basis for a management algorithm. Eur J Neurol 8(Suppl 5):98–108. https://doi.org/10.1046/j.1468-1331.2001.00042.x

Romkes J, Peeters W, Oosterom AM, Molenaar S, Bakels I, Brunner R (2007) Evaluating upper body movements during gait in healthy children and children with diplegic cerebral palsy. J Pediatr Orthop B 16(3):175–180. https://doi.org/10.1097/BPB.0b013e32801405bf

Rosenbaum P, Paneth N, Leviton A, Goldstein M, Bax M, Damiano D, Dan B, Jacobsson B (2007) A report: the definition and classification of cerebral palsy April 2006. Dev Med Child Neurol Suppl 109:8–14. Erratum in: Dev Med Child Neurol (2007) 49(6):480

Santos MJ, Kanekar N, Aruin AS (2010) The role of anticipatory postural adjustments in compensatory control of posture: 2. Biomechanical analysis. J Electromyogr Kinesiol 20(3):398–405. https://doi.org/10.1016/j.jelekin.2010.01.002

Sato H (2020) Postural deformity in children with cerebral palsy: why it occurs and how is it managed. Phys Ther Res 23(1):8–14. https://doi.org/10.1298/ptr.R0008

Schmidt RA (1975) A schema theory of discrete motor skill learning. Psychol Rev 82(4):225–260. https://doi.org/10.1037/h0076770

Schmidt RA (1988) Chapter 1: Motor and action perspectives on motor behaviour. In: Meijer OG, Roth K (eds) Complex movement behaviour. 'The' motor-action controversy. Advances in psychology, vol 50. North-Holland, pp 3–44. https://doi.org/10.1016/S0166-4115(08)62551-0

Surveillance of Cerebral Palsy in Europe (SCPE) (2000) Surveillance of cerebral palsy in Europe: a collaboration of cerebral palsy surveys and registers. Dev Med Child Neurol 42(12):816–824. https://doi.org/10.1017/s0012162200001511

Segal M (2018) Muscle overactivity in the Upper Motor Neuron syndrome: pathophysiology. Phys Med Rehabil Clin N Am 29(3):427–436. https://doi.org/10.1016/j.pmr.2018.04.005

Sheperd RB (2014) Cerebral Palsy in Infancy: targeted activity to optimize early growth and development, Cap.11, 1st edn. Elsevier Publ.

Shepherd RB (2014) Annotation A. aspects of motor training. In: Shepherd RB (ed) Cerebral palsy in infancy. Churchill Livingstone, Elsevier, St. Louis, pp 29–50

Shevell MI (2010) The terms diplegia and quadriplegia should not be abandoned. Dev Med Child Neurol 52:508–509. https://doi.org/10.1111/j.1469-8749.2009.03566.x

Shrader MW, Wimberly L, Thompson R (2019) Hip Surveillance in children with cerebral palsy. J Am Acad Orthop Surg 27(20):760–768. https://doi.org/10.5435/JAAOS-D-18-00184

Simon AL, Ilharreborde B, Megrot F, Mallet C, Azarpira R, Mazda K, Presedo A, Penneçot GF (2015) A descriptive study of lower limb torsional kinematic profiles in children with spastic diplegia. J Pediatr Orthop 35(6):576–582. https://doi.org/10.1097/BPO.0000000000000331

Sutherland DH, Davids JR (1993) Common gait abnormalities of the knee in cerebral palsy. Clin Orthop Relat Res 288:139–147

Takakusaki K, Chiba R, Nozu T, Okumura T (2016) Brainstem control of locomotion and muscle tone with special reference to the role of the mesopontine tegmentum and medullary reticulospinal systems. J Neural Transm 2016(123):695–729. https://doi.org/10.1007/s00702-015-1475-4

Woollacott MH, Shumway-Cook A (2005) Postural dysfunction during standing and walking in children with cerebral palsy: what are the underlying problems and what new therapies might improve balance? Neural Plast 12(2–3):211–9; discussion 263–272. https://doi.org/10.1155/NP.2005.211

Woollacott MH, Burtner P, Jensen J, Jasiewicz J, Roncesvalles N, Sveistrup H (1998) Development of postural responses during standing in healthy children and children with spastic diplegia. Neurosci Biobehav Rev 22(4):583–589. https://doi.org/10.1016/s0149-7634(97)00048-1

Xie L, Wang J (2019) Anticipatory and compensatory postural adjustments in response to loading perturbation of unknown magnitude. Exp Brain Res 237(1):173–180. https://doi.org/10.1007/s00221-018-5397-x

Yokochi K, Inukai K, Hosoe A, Shimabukuro S, Kitazumi E, Kodama K (1991) Leg movements in the supine position of infants with spastic diplegia. Dev Med Child Neurol 33(10):903–907. https://doi.org/10.1111/j.1469-8749.1991.tb14800.x

Yong-Gu H, Chang-Kyo Y (2020) Effectiveness of treadmill training on gait function in children with cerebral palsy: meta-analysis. J Exer Rehabil 16(1):10–19. https://doi.org/10.12965/jer.1938748.374

The Child with Unilateral Spastic Cerebral Palsy

3

Liliana Zerbino and Psiche Giannoni

According to the Surveillance of Cerebral Palsy in Europe (SCPE), the hemiplegic form is classified as unilateral spastic cerebral palsy (USCP). Among the various forms of cerebral palsy (CP), this is one of the most common affecting about 30% of children (Stanley et al. 2000; SCPE 2000). Its frequency has not changed significantly over time (Krägeloh-Mann and Cans 2009). Despite the good level of independence usually reached by these children, this form is characterized by many postural-kinetic problems and by the spontaneous use of only the unaffected hand with consequent difficulty in bimanual coordination. Furthermore, numerous studies report that children with USCP present sensory deficits that, in their upper extremities, cause limitations in stereognosis, proprioception and tactile discrimination (Wingert et al. 2008; Riquelme and Montoya 2010). (See also Chap. 9 Sect. 9.2 and Chap. 13 Sect. 13.2.5.).

Hemiplegia can be a congenital form, caused by prenatal or perinatal damage, or an acquired form, secondary to damage occurring within the first years of life. Thanks to the use of magnetic resonance imaging and its relative classification system, the position, size and timing of insult can be identified, better focusing the type and extent of the impairment (Niemann 2001; Himmelmann et al. 2016). Based on these criteria, Cioni et al. (1999) propose a classification of hemiplegia in four forms:

- Form I: the lesion occurs in the first and second trimester of pregnancy due to brain malformations linked to early disorders of neuronal migration (cortical dysplasia, lissencephaly, arachnoid cysts, etc.).
- Form II: the lesion is in the third trimester of pregnancy or the preterm infant, due to periventricular leukomalacia or haemorrhages of the periventricular white

L. Zerbino
DSS, University of Florence, Florence, Italy

P. Giannoni (✉)
DIBRIS, University of Genoa, Genoa, Italy

© The Author(s), under exclusive license to Springer Nature Switzerland AG 2022 127
P. Giannoni, L. Zerbino (eds.), *Cerebral Palsy*,
https://doi.org/10.1007/978-3-030-85619-9_3

matter, the possible presence of cysts and areas of gliosis in the contralateral periventricular white matter.

- Form III: the lesion occurs around the end of pregnancy; therefore, it concerns full-term infants, who have had perinatal difficulties and present cortico-subcortical lesions from a stroke in the territory of the middle cerebral artery. If the lesion also affects basal ganglia, dyskinesia could be observed (Cioni et al. 2010), although this hemidystonic form is rare.
- Form IV: the lesion is acquired after birth; it can be caused by infections of the nervous system or by head injuries or vascular malformations, etc.

The prognosis of the child with USCP is favourable for the acquisition of functional autonomy in daily life activities (ADLs), walking, sports activities and social participation. But comorbidity is present, which can influence these self-sufficiency outcomes. The children can have visual abnormalities (see also Chap. 11) for which they need an accurate assessment of visual function (Guzzetta et al. 2001); they may present attentional and executive impairments (Bottcher et al. 2010), disturbance of sensation, as poor tactile perception (Auld et al. 2012), deficits of somatosensory discrimination (McLean et al. 2017) and behavioural problems (Goodman and Graham 1996; Parkes et al. 2009). It is also common for children with USCP and mental retardation, microcephaly or severe neurological injury to develop epilepsy, a complication which can negatively affect the prognosis and the results of the rehabilitation interventions (Karimzadeh et al. 2010).

Secondary musculoskeletal problems often start emerging in the toddler and pre-schooler age group, and they may require the use of orthoses, drug treatment and/or corrective orthopaedic surgery later on.

Considering the wide variety of problems that these children can present, the participation of a multi-disciplinary team who work together with the family will be necessary throughout the clinical decision-making process.

The child with hemiplegia is very active and can reach independently the various stages of the neuro-development. Consequently they are classified as level I in the Gross Motor Function Classification System (GMFCS) (Rosenbaum et al. 2002). The main goal of the therapy is to improve the functional repertoire of the child, both with regard to walking and the use of the affected upper limb, including in bimanual activities, as widely reported in Sect. 9.2. of the Chap. 9).

Family members of the small baby are often the first to suspect that something is wrong with the child's motor development, referring to the paediatrician that the infant uses one hand less than the other to reach for toys and that the hand least used is often kept semi-closed or fisted. They also report that the head is rotated more towards the side of the most used hand or that one leg kicks with less force than the other.

The professional detects other signs such as hypokinesia in the hemi-side, abnormal general movement (absence of fidgety movements on the affected side—Prechtl 1997). In this regard, many authors report that the lack of fidgety movements is a predictive and reliable element for the diagnosis of CP (Hadders-Algra 2004; Bosanquet et al. 2013; Cioni et al. 2014). Other signs of concern are the asymmetry between the two body sides, the alteration of muscle stiffness and strength and sometimes the presence of epilepsy. These asymmetrical impairments cause early posturo-kinetic, visuo-perceptive orientation of the infant towards the unaffected side, contributing to the creation of important perceptual conflicts between the two sides of the body in the future. For example, the fact that the supine child remains for a long time with the head turned towards the most valid side affects both their sensory experience and their exploration and relationship with the environment. All this is involuntarily emphasized even by the caregivers, who often place themselves on the most active side of the child, e.g. during relational exchanges, at the time of feeding, changing diapers, baby bathing, etc.

Characteristics of the Child with USCP
- Muscle weakness on the impaired side, with hypokinesia
- Asymmetry between the two sides of the body and impaired movement coordination
- Increased stiffness recruitment, mainly in the distal parts of the body
- Sensorial and perceptive disorders
- Lack of synchronization between limb movements
- Reduced weight-bearing on the affected side
- Neuropsychological disturbances
- Possible epilepsy

3.1   Natural Clinical Development of Unilateral Spastic Cerebral Palsy

3.1.1   Supine

Despite their hemiplegic impairment, the child is still able to move using both sides, but, on the affected one, there is less range of movement (RoM) at the level of the scapulohumeral joint, and the girdles are misaligned. Difficulty in activating the proximal limb muscles impedes the emergence of functional distal movements in the hand, which, as described above, is often the early sign observed first by family members.

In this child's neuro-development process, some important functional appointments are missed, for example, the ability to orientate on the midline to reach and grasp an object during the second trimester of the first year. Reaching may be possible, but with an inaccurate movement sequence conditioned by both posturo-kinetic and sensory-perceptual problems as well as by weak stabilizing muscles at the shoulder. This means that the infant will have difficulty organizing bimanual activities on the midline, a skill that a child usually develops around 4 months of age, when the asymmetrical tonic neck reflex (ATNR) recedes.

The Importance of Midline Orientation and Control

The ability to remain in midline allows the infant to organize many important basic abilities and acquire new skills:

- Free movements of the head, both in anterior flexion and rotation, also activate the muscles of the anterior and lower trunk.
- Stability of the shoulder girdle facilitates eye-hand coordination and the anterior flexion of the glenohumeral joints in reaching and grasping.
- Variability of kicking, assisted by central pattern generators, strengthens the muscles of the lower limbs and the abdomen, increasing core stability.
- Haptic experiences lead to greater body knowledge: the child, who stays on the midline, can touch their hands, legs and feet more easily and bring them to their mouth in a *crescendo* of haptic inputs. Enthusiasm for movement, emphasis on visual exploration and interactions with the adult and cognitive and communicative curiosity all lay the foundations for the functions of eye-hand-mouth-foot coordination and bimanual activities.
- Stability on the midline enables rotation between the two girdles; the activation of the *obliquus abdominis* muscles facilitates postural transfers such as rolling to both sides and back to the starting positions of supine or prone.

In children with USCP, the same misalignment present in the shoulder girdle is also observed at the pelvic girdle, both on the horizontal and frontal planes which causes an alteration of kicking. During intrauterine life, the foetus is already experiencing and training their kicking abilities with its natural rhythmic and synchronic characteristics. After birth, supported by the central pattern generators, spontaneous kicking activity of the young infant exercises the abdominal and lower limb muscles, trains spontaneous motor skills with its alternations of pause and activity and favours the haptic experiences through the movement of the legs, which the child also learns to move for exploratory purposes (Thelen 1994).

In the child with hemiplegia, experiences of kicking in the supine position will be incomplete and altered due to:

- Alteration of muscle strength and consequent increase in stiffness on the affected side during the activity of the unimpaired side
- Consequent reduction of RoM at the joint level and less fluidity and selectivity of movement seen, for example, in the tibiotarsal joint
- Misalignment in all segments of the body, with both upper and lower girdles on the hemiplegic side rotated backwards, resulting in difficulty in reaching forwards with the upper limb and in bringing the leg forwards. This can cause future contractures of the pectoral muscles, consolidated misalignment of the pelvis with the hip first in external rotation and, then later, when the child becomes more active, in internal rotation.

3.1.2   Prone

This is a position that the child does not enjoy, even if family members propose it often when the infant is awake, e.g. on the changing table and on a rug or mat on the floor to play. They experience difficulty in supporting on forearms and hands to keep their head up, using the extension of the trunk and hips, and transfer weight from one side to the other. The child tends not to lean on the hemiplegic side (Fig. 3.1), which remains immobile and sometimes blocked under the weight of their body. They will begin to use almost exclusively the unaffected arm and that side of the body which becomes more and more competent in compensating for the motor and sensory limitations on the affected side.

3.1.3   Crawling

The child without cognitive problems is strongly motivated to move. They learn to change position by "transporting" their "different" affected side like bulky luggage (Fig. 3.2). The hemiplegic side is always pulled along behind, with the lower limb fixed in extension and the hip in intra-rotation, recruiting greater stiffness that limits joint RoM, whereas the able-bodied child alternates flexion and extension of the lower limbs with the abduction and external rotation of the hips.

The child with hemiplegic impairment learns to compensate by moving more quickly to avoid the need of controlling the numerous environmental variables that they would be obliged to manage if they moved slowly. Weight-bearing and balance are well perceived on the able side but approximate and confused on the other. The head, "container" of tele-receptors, is oriented mainly from information arriving from the unaffected side, and so it functions with only a partial input, not an all-round, comprehensive viewpoint.

Fig. 3.1 Difficulty to support on the hemiplegic side

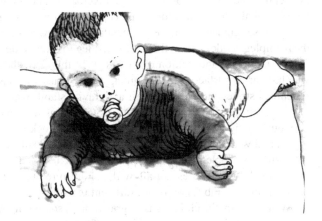

Fig. 3.2 Crawling without
involving the
hemiplegic side

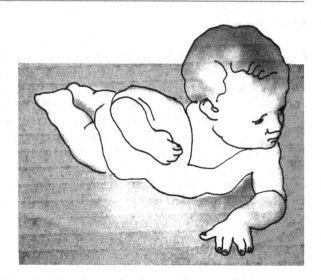

3.1.4 Rolling onto the Side

From a supine position, the child can spontaneously rotate towards the hemiplegic side because the movement is from the most active one. However, the child does not make an actual turn onto the affected side and therefore cannot reach the prone position with full extension in the trunk and alignment between the two girdles.

3.1.5 Sitting

When the young infant is initially put into sitting by an adult, they have scarce activity in the trunk muscles on the affected side, which prevents them from organizing and orienting properly towards the midline. The infant/toddler/child passes independently from supine to the sitting position in a very asymmetrical way, transferring their entire body weight towards the unaffected side, not only because of the bilateral muscle imbalance but also for the perceptive disturbances on the impaired side.

The misalignment of the pelvis, positioned backwards on the horizontal plane on the hemiplegic side, allows the unaffected leg to easily extend and move, but it constrains abduction and flexion of the other. In this way, the child can have a wider weight-bearing surface, and they quickly learn to use this posture as a compensatory functional strategy to increase their antigravity stability and feel safer.

While on the floor, the child with USCP learns to move in the sitting position very quickly by weight-bearing mainly on the buttock of the unaffected side, moving around with great enthusiasm, with the impaired side lagging behind.

A similar problem happens with the retraction of the shoulder girdle on the affected side, which does not allow the child to rotate their trunk properly and so bring the upper limb forwards for efficient reaching.

Even to sit up, the child leans or grasps on to something with the unaffected arm, and, once seated, this same hand is used for the various exploration and manipulation activities, becoming the child's expert and super-specialized hand.

Fig. 3.3 Typical posture
in the right side caused by
associated reactions and
increased stiffness

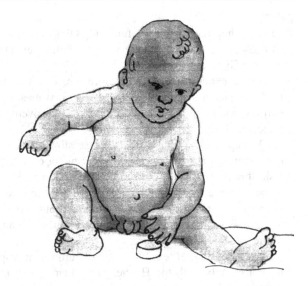

The precarious motor capacity on the hemi-side and the hyperactivity of unaffected side gradually consolidate two different functions for the two sides: the unaffected side increasingly becomes the most active, and the hemiplegic side assumes a function of stabilizing with very little RoM variability.

This inequality of motor function increases the muscle tonic recruitment on the impaired side, giving way to associated reactions, which the child will soon adopt as anticipatory strategies to stabilize the posture and so they are activated before beginning any movement (Fig. 3.3).

Many studies have been published on the functional abilities in the unaffected upper limb of these children (Williams et al. 2012; Tomhave et al. 2015; Picelli et al. 2017; Hawe et al. 2020; Burn and Gogola 2021). Moreover, other studies on adults with stroke and severe upper limb involvement point out that the unaffected arm is not as skilled as one might think and therefore requires attention as well as the impaired limb (Sainburg et al. 2016; Maenza et al. 2020; Pellegrino et al. 2021).

What Is an Associated Reaction?
Often no distinction is made between the terms "associated movement" and "associated reaction". But, even though both have some aspects in common, they do not have the same meaning. *Associated movements* can be observed mainly during the period when a person is learning a new skill.

On the other hand, *associated reactions* (sometimes also called *dyssynergic patterns of movement*) occur in situations that require motor control, that the person has not yet perfected. They are a positive sign of reorganization of the central nervous system and manifest as stereotypical patterns. These patterns recruit motor units that would normally not be used to perform a certain task, such as maintaining an upright position or walking, that requires good balance skills. If used frequently these patterns can become consolidated because they are functional for completing the task, so much so that they sometimes occur even a few seconds before effectively starting the task (Bassøe Gjelsvik 2008).

An associated reaction is therefore considered the visible result of the difficulty in postural adaptation, and it manifests itself by an increase in muscle stiffness and temporary decrease in range of movement, e.g. showing a more tonic and flexed upper limb.

On this basis, during a treatment session with children with USCP, who often manifest associated reactions during, or even before, the execution of a task, it does not make sense to ask the child to control or even "inhibit" an associated reaction. Instead, it is necessary to understand the cause that induces it (e.g. muscle weakness and/or proprioceptive problems) and then work on both motor and perceptual components to improve the performance of the same task in the future.

Moreover, like all excessive tonic recruitment responses, these reactions do not comply with the Henneman principle, that is, with the progressive innervation law (see Chap. 7 Sect. 7.2).

Associated reactions in neurological pathologies can be triggered by different factors, such as antigravity tasks (balance, transfers, weight-bearing, etc.), selective and fine movements and highly emotional states (fear of falling or excitement).

Advantages of sitting
- First autonomous transfer in an antigravity position
- Increase in visual exploration of the surrounding environment
- Increased possibility to use hands for manipulation
Disadvantages of sitting
- Increase of asymmetry
- Increased muscle/joint stiffness (contractures, future retractions)
- Possible perceptual exclusion of the hemiplegic side
- Reinforcement of compensatory strategies

3.1.6 Kneeling

The child with USCP easily transfers into kneeling from the sitting position, by grasping a support with the unaffected hand and then pulling up. It is more difficult for them to carry out the prone to kneeling transfer through the quadruped position as the latter involves support on the four limbs and a complex sequence of weight shifts, rotations, uprighting reactions and balance.

Most of the signs described above can be easily observed as the child with USCP moves and self-organizes:

- Retroposition of the hemiplegic side
- Uneven distribution of weight-bearing between the two sides of the body
- Misalignment of the two girdles on the frontal plane
- Flexion of the impaired hip, with weakness of the extensor muscles of the hip and reduction of selective movements on all three planes
- Presence of associated reactions, involving the upper limb and sometimes the mouth, caused by difficulty in performing the upright transfer

3.1.7   Half-Kneeling

The child with USCP who is kneeling and wants to stand up automatically takes hold of some anterior support only with the hand of the unaffected arm, shifting their weight totally onto that side (Fig. 3.4). This will position them to pull up using the flexor synergy, thus limiting the uprighting extension of the trunk. They then half-lift the affected leg forwards, just enough to obtain a minimal support on the ground of the forefoot. They weight-bear here briefly as they quickly bring the unaffected leg forwards, which, from then on, effectively becomes the weight-bearing leg to stand up. In this way, the child remains completely oriented only their sound side, dragging up the hemiplegic leg last.

Fig. 3.4 The typical "pseudo half-kneeling" transfer to standing of the child with USCP

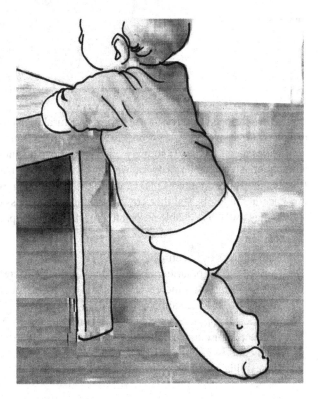

Fig. 3.5 Typical standing
posture of the child
with USCP

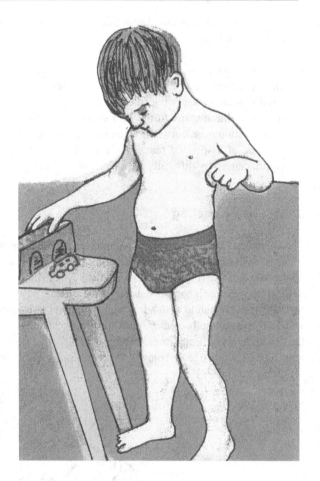

The use of speed in carrying out various postural transfers is a functional strategy of this child, to overcome their posture-kinetic difficulties.

Besides the "fast speed" strategy described above, to stand up the unaffected side simultaneously takes on tasks of weight-bearing, stabilization and mobility (performing the functional movement), while the affected leg, with reduced RoM at the hip-knee-ankle joints, stabilizes by increasing the stiffness of the whole lower limb and displays with a probable associated reaction in the upper limb (Fig. 3.5).

Disadvantages of kneeling
- Lack of perceptual experience regarding the differentiated load between the two limbs and therefore problems to control the centre of mass (CoM) inside the base of support (BoS)
- Reduced support base and consequent problems with balance
- Reduced muscular recruitment of the hip extensor muscles, increased stiffness of the *iliopsoas* muscle, to stabilize the affected joint
- Consolidation of compensation strategies

3.1.8   Standing

The child with USCP acquires the standing position with a slight chronological delay with respect to an able-bodied child. Thanks to their unimpaired hand, they have already experienced every type of hold, grip and support onto which they can cling, push or pull on to stand up.

In standing, some typical features can be observed:

- Shifting of body weight towards the sound side of the body.
- Retroposition of the affected side, semiflexion of the hip joint and abduction of the lower limb which supports less weight.
- Increase in muscle and joint stiffness, mainly in distal parts.
- Perceptive disorder of the lower impaired limb, in particular the foot, which shows a grasping reaction and supports precariously on the ground (see Chap. 6 Sect. 6.4.3).
- Associated reactions of the upper limb in shoulder abduction, elbow flexion, ulnar deviation and with a fisted hand (Fig. 3.5). In the presence of a dyskinetic component, the upper limb is extended, abducted and inward rotated with flexed wrist and half-closed hand.

If the child manages to play a game while standing, they are most likely to use their unaffected hand, and, if they have difficulties maintaining the upright position, they lean on a support surface with their trunk bent forwards.

3.1.9   Squatting

The transfer from the standing position to squatting (e.g. used functionally to pick up objects from the floor) occurs with completely different muscle control to standing up, because the movement is towards gravity and so the task requires precise control of eccentric muscle work to regulate the speed during the changes of position.

The child with USCP will spontaneously activate various compensation strategies to be able to carry out this transfer:

- Increase the BoS width to get more stability
- Shift their weight more to the unaffected side
- Use the impaired leg in internal rotation and adduction at the hip, caused by weak activity of the hip abductor and stabilizer muscles at the hip joint
- Display associated reactions of the upper limb to control the postural variables during the transfer (Fig. 3.6)

All these compensations increase the misalignment between the various parts of the body on both sides, and they make all postural shifts more precarious.

Fig. 3.6 Associated
reaction arm posture
during the stand-to-
squatting transfer

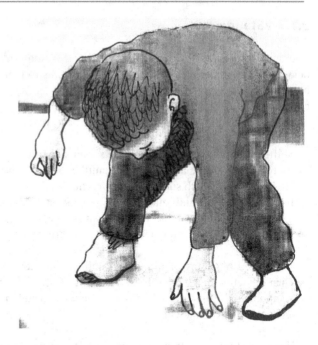

3.1.10 Walking Sideways

As with walking forwards, sideway walking implies shifts in weight-bearing from
one leg to the other but with the difference here that the transfer calls for alternate
activation of hip abduction and adduction maintaining the hip in extension, whereas
the child with USCP organizes their first upright sideway movements searching for
any kind of anterior support to hold on to (sofas, tables, chairs, etc.), moving always
in the direction of the unaffected side, with the hemiplegic side lagging behind.

The effort of controlling all the various components involved in the weight-
bearing shifts increases muscle stiffness because, unless guided by the therapist, the
child will avoid moving their body weight onto the compromised side. This difficulty can be caused not only by the motor components of the impairment but also
by sensory-perceptual disturbances that create confusion regarding environmental
inputs, and so the child prefers to rely on visual, auditory and tactile-proprioceptive
information coming from the sound side.

3.1.11 Walking

Clinical experience reports that children with USCP walk a few months later than
the norm (around 17/24 months), even though they then acquire the ability in a short
time. The therapist will have to take this into account in their work plan, knowing
that, just as the youngsters are quick in learning to walk, they will soon learn to run
and get away, using too many compensatory strategies.

It is rare that these youngsters do not reach these levels of function, although they can
be compromised in the presence of severe epilepsy and/or cognitive-relational disorders.

The child with USCP manifests different types of gait deviations, as reported by many scientific studies. Winters Jr et al. (1987) were among the first authors to propose the kinematic classification of walking in this form of CP. They describe four types of gait patterns based on the sagittal plane kinematics of the pelvis, hip, knee and ankle and the muscles more involved in each type:

- Type 1: foot drop in swing phase
- Type 2: true equinus, with excessive ankle plantar flexion in both stance and swing phase
- Type 3: *triceps surae* spasticity or contracture, ankle dosiflexion in swing phase, "stiff knee gait" as the result of hamstring/quadriceps co-contraction
- Type 4: more severe form involving the hip that does not extend in the terminal stance phase

Later Rodda and Graham (2001) propose a kinematic classification that analyses further patterns considering the other kinematic planes in addition to the sagittal one. For example, they focus on the internal rotation and adduction of the impaired limb as well as pelvic rotation, often observed in severe USCP. Moreover, these authors describe a very frequent pattern with knee in hyperextension (*genu recurvatum*) in the terminal stance phase. Furthermore, for each pattern identified, Rodda and Graham give indications for the most suitable therapeutic intervention.

Indeed, during the swing phase, the child with hemiplegia often has the pelvis tilted upwards which causes them to drag their affected leg forwards in circumduction which is very similar to the hemiplegic gait in the adult.

Moreover, during the various stages of walking, the impaired upper limb plays an important role in maintaining stability and balance. In particular, when the child walks, evident associated reactions, similar to the physiological middle guard position, can be observed, with shoulder in abduction, external rotation, elbow flexion, forearm pronation, wrist flexion, thumb adduction and ulnar deviation (Gage 2004; Galli et al. 2012; Bonnefoy-Mazure et al. 2014).

The continual use of the same compensation strategies for walking causes early retractions in certain muscle groups, mainly in the affected lower limb, which can require corrective orthopaedic surgery with benefits from the functional point of view.

Advantages of walking
- Acquisition of autonomy in moving around
- Experience of peri-personal space
- Improvement in social interaction

Disadvantages of walking
- Increase in muscle stiffness with early contracture/retraction of lower limb muscles
- Reduced RoM at the main lower limb joints
- Poor perceptual elaboration of inputs on the hemiplegic side
- Reduced variety of motor patterns in the affected upper limb, hampered as well by associated reactions

3.2   Practical Suggestions

The problems of the child with USCP are related not only to the motor impairments but also to the sensory/perceptual/praxis and cognitive deficits. Therefore, it is necessary to focus on different aims that require a careful multidisciplinary intervention.

Different aims of intervention of the therapist:
- *For the child (autonomy and quality of life)*
  - Favour the functional integration of all parts of both sides of the body
  - Promote the functional use of the impaired upper limb, even with a secondary support role in carrying out motor skills
  - Facilitate the acquisition of more selective movements at the hip and in the rest of the impaired lower limb
  - Support the older children and adolescents in self-management to maintain the intrinsic properties of the soft tissues, including muscles
  - Support the child (also with verbalization) to manage their emotions of anger and frustration emerging from the confrontation between the different abilities in the two sides of their body
  - Enhance support through the involvement of different professional where necessary, both for psychological and educational aspects
  - Encourage the participation in sports activities, like swimming, volleyball, canoeing, skiing, etc.
- *For the parents and caregivers (everyday management)*
  - Provide education and counselling on the daily home management the handling of the child: how to support and move the infant in one's arms (holding and handling techniques), how to position them in sitting in the various seats (baby chair, highchair stroller, car seat, parent's bicycle) and later on tricycles, etc.
  - Advise on how to facilitate the alignment of the various body areas during the day and to foster exploratory experiences of the impaired side (e.g. touch the dad's beard, the foot in contact with the surface of the bathtub, use of both limbs for playing with big toys, etc.), motivating the child gently and avoiding impossible requests
  - Activate the necessary support from professionals (e.g. psychologist, family therapist, psychiatrist) to process the distress of the birth of a problematic child and the relationship with siblings
  - Address some educational aspects such as respect of the child's possibilities, to avoid asking for impossible performances
- *For the treatment session*
  - Assess the relationship among the various parts of the body and strengthen weak muscles, to obtain more functional symmetrical postural alignment
  - Promote functional tasks that involve and integrate all parts of both sides of the body

- Monitor any associated reactions and find out what causes them
- Introduce activities of care of connective, muscular and neural tissues, to prevent or delay their intrinsic modifications (see Chap. 7)
- Assess the child's praxic skills and eventual perceptual sensory problems
- Set up a personalized home program to support the therapeutic goals
- Assess and plan with the multidisciplinary team the needs for orthoses and pharmacological and/or surgical interventions to prevent/reduce muscular skeletal deformities
- Select and adapt equipment to facilitate ADLs, written communication, etc. (see Chap. 9, Sect. 9.2)
- Support visual development by collaborating with ophthalmologists and visual rehabilitators for visual functional disorders (see Chap. 11)
- Provide support to teachers of visual, praxic, learning problems of the child

3.2.1   Holding Infant/Toddler in Adult's Arms

When educating parents and caregivers in holding and handling techniques, the therapist should first explain the importance of alignment on the three kinetic planes of the various parts of the child's body.

Suggestions
- Various positions and ways of holding the infant in one's arms are described as follows:
  - *The parent and other caregivers can hold the infant vertically, with the unaffected side against their body and the affected side positioned on the outside. One hand of the adult is put over the child's affected hip, while the other is under the armpit on the same side, with their fingers on the medial margin of the scapula to favour abduction and to counteract the retroposition of the shoulder. To gain the symmetry of the trunk, the adult uses that hold to elongate and align that side of the trunk by increasing the distance between the two girdles.*
  - *The infant can be held on the side of the parent's body, with the lower limbs abducted and flexed over their hips, and the parent acts as previously.*
  - *The infant can also be held vertically with the impaired side resting against their parent's body, and the arm and shoulder of the child remain resting on parent's shoulder, who manually aligns the body as before.*
  - *The infant can be held with their back leaning against their parent's chest. Here, the parent needs to support the child's pelvis with one arm and with the other bring the affected shoulder girdle forwards* (Fig. 3.7).

Fig. 3.7 Baby carried
with their back against
their parent's chest

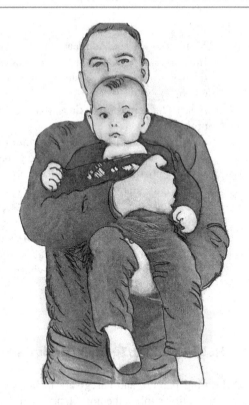

— *Another position is to sit the infant on the parent's lap, with a table placed in front of them. The parent can abduct their legs so they open the child's thighs too. The height of the table should be at the level of the child's armpits, to favour the support of the upper limbs with a 90° forward flexion of the shoulders. Once well positioned, the parent can propose various play activities with the child's hands, favourite toys, exploring the surrounding environment with eyes and hands, etc.*

— *As in the previous situation, the parent puts their arm across the baby's chest and, passing under the armpits, places their hand behind the shoulder joint on the impaired side, checks the alignment of the trunk, increases the forward position of the impaired arm and introduces some rotation between the two girdles. The child is then encouraged to look around for a game, a person, etc., while the shoulder girdle remains aligned horizontally.*

— *The therapist can consult the parent to decide other postural systems for carrying the child, such as kangaroo wrap, baby carriers, backpacks, etc.*

3.2.2 Supine

The main goals of therapy for the young child in the supine lying are active orientation on the midline, maturation of eye-hand-mouth-foot coordination and acquisition of balance skills that prepare for independent sitting.

Suggestion
- Facilitate good postural alignment:
    1. *Position the infant in a U-pillow or on a small wedge, to obtain:*
        - *Release of the posterior muscles of the neck and trunk*
        - *Alignment of head and trunk and the forward position of the scapula*
        - *Organization of upper limbs towards the midline*
    2. *Facilitate the release of the posterior muscles of the trunk by flexing the hips, lifting the pelvis off the floor and introducing activities which involve the abdominal muscles.*
- Improve visual exploration of the surroundings:
    1. *Facilitate face-to-face interaction and eye-to eye contact with the child.*
    2. *Improve the quality and duration of the child's eye-to-eye contact prolonging the use of facial gestures, expressions and mimicry, auditory input and verbal communication strategies.*
    3. *Practise eye-to-eye tracking skills towards the impaired side, slowly moving sideways and then back to midline.*
    4. *Solicit saccadic sideway movements especially towards the problematic space by the therapist moving their face with small rapid movements.*
- Promote sensory motor initiatives and coordination of the limbs:
    1. *Activate movements that recruit important muscles such as the* transversus abdominis *and the* recti abdominis*:*
        - *Encourage the child to look at and touch various parts of their body: e.g. help them to touch the unaffected hand with the affected one and move them together or to take their foot from the contralateral side and bring it to the mouth.*
        - *Facilitate eye-hand-foot-mouth coordination, suggesting games with the various segments of body, e.g. the infant holds their foot, takes off their sock, claps their hands or feet, holds a large and light ball with all their limbs, etc. (Fig. 3.8).*

Fig. 3.8 Sensory motor facilitation in supine (Modified from European Bobath Tutors Assoc., with permission)

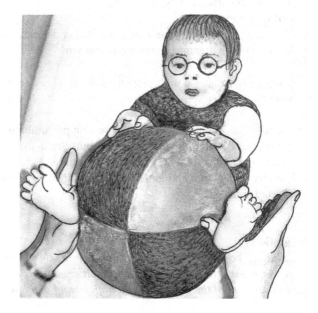

 – *Encourage active kicking with the lower limbs moving together and/or with alternated and rhythmic flexion/extension; if necessary, give some initial sensory inputs to obtain a more appropriate active pattern.*
2. *Offer the infant various tactile-proprioceptive experiences:*
   – *Propose tactile interaction of all areas of both feet with a variety of surfaces, objects and games involving different types of touch (pressure, vibration, etc.), textures, mediums, shape, temperature and so on.*
   – *Propose all the same types of activities for the hands, like playing with sponges (such as kitchen ones) or shower gloves, that have different roughness.*

3.2.3 Rolling to Side and Prone

Starting from the supine position, the therapist can motivate the child with tasks that attract their curiosity and induce them to move actively. For example:

– Supine → half-side and side
– Supine → prone
– Supine → rolling over in adult's arms to change position
– Supine → sitting
– Supine → side → prone → side sitting
– ......

These changes of position proposals do not have a rigorous sequence, but the order depends on many factors:

– Curiosity of the child towards their surroundings
– Perceptive characteristics of the child
– Motivation to move
– Characteristics of the relationship between child and adult
– Abilities of the therapist to induce movement

Every motor proposal in the supine position allows several goals to be achieved, including:

– Recruitment of more motor units to sustain postural muscle activation
– Involvement of all *obliquus abdominis* muscles in the rotations between the two girdles and all the muscles of the impaired limbs
– Enhancement of perception with tactile/proprioceptive inputs, particularly on the affected side

Suggestion
• Facilitate the transfer from supine to side lying by rolling over the impaired side:
   1. *Verify the relationship between the different parts of the body and the correct alignment of the two girdles on both frontal and horizontal planes.*

2. *Prepare for the roll and the weight-bearing experience by maintaining the affected hip in extension with one hand on the child's upper internal thigh and elevating and externally rotating the affected upper limb with the other (Fig. 3.9). Sustain the child's initiative also when they are in intermediate positions.*

3. *Motivate the child to roll activating the unaffected side and to remain in intermediate positions as well; for example, the child turns to half-side and/or goes back and forwards between the supine and prone position.*

4. *Verify that the affected hip remains well extended and that the hand is not fisted.*

- Facilitate the transfer from supine to side lying by rolling over the unaffected side:
    1. *Verify again the alignment between the two girdles, as before.*
    2. *Verify the mobility of the affected scapula and shoulder releasing any tight muscles and facilitating the scapula to protract and the arm move forwards.*
    3. *Solicit the child to actively move and rotate the affected side and so turn onto the unaffected side.*
    4. *Be sure that the child arrives in the prone position with the hips extended and a correct alignment between the two girdles (Fig. 3.10).*

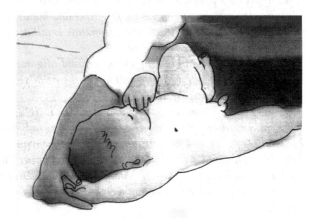

Fig. 3.9 Preparing to roll over on the affected side

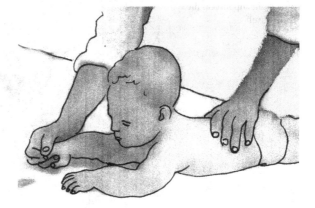

Fig. 3.10 The prone position after rolling from supine

3.2.4 Prone

The prone position is important because it represents the child's first significant antigravity task to manage independently. It involves uprighting of the head and trunk, extension of the hip and support on both upper limbs.

As described above, even though the child with USCP spontaneously moves from supine into the prone position by activating their "best" side and rolling towards and over the affected one, it is useful for the therapist to train the movement towards both sides.

Suggestion
- Work for valid support on the child's forearms in the prone position:
  1. *Verify the alignment between the parts of the body and the uprighting of the head and trunk.*
  2. *Verify the position of the scapula, and release the muscles of the shoulder joint to wide increase RoM of the glenohumeral joint.*
  3. *Facilitate the support on both forearms, by checking that the elbow is flexed at 90° and the affected hand is well open, ready to sustain the weight of the upright trunk.*
  4. *Apply light pressure through the shoulder joint to the elbow to further emphasize the weight perception on forearms and hands.*
  5. *Propose simple play activities, stimulate small active weight transfers on the frontal plane, and then return.*
  6. *If necessary, facilitate the extension and alignment of the trunk initially by inserting a small wedge or roll under the child's shoulder girdle.*
- Work for improving balance:
  1. *Involve the impaired upper limb in active weight-bearing by facilitating the child to rotate their head, and so move slightly from one forearm and the other, e.g. to look at their parent's face or a favourite toy.*
  2. *Propose reaching tasks with the unaffected upper limb with objects at different positions, heights and distances to solicit active recruitment of the extensor muscles of the trunk and weight-bearing on the affected side (Fig. 3.11).*

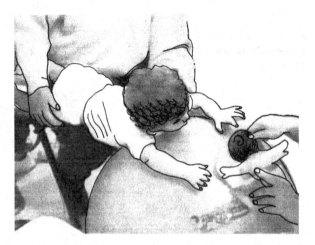

Fig. 3.11 Reaching task with weight support on the affected limb

Fig. 3.12 Prone on a table with feet over the edge (Modified from European Bobath Tutors Assoc., with permission)

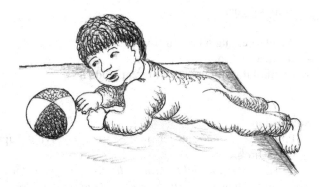

3. *Favour reaching forwards with the affected arm, first recruiting the external rotator muscles, the shifting of the scapula on the rib cage and the extension forwards of the arm* (see also Sect. 7.2.1.2. in Chap. 7).
4. *Foster motor initiative of the upper limb with wrist extension, hand opening and thumb abduction by proposing appropriate interactive play with objects and people.*
5. *Adapt the therapeutic proposals to the personal initiatives of the child:* e.g. *push on hands, lean on flexed elbows, touch face with hemiplegic hand or both hands, build a tower,* etc.
6. *During all these activities, verify that the child's weight is well distributed on the limbs and pelvis and that the impaired hip is extended.*
7. *If the child is on a treatment table, pay attention that their feet are over the edge to counteract the equinus, and facilitate selective movements at the tibiotarsal joint* (Fig. 3.12).

Note
- For all therapeutic activities, it is best for the child to be undressed so that the therapist has direct visual and manual feedback of the activity of the muscles which may be too weak or too tight and/or hyperactive. If the child is very small or fragile, they can wear a tight-fitting bodysuit.

3.2.5   Sitting Up Independently

Even though in a very asymmetrical way the child with USCP organizes their movements independently, they encounter difficulties in the prone → sitting transfer because they do not spontaneously use the affected arm. During this transfer, the child receives different inputs when they lean on the two different sides of the body. Therefore it is advisable that the therapist first manually guides this position change so that the child can dwell on certain sensorial perceptions that they would otherwise inevitably lose in the haste to carry out the movement. Later, the therapist should gradually reduce their guidance as the child acquires new abilities.

Proposal goals:

- Weight-bearing on forearm-wrist-hand
- Balance control
- Postural transitions with different modalities

Suggestion
- Proposal of the transfer into sitting, involving support on the impaired upper limb:
    1. *Verify that the child's arm is effectively in contact with the surface to be used for pushing up to sitting (internal side of the forearm on the support, hand open ready for more contact on finger tips and hypothenar eminence) and that the hip is in position ready for active weight-bearing.*
    2. *Solicit the child to sit up actively, using verbal encouragements and tactile/ proprioceptive inputs, always verifying the weight-bearing and the balance reactions of the lower limbs* (Fig. 3.13).
    3. *Moving towards a more anti-gravity position, the child should have time to gradually adapt to their new relationships with the surrounding environment. The therapist can let the child stay in half sitting and/or go straight to sitting back again, to vary the sequence and so motivate their collaboration.*
- Proposal of transfer to sitting with support on the unimpaired upper limb:
    1. *Verify the muscle weakness or excessive stiffness in the shoulder and trunk, and, if necessary, work on these components.*
    2. *Verify the position of the head of the humerus into the glenoid, counteracting any protraction and internal rotation.*
    3. *With a proximal grip, facilitate the child to begin the transfer by protracting the affected arm forwards in the direction of the opposite hip as they push up on the unaffected arm.*

Fig. 3.13 Transfer to sitting with weight-bearing on affected side and use of impaired upper limb for support

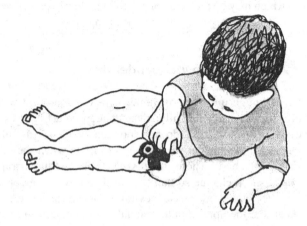

4. *Motivate the child to move as actively as possible, and check for balance reactions in extension and abduction in impaired lower limb.*
- Support and motivate the child to experiment the different postural transfers to sitting:
  - *Prone → side-sitting, with support on the impaired side*
  - *Side-sitting on one side → rotation → sitting on the other side*
  - *Supine → prone → rotation → long-sitting*
  - *.........*

3.2.6 Sitting

The sitting position can be reached and maintained in several ways, and the therapist should be open to any initiative from the child and be ready to quickly seize the opportunity to support it. It is not mandatory to treat them in a "symmetrical" way. The child can sit differently, and every type of position can become functional and be used in therapy.

For example, the child can sit:

- In side-sitting
- In long-sitting, not necessarily symmetrically
- On a table, along the side or on the corner
- On a bench or a stool
- Held in the adult's arms, on the lap or piggyback
- On a ball
- Astride a toddler bike, tricycle, roll, bench, chair, etc.
- ......

Goals of these sitting proposals:

- Improve uprighting extension of the trunk and balance reactions in a more complex antigravity position
- Practise weight-bearing on lower limbs and feet
- Facilitate midline orientation and bimanual activities for functional independence
- Broaden spatial orientation and exploration

Suggestion
- Prepare the conditions for a good BoS that will enhance the child's stability in sitting:
  1. *Get the child to sit on a bench or a sturdy stool, with both feet well supported on the ground; if the trunk is too flexed, insert a small wedge with the high part under the child buttock to induce anterior tilting of the pelvis and more extension of the spine.*

2. *Verify the position and weight-bearing of the pelvis on the sagittal and horizontal plane, so that the feet are aligned at the same level.*
3. *Check that both feet, particularly the impaired one, are in good contact with the ground and taking some weight; a usually previous manual releasing of the soft tissues and/or muscle activation is necessary to get adequate contact of the impaired foot on the ground (see also Chap. 6 Sect. 6.4.3).*
4. *Enhance the perception of weight-bearing on the feet by applying light manual pressure through the knee to the heel.*

- Propose sensory motor tasks in the space around the child:
  1. *Focalise the child's interest towards their anterior space, forwards and slightly downwards.*
     Examples:
     - *Invite the child to pick up a large ball off the ground, hold it and lift it a little higher.*
     - *Ask the child to feel some small objects under their feet that they have not seen, and then look at them and pick them up* (Fig. 3.14).
  2. *Vary the characteristics of surface area: cold, rough/smooth/dry/wet surfaces, surfaces inclined up and down.*

Note

- Requests of activities which are too demanding and too difficult for the child should be avoided because they are not helpful and can evoke associated reactions and cause unnecessary, strong emotional feelings like anxiety, anger and frustration.

Fig. 3.14 Sensory motor tasks involving feet

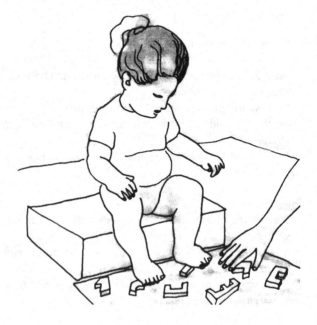

3.2.7   Sitting in Front of a Table

Doing activities sitting in front of a table is important because it prepares the child for future everyday functions, such as eating, dressing, playing and writing. It also facilitates participation in social, educational and community life, e.g. playgroups, kindergarten and school.

Suggestion
- Work for good support of the upper limbs on the table surface:
  1. *First check the alignment of the trunk and the two girdles as well as the position of the scapula.*
  2. *If necessary, release the internal rotation muscles of the shoulder, and train the activity of weak external rotation muscles; mobilise the scapula on the rib cage.*
  3. *Guide the positioning of the upper limb on the table, as suggested in Chap. 2 Sect. 2.2.2 and Chap. 9 Sect. 9.2.3, in such a way that the limb is not in the typical pattern of forearm pronation, ulnar deviation at the wrist and closed hand*
  4. *Pay particular attention to the initial contact of the hand with the surface: the frictional contact of the hand on the surface helps to stabilize the position of the arm, favouring orientation on the midline and balance (see Contactual Hand-Orienting Response in Chap. 6).*
- Propose differentiated sensory experiences:
  - *Propose activities that favour haptic exploration of objects, aimed at discovering possibilities for functional manipulation (about the concept of affordance:* Gibson 1979, 1988) *(Fig. 3.15).*
  - *propose activities that stimulate the child to touch the affected arm and hand, to hold both hands and move them together* (Figs. 3.16 and 3.17).

Fig. 3.15 Haptic exploration

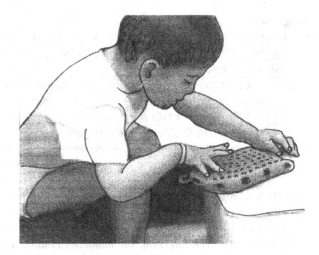

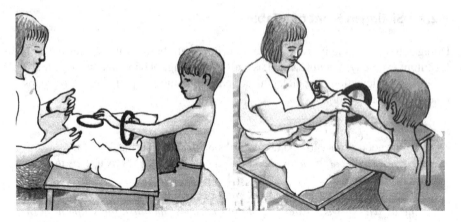

Figs. 3.16 and 3.17 Training for dressing and undressing

- *Propose activities with large toys that inevitably require the use of both the upper limbs.*
- *Encourage the child to involve the impaired upper limb in functional and play activities.*

3.2.8 Sitting Without Feet Support

While the sitting position with support on the feet favours the active uprighting of the trunk and the body stability, sitting without this support is challenging and requires many more balance skills.

If this activity triggers fear and perceptual difficulties and provokes associated reactions, provide the child with proprioceptive inputs, such as weight-bearing facilitation over a joint area.

Suggestion
- Let the child feel weight-bearing shifts on the three planes of motion:
    1. *Get the child to sit on the long side of a treatment table, and stay close so that they feel more secure.*
    2. *Check that the trunk maintains upright alignment and if any muscle tension or weakness is present.*
    3. *Check the position of the humerus head into the glenoid and that the forearm is not pronated; facilitate dorsiflexion of the wrist and opening of the hand.*
    4. *Work for contact of the hand on the surface, so that it becomes a reference point for support; prepare the pelvis on the impaired side for the weight-bearing shifts (Fig. 3.18).*
    5. *Induce slight transfer of weight onto the impaired limb, asking the child to reach for a toy in front of them with their sound arm. Make sure that their shoulder girdle still remains aligned with the surface of the table.*
    6. *Reduce, or even interrupt, the manual guidance as soon as support on the arm and balance reactions are effectively in action.*

Fig. 3.18 Arm support and balance reactions in sitting

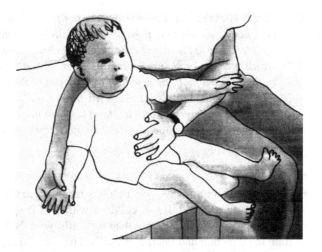

- Gradually introduce more dynamic and challenging activities:
  - *As suggested by Schmidt's theory on motor learning* (Schmidt 1975), *propose activities with similar tasks but with characteristics of variability, which require different problem-solving strategies and the involvement of other parts of the body. For example, propose playing with similar objects but with different characteristics of weight, consistency, texture and position, which the child can also use imaginatively.*

3.2.9   Sitting Astride

When sitting astride a mobile support like a toddler "balance bike" or a tricycle without pedals, the young child can practise balance and weight-bearing on the impaired lower limb and also learn to use alternating rhythmic lower limb movements to move around and explore the environment, a "pre-walking" functional activity useful to prepare skills for future walking.

Suggestion
- Train rhythmic movements of the lower limbs:
  - *Have the child sit astride a balance bicycle or similar car/animal-shaped toy on wheels so that, under a caregiver's supervision, the child can learn and enjoy moving around.*
  - *Choose the best stable model of the object on wheels, and carry out any needed regarding the height and width of the seat and the height of the handlebar, to have the appropriate angular relationship between hip, knee and ankle joints.*
- Check/create the conditions for the child to move around:
  1. *Check and, if necessary, modify the handlebar to facilitate the child's grip: U shape, increase diameter, regulate width of handles, use fastener or glove with Velcro[1] (Fig. 3.19).*

---

[1] Velcro Ltd., Knutsford (UK), www.velcro.uk

2. *Verify effective weight-bearing on both lower limbs, and, if necessary, enhance it on the impaired side with slight manual pressure through the affected knee to the foot. As the child experiments moving forwards and backwards pushing on their feet, facilitate and practise the heel-to-toe movement in the affected foot, the essential mechanism of the push-off phase of gait.*
3. *Support all the child's interests, intentions and attempts to move, including initiatives to move around, to stand up from this astride sitting position, sitting down again and getting off the object climb over, go back, etc.*

Note
- When seated on a mobile toy, toddlers usually learn to go backwards first and then later forwards. Instead, children with USCP spontaneously tend to keep moving only backwards rather than forwards, with the hip of the impaired lower limb in adduction and internal rotation. The use of this pattern increases muscle stiffness. Therefore, the therapist needs to intervene and be sure that the child learns to move forwards, sharing the necessary training indications to the caregivers.

3.2.10 Half-Kneeling

There are various ways to perform the transfer to standing. Most often a younger child stands up from the floor passing through the half-kneeling position, while an older child stands up from many different positions, although the most frequent transfer becomes from the sitting position (see also Chap. 2 Sect. 2.2.2). Before working with the child with USCP on the transfer through half-kneeling, the therapist should verify

Fig. 3.19 Adaptation of a toddler bike

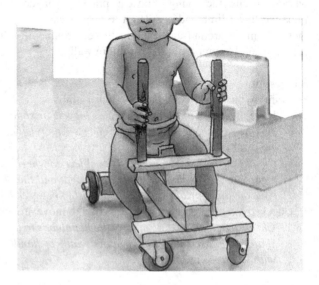

the presence of a straight trunk, appropriate pelvic tilting and good feet support, the fundamental components for efficient final linear acceleration of the trunk.

Training in standing up through half-kneeling is particularly worthwhile in these children, because it requires the use of an extended hip in the leg that first bears the body weight, while the other in flexion then takes on the task of supporting the body load during uprighting. This is excellent practice for the impaired lower limb because it is engaged in functions of support both on an extended and a flexed hip.

It is recommended to work first in the position which requires hip extension on the impaired side because that means releasing the hip flexor muscles and recruiting all the extensor postural muscles of that side, particularly the *glutei*.

Suggestion
- Create a setting that facilitates the half-kneeling transition:
  - *The half-kneeling position may be perceived by the child as very unstable, if any perceptual problems are present. Therefore, the therapist should stay close to the child and use their body as containment or a proprioceptual reference point.*
  - *If necessary, create a semi-closed environment with more boundaries, like a corridor-like space between chairs or benches where the child can stand up feeling more at ease.*
- Train the transfer kneeling → half-kneeling → standing:
  1. *Prepare for the transfer by establishing a functional/play goal that motivates the child to stand up. Position yourself on your knees behind or in front of the child.*
  2. *Verify the position of the trunk and the pelvis on the three planes with the child in kneeling; activate extension in the hips (gluteus major and minor muscles) to assure alignment and hip stability throughout the transfer.*
  3. *Propose the first transfers with the unaffected limb moving into flexion, while the impaired leg weight-bears on the extended hip.*
  4. *Take care that, during uprighting to standing with the sound leg forwards, the impaired limb arrives in standing next to the other mainly with a inertial action, not through tight flexor muscles; support this type of movement by first facilitating the release and elongation of the psoas major muscle and the long head of rectus femoris.*
  5. *When the child reaches the standing position, regain the active extension in the affected hip.*
  6. *If the child is more skilled and confident, let them experience the transfer with the impaired leg as the first mover. In this case, check the starting movement by recruiting first the gluteus medium and the tensor fasciae latae to facilitate the weight shift to the unaffected and also the rectus femoris, iliacus and sartorius; secondly verify the tension of the gracilis and adductor longus to align the femur and begin the weight transfer on the affected leg towards the standing position (Fig. 3.20).*
  7. *If the child still does not manage the transfer well, try facilitating their confidence and ability by placing a ball of adequate size under their flexed hip, and let them experiment small weight shifts in different directions.*

Fig. 3.20 Transfer
through half-kneeling

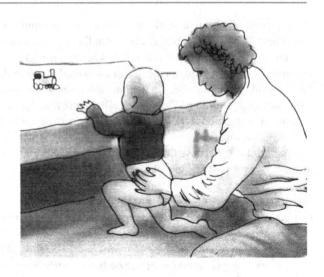

Note
- It is very important that the training experiences regarding the half-kneeling position are finalized to moving into standing, so that the child links the transition to a functional goal which has a clear meaning for them.

3.2.11 From Squatting to Standing and Back

Mastering transitions from a low to a more erect antigravity position is a great functional achievement for the child. However, it is equally important that the child learns to lower themselves to the ground while maintaining good control during the transition, as it means engaging most muscles in eccentric contraction. Moving down to squatting is particularly challenging because it requires that all the posterior trunk muscles, the quadriceps and the calf muscles work eccentrically.

Just as a child with physiological development often lowers themself to play, to pick up objects from the floor, to sit on the potty or to pet the cat, the same functional activities can be proposed to the child with USCP. As in the half-kneeling transition, this child may be able carry out the transfer by themself but in a very imprecise way, and so it is important to train them to do it with more alignment and appropriate weight-bearing.

Suggestion
- Train the transition from squatting to standing:
  1. *Before starting the transfer to the standing position, verify the full support of both the feet on the ground, and, if necessary, release the* triceps surae *of the impaired leg to improve support on the foot.*
  2. *Encourage the child to return to a full squatting position, adding slight but perceptible pressure stretching of the quadriceps along the longitudinal axes of the two femurs, to enhance the weight-bearing on the lower limbs.*

3. *In the same way, facilitate the transfer forwards of the child's CoM.*
4. *Motivate the child to stand up, and at the same time facilitate the contraction of the less-able* quadriceps *with a light pressure, this time towards its muscle belly.*

- Train the transition from standing to squatting:
  1. *Facilitate the descent using the same manual guidance used in other CP forms for the stand-to-sit transfer: as in point 2, accompany the descent of the child to the full squatting position, checking that an even distribution of weight is maintained on both feet.*
  2. *Based on the child's abilities, propose tasks that require stopping the descent at different heights from the ground, for example, by placing a toy on the floor or on a bench, so that the child can feel and manage the different RoMs of hip/knee/ankle joints.*
  3. *If the child is skilled and motivated, propose they lean forwards from squatting to get a toy in front of them with the unaffected arm so that they can mainly support their weight on the impaired side.*

3.2.12 Standing

As described above, the impairment of the child with USCP still allows them to acquire independent walking, even if later than a well-bodied child and with the use of compensatory strategies. Knowing this, the therapist should foresee and counterbalance the overuse of these strategies, working early on those components that allow a more appropriate erect position and a more functional and efficient walk:

- Alignment of the two girdles with each other, both on the horizontal and frontal plane, paying particular attention that the impaired side is not positioned backwards.
- Mobility of the pelvis on all three planes.
- A good contact of the impaired foot with ground, to receive sensory inputs to properly organize the linear acceleration of the body and acquire a good balance

Note
- When learning to walk, the child with USCP uses speed to avoid the accuracy required in the different phases of the movement. The therapist has needs to concentrate on a selection of critical components rather than on all of them indiscriminately, knowing that the child will acquire some of these abilities by themself.

Suggestion
- Prepare the affected foot for efficient support on the ground:
  1. *If the child is already standing, verify the position of the pelvis, limb and foot, and intervene to release tight muscles* (e.g. triceps surae) *and strengthen weak groups* (e.g. tibialis anterior). *To do this, return to a lower position that*

allows to work on the appropriate recruitment of the muscle groups, which otherwise could not be achieved while they are excessively involved in maintaining the higher antigravity posture.

2. *Align the foot and leg, release the tight muscles of the foot, and facilitate the activity of muscles useful for widening the support base (*e.g. abductor digiti quinti*) and so improve stability* (see also Sect. 6.4.3. of Chap. 6).

- Improve weight-bearing shifts on the three planes:
  1. *Stand in front of the child, and propose play/functional activities that require small weight shifts on the frontal and sagittal plane, checking the active recruitment of the* gluteus major *and* minor *as extensor and abductor muscles of the affected hip.*
  2. *Introduce proposals requiring rotations between the two girdles, to improve the forward rotation of the affected pelvis on the horizontal plane, and maintaining of an efficient weight-bearing stability when the best side is moving.*
  3. *Emphasize the shifting of the bodyweight on the frontal plane by offering the child activities that require reaching an interesting object placed on the side or just looking at it if the task is too difficult. During these transfers, the extensor and abductor muscles of the hip should be recruited.*
  4. *A big gym ball can facilitate the weight shifts, if the child is not afraid to interact with a large mobile object* (Fig. 3.21).

3.2.13 Standing on One Leg

It is important to train weight-bearing on one leg because it is essential for many functional situations:

Fig. 3.21 Transfers of weight-bearing, using a big gym ball

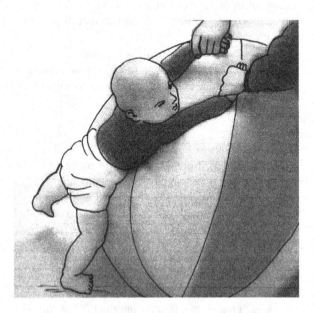

- Supporting on one leg during the full stance phase of the gait cycle
- Going up and down stairs or stepping up and down
- Getting over obstacles, getting on a tricycle or rocking horse, etc.
- Getting in and out of a container (a box, a big basket, etc.)
- Stepping from one object to the other (Fig. 3.22)
- Skipping and jumping on alternate feet

In particular, the child should be able to support the weight alternatively on both lower limbs and to cope with the different sensory perceptual experiences.

Suggestion
- Evaluate the effective shifting of the weight-bearing on the affected lower limb:
  1. *Stand in front of the child, and verify the aligned position of the pelvis on the horizontal plane and that the hips are both extended with maximum recruitment of the* gluteus major and minor *muscles.*
  2. *Check the presence of active weight-bearing on both limbs, and propose activities with small movements that allow to verify the actual change of weight-bearing alternately, first on the impaired leg and then on the other, e.g. shift the weight onto the affected side, and then ask the child to place their sound foot lightly on the therapist's thigh. Remember to check the recruitment of the hip extensor muscles during these performances.*
  3. *By moving the raised lower limb slightly forwards, back and to the side, the child is challenged to maintain stable postural control by adapting their body to these small changes* (Fig. 3.23).
  4. *Create a setting with tasks such as climbing with the unaffected limb onto a step/platform getting into a large box with interesting objects; the affected hip should remain extended in the phase of full support.*
  5. *Motivate the child reverse these movements with the sound leg, stepping down from the step and getting out of the box sideways, forwards and backwards.*
- Train the child to move and lift the impaired limb as the first mover:
  1. *As done before for the sound limb, create a setting with tasks that this time require stepping onto a stair or climbing over an obstacle.*
  2. *Use manual facilitations to recruit effectively the* gluteus medius, peronei *and the* abductor digiti quinti *muscles, releasing at the same time the* triceps surae

Fig. 3.22 Stepping from one object to another

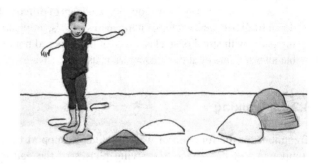

Fig. 3.23 Balance training
on one leg

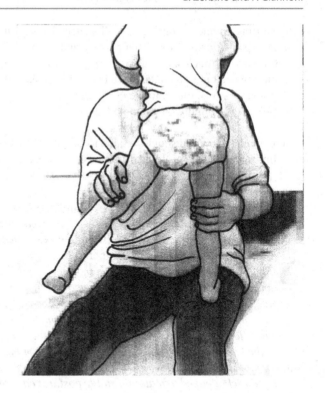

and tibialis posterior; *with a hold on the child's fifth toe, guide a slight external rotation of the leg and the placing of the foot on the ground.*

3. *As soon as the heel touches the ground and during the full stance phase, control the extension of the hip and the knee to facilitate the weight-bearing on the whole foot.*

Note
- If the knee is hyperextended under full weight-bearing on the affected leg, consider that, in this situation, it will be combined with flexion at the hip so that, almost always, it is necessary to realign and extend the hip joint to properly realign the knee.
- The activities of getting in and out of containers of different heights, stepping up and down from benches, walking on inclined surfaces, going up and down steps, following paths with small obstacles, etc. can be proposed not only in treatment sessions but also at home or at the kindergarten, as interactive games with other children.

3.2.14 Walking

Treatment for the function of walking aims to support the acquisition of the basic components of the stance and swing phases of the gait cycle, i.e. valid weight-bearing, balance and propulsion. Training should then be directed towards real, functional and challenging walking situations where the child moves with a purpose and in environments other than the treatment setting.

Functional walking also requires walking for different durations, at different speeds and with good endurance, doing other things while walking, like carrying something or talking, for example.

During the various phases of gait, the therapist should observe and guide the child's performances as necessary. The techniques to guide and train the sequence of walking are discussed in Chap. 2 and Chap. 7 Sect. 7.2.1.

The therapist can facilitate the child with hemiplegia in their first attempts of walking by proposing a mobile aid (a chair, stable cart or walker) to push, which gives them a wider BoS that increases their stability and helps them to cope with the open space in front. The pushing surface of the aid should be at the height of the child's shoulders, not lower which could cause flexion of the hips and the loss of the trunk uprighting and not higher, to avoid excessive extension and the increase in stiffness which would hamper forward progression.

Suggestion
- Verify the postural alignment, for initiating functional walking:
  1. *Verify the position of the shoulder and pelvic girdles on the three planes and the alignment between them.*
  2. *Establish a functional walking goal with the child to motivate the activity,* e.g. *carry a large toy with both arms to give to someone or to put away* (Fig. 3.24).
  3. *Verify first the mobility of the scapula and the RoM of the glenohumeral joint, and then guide, as necessary, the extension of the upper limb and opening of the hand, depending on the task and the characteristics of the object to be carried.*
  4. *Prepare the contactual hand response with the object, exerting a light pressure on the child's hand, as they may have an avoiding reaction to tactile input. Check for this, and make sure that the effort of the task does not evoke an associated reaction.*
- Start the sequence of gait:
  1. *Training for functional walking has the same characteristics of training proposed to children with BSCP (see Sect. 2.2.2). However, for a child with USCP, it is even more important that they initiate the sequence of strides taking the first step with the unaffected limb, to carry out the second step with the affected one with an inertial return of the long head of the* biceps femoris *and not with its active concentric recruitment that would trigger an altered swing pattern.*
  2. *Check for effective forward rotation of the pelvic girdle on the impaired side and for the appropriate length of the step.*
- Train the child to manage many variables while walking:
  1. *Propose different activities and games aimed at giving the child different walking experience with different sequences of movement that may concern:*
     (a) *Specific procedures of execution, based on a task:*
         - *Walk sideways, with or without support, in both directions*
         - *Cross-stepping, alternating both lower limbs*

Fig. 3.24 Walking
carrying a large toy

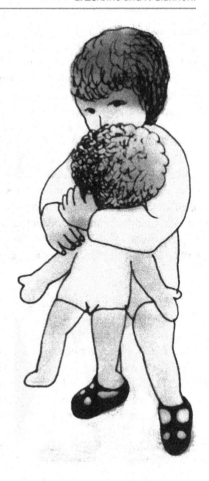

- – *Walk backwards*
- – *Tandem gait*
- – *Walk in circles*
- – *Carry out U-turns*
- – *The diagonal crossing of a room*
- – *Carry out steps of different lengths: long (as a giant) and short (as a hant)*
- – *Walk silently with light footsteps and* vice versa *noisily with heavy footsteps*
- – *Walk quickly and slowly*
- – *Walk with eyes closed*
- – *Jump and run*
- (b) *Based on environmental constraints to be respected:*
  - – *Climb over obstacles along the path*
  - – *Go up and down stairs*
  - – *Walk along a very narrow base*
  - – *Walk uphill and downhill*
  - – *Walk on different types of surfaces*

Note
- Age, level of impairment and subjective needs greatly influence the type and difficulty of the activities that the therapist can propose. A teenager and an adult can benefit from the challenge of running to catch a bus and doing two tasks at once, like talking on the phone while walking, dancing with a friend or walking with an open umbrella in the rain.

3.2.15 Going Up and Down Stairs

- Prepare the child to go up a step in front of them:
  1. *Propose the step experience in a real context, like the home environment if possible, using stairs and steps that lead to a significant place for the child.*
  2. *With an older child, go directly to the front of a stair; with a toddler offer a platform that they can cope with easily. Check their postural alignment before starting the step practice.*
  3. *Stand beside the affected side of the child, and ask them to place their sound foot on the step, simultaneously verifying the active recruitment of the two* glutæi *for the extension of the affected hip.*
  4. *Facilitate the step up so the impaired foot reaches the other foot on the platform/stair with the same modalities as for starting the swing phase of the gait cycle: use distal manual facilitation to recruit the active involvement of the* tibialis anterior *and* peronæi, *to place the foot on the platform.*
  5. *As the foot is on the surface, apply a manual pressure along the axis of the femur, and assist them in transferring the bodyweight forwards onto the supporting foot; during this transfer, the trunk should also be active with an uprighting linear acceleration.*
  6. *To facilitate the full stance phase on the step, assist the concentric activity of the* quadriceps, *with slight but precise manual pressure towards the muscle belly, and at the same time, solicit the recruitment of the* gluteus maximus.
  7. *Based on the ability of the child, their age and their motivation, take into consideration that the child cannot always perform the sequence of the two steps in succession, so also plan to work only on part of the sequence for some time.*
- Train the child to backstep, going down the stairs:
  1. *Ask the child to backstep going down, alternating their lower limbs in the descent.*
  2. *Have the child descend with the unimpaired limb as the first mover, and accompany the descent by exerting a slight pressure on the impaired leg to help the child keep the weight-bearing on the foot remaining on the step until the other foot reaches the support.*
  3. *Propose also that the child descends with the impaired leg first, keeping in mind that the movement of the back leg occurs with hip extension, the elongation of the* iliopsoas *and the* rectus femoris *muscles and the activation of the* gluteus maximus *and* hamstrings. *Pay attention as well to the initial contact of the forefoot with the ground, which occurs without visual control and requires greater perceptual attention* (Fig. 3.25).

Fig. 3.25 Stepping down
with the impaired leg

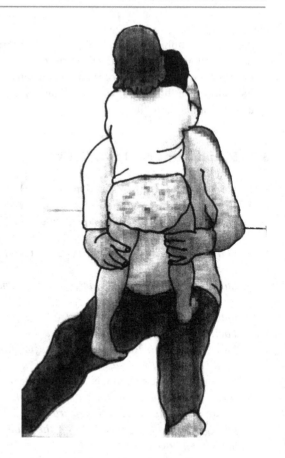

- Train the child to go down with the stair backward:
  1. *As the child could have spatial perceptual disturbances, ask the caregiver to stay in front of the child but a little further down.*
  2. *Stand beside their affected side, and ask them to place their sound foot first down onto the step.*
  3. *Because weight-bearing on the impaired foot is difficult at first, apply some manual pressure over the child's knee to stabilize their limb while the other is descending.*
  4. *As the sound foot arrives on the surface, guide the child's leg to reach the lower step in different ways:*
     - *If the child wears shoes, guide their affected leg to place the foot on the surface.*
     - *If the child is barefoot, facilitate the dorsiflexion of the ankle with manual distal guide at the metatarsophalangeal joint, and then guide the child's foot onto the step.*

Note

- If the task of the stairs is proposed to a toddler, it is important to remember that, age-wise, they go up and down one step at a time; the sequence of alternating steps comes later.
- With an older child and adolescent, training on stairs should include a rigorous sequence of patterns to improve proprioceptive inputs on the impaired side. Therefore it is important that, in therapy, they avoid clinging to handrails or other supports around them. It will be different in daily life and working environments where it is just important to perform functionally.

3.3   Other Therapeutic Approaches

3.3.1   Constraint-Induced Movement Therapy

Constraint-induced movement therapy (CIMT) was initiated in the early 1980s in the USA, based on behavioural research on primates conducted by Taub (1980). This technique was then applied to adults with hemiparesis resulting from stroke or head injury (Wolf et al. 1989; Taub and Wolf 1997). Since then, it has become a rehabilitation intervention used in asymmetrical motor impairment involving the upper limb that consists in facilitating the obliged, intensive use of the impaired hand by constraining the use of the less affected arm, with the application of a rigid plaster cast, a glove with rigid insert, a mitt, sling, splint, hand support, etc. CIMT has been applied in children with unilateral neuro-motor damage, with the aim of counteracting the "learned non-use" or "developmental non-use" of the impaired upper limb by promoting motor and manipulation activities with the more affected upper limb while the less-affected side is immobilized (Taub et al. 2004, 2006; Deluca et al. 2006; Eliasson et al. 2011, 2018; Hwang and Kwon 2020).

Various scientific publications regarding CIMT report various proposals for the application of the method with regard to the type of constraint, the intensity of the application, the proposed environment, etc. Originally, CIMT was a very demanding therapy for the child and the family, with the indication to use a type of brace restraint for 90% of the waking time, for 2 weeks, with 6 h of training in a therapy session with specialized personnel. Since then, a modified form (mCIMT) has been proposed indicating the daily application of the constraint for 2–3 h per day, for 1–2 months, requiring intense activity of the impaired hand with tasks of stretching and grasping (Charles et al. 2006; Aarts et al. 2010).

Applying CIMT implies a great commitment to using the impaired limb, but it is also likely that the child themself is not motivated to collaborate and that they experience frustration for their difficulties and failures. Moreover, the child with USCP may have problems in the cognitive and attentional areas, and the therapist will know if it is the case to involve and motivate them for this kind of intervention and how to calibrate the therapeutic proposal to the child's level of collaboration and abilities.

A 2019 Cochrane review compared the results of various CIMT applications, with different amounts and combinations with other forms of intervention, e.g. hand arm bimanual intensive care, bimanual therapy and occupational therapy. The conclusion reports some good results with more intense applications, but not relevant compared with other types of rehabilitation approaches (Hoare et al. 2019).

3.3.2   Hand Arm Bimanual Intensive Therapy

Hand arm bimanual intensive therapy (HABIT) is an intensive treatment to use in asymmetrical upper limb impairments that aims at improving bimanual use of the upper limbs and the collaboration of both the affected and unaffected hands, as "two hands are better than one" to achieve better functioning (Gordon 2010; Gordon et al. 2011). HABIT does not contemplate constraints, but training with play proposals that facilitate bimanual activities, paying particular attention to the movements of the affected limb, such as stabilization, cooperation and manipulation activities.

Sakzewski et al. (2014) report HABIT as valid as a CIMT. Similarly, a multicentre clinical trial (Fedrizzi et al. 2013) compared mCIMT and HABIT to standard treatment in 105 children with USCP. Those treated with mCIMT or HABIT showed an improvement in the function of the affected upper limb as to grip and spontaneous use of hands for play and ADL in both groups. These improvements were maintained in the follow-up phase after 6 months. Such intensive treatment methods can be applied simultaneously.

Bilateral arm training has emerged as an approach that leads to positive outcomes in treating upper extremity paresis after stroke. However, most studies have not sufficiently evaluated the fact that interhemispheric inhibition is dynamically task-dependent and has a direct implication for the neurorehabilitation of stroke patients (Murase et al. 2004). Furthermore, the rationale for using this type of training has not been completely explained. McCombe Waller and Whitall (2008) suggest that bilateral training can improve unilateral paretic limb functions of the upper extremity after stroke, provided that specific training approaches are carefully matched to baseline characteristics of the patients.

3.3.3   Action Observation Treatment

Just over 20 years ago, the mirror neuron system (MNS) in the ventral premotor cortex (area F5) and the inferior parietal lobule (area PFG) of monkeys were discovered (di Pellegrino et al. 1992; Rizzolatti et al. 1996). It is theorized that a class of visuomotor neurons is activated when the primate performs a goal-directed motor action and when it observes an individual performing the same or a similar act, thus suggesting that the MNS has an important role in the recognition of the observed actions and the learning of motor functions. Based on these studies, the rehabilitation method of action observation treatment (AOT) has been developed, which proposes a combination of observations of daily actions (e.g. picking up an object, drinking from a glass, etc.) and motor training of the same actions that have been previously observed (Ertelt et al. 2007).

This technique has been applied both to adults with chronic stroke, showing an improvement in the motor functions of the hemiplegic upper limb and to school-aged children with USCP (Sgandurra et al. 2011; Kirkpatrick et al. 2016). Given the positive results of the application of AOT in children with CP, some studies hypothesize an early intervention even in very young infants with suspect signs of CP (Burzi et al. 2016), facilitating observation and learning of reaching and grasping. The feasibility of the intervention depends on the ability of clinicians to make an early diagnosis and therefore direct the infants to rehabilitation before the age of 6 months (Guzzetta et al. 2013).

While several studies have shown the benefits of this therapy, others are less favourable, indicating a lack of scientific clarity and suggesting that new and different studies on AOT need to be performed to properly identify its role in the rehabilitation therapy of neurological disorders (Plata-Bello 2017).

3.3.4 Motor Imagery

Motor imagery (MI) is the mental simulation of a movement, i.e. imagining a movement without actually performing it. Many studies have demonstrated that real actions and imagined actions activate the same areas in different parts of the brain (Jeannerod 2001): the prefrontal cortex, the premotor cortex, the supplementary motor area, the cingulate gyrus, the parietal cortex and the cerebellum. Moreover, the timing of real and imagined actions is also quite similar (Karlinksky and Flash 2015). These studies suggested, for example, that mental training of skilled activities was useful and, in particular, "motor learning without movement" was possible (De Vries and Mulder 2007). The person involved can imagine a movement of the body without actually performing the movement (motor imagery), or they may imagine an object that is moving (movement imagery) (Decety 1996). Some studies demonstrate that in these situations, there is also a participation of the autonomic system (Sommerville and Decety 2006): cardiac and respiratory activity changes when, for example, one imagines oneself running or someone is observed running (Paccalin and Jeannerod 2000).

Application of these methods in children with CP should be evaluated carefully, considering that both cognitive problems and impaired motor planning often coexist.

For example, in a child with USCP, motor planning may be compromised also by an inability to use motor imagery, so MI training could be a useful starting point for the rehabilitation of motor planning problems (Steenbergen and Gordon 2006; Crajé et al. 2010).

MNS seems to work more effectively through training with AOT rather than MI, which requires cognitive participation that is not always possible to obtain in children with CP (Cuenca-Martínez et al. 2020).

References

Aarts PB, Jongerius PH, Geerdink YA, Van Limbeek J, Geurt AC (2010) Effectiveness of modified constraint-induced movement therapy in children with unilateral spastic cerebral palsy: a randomized controlled trial. Neurorehabil Neural Repair 24:509–518. https://doi.org/10.1177/1545968309359767

Auld ML, Boyd R, Moseley GL, Ware R, Johnston LM (2012) Tactile function in children with unilateral cerebral palsy compared to typically developing children. Disabil Rehabil 34(17):1488–1494. https://doi.org/10.3109/09638288.2011.650314

Bassøe Gjelsvik BE (2008) The Bobath Concept in adult neurology. Thieme Verlag. https://doi.org/10.1055/b-002-59217

Bonnefoy-Mazure A, Sagawa Y Jr, Lascombes P, De Coulon G, Armand S (2014) A descriptive analysis of the upper limb patterns during gait in individuals with cerebral palsy. Res Dev Disabil 35(11):2756–2765. https://doi.org/10.1016/j.ridd.2014.07.013

Bosanquet M, Copeland L, Ware R, Boyd R (2013) A systematic review of tests to predict cerebral palsy in young children. Dev Med Child Neurol 55(5):418–426. https://doi.org/10.1111/dmcn.12140

Bottcher L, Flachs EM, Uldall P (2010) Attentional and executive impairments in children with spastic cerebral palsy. Dev Med Child Neurol 52(2):e42–e47. https://doi.org/10.1111/j.1469-8749.2009.03533.x

Burn MB, Gogola GR (2021) Dexterity of the Less Affected hand in children with hemiplegic cerebral palsy. Hand (N Y). https://doi.org/10.1177/1558944721990803

Burzi V, Tealdi G, Boyd RN, Guzzetta A (2016) Action observation in infancy: implications for neuro-rehabilitation. Dev Med Child Neurol 58(S4):74–77. https://doi.org/10.1111/dmcn.13048

Charles JR, Wolf SL, Schneider JA, Gordon AM (2006) Efficacy of a child-friendly form of constraint-induced movement therapy in hemiplegic cerebral palsy: a randomized control trial. Dev Med Child Neurol 48(8):635–642. https://doi.org/10.1017/S0012162206001356

Cioni G, Sales B, Paolicelli PB, Petacchi E, Scusa MF, Canapicchi R (1999) MRI and clinical characteristics of children with hemiplegic cerebral palsy. Neuropediatrics 30:249–255. https://doi.org/10.1055/s-2007-973499

Cioni G, Sgandurra G, Muzzini S, Paolicelli PB, Ferrari A (2010) Forms of hemiplegia. In: The spastic forms of cerebral palsy. Springer ed., Milano

Cioni G, Belmonti V, Einspieler C (2014) Early diagnosis and prognosis in cerebral palsy. In: Sheperd RB (ed) Crebral palsy in infancy. Elsevier Ltd, Edinburgh, pp 179–187

Crajé C, van Elk M, Beeren M, van Schie HT, Bekkering H, Steenbergen B (2010) Compromised motor planning and Motor Imagery in right hemiparetic cerebral palsy. Res Dev Disabil 31(6):1313–1322. https://doi.org/10.1016/j.ridd.2010.07.010

Cuenca-Martínez F, Suso-Martí L, León-Hernánde JV, La Touche R (2020) The role of movement representation techniques in the motor learning process: a neurophysiological hypothesis and a narrative review. Brain Sci 10:27. https://doi.org/10.3390/brainsci10010027

De Vries S, Mulder T (2007) Motor imagery and stroke rehabilitation: a critical discussion. J Rehabil Med 39:5–13. https://doi.org/10.2340/16501977-0020

Decety J (1996) The neurophysiological basis of motor imagery. Behav Brain Res 77:45–52. https://doi.org/10.1016/0166-4328(95)00225-1

Deluca SC, Echols K, Law CR, Ramey SL (2006) Intensive pediatric constraint-induced therapy for children with cerebral palsy: randomized, controlled, crossover trial. J Child Neurol 21(11):931–938. https://doi.org/10.1177/08830738060210110401

di Pellegrino G, Fadiga L, Fogassi L, Gallese V, Rizzolatti G (1992) Understanding motor events: a neurophysiological study. Exp Brain Res 91:176–180. https://doi.org/10.1007/BF00230027

Eliasson AC, Shaw K, Berg E, Krumlinde-Sundholm L (2011) An ecological approach of constraint induced movement therapy for 2–3 year-old children: a randomized control trial. Dev Disabil 32:2820–2282. https://doi.org/10.1016/j.ridd.2011.05.024

Eliasson AC, Nordstrand L, Ek L, Lennartsson F, Sjöstrand L, Tedroff K, Krumlinde-Sundholm L (2018) The effectiveness of Baby-CIMT in infants younger than 12 months with clinical signs of unilateral-cerebral palsy; an explorative study with randomized design. Res Dev Disabil 72:191–201. https://doi.org/10.1016/j.ridd.2017.11.006

Ertelt D, Small S, Solodkin A, Dettmers C, McNamara A, Binkofski F, Buccino G (2007) Action observation has a positive impact on rehabilitation of motor deficits after stroke. Neuroimage 36:T164–T173. https://doi.org/10.1016/j.neuroimage.2007.03.043

Fedrizzi E, Rosa-Rizzotto M, Turconi AC, Pagliano E, Fazzi E, Pozza LV, Facchin P, GIPCI Study Group (2013) Unimanual and bimanual intensive training in children with hemiplegic cerebral palsy and persistence in time of hand function improvement: 6-month follow-up results of a multisite clinical trial. J Child Neurol 28(2):161–175. https://doi.org/10.1177/0883073812443004

Gage JR (2004) The treatment of gait problems in cerebral palsy. Mac Keith, Cambridge University Press, London

Galli M, Cimolin V, Crivellini M, Romkes J, Albertini G, Brunner R (2012) Quantification of upper limb motion during gait in children with hemiplegic cerebral palsy. J Dev Phys Disabil 24:1–8. https://doi.org/10.1007/s10882-011-9250-4

Gibson JJ (1979) The ecological approach to visual perception. Houghton Mifflin Harcourt (HMH), Boston

Gibson EJ (1988) Exploratory behaviour in the development of perceiving, acting, and the acquiring of knowledge. In: Rosenzweig MR, Porter LW (eds) Annual review of psychology, vol 39. Annual Reviews, Palo Alto, pp 1–41

Goodman R, Graham P (1996) Psychiatric problems in children with hemiplegia: cross sectional epidemiological survey. BMJ 312(7038):1065–1069. https://doi.org/10.1136/bmj.312.7038.1065

Gordon AM (2010) Two hands are better than one: bimanual skill development in children with hemiplegic cerebral palsy. Dev Med Child Neurol 52(4):315–316. https://doi.org/10.1111/j.1469-8749.2009.03390.x

Gordon AM, Hung YC, Brandao M, Ferre CL, Kuo HC, Friel K, Petra E, Chinnan A, Charles JR (2011) Bimanual training and constraint-induced movement therapy in children with hemiplegic cerebral palsy: a randomized trial. Neurorehabil Neural Repair 25(8):692–702. https://doi.org/10.1177/1545968311402508

Guzzetta A, Fazzi B, Mercuri E, Bertuccelli B, Canapicchi R, Duin J, Cioni G (2001) Visual function in children with hemiplegia in the first years of life. Dev Med Child Neurol 43:321–329. https://doi.org/10.1111/j.1469-8749.2001.tb00212.x

Guzzetta A, Boyd R, Perez M, Ziviani J, Burzi V, Slaughter V, Rose S, Provan K, Findlay L, Fisher I, Colombini F, Tealdi G, Marchi V, Whittingham K (2013) UP-BEAT (Upper Limb Baby Early Action-observation Training): protocol of two parallel randomised controlled trials of action-observation training for typically developing infants and infants with asymmetric brain lesions. BMJ Open 3(2). https://doi.org/10.1136/bmjopen-2012-002512

Hadders-Algra M (2004) General movements: a window for early identification of children at high risk for developmental disorders. J Pediatr 145(2 Suppl):S12–S18. https://doi.org/10.1016/j.jpeds.2004.05.017

Hawe RL, Kuczynski AM, Kirton A, Durkelow SP (2020) Assessment of bilateral motor skills and visuospatial attention in children with perinatal stroke using a robotic object hitting task. J Neuroeng Rehabil 17:18. https://doi.org/10.1186/s12984-020-0654-1

Himmelmann K, Horber V, De La Cruz J, Horridge K, Mejaski-Bosnjak V, Hollody K, Krägeloh-Mann I, SCPE Working Group (2016) MRI Classification System (MRICS) for children with cerebral palsy: development, reliability and recommendations. Dev Med Child Neurol 59(1):57–64. https://doi.org/10.1111/dmcn.13166

Hoare BJ, Wallen MA, Thorley MN, Jackman ML, Carey LM, Imms C (2019) Constraint-induced movement therapy in children with unilateral cerebral palsy. Cochrane Database Syst Rev 4(4):CD004149. https://doi.org/10.1002/14651858.CD004149.pub3

Hwang YS, Kwon JY (2020) Effects of modified constraint-induced movement therapy in real-world arm use in young children with unilateral cerebral palsy: a single-blind randomized trial. Neuropediatrics 51(4):259–266. https://doi.org/10.1055/s-0040-1702220

Jeannerod M (2001) Neural simulation of action: a unifying mechanism for motor cognition. Neuroimage 14:103–109. https://doi.org/10.1006/nimg.2001.0832

Karimzadeh P, Agha Mohammad Pour M, Amirsalari S, Tonekaboni SH (2010) Risk factors and prognosis of epilepsy in children with hemiparetic cerebral palsy. Iran J Child Neurol 4(3):25–32. https://doi.org/10.22037/ijcn.v4i3.2005

Karlinsky M, Flash T (2015) Timing of continuous motor imagery: the two-thirds power law originates in trajectory planning. J Neurophysiol 113(7):2490–2499. https://doi.org/10.1152/jn.00421.2014

Kirkpatrick E, Pearse J, James P, Basu A (2016) Effect of parent-delivered action observation therapy on upper limb function in unilateral cerebral palsy: a randomized controlled trial. Dev Med Child Neurol 58(10):1049–1056. https://doi.org/10.1111/dmcn.13109

Krägeloh-Mann I, Cans C (2009) Cerebral palsy update. Brain Dev. 31(7):537–544. https://doi.org/10.1016/j.braindev.2009.03.009

Maenza C, Good DC, Winstein CJ, Wagstaff DA, Sainburg RL (2020) Functional deficits in the less-impaired arm of stroke survivors depend on hemisphere of damage and extent of paretic arm impairment. Neurorehabil Neural Repair 34(1):39–50. https://doi.org/10.1177/1545968319875951

McCombe Waller S, Whitall J (2008) Bilateral arm training: why and who benefits? Neurorehabilitation 23(1):29–41. https://doi.org/10.3233/NRE-2008-23104

McLean B, Taylor S, Blair E, Valentine J, Carey L, Elliott C (2017) Somatosensory discrimination intervention improves body position sense and motor performance in children with hemiplegic cerebral palsy. Am J Occup Ther 71(3):7103190060p1–7103190060p9. https://doi.org/10.5014/ajot.2016.024968

Murase N, Duque J, Mazzocchio R, Cohen LG (2004) Influence of interhemispheric interactions on motor function in chronic stroke. Ann Neurol 55(3):400–409. https://doi.org/10.1002/ana.10848

Niemann GA (2001) New MRI-based classification. In: Neville B, Goodman R (eds) Congenital hemiplegia. Clinics in developmental medicine. Mac Keith Press, London, pp 37–52

Paccalin C, Jeannerod M (2000) Changes in breathing during observation of effortful actions. Brain Res 862(1–2):194–200. https://doi.org/10.1016/s0006-8993(00)02145-4

Parkes J, White-Koning M, McCullough N, Colver A (2009) Psychological problems in children with hemiplegia: a European multicentre survey. Arch Dis Child 94(6):429–433. https://doi.org/10.1136/adc.2008.151688

Pellegrino L, Coscia M, Pierella C, Giannoni P, Cherif A, Mugnosso M, Marinelli L, Casadio M (2021) Effects of hemispheric stroke localization on the reorganization of arm movements within different mechanical environments. Life 11(5):383. https://doi.org/10.3390/life11050383

Picelli A, La Marchina E, Vangelista A, Chemello E, Modenese A, Gandolfi M, Ciceri EFM, Bucci A, Zoccatelli G, Saltuari L, Waldner A, Baricich A, Santamato A, Smania N (2017) Effects of robot-assisted training for the unaffected arm in patients with hemiparetic cerebral palsy: a proof-of-concept pilot study. Behav Neurol 2017:8349242. https://doi.org/10.1155/2017/8349242

Plata-Bello J (2017) Chapter 1: The study of Action Observation Therapy in neurological diseases: a few technical considerations. In: Neurological physical therapy. Intech Publ., pp 1–12. https://doi.org/10.5772/67651

Prechtl HFR (1997) State of the art of a new functional assessment of the young nervous system. An early predictor of cerebral palsy. Early Hum Dev 50(1):1–11. https://doi.org/10.1016/S0378-3782(97)00088-1

Riquelme I, Montoya P (2010) Developmental changes in somatosensory processing in cerebral palsy and healthy individuals. Clin Neurophysiol 124(8):1314–1320. https://doi.org/10.1016/j.clinph.2010.03.010

Rizzolatti G, Fadiga L, Gallese V, Fogassi L (1996) Premotor cortex and the recognition of motor actions. Brain Res Cogn Brain Res 3(2):131–141. https://doi.org/10.1016/0926-6410(95)00038-0

Rodda J, Graham HK (2001) Classification of gait patterns in spastic hemiplegia and spastic diplegia: a basis for a management algorithm. Eur J Neurol [Case Reports Review] 8(Suppl 5):98–108. https://doi.org/10.1046/j.1468-1331.2001.00042.x

Rosenbaum PL, Walter SD, Hanna SE, Palisano RJ, Russell DJ, Raina P, Wood E, Bartlett DJ, Galuppi BE (2002) Prognosis for gross motor function in cerebral palsy: creation of motor development curves. JAMA 288(11):1357–1363. https://doi.org/10.1001/jama.288.11.1357

Sainburg RL, Maenza C, Winstein C, Good D (2016) Motor lateralization provides a foundation for predicting and treating non-paretic arm motor deficits in stroke. Adv Exp Med Biol 957:257–272. https://doi.org/10.1007/978-3-319-47313-0_14

Sakzewski L, Ziviani J, Boyd RN (2014) Efficacy of upper limb therapies for unilateral cerebral palsy: a meta-analysis. Pediatrics 133(1):e175–e204. https://doi.org/10.1542/peds.2013-0675

Schmidt RA (1975) A schema theory of discrete motor skill learning. Psychological Review, 82(4),225-260. https://doi.org/10.1037/h0076770

SCPE (Surveillance of Cerebral Palsy in Europe) (2000) A collaboration of cerebral palsy surveys and registers. Dev Med Child Neurol 42:816–824. https://doi.org/10.1017/S0012162200001511

Sgandurra G, Ferrari A, Cossu G, Guzzetta A, Biagi L, Tosetti L, Fogassi L, Cioni G (2011) Upper limb children action-observation training (UP-CAT): a randomised controlled trial in hemiplegic cerebral palsy. BMC Neurol 11:1–19. https://doi.org/10.1186/1471-2377-11-80

Sommerville JA, Decety J (2006) Weaving the fabric and social interaction: articulating developmental psychology and cognitive neuroscience in the domain of motor cognition. Psychon Bull Rev 13:179–200. https://doi.org/10.3758/bf03193831

Stanley FJ, Blair E, Alberman E (2000) Cerebral palsies: epidemiology and causal pathways. Mac Keith Press, London

Steenbergen B, Gordon AM (2006) Activity limitation in hemiplegic cerebral palsy: evidence for disorders in motor planning. Dev Med Child Neurol 48:780–783. https://doi.org/10.1017/S0012162206001666

Taub E (1980) Somatosensory deafferentation research with monkeys: implications for rehabilitation medicine. In: Ince LP (ed) Behavioral psychology in rehabilitation medicine: clinical applications. Williams & Wilkins, New York, pp 371–401

Taub E, Wolf SL (1997) Constraint induced movement techniques to facilitate upper extremity use in stroke patients. Top Stroke Rehabil 3:38–61. https://doi.org/10.1080/10749357.1997.11754128

Taub E, Ramey SL, De Luca S, Echols K (2004) Efficacy of constraint-induced movement therapy for children with cerebral palsy with asymmetric motor impairment. Pediatrics 113:305–312. https://doi.org/10.1542/peds.113.2.305

Taub E, Uswatte G, Mark VW, Morris DM (2006) The learned non use phenomenon: implications for rehabilitation. Eura Medicophys 42(3):241–256

Thelen E (1994) Three-month-old infants can learn task-specific patterns of interlimb coordination. Psychol Sci 5(5):280–285. https://doi.org/10.1111/j.1467-9280.1994.tb00626.x

Tomhave WA, Van Heest AE, Bagley A, James MA (2015) Affected and contralateral hand strength and dexterity measures in children with hemiplegic cerebral palsy. J Hand Surg Am 40(5):900–907. https://doi.org/10.1016/j.jhsa.2014.12.039

Williams J, Anderson V, Reid SM, Reddihough DS (2012) Motor imagery of the unaffected hand in children with spastic hemiplegia. Dev Neuropsychol 37(1):84–97. https://doi.org/10.1080/87565641.2011.560697

Wingert JR, Burton H, Sinclair RJ, Brunstrom JE, Damiano DL (2008) Tactile sensory abilities in cerebral palsy: deficits in roughness and object discrimination. Dev Med Child Neurol 50(11):832–838. https://doi.org/10.1111/j.1469-8749.2008.03105.x

Winters TF Jr, Gage JR, Hicks R (1987) Gait patterns in spastic hemiplegia in children and young adults. J Bone Joint Surg Am 69(3):437–441

Wolf SL, Lecraw DE, Barton LA, Jann BB (1989) Forced use of hemiplegic upper extremities to reverse the effect of learned non use among chronic stroke and head-injured patients. Exp Neurol 104(2):125–132. https://doi.org/10.1016/S0014-4886(89)80005-6

The Child with Dyskinesia

4

Liliana Zerbino and Psiche Giannoni

In 1871, Hammond first described dyskinesia, using the term athetosis (from the Greek for "without a fixed position"), as a condition "characterized by an inability to retain the fingers and toes in any position in which they may be placed, and by their continual motion".

The dyskinetic form constitutes about 15% of all CP cases (Himmelmann et al. 2005), and it presents as a motor disorder characterized by involuntary, uncontrolled, recurrent, occasionally stereotyped movements, with a predominance of primitive reflex patterns and fluctuation of the muscle tone (Cans 2000). The involuntary movements can increase in relation to the emotional states of the child, intolerance of specific tactile experiences, pain and digestive and constipation problems. The involuntary movements usually decrease during sleep.

The term dyskinesia is used when referring to both dystonia and choreoathetosis, which can sometimes be present simultaneously, as reported by many authors (Bobath 1977; Cans et al. 2007; Sun et al. 2018). Traditionally they have been included in a mixed group of CP. Choreoathetosis is a combination of choreic and athetoid movements, in which the chorea shows rapid, involuntary, jerky, often fragmented movements which usually begin to manifest proximally, while athetosis is comprised of movements that are slower, constantly changing, writhing or contorting and mostly distal.

Dystonia is characterized by sustained or intermittent muscle contractions, which lead to abnormal, often repetitive, movements and postural attitudes (Cans et al. 2007). Usually, children with dystonia have more functional problems than children with choreoathetosis (Sun et al. 2018), but both defects increase during activity and their presence interferes with and severely limits the child's functional abilities.

L. Zerbino
DSS, University of Florence, Florence, Italy

P. Giannoni (✉)
DIBRIS, University of Genoa, Genoa, Italy

P. Giannoni, L. Zerbino (eds.), *Cerebral Palsy*,
https://doi.org/10.1007/978-3-030-85619-9_4

Dystonia is mainly due to hypoxic/ischemic damage to the basal ganglia, thalamus and/or brainstem, occurring during the prenatal, perinatal or childhood period (Sanger et al. 2010), while athetoid movements are observed with a lesion of the thalamus and basal ganglia (Krageloh-Mann et al. 2002; Monbaliu et al. 2016). White matter damage in the brain can also cause spasticity (Krägeloh-Mann and Cans 2009; Himmelmann and Uvebrant 2011).

Dyskinesia usually involves the child's entire body, but, although it is rare, some athetoid or dystonic features may sometimes be noted in unilateral spastic CP or mixed ataxic-athetoid forms (Bobath 1966).

Additionally, babies with medulla oblongata damage may have difficulty in swallowing, which in turn can affect their nutrition and cause excessive drooling. Speech is usually hampered by dysarthria, due to the involvement of the phonatory muscles (Scrutton et al. 2004).

In contrast to the bilateral and unilateral spastic forms, epilepsy is rare in children with dyskinetic CP (Mesraoua et al. 2019).

The rehabilitation approach for children presenting the dyskinetic CP is distinct from the treatment for the bilateral spastic form because the types of motor impairment are completely different. The latter involves limited movement patterns and increase of muscle stiffness, while the athetoid and dystonic forms present the following features:

- Extremely variable muscle tone with continual fluctuations of stiffness
- Difficulty in the maintenance of body alignment
- Non-functional, disorganized movements
- Presence of primitive reflexes (ATNR, STNR, Galant, etc.)
- Difficulty in movement control and coordination
- Difficulty in the functions of the upper limbs on the midline (e.g. eye-hand-mouth incoordination)
- Righting reaction strategies from distal to proximal (Ferrari and Cioni 2010)
- Perceptual disorders

The athetosis usually involves every body segment, and, as said before, athetoid or dystonic hemiparesis and the mixed ataxic-athetoid forms are rare.

4.1 Natural Clinical Development of the Dyskinetic Form

In the beginning, the baby and young infant with a suspected diagnosis of CP sometimes present with severe hypotonia, and some authors refer to them as a "floppy child", unable to react to gravity (Dubowitz 1969; Bobath and Bobath 1975). Milani Comparetti (1978) describes the child as "puppet-like", with an absence or lack of postural and motor patterns. At first, this form is not distinctive from the initial state of the other types of CP, but later it usually evolves in the typical dyskinetic or ataxic form.

As the child becomes more active and responsive to the environmental experiences, there is gradual activation of motor activity, characterized by the presence of involuntary movements. The child starts to move, first with small fluctuating and redundant movements at the proximal and/or distal joints that make it difficult to acquire functional skills. The coexistence of dystonia is an additional problem for this child.

The presence of these numerous involuntary movements makes it difficult for the child to perceive the characteristics of the environment and understand their relationship with it. The child can have perceptual problems, as when situations of being moved evoke fear and/or hyper-alertness, like being picked up from their cot or moving in a stroller or a caregiver's arms. While moving, this child is generally overwhelmed by visual, tactile, proprioceptive, vestibular, auditory, olfactory and emotional stimuli which they are unable to filter nor maintain within a reasonable threshold of perceptual tolerance.

4.1.1 The Child with Hypotonia

During their first year of life, this child is quiet, generally sleeps more, does not cry vigorously and has poor social interactive abilities and scarce antigravity head and trunk control. Many parents refer that they have difficulty containing their baby gently and safely in their arms. Indeed, embracing these children can be difficult, and they need help to adapt to new positions. The affective tonic-body attunement of the triadic baby-parent relationship will need special attention. The Brazelton behavioural observation model can be a useful tool for building baby and parent attachment (Brazelton and Nugent 2011). Parents need guidance to experience cuddliness and other basic interactions to build the baby-parent attachment.

The hypotonic phase is transient and of variable and unclear duration. Usually, a child who develops the athetosis form starts to modify their motor behaviour around the age of 18–24 months, when they attempt to move actively, and therefore the first athetoid and/or dystonic movements appear. Frequently, the longer the hypotonic phase, the more severe the motor and cognitive impairment.

It is essential to make a differential diagnosis during the first year of life, as hypotonia can be the clinical expression not only of CP but also of other important pathologies, which include metabolic, genetic neuromuscular disorders and particular syndromes (Peredo and Hannibal 2009). A prompt diagnosis is not always easy and requires numerous clinical and instrumental examinations and hospitalizations, which negatively affect the child's development and the already fragile equilibrium within the family.

4.1.1.1 Supine

The child is usually quite immobile and shows a "frog-like" posture (Fig. 4.1) with the lower limbs in flexion, abduction and externally rotated, with feet in inversion.

The tactile pressure is mainly on the same areas of the body, as the baby is not able to change their position, so all sensory information comes to them from the back of their body.

The control of the head is extremely poor, and it often lies rotated towards one side which becomes the preferential one. This posture can lead to future malalignment problems of the spine. A weak asymmetrical tonic neck reflex (ATNR) can be

Fig. 4.1 Child in a
"frog-like" posture in
the legs

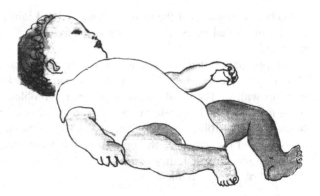

observed, sometimes associated with weak grasping at the hand and ipsilateral Galant reaction. Kicking in the lower limbs is not present, but there are some weak, rarely simultaneous flexion movements on both sides. The hypotonia causes the joints to be hypermobile, and excessive ankle dorsiflexion is sometimes noticed where the toes even touch the shin.

The child has abdominal breathing with a superficial, short paradoxical breathing pattern. The lateral diameter of the ribcage is wider than the anterior, excessively opened and flattened; the intercostal spaces are dilated due to hypotonia (Seddon and Khan 2003).

Eye contact with the caregiver is affected by the postural stillness of the child and from visual incoordination like the erratic gaze or hyper-fixation. The primary relationship between parent and child is early altered by the passive attitude of the baby, which makes any interpersonal sharing difficult. Also, hypotonia associated with joint hypermobility usually worries the parents as they fear they can hurt their baby during everyday caring.

4.1.1.2 Prone

The child does not like this position as they cannot move the head to clear their airways, as every newborn does automatically, and they do not attempt to raise the head (Fig. 4.2). Moreover, the weight of the body is too heavy for this floppy child. The posture is the same frog-like as in supine, and this time the sensorial inputs constantly come from the anterior part of the body. The upper limbs are in flexion and abduction, and the hands can be opened and rest on the surface, without any explorative contact with the environment.

> **The skin of the child**
> The connective tissue is a very important access point in the interaction between the child and the environment. When it is altered, the reception, processing and integration of the stimuli are compromised (see Chap. 7). The hypotonic child's skin is diaphanous, thin and fragile, often excessively

sweaty or cold, which are symptoms of neurovegetative disorders. For this reason, this child has a very low tolerability threshold to tactile stimuli that requires close attention from caregivers during daily care. Due to such perceptual disturbance, the child could feel clothes as their "second skin", promoting them as their natural borders with the environment, and, for this reason, when undressed, they may show discomfort and distress and weakly cry.

The nutrition of the child

Nutritive and non-nutritive sucking can be difficult in infant with hypotonia because of the extreme muscle weakness around their mouth, and it is not possible to evoke the sucking and rooting reflexes. The mouth is usually half-open, causing drooling, also when the baby will be put in a sitting position. For the same reason as not closing the lips, swallowing will be impaired: lips and tongue have weak functional movements, and the food remains inside the mouth for long. Sometimes, severe aspiration pneumonia is detected and hospitalization is needed. When small children with hypotonia have significant eating, drinking and swallowing difficulties, gastrostomy is used. This is a form of enteral feeding where food is delivered directly into the stomach and ensures the necessary amount of food and drink. Consequently, lunch and dinner time often becomes a reason for anxiety and worrying, instead of happiness and satisfaction, and parents will prefer postures that are more effective from their point of view for feeding, but highly inadequate and dangerous. In this case, it is crucial to get in touch with a speech therapist specialized in dysphagia, for proper suggestions about an appropriate positioning (see Chap. 10).

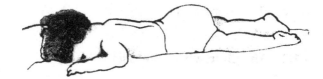

Fig. 4.2 Child lying in a prone position

4.1.1.3 Infant in the Adult's Arms

The muscle weakness does not allow the natural postural adjustment between child and mother in a mutual tonic dialog (de Ajuriaguerra 1970). Parents try to find strategies to contain the child, but having difficulty respecting their fragility, when instead the approach should be gentle and without sudden movements. The child should be lifted slowly and should have the opportunity to catch the adult's gaze and predict what will happen around them (Fig. 4.3).

Fig. 4.3 Child with
hypotonia in parent's arms

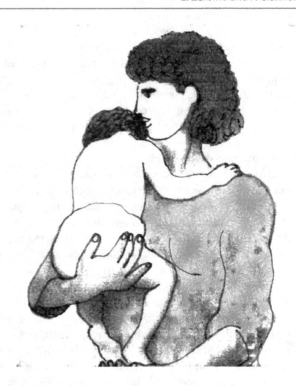

4.1.1.4 Sitting

When the child is transferred from the lying position to sitting, the head control is lacking in the intermediate positions. When seated, the head often falls backwards or forwards, where it will worsen the child's flexed posture (Fig. 4.4). When the child is not adequately supported in sitting, the body can fall in all directions, and therefore it is crucial to consider a good postural system, to guarantee the alignment of the various segments of the body.

4.1.2   The Child with Athetosis

4.1.2.1 Child's First Movements

Due to their poor movement experience and interaction with the environment, the child with hypotonia cannot use feedforward strategies. The child who will develop athetosis could occasionally produce some involuntary movement with intermittent spasms, which the caregiver can interpret as a sign of discomfort or an initial attempt to change position. They pass a lot of time in the supine position, and when they are lying on their back, they can begin to experiment with some basic movements. In this situation one of the easiest movements for them is bridging, propping up only on the upper body and heels, giving them satisfaction because they can begin to explore the floor around.

Advantages of moving in supine
- Initiative to move, increasing motivation
- New sensorial and perceptual experiences
- Satisfaction for the family

Disadvantages of moving in supine
- Strengthening of the extension synergy and misalignment
- Increased stiffness at neck and shoulder girdle
- Opening of the mouth with the involvement of the lower jaw, with possible future dislocations
- Drooling
- Severe difficulty in the acquisition of eye-hand-mouth coordination

4.1.2.2 Side Lying

From the supine position, the child reaches the side lying using a simplified strategy as half-rolling, which exploits the global flexion of the lower limbs (Fig. 4.5). However, they are not able to reach the prone position by themselves, due to the

Fig. 4.4 Child with poor antigravity reactions

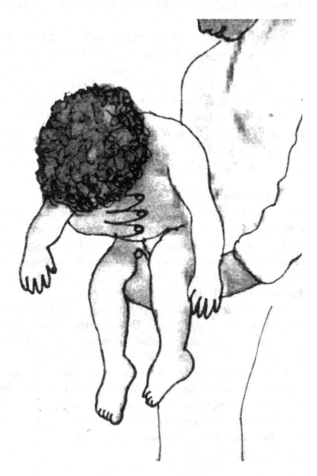

Fig. 4.5 Transfer "en bloc" to sideway

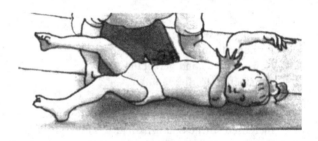

Fig. 4.6 Hip flexion shift weight-bearing on the upper body

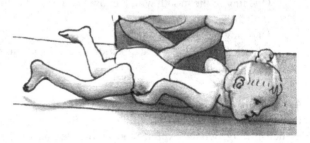

difficulty to gradually realign their body segments and upright the upper part of their body.

In side lying, the child can engage with the objects exploiting the ATNR. They reach the toy extending their arm, experiencing a first distal contact without using the visual cues. They could even learn to selectively use their feet to gain further sensorial information and perform more complex functions. Then, the child will learn to roll from supine to the prone position, moving first their less impaired side, with the pelvis and flexed lower limbs moving first to counteract the extension of the shoulder girdle and neck. With the effort, involuntary contractions of the muscles of the face and oral cavity can be appreciated, such as grimaces, tongue protrusion, lip-smacking, puckering and pursing.

4.1.2.3 Prone

In this position, more tonic activity in flexion at the pelvis girdle level emerges, which reduces weight-bearing on the lower limbs and shifts it to the upper parts of the body (Fig. 4.6). The child finds themself in a very uncomfortable situation: the organization of moving forwards in creeping is difficult, unless they learn to use some intermittent tonic contractions, one against the other, both in flexion and in extension (Bobath and Bobath 1975).

Being mainly in horizontal positions, the child begins to move often in a chaotic way, without any specific goal. The important emotional component and the excitement for environmental experiences, which the child is unable to filter, can cause abnormal movements, especially in the face and limbs.

Excessive movements and various fluctuations in tonic recruitment become a predominant means that the child uses to express their emotions and to communicate with the environment. Everyday caregivers realize this and come to understand the moods and needs of the child. This can foster a privileged relationship mainly with these caregivers, who will need to help external people understand what the child is communicating.

4.1.2.4 Sitting

From the prone position, always with tonic contractions at the level of the pelvic girdle, the child first learns to flex the lower limbs and then, with the support of an elbow, straightens and sits between their heels. Some children even use the forehead as a support point for this transfer. The new wide base of support between the heels gives the stability necessary to maintain the position and use the upper limbs for some functional activities.

The child can choose to sit like this, with their hands in a fisted position on the surface to reduce excessive oscillation of the upper body or with the upper limbs in open kinetic chain for some functional use, often taking advantage of the ATNR.

In this position, the child can also learn to "bunny hop" around on the floor with skill. This motor strategy becomes so efficient and satisfying that the child often adopts it for a long time and is not be motivated to walk.

Advantages of sitting between the heels
- First functional antigravity position
- Moving around independently (bunny hop) and exploring the surroundings
- Visual exploration of the environment
- Better functional use of the upper limbs

Disadvantages of sitting between the heels
- Increase of the dyskinetic movements, worsening the internal rotation/adduction of the femurs, to stabilize the posture
- Difficulty in choosing alternative strategies
- Excessive physical effort, frustration and helplessness in case of failures
- Risk for dislocation of the hip joints
- Possible pain

The child rarely sits with the lower limbs in extension because it is a very uncomfortable situation for them, as the centre of gravity (CoG) is too far behind the support base due to the extension of the upper body (Fig. 4.7). Children with less stiffness may instead maintain the position in long sitting with hip flexion and abducted lower limbs, to widen the support base and feel more stable (Fig. 4.8). Even though the head and upper limbs are not in the midline, which negatively affects hand-eye coordination, manipulation and visual functions, athetoid children are very resourceful and imaginative, and their unusual strategies for moving while sitting on the floor can be amazing.

Disadvantages of long sitting
- Further consolidation of the abnormal posture
- Lack of bimanual activities
- Difficulty in eye-hand coordination, particularly on midline.

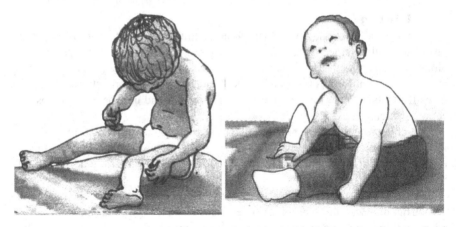

Figs. 4.7 and 4.8 Different strategies for long sitting

Because of the alternating movements from excessive flexion to extension, it is difficult for a very compromised child to sit safely in a chair, but a more experienced child may use more efficient strategies by stabilize on the chair with one lower limb or the backrest with one arm (using the ATNR), while the other arm approaches an object and explores it.

Advantages of sitting on a chair
– Better participation in social life
– Improvement of visual strategies in an upright position
Disadvantages of sitting on a chair
– Increase of postural misalignment
– Increase of involuntary movements to stabilize the posture
– Difficulty in manipulation and functional use of upper limbs, engaged for safety

4.1.2.5 Standing

The strategies to stand up from the floor are variable and extremely personalized. Each child moves from a synergy to another through sudden fluctuations of the muscle tone.

For the dyskinetic child, it is difficult to maintain a stable standing position, because the centre of mass (CoM) is higher than in the other positions and there is more body sway. Having to solve so many instability problems, these children usually achieve the autonomous standing position late in the preadolescent or adolescent period.

The child uses several strategies to stabilize the different parts of their body so they have to control fewer movement variables. Examples:

- "Freezing" the pelvic girdle and the joints of lower limbs, thus reducing their motion and allowing a better movement of the upper body
- Abduction of the lower limbs to create a wider base of support and better control the shifting of the CoM

- Stabilization of the head by hyperextending the cervical spine and protruding the chin to counterbalance the global attitude of extension and ensure moderate visual control
- Stretching and abduction of the arms to stabilize the body by increasing the momentum of inertia or stretching the upper limbs forwards, with elbow extension and clasped hands, to explore the anterior space

Despite these strategies, the standing position continues to be unstable, due to the presence of involuntary movements, particularly at the head, and it requires continual control to keep the CoM inside the base of support. To overcome these problems, the child often keeps the pelvis forwards, with the hip joints at the limit of their maximum range in abduction-extension and extension at the knees to control the postural oscillation.

4.1.2.6 Walking

Children who have a higher degree of stiffness have a better chance of achieving the function of walking because the stiffness is used for stability. However, the gait pattern remains uncertain, asymmetrical, arrhythmic and with excessive flexion-extension movements of the lower limbs. There is zigzag, not linear, progression forwards, with no rotation between the two girdles.

To facilitate the task of walking and to simplify the control of the multi-joint movements of the lower limbs, the child uses the strategy of keeping the most of joints up to the physiological limit (see the "Barrier" Concept, in Chap. 7) or working hard to co-contract the antagonist muscle groups, through continual adjustments.

Sometimes, other unusual strategies are noted for overcoming functional difficulties, such as walking quickly or keeping the upper limbs stabilized by the sleeves of their sweater or throwing a quick glance at a reference point somewhere in space and then advancing towards it even when the eyes are no longer on the target because of the involuntary movements of the head.

For all these reasons, the athetoid child finds it easier to move in a closed environment, with few variables, or in a known, controlled and foreseeable space.

Associated Problems

    Cognitive

        The cognitive level of children with dyskinetic CP varies, depending on the different motor features: the more severe the impairment, the greater the cognitive problems (La Porta-Oyos et al. 2019).

    Social relationships

        The child is usually on good terms with the adult and cooperates with those they trust. One can notice curiosity and stubbornness, as well as behaviours of helplessness, anger and frustration towards the outside world. The child struggles to manage their own emotions and often needs some kind of mediation from the caregiver in case of situational changes.

Communication

Difficulties in the facial and oral motor control (mimicry with presence of grimaces, excessive opening of the mouth, tongue protrusion, drooling) and in gesturing with the upper limbs (presence of ATNR, distal involuntary movements, impossibility to differentiate finger movements). Verbal language can appear very late and have dysarthric and dysphonic characteristics. The child usually speaks very slowly, with no modulation, sometimes with explosive sounds and without consonants, because of being produced during the inspiration phase. Communication is often so slow and strenuous that the person listening is tempted to interrupt and interpret the content of the communication.

Sensory disorders

The child with dyskinesia caused by kernicterus can often present neurosensorial deafness (Weir et al. 2018).

Perceptual disorders

The athetoid child has many perceptual problems. They easily feel overwhelmed by the environmental stimuli that they cannot manage them all and they find it hard to concentrate on a single one and shut out the background noise. It is difficult for them to use multimodal strategies, such as observing and touching at the same time. To approach an interesting target and explore it visually, the child excludes the foveal vision and stresses the peripheral one. When they touch or look at an object, avoiding reactions appear, characterized by an avoiding gaze and/or pulling the hand/foot back from the stimulus (Twitchell 1961; Bobath and Bobath 1975).

Visual impairments

The child with dyskinesia is constantly struggling with involuntary movements in their eyes, trunk and limbs. Since eye movements depend on those of the head, visual coordination, scanning ability, visual pursuit and focus are not easy for them (Jan et al. 2001). As written before, the child prefers to use the peripheral rather than foveal vision and adopt a glance strategy. Moreover, they use the "squeeze gaze strategy" to maintain the focus on a moving target (see Chap. 11). Eye-hand-mouth coordination is difficult due to body misalignment. For all these reasons, early ocular, visual, oculomotor and visuoperceptual evaluation is very important and recommended.

Seizures

Dyskinetic children with basal ganglia lesions are very unlikely to have seizures unless they also have a cortical lesion. On the other hand, seizures can occur in full-term infants, who have had acute hypoxia or anoxia. In this case, the lesion is also present in the rolandic areas which are highly epileptogenic (Sellier et al. 2012). Initially, it can be very difficult for caregivers to differentiate seizures from the involuntary movements that the child with CP dyskinesia presents.

4.1.2.7 Evaluation Scales

To assess dystonia and/or choreo-athetosis, many scales are proposed. Some of them are listed below, from the earlier to the more recent (Stewart et al. 2017).

Scales to measure dystonia and choreoathetosis in children with dyskinetic CP are the following:

- Burke-Fahn-Marsden Dystonia Rating Scale (BFMDRS) (Burke et al. 1985)
- Barry-Albright Dystonia Scale (BADS) (Barry et al 1999)
- Unified Dystonia Rating Scale (UDRS) (Comella et al. 2003)
- Movement Disorder-Childhood Rating Scale (MD-CRS 4–18) (Battini et al. 2008)
- Movement Disorder-Childhood Rating Scale 0–3 Years (MD-CRS 0–3) (Battini et al. 2009)
- Dyskinesia Impairment Scale (DIS) (Monbaliu et al. 2012)

4.2 Practical Suggestions for the Child with Hypotonia

The management and treatment of the small child with hypotonia should be focused on improving the antigravity control and the tolerance to sensory information.

Different aims of intervention of the therapist:
- *For the child (autonomy and quality of life)*
  - Improve autonomic control
  - Support respiratory function
  - Increase the perceptual tolerance to stimuli
  - Facilitate adaptations for postural transfers
  - Promote feeding abilities (mouth closure, swallowing, tolerance of different food textures, tastes, etc.)
- *For the parents and caregivers (child management)*
  - Offer counselling for the everyday management of the child (hygiene, dressing, postural transfers, etc.)
  - Share holding modalities that make the baby feel safe
  - Assess and provide personalized postural and positioning aids, such as customized postural systems, elastic bands, elastic close-fitting suits, baby nursing pillows, etc.
  - Educate on early communication facilitations (parent's gaze, voice, smile, proprioceptive tactile contact, etc.)
- *For the treatment session*
  - Improve perceptual tolerance of selected sensorial inputs (touch, sight, proprioception, etc.)
  - Increase muscle stiffness by recruitment of motor units
  - Introduce prompt gradual antigravity experiences
  - Improve oro-motor control as support to feeding
  - Identify useful aids and orthoses for postural containment

4.2.1 Infant in the Parent's Arms

The baby with hypotonia will have many benefits by being held by the parents:

- Sensation of safe perceptual containment
- Opportunities to experience and learn to adapt to the first natural environment of the hands and bodies of mother and father
- Maturation of perceptual knowledge and interactive abilities through the intimate, tactile and proprioceptive relationships with both parents
- Facilitation by the parents of eye-to-eye contact and exchanges using all the early communication modalities (like smiles, cuddles, cradling, cooing, chatting, singing and imitating each other)

Suggestion
- Discover with the parents, the best modalities to hold and support the infant appropriately in different positions:
- *Examples:*
  - *The child is held with one side in contact with their parent, supported in slight flexion of the shoulder girdle* (Fig. 4.9), *upper limbs towards midline and lower limbs flexed. In the first month of life, the distance at which the newborn can focus is about 25–30 cm. (the distance from the breast to mother's face), so it favours eye-to-eye contact and facial exploration immediately after birth and social smiling at around 2 months of age.*

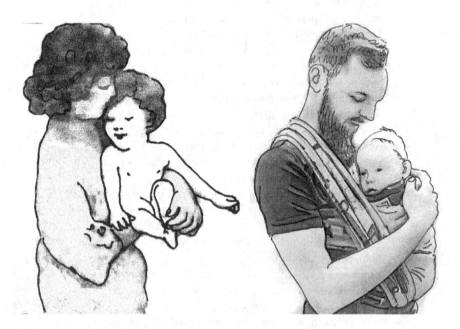

Figs. 4.9 and 4.10 Different modalities to carry the baby

- *Later on the infant is held directly facing the parent, who supports them safely with one arm around their shoulders, while the other arm stabilising the pelvis.*
- *When the infant is older, they can be held in the parent's arms, facing outwards: one arm transversely supports the upper trunk of the child under their arms, while the other holds the pelvic area with the lower limbs aligned. In this position the infant can begin to explore the surroundings.*
- *In the first months, caregivers can use a baby pouch or sling* (Fig. 4.10). *The baby is in a safe space with boundaries and experiences the body contact and the vertical posture. This can be comfortable for the adult as well, as the baby cannot fall, the parent's hands are free, they can make eye contact with the baby, the mother can breastfeed them,* etc.

4.2.2   Supine

As the floppy child is often inactive, they spend some of the time supine, are not able to change position and receive limited perceptual inputs. During a treatment session, the therapist can propose some different postural experiences, and, as the child adapts to the new inputs, they can work on facilitating some first antigravity midline control of the head and upper trunk.

Suggestion
- Propose perceptual experiences in supine position:
  1. *Align the different parts of the body: the head should be straight on the midline, and the muscles of the posterior chain should be elongated.*
  2. *See if a U-shaped pillow (with noiseless padding) could be useful to maintain the infant in a well-aligned position or otherwise a wedge which supports both head and trunk.*
  3. *Slightly flex the child's shoulders and bring their hands onto the midline* (Fig. 4.11), *in contact with each other touching their body (preliminary body schema experiences). Extend and align the lower limbs, or flex them and put their feet on the surface, to have some first foot contact input.*
  4. *Use tapping facilitation to activate some muscle recruitment, from distal to proximal in some specific segments of the body, which the child is not yet able to control against gravity (e.g. upper or lower limbs).*
  5. *Facilitate eye-to-eye contact with the infant and promote fixation, focalization and smooth tracking to look at their own hands or a favourite toy.*
  6. *Use simple infant positioning equipment for the child during the day, for example, semi-inclined baby chair or stroller (semi-supine position) with lateral trunk supports or U-cushion.*

Note
- The therapist's hands should always touch the infant in a way to convey precise, definite and pleasurable sensations, considering that light and uncertain tactile stimulation gives unclear information.

Fig. 4.11 Child with their hands in midline

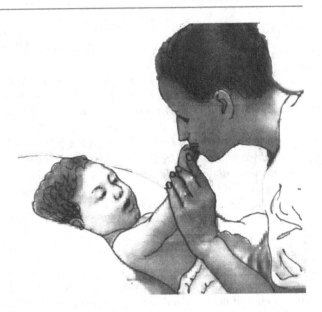

- The positive touch experience of infant massage (McClure 2017) would be extremely beneficial to increase the child's tolerance to tactile-perceptive stimuli and their knowledge of their physical boundaries.
- Dressing and undressing time is also an important opportunity for the infant to have pleasant and reassuring containment, though early neurovegetative instability can while sometimes being naked can distress the baby, who may show discomfort by crying faintly.

Tapping and Manual Pressure Techniques

Tapping is a specific manual proprioceptive facilitation, developed by Margaret Rood (1954, 1956) to enhance muscle activity. Although being disregarded in recent years, this technique remains useful in certain situations (Bordoloi and Deka 2018).

According to Rood, tapping stimulation applied on the belly of a muscle activates its spindles as a stretch excites the alpha motor neurons at the spinal level.

Tapping has been applied by Berta Bobath in the treatment of CP children with hypotonia, e.g. in a floppy or ataxic child, to recruit more muscular activity (Bobath 1977).

The therapist should be always aware that this technique is applied to children with CP only to enhance muscle activity where low muscle tone is present and never where the amount of stiffness is within normal levels or even higher.

Pressure and joint compression are two other different techniques, the latter often called "push-pull". A pressure/compression input applied through the long axis of the bones at one or more joints involved simultaneously in a motor function facilitates the co-activation of the muscle contractions and the enhancement of antigravity postural stability.

As the joint compression technique facilitates motor control when jerky movements are present, it is successfully applied in cases of dyskinesia.

The therapist should use all these facilitation techniques very carefully, not only verifying their effect in real time but also anticipating what the child's reaction might be and what muscle recruitment can occur based on the amount of sensory input received. The therapist should always attune their manual facilitations to the single situations and, as with all therapy, apply them only when and as needed, and verify that they provide the desired effects. When used in CP, any unwanted and/or excessive increase in stiffness is to be avoided.

4.2.3 From Supine to Sitting

The transfer from supine to the sitting position has the objective of accustoming the child to participate in a sequence that involves many parts of their body and happens many times in a daily routine, e.g. getting up from bed.

Suggestion
- Prepare the first antigravity activity reactions in supine position:
  1. *Put the baby on a U-shaped pillow or wedge, and stand in front of them, and then place gently one hand on the child's sternum, to give them a perceptual reference point; follow their breathing rhythm, emphasizing the exhaling phase and maintaining visual contact with the child.*
  2. *Slightly externally rotate the humeri in the glenoid joints, and then bring the child's upper limbs forwards to the midline.*
  3. *Make eye contact with the child, and stimulate them to gradually raise their head, facilitating with vocal input, gentle tractions, etc.*
  4. *Slowly guide the transfer (Fig. 4.12), to foster head control and giving the child time to appreciate the new perceptual information. Be careful when facilitating the return back to supine too.*

4.2.4 Prone

Knowing that this small child will not feel comfortable in this position, the therapist should work gradually here and find ways to make it more acceptable like lying prone on the parent's body (Pumerantz and Zachry 2018).

Thanks to this position, the child begins feeling some weight-bearing on the upper limbs with hands opened and on the extended hips, and they can start organizing their first antigravity postural reactions. This position favours the emergence of head control, fundamental for basic functions as visual control of the environment, feeding, eye-hand function, etc.

Fig. 4.12 Transfer from
supine to sitting

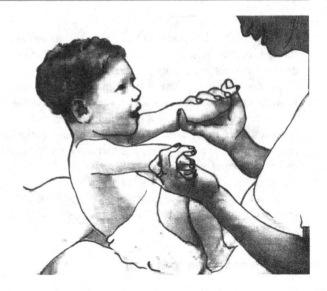

Suggestion

- Provide a proper alignment:
  1. *Lay the child prone on a wedge, and place two draft-stopper rolls along each side; the height of the wedge should allow the hands and/or the forearms to be in contact with the base support.*
  2. *Align all parts of the body, paying attention to the lower limbs, which should be well-positioned and not in the typical hypotonic posture. Their feet should be off the edge of the surface.*
- Evoke the first active antigravity reactions:
  1. *Search for the first antigravity extension reactions at the head and shoulder girdle: the child should support on their forearms and open hands. In case the task of raising the head is too difficult and the head remains on the child's hands, let them first adapt to this new position and have a hand-mouth contact experience. After that, use the gentle tapping technique, and work specifically on that first lifting of the head from the support and rotating the head side to side.*
  2. *Once head lifting against gravity is gained in the semi-inclined prone position, advance to facilitating head control in slightly different situations, e.g. lying flat without the wedge.*
  3. *Afterwards, try to get the baby to rest their face on their open hands; this task not only reduces the base of support but requires bending of the elbows and supports the head weight on the hands.*
  4. *Use the tapping and pressure techniques to increase the muscle contraction activity in the neck and shoulders: place one hand on the child's head, while holding their wrists together with the other hand. Gently press repeatedly towards the linear direction head → elbows, looking for some active antigravity reaction at the upper body. In this position, the child can receive a lot of sensorial information (load, pressure, etc.).*

5. *Reinforce the antigravity extension of the head by involving visual contact: e.g. have a caregiver face-to-face in front of the child or attract the child's attention with an interesting toy, to evoke the visual coupling and, therefore, the maintenance of the antigravity head position.*

- Prepare the child to deal with other postural changes:

  1. *Position the small child in prone on a small roll or wedge, where they can support on forearms and open hands.*
  2. *Facilitate weight-bearing on their upper limbs and head uprighting by applying:*
     - *Gentle pressure and/or joint compression techniques, acting along the humerus axis, from shoulder girdle to forearms*
     - *Manual trunk stability by supporting the child with one hand in front of the sternum and the other at the thoraco-lumbar level and applying pressure by tapping*
  3. *Induce minimal weight shifts from side to side, enhancing the perception of the weight support rather than focusing on the motion itself.*
  4. *Transfer the weight onto one forearm, and guide the other to move forwards to touch an object in front: first work for the stability of the muscles around the shoulder girdle, and then facilitate the extension of the upper limb for a reaching task, engaging the activity of the* brachial triceps (see also Sect. 7.2.1.2. of Chap. 7).
  5. *Let the infant experience some changes of positions: half side lying, side lying, supine and return; if possible, move them towards the sitting position.*

Note

- The baby can also be kept lying on the therapist's lap and with the parent in front, in such a way as to favour some head control and the relationship with their parent at the same time.

4.2.5 Supported Sitting

The infant might be too hypotonic to react to the antigravity forces in the sitting position. It is important that the caregiver let the child perceive the inputs coming from this new position and that they catch every little reaction coming from them.

When the infant is in supported sitting, the following functions can be improved:

- Head control
- Visual function
- Antigravity uprighting of the trunk
- Weight-bearing perception on the pelvis
- Tactile and proprioceptive awareness of the lower limbs
- Foot support on the surface

Suggestion
- Propose the sitting experiences in therapy on your lap:
  1. *Ask the parent or caregiver to sit in front of the infant.*
  2. *In this position your body is in contact with the infant's back, supporting them firmly to convey security and tactile-proprioceptive inputs, and facilitate anti-gravity muscle activity.*
  3. *Verify that the trunk is aligned and uprighted.*
  4. *If the infant has difficulty maintaining trunk righting reaction, apply gentle compression techniques downwards from the top of the head through the spine to recruit more extensor muscle activity, checking that the trunk remains properly aligned* (Fig. 4.13).
- Use tapping techniques on other segments of the body:
  Examples:
  - *Tap the shoulder girdle with gentle pressure along the spinal axis; check that the trunk is well extended and the pelvis is tilted forwards.*
  - *Hold the child's hands together* (Fig. 4.14), *and tap from distal to proximal, occasionally varying the degree of shoulder anterior flexion* (Fig. 4.15).
  - ....
- Core stability: prepare the trunk to interact with gravity:
  1. *Move slightly away from the back of the child's body, and observe if they can maintain some active trunk extension with the help of a visual facilitation, like looking at a parent or an interesting toy.*
  2. *If the child has difficulty maintaining the upright position, give some tactile-proprioceptive inputs with one hand across the front of their rib cage and the other giving pressure at the thoracic-lumbar level to induce the anterior tilting of the pelvis.*
- Verify trunk extension in different postural settings:
  Examples:

Fig. 4.13 Compression technique from top of the head

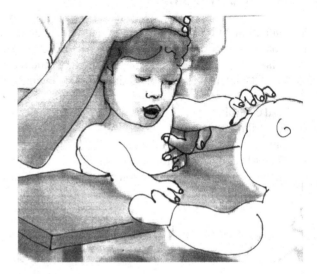

Fig. 4.14 Child's
wrist hold

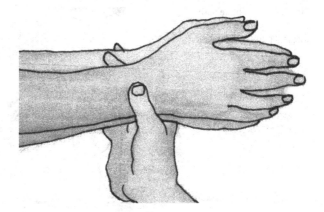

Fig. 4.15 Tapping
techniques through the
arms from distal to
proximal

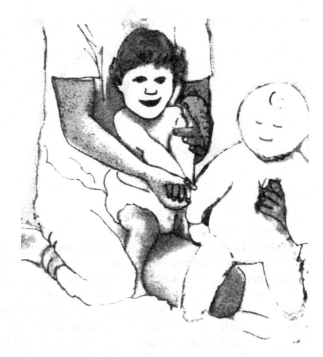

- *Sit the child on a treatment table and sit in front of them; the table should be high enough for them to rest their feet on your lap; facilitate active antigravity uprighting in extension by giving manual stability at the lower trunk, which will increase weight-bearing on their thighs and feet.*
- *Sit the child with their legs astride on your lap, in front of a recessed table on which they can rest their forearms, and open hands facilitate the perception of the weight-bearing on the upper limbs, by using tapping techniques from proximal to distal.*
- *Sit the child on a small bench, and verify that their feet rest on the floor and hips not excessively abducted; stay in front of or behind them, and elicit some active upper limb movements (Fig. 4.16).*

Fig. 4.16 Facilitate active
upper limb movements
through playing activities

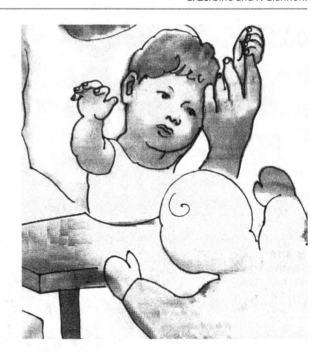

Fig. 4.16 Facilitate active upper limb movements through playing activities

_ ....

4.2.6 Standing

The standing position with the higher CoM will be particularly demanding for this small child. They could be in the transition phase from hypotonia to the emergence of involuntary movements, finding themself having to manage not only the motor components of their impairment but also perceptive problems with the environment.

The child may not yet be able to maintain the new anti-gravity position and therefore benefit from leg braces to increase their stability. There are excellent orthoses available, but temporary knee splints made of rigid cardboard could be useful. For the same goal, a neoprene band wrapped around the abdominal muscles could prove helpful in improving core stability. In recent years, commercially available Lycra garments are being used for dyskinetic children for similar purposes.

Suggestion
- Putting the child in the erect position using lower limb braces:
  1. *Apply suitable braces in supine.*
  2. *The transfer from supine to standing cannot be active, so first rotate the child to the side lying position, and then hold both the shoulder girdle and the lower limbs to put them into standing. This transfer has to be carried out carefully and gradually.*
  3. *Sit behind them, and keep close to the child's body, to convey the perception of having a boundary and being safe despite the surrounding "empty" space.*

Fig. 4.17 Pressure
tapping from the head

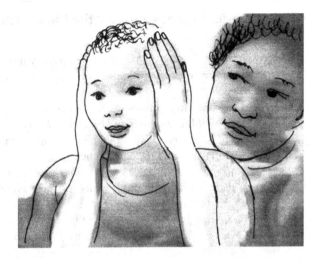

4. *If necessary, fill the "void" with objects such as tables, chairs, benches,* etc.
- Working from behind to obtain the postural reactions in standing:
  1. *Verify the adequate alignment of the child's body, and, from behind, apply gentle tapping facilitation along the longitudinal axis of the body, to get an active uprighing reaction.*

     Examples of tapping in different parts of the body:
     - *Pressure tapping from the head: place hands on the child's temples, first passing under their armpits, taking care not to overcompress the ears* (Fig. 4.17).
     - *Pressure tapping from the shoulder girdle: use when the child already has some head control.*
     - *Pressure tapping at the trunk (use when the child has developed some trunk control): first separate from child's body, and position your hands on the youngster's trunk area, and then start tapping in a centripetal way to improve the stability of the core.*
     - ....

Note
- To help the child become accustomed to the standing position, they can be temporarily placed—for example, at home—on a prone-standing table, with the inclination personalized to their individual needs. This situation is quite constrained and passive for the child, but, taking advantage of the postural alignment, the therapist can intervene emphasizing the contact of the forearms and hands on the surface of the anterior recessed table and introduce activities with the upper limbs. These proposals facilitate some active uprighting reactions enhancing head control and the activation of the posterior muscle chain. This passive type of standing should be suspended as soon as the child improves their core stability and starts supporting weight on their lower limbs.

4.3   Practical Suggestions for the Child with Athetosis

It is important to help the child control involuntary movements and filter sensory inputs from the environment, so that to increase their repertoire of functional skills.

Different aims of intervention of the therapist:

- *For the child (autonomy and quality of life)*
  - Increase the perceptual tolerance to inputs, in order to improve the relationship with the environment
  - Improve emotional self-regulation, so that it does not excessively affect the quality of movements and the possibility to communicate
  - Promote functional transfer modalities
  - Train independent activities of the daily life, introducing aids, which have been assessed by the therapist together with the child and/or the caregivers
- *For the parents and caregivers (child management)*
  - Identify communication modalities, e.g. gaze, gestures, vocal expressions, communication aids, such as AAC, etc. (see Chap. 12)
  - Share suggestions to help the child carry out simple activities of daily living, such as washing hands, hold a glass, dressing and undressing, etc.
  - Educate regarding appropriate handling, during everyday care, to avoid overstimulate the child with many sensory inputs (e.g. excessive tactile inputs, sudden postural changes, loud noise, etc.)
  - Educate parents and caregivers in the application, and use aids and orthoses to maintain adequate postural alignment of the child during transfers
  - Help them recognize the child's needs, including their need to have rest periods
- *For the treatment session*
  - Promote postural control, containing the fluctuations of muscular tonic activity
  - Install the habit that the child seeks better postural alignment, to feel more stable
  - Introduce appropriately timed upright positions, knowing that early weight-bearing facilitates the recruitment of muscular activity and improves stability
  - Improve breathing and oro-motor control (see also Chap. 10)
  - Improve perceptual control and filtering of environmental inputs to improve the child's decoding abilities
  - Facilitate eye-hand-mouth coordination, to promote functions such as manipulation, self-feeding, writing, use of hand devices, etc.
  - Evaluate equipment and assistive devices, such as postural systems, transfer aids, communication aids, etc. (see Chap. 13)

4.3.1 Supine

This child may have a history of prolonged hypotonia or already exhibit fluctuations in muscle activity or even high stiffness, if athetosis is associated with dystonia.

The child with athetosis does not like the supine position, as many parts of the body are in contact with the supporting surface and it is difficult for them to tolerate so many inputs. Moreover, sensory channels such as the visual and vestibular systems are very disturbed by the continuous involuntary movements of the head and all the body.

However, the supine position can be proposed during treatment, to reach some goals, such as:

– State of calmness
– Perceptual tolerance
– Postural alignment
– Eye-hand coordination and visual coupling
– Better breathing rhythm
– Oro-motor control

Suggestion
- Seek postural alignment:
  1. *Align the child in the supine position, using a wedge or a U-shaped pillow; if a child has a low perceptual threshold, remember to filter the inputs in the surrounding environment.*
  2. *Stay in front of the child, flex their lower limbs with feet on the surface, and stabilize the position by applying manual pressing towards the feet.*
  3. *Gain eye-to-eye contact with the child, gently holding their head still, to facilitate the visual fixation and focusing. Approach the child slowly so as not to provoke visual or body avoiding reactions provoked by sudden and unexpected activities.*
- Facilitate a good breathing rhythm:
  1. *Verify that the child's nasal airways are clear and that the child can breathe through their nose when their mouth is closed.*
  2. *Put one or both hands on the child's sternum or on the sides of the ribcage, follow the exhaling in sync with the child, and then try gradually to prolong the expiration phase (Fig. 4.18).*
  3. *Encourage the child to make vowel sounds that have some small expressive meaning, e.g. "aaaa" → satisfaction, "ooo" → amazement, etc.*
  4. *Accompany the exhaling phase by flexing both legs towards the sternum, and then extend them back down slowly during inspiration.*
- Propose some active movements, maintaining the alignment of the body:
  1. *Encourage the child to lift their upper limbs up towards the midline, for example, to touch your hair and to point, reach or hold a ball.*
  2. *Create some boundary in the anterior space, for example, with your arms, so that the child can move their upper limbs within this limited action area.*

Fig. 4.18 Facilitation of
the breathing rhythm

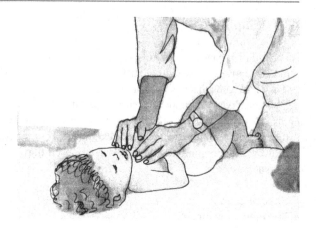

3. *Propose some simple activities to be able to observe the quality of spontaneous movements of the upper limbs and eye-hand-mouth coordination when they touch their face, visually explore their own hands, touch their mouth, etc.*
4. *Offer the child a small coloured enjoyable toy or object, for example, a piece of cloth, or a doll.*
5. *Ask the child to grasp and hold a small object, maintaining their upper limbs and wrists extended; if necessary, recruit some more muscle co-activation at the proximal girdle, using a distal to proximal tapping technique.*
6. *Encourage the child to move the same object in different directions, to put it somewhere or to give it to someone.*
7. *Verify that the child can interrupt the action they are performing at various stages, to evaluate their ability to maintain muscle co-contraction at the various joints involved in the movement, for example, that the child can hold the toy still in the air near them or near you.*

4.3.2 From Supine to Sitting

Most likely, this child needs help to move from the supine to the sitting position, because the transfer will be difficult as it requires the simultaneous control of many different parts of the body as well as many antigravity adaptive reactions:

– Stability of the head and trunk
– Maintenance of several joints in flexion during the upright transfer
– Postural adjustment and realignment when in sitting
– Tolerance of the intense and differentiated sensory inputs in the new position

Suggestion
• Prepare the child to move towards the position characterized by a higher CoM:
  1. *Verify the alignment of the different parts of the body.*

2. *Guide the child to find a good breathing rhythm.*
3. *Propose to the child some activities with the upper limbs in a closed kinetic chain, so that they can better control their involuntary movements and body alignment: e.g. stay in front of the child and hold their hands, or ask them to hold with both hands an object like a stick or a ring.*
4. *If necessary, use a tapping technique from distal to proximal, to activate the shoulder girdle.*
5. *Get the child to practise prolonged periods of active eye coupling to improve their visual fixation and control of ATNR.*
6. *Facilitate the child to gradually raise first their head and then their trunk.*
7. *If the child has problems performing this task adequately, interrupt the sequence, and concentrate on practising the initial part of the transfer first; it is important to train the sequence of returning to the starting position as well.*
8. *During the transfer to sitting, facilitate the child to control their performance, giving them a precise visual reference point.*
9. *As soon as the child reaches the sitting position, stabilize the posture with slight manual pressure on their shoulder or pelvic girdle.*

Note

- The therapist can guide the first sitting experiences of the child with dyskinesia in many different ways:
  - Facilitate the child's concentration by directing their attention, even visually, to a specific target.
  - Prepare the environmental setting carefully to make it perceptually less "busy".
  - Create a boundary in the perceptual void surrounding the child using the therapist's body and/or shaped pillows, wedges, towels, etc. (Fig. 4.19).

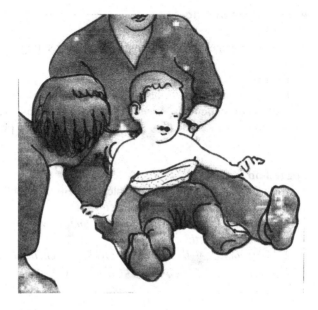

Fig. 4.19 Providing boundaries in the perceptual space around the child

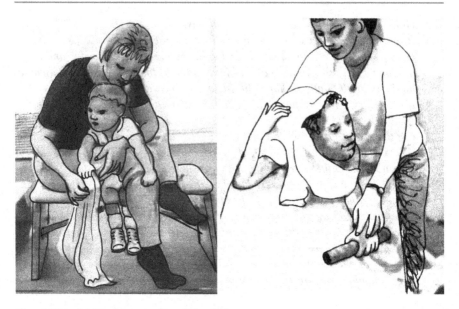

Figs. 4.20 and 4.21 Strategies for solving ADLs

- In particular, when the baby is still floppy, facilitate the transition by initiating the transfer with the infant in a semi-lying position on a wedge.
- Advise the caregivers on the most suitable positions to dress and undress the child and control the excess of involuntary movements (Fig. 4.20).
- Guide the child to find the right strategies to deal with ADLs, for example, to take a sweater off (Fig. 4.21).

4.3.3   Long Sitting

The child can benefit from learning to sit in long sitting for the following reasons:

- The BoS is wider and they are more stable.
- They can consolidate the ability to maintain the midline position.
- It allows the child to experience some body rotations, to reach for objects at their side, to move to a side lying position or to go back to prone.

Suggestion
- Work for stabilization at the girdles, to help the child to actively control their posture and upper limb distal movements:
  1. *Sit behind the child, their body in contact with your's and with their lower limbs in abduction.*
  2. *Your contact with the child provides an environmental boundary and can induce an anterior pelvic tilt if necessary, and control the position of the*

Fig. 4.22 Touching objects with different textures

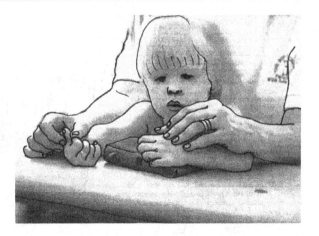

shoulder girdle in flexion (in case of excess extension) and the upper limbs to act in the midline.

3. *Train the child to sit with extended upper limbs and open hands in front.*
4. *If necessary, give the child more stability using tapping techniques from proximal to distal.*

- Gradually introduce sensory inputs to improve child's interaction with the environment:
  1. *Initially ask the child to look at a target (e.g. a picture on a book) without touching it.*
  2. *When the child is capable of maintaining both eye contact and postural control, move the target, and ask them to keep looking at it.*
  3. *Modify the task level in one of the suggested way:*
     - *Ask the child to touch the object target which could have different textures (Fig. 4.22).*
     - *Ask them to hold the object with both hands, and move it in different directions with a functional purpose.*
     - *If the child is very skilled, ask them to move a ball towards a person in front or to try to catch it while maintaining postural control.*
- Reduce the manual support to the child as soon as possible:
  1. *Gradually reduce your body contact with the child, substituting it, if necessary, with some alternative like a towel (Fig. 4.19) or a draft-stopper.*

4.3.4   Sitting with Feet on the Floor

The child with athetosis should learn to keep their feet on the ground while sitting, even if the standing position is not among the current functional goals. Improving their tolerance to the sensory inputs arriving through the feet helps them to maintain a more stable sitting posture and prepares for the transfer to the upright position later on.

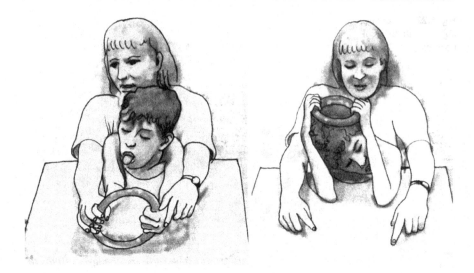

Figs. 4.23 and 4.24 Improvement of perceptual tolerance

During therapy dedicated to improving perceptual function, the child should be barefoot! If, instead, the goal is the transfer from sitting to standing and then walking, it is best to have them wear shoes.

A proper sitting position promotes improvement in the following functions:

- Weight-bearing on the lower limbs and tolerance of foot-to-floor contact
- Control the displacement of the CoM with an adequate tilting of the pelvic girdle without exploiting a pathological strategy in extension synergy
- Perceptual tolerance and reduction of avoiding reactions of the head, eyes, tongue, hands, etc. (Figs. 4.23 and 4.24)
- Head control with improvement of visual scanning
- Ability to move the arms forwards to carry out functional ADL, e.g. feeding, writing, undressing

Suggestion
- Work for the proper posture in sitting:
  1. *Make sure that the child has a mental image of the new setting, using verbal descriptions and other modalities, giving them time to understand and making it easier to adapt.*
  2. *Start by asking the child to sit on a small bench or stool without a back which could stimulate trunk extension.*
  3. *Use a stable chair, i.e. with a wide base and adequate height, and consider offering them a chair with handholds which the child can grasp to maintain an adequate position.*

Fig. 4.25 Gentle manual pressure on the sternum to limit avoiding reactions

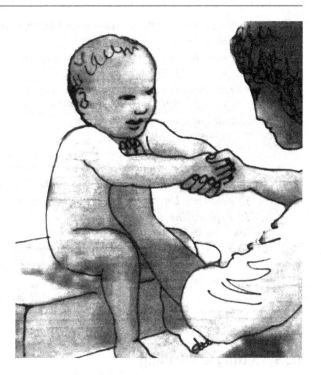

4. *Verify the alignment of the child's head and trunk and the anterior tilting of the pelvis; if necessary, apply slight manual pressure through the knee to the heel to enhance the perception of the weight-bearing on their feet.*

5. *As described before, if the child has important perceptive problems, provide a special boundary with your arms, and/or "fill" the space around them with small tables, chairs with backrest, etc.*

- Propose activities that require the CoM displacement forwards:
  1. *Guide the child to maintain their sitting position properly, by exerting light pressure on their shoulder girdle to improve uprighting.*
  2. *When a child is hesitant to move the trunk forwards due to a low perceptual tolerance threshold, apply gentle pressure to their sternum while holding their arms together, to counteract a possible avoidance reaction* (Fig. 4.25).
  3. *To facilitate the control of involuntary movements, invite the child to rest their hands on your knees or to hold something like a stick; the transfer of the CoM forwards improves the weight-bearing too.*
  4. *Propose more complex activities, for example, a task that requires the child to rotate their head to explore the surroundings while maintaining their current posture.*
- Prepare the child to sit more independently, and improve their functional (bi) manual abilities:

1. *Sit the child in front of a recessed table where they can support their forearms on the table surface.*
2. *Verify that the feet are in contact with the floor, and, if necessary, place a non-slip mat under their buttocks and/or feet.*
3. *Propose functional manual activities that are part of the child's everyday life, providing simple aids preferably adapted hand-made everyday objects.*
    Examples of simple manual aids:
    (a) *To allow more stability during grasping and/or manipulation:*
        - *Handles with suction cups, easily found commercially in stores*
        - *Small sticks or handles fixed in vertical positions on the table*
        - *An old-style plunger positioned on the surface*
    (b) *To guarantee better friction: non-slip mats*
    (c) *To improve the connect with the work surface: weighted wristbands, small sacks filled with sand or marbles*
    (d) *To increase the perceptual context:*
        - *Mark a perceptual track on the table, and ask the child to follow it with some toys.*
        - *Position the child's feet inside a small box to provide distal spatial borders.*

4.3.5 Sitting to Standing

This is a critical transfer for child because they need to maintain a good reference point on their feet while they are moving upwards and at the same time manage their involuntary movements. The other motor component to cope with is the gradual body uprighting managing the change of CoM to the smaller standing BoS without sudden jerky movements.

It is equally important that the child learns to return to the sitting position (BTS), a transfer that is challenging because it requires the child to control their posture while moving towards gravity without visual feedback.

Suggestion
- Prepare the child for the sit-to-stand (STS) transfer:
    1. *Have the child in front, seated on a small bench or a chair without a backrest (Fig. 4.26).*
    2. *Verify the effective foot-to-floor contact, and emphasize weight-bearing through slight manual pressure along the leg axis, if needed.*
    3. *Train the child to control their upper limb involuntary movements, which otherwise could interfere with the efficiency of the transfer.*
    For example:
    - *Ask them to bring their arms forwards with clasped hands, to touch your chest.*
    - *Ask the child to rest their hands on your shoulders, maintaining the contact on them, to control various haptic inputs.*

Fig. 4.26 Child
maintaining midline during
sitting

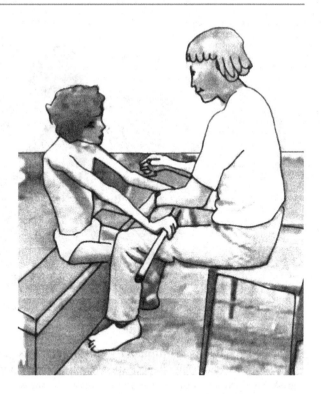

- During the STS transfer, guide the child in controlling the upper limb involuntary movements:
    1. *Verify that the child moves forwards and then upwards, taking care that their head and shoulders move forwards first and then the buttocks are lifted off the surface.*
    2. *This phase can trigger an increase in involuntary movements in the upper limbs, so some strategies are necessary to control these interferences:*
        Examples:
        – *The child can clasp their own hands together; if needed, help them by holding their wrists using a fork-like hold.*
        – *The child holds an object with both hands (small stick, scarf, ring).*
        – ....
    3. *Complete the STS sequence, applying manual pressure to the pelvis to enhance weight-bearing in standing.*
    4. *After practising STS transfer, ask the child to interrupt the sequence pausing in intermediate positions.*
    5. *Likewise, propose the child to return from standing to sitting (Fig. 4.27).*

Note
- During this difficult transfer, the therapist should avoid any background "noise", for example, excessive acoustic, visual or tactile inputs.

Fig. 4.27 The back-to-sit transfer

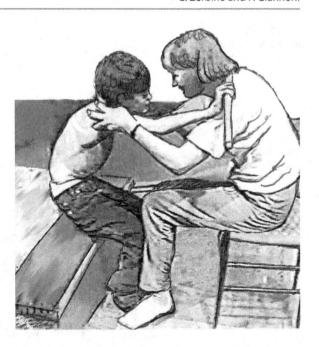

- The child could transfer from STS or BTS too quickly, missing the accuracy of the sequence and losing their postural control. The therapist should foresee these risks, and even that of falling, and be ready to slow the sequence down: the child could receive some manual pressure and alignment facilitation to the critical parts of the body to help control the shifting of COM and the maintenance of appropriate weight-bearing.

4.3.6 Standing

The ability to maintain the upright position is very demanding for the child with athetosis who usually learns and uses some strategies to achieve postural stability and reduce the sway of the body. For example:

- They adopt a pelvic strategy that exploits the RoM of the hip joints, choosing a position in maximal extension to give more stability to the pelvic girdle and, indirectly, to lower limbs.
- They abduct their lower limbs and widen their BoS, to control the CoM displacement.
- They stare at a fixed point in the environment and, unlike the ataxic child, use it to refocus again, if their head movements disorganize their stability.
- They use peripheral vision and the glance strategy to understand what is going on around them, without moving their head.

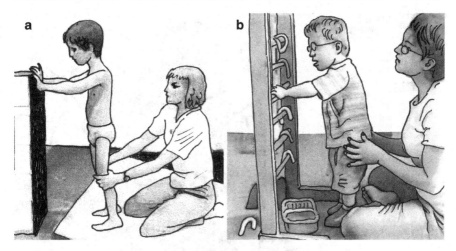

Fig. 4.28 Standing (**a**) with open hand support, (**b**) holding onto a support

Suggestion
- Let the child gradually adapt to the new antigravity position, dealing with the sensory inputs coming from the feet:
    1. *First, to increase the child's stability, ask them to hold onto the high backrest of a chair with both hands or to place their hands on another surface in front of them* (Fig. 4.28a, b).
    2. *Tolerate the abduction of the lower limbs at the beginning, and train them to actively reduce the BoS later on.*
    3. *Facilitate the maintenance of alignment in the standing position by suggesting they focus on an interesting object target placed on the midline in front of them.*
    4. *If necessary, improve their unstable core with some tapping technique on the abdominal muscles* (Fig. 4.29).
    5. *Later on, propose the child maintain the focus and pursuit a moving target, without losing their postural alignment.*
- Propose some functional tasks that require simple activities with the upper limbs while maintaining the standing position:
    1. *Draw attention to an object target, and ask the child to follow it with their eyes while maintaining their stance.*
    2. *Propose to the child to move one hand slightly to reach and touch an interesting object, while they are still supported on the other hand*
    3. *If the child is able, ask them to go back to the starting position, and/or ask them to do the same movement with the other arm.*
    4. *If the child is even skilled, ask them to grasp the object, and move it somewhere for a functional purpose.*

Fig. 4.29 Tapping
technique to improve the
core stability

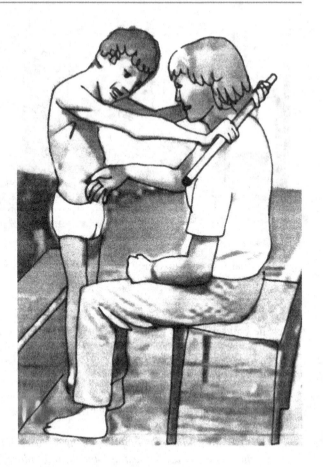

5. *Try to introduce a body-knowledge play, which involves the child's emotional participation, by asking them to touch some parts of their body with one hand (face, shoulder, tummy, etc.).*
- Verify the ability of the child to manage the standing position without using the upper limbs for support:
    1. *Act as the child's stability reference point by just standing in front of them without any physical contact.*
    2. *Gradually propose more functional tasks (looking around, holding a big toy with both hands, talking, etc.) while they control their postural stability.*

4.3.7 Walking

While a child with spastic CP has an advantage of being able to practise every single phase of gait, this is not the case with the child with athetosis who needs to construct

Fig. 4.30 Therapist as a
reference point during gait

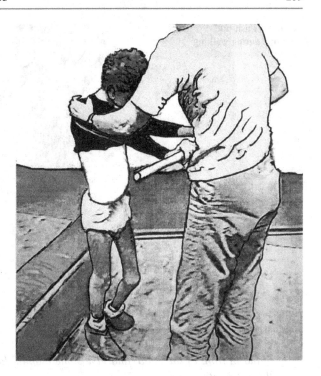

their own learning patterns. They are intolerant to any constraint, which does not give them the freedom to manage their continuous movements.

They are usually uncomfortable with an excess of sensory inputs, and therefore the adult should limit touch during motor tasks. Nevertheless, the child can benefit from specific manual guidance and pressure for stability applied at the right time and in the right part of the body.

Suggestion
- Allow the child to train their own walking patterns:
  1. *Help the child control the possible trunk and hip extension by acting as a reference point in the space to walk towards; for example, propose they hold a stick and start walking towards you* (Fig. 4.30).
  2. *If necessary, use some pressure technique to elicit more stability, particularly at the core.*
  3. *Give pressure inputs during single steps as well to improve weight-bearing in full stance.*
  4. *As soon as possible, gradually reduce the manual facilitations, still remaining close and in front to help out in case of specific needs, like very unstable walking conditions.*

Fig. 4.31 Push-pull
technique during walking

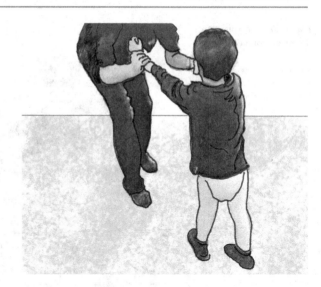

Suggestion

- Give more manual facilitation, if needed:
  1. *Stand in front of the child, and give some manual facilitation for improving their stability:*
- *Apply some manual pressure on their shoulders or humeri with slight flexion at the shoulder joint, to counteract the posture in extension.*
- *With a more skilled child, grasp the upper limbs distally, keeping their hands open and wrists extended, and then ask the child to move while applying some manual compression tapping* (Fig. 4.31).
  2. *At the same time, facilitate the shifting of the body weight, to activate the central pattern generators and elicit the first step.*

References

Barry MJ, VanSwearingen JM, Albright AL (1999) Reliability and responsiveness of the Barry-Albright Dystonia Scale. Dev Med Child Neurol. 1999 Jun;41(6):404–11. https://doi.org/10.1017/s0012162299000870

Battini R, Sgandurra G, Petacchi E, Guzzetta A, Di Pietro R, Giannini MT, Leuzzi V, Mercuri E, Cioni G (2008) Movement disorder-childhood rating scale: reliability and validity. Pediatr Neurol. 2008 Oct;39(4):259–65. https://doi.org/10.1016/j.pediatrneurol.2008.07.002.

Battini R, Guzzetta A, Sgandurra G, Di Pietro R, Petacchi E, Mercuri E, Giannini MT, Leuzzi V, Cioni G (2009) Scale for evaluation of movement disorders in the first three years of life. Pediatr Neurol. 2009 Apr;40(4):258–64. https://doi.org/10.1016/j.pediatrneurol.2008.11.003

Bobath K (1966) The motor deficit in patients with cerebral palsy. Clinics in developmental medicine, No. 23. W. M. Heinemann Medical Books, London

Bobath B (1977) Facilitation techniques for the treatment of children with cerebral palsy. Lecture given at a post graduate course on Bobath concept, Londo

Bobath B, Bobath K (1975) Motor development in the different types of cerebral palsy. W. Heinemann Medical Books Ltd

Bordoloi K, Deka RS (2018) Scientific reconciliation of the concepts and principles of Rood approach. Int J Health Sci Res 8(9):225–234

Brazelton TB, Nugent JK (2011) Neonatal behavioral assessment scale, 4th edn, Clinics in developmental medicine, No. 190. Mac Keith Press, London

Burke RE, Fahn S, Marsden CD, Bressman SB, Moskowitz C, Friedman J (1985) Validity and reliability of a rating scale for the primary torsion dystonias. Neurology. 1985 Jan;35(1):73–7. https://doi.org/10.1212/wnl.35.1.73

Cans C (2000) Surveillance of cerebral palsy in Europe: a collaboration of cerebral palsy surveys and registers. Dev Med Child Neurol 42:816–824. https://doi.org/10.1111/j.1469-8749.2000. tb00695.x

Cans C, Dolk H, Platt M, Colver A, Prasauskiene EA, Krageloh-Mann IK (2007) Recommendations from the SCPE collaborative group for defining and classifying cerebral palsy. Dev Med Child Neurol 49:35–38. https://doi.org/10.1111/j.1469-8749.2007.tb12626.x

Comella CL, Leurgans S, Wuu J, Stebbins GT, Chmura T; and The Dystonia Study Group (2003) Rating scales for dystonia: a multicenter assessment. Mov Disord. 2003 Mar;18(3):303–312. https://doi.org/10.1002/mds.10377

de Ajuriaguerra J (1970) Manuel de psychiatrie de l'enfant, 2nd edn. Masson Paris

Dubowitz V (1969) The floppy infant. Clinics in developmental medicine No. 31. London, Spastics International in Association with Heinemann Medical, pp 10–15

Ferrari A, Cioni G (2010) The spastic forms of cerebral palsy: a guide to the assessment of adaptive functions. Springer, Milan. https://doi.org/10.1007/978-88-470-1478-7

Hammond WA (1871) Athetosis, a treatise on diseases of the nervous system. Appleton and Co., D. New York, pp 654–662

Himmelmann K, Hagberg G, Beckung E, Hageberg B, Uvebrant P (2005) The changing panorama of cerebral palsy in Sweden. IX. Prevalence and origin in the birth-year period 1995-1998. Acta Paediatr 94(3):287–294. https://doi.org/10.1111/j.1651-2227.2005.tb03071.x

Himmelmann K, Uvebrant P (2011) Function and neuroimaging in cerebral palsy: a population-based study. Dev Med Child Neurol 53(6):516–521. https://doi.org/10.1111/j.1469-8749.2011.03932.x

Jan JE, Lyons CJ, Heaven RK, Matsuba C (2001) Visual impairment due to a dyskinetic eye movement disorder in children with dyskinetic cerebral palsy. Dev Med Child Neurol 43(2):108–101. https://doi.org/10.1017/s0012162201000184

Krägeloh-Mann I, Cans C (2009) Cerebral palsy update. Brain Dev 31(7):537–544. https://doi.org/10.1016/j.braindev.2009.03.009

Krägeloh-Mann I, Helber A, Hagberg G, Mader I, Staudt M, Wolff M, Groenendaal F, De Vries L (2002) Bilateral lesions of thalamus and basal ganglia: origin and outcome. Dev Med Child Neurol 44:477–484. https://doi.org/10.1111/j.1469-8749.2002.tb00309.x

La Porta-Oyos O, Ballester-Plané J, Leiva D et al (2019) Executive function and general intellectual functioning in dyskinetic cerebral palsy: comparison with spastic cerebral palsy and typically developing controls. Eur J Paediatr Neurol 23(4):546–559. https://doi.org/10.1016/j.ejpn.2019.05.010

McClure V (2017) Infant Massage: A handbook for loving parents. 4th ed Bantam Pub

Mesraoua B, Ali M, Deleu D, Al Hail H et al (2019) Epilepsy and cerebral palsy. In: Neurodevelopment and neurodevelopmental disease. https://doi.org/10.5772/intechopen.82804

Milani Comparetti A (1978) Classification des infirmités motrices cérébrales. Méd Hyg 36:2024–2029

Monbaliu E, Ortibus E, De Cat J, Dan B, Heyrman L, Prinzie P, De Cock P, Feys H (2012) The Dyskinesia Impairment Scale: a new instrument to measure dystonia and choreoathetosis in dyskinetic cerebral palsy. Dev Med Child Neurol. 2012 Mar;54(3):278–83. https://doi.org/10.1111/j.1469-8749.2011.04209.x

Monbaliu E, de Cock P, Ortibus E, Heyrman L, Klingels K, Feys H (2016) Clinical patterns of dystonia and choreoathetosis in participants with dyskinetic cerebral palsy. Dev Med Child Neurol 58(2):138–144. https://doi.org/10.1111/dmcn.12846

Peredo DE, Hannibal MC (2009) The floppy infant: evaluation of hypotonia. Pediatr Rev 30(9):e66–e76. https://doi.org/10.1542/pir.30-9-e66

Pumerantz C, Zachry A (2018) Establishing Tummy Time Routines to Enhance your Baby's Development. https://www.aota.org/aboutoccupational-therapy/patients-clients/childrenandyouth/tummy-time.aspx

Rood MS (1954) Neurophysiological reactions as a basis for physical therapy. Phys Ther Rev 34:444–449

Rood MS (1956) Neurophysiological mechanisms utilized in the treatment of neuromuscular dysfunction. Am J Occup Ther 10:220–225

Sanger TD, Chen D, Fehlings DL, Hallett M et al (2010) Definition and classification of hyperkinetic movements in childhood. Mov Disord 25(11):1538–1549. https://doi.org/10.1002/mds.23088

Scrutton D, Damiano D, Mayston M (2004) Management of the motor disorders of children with cerebral palsy. In: Clinics in developmental medicine, 2nd edn. Mac Keith Press

Seddon PC, Khan Y (2003) Respiratory problems in children with neurological impairment. Arch Dis Child 88:75–78. https://doi.org/10.1136/adc.88.1.75

Sellier E, Uldall P, Calado E, Sigurdardottir S, Torrioli MG, Platt MJ, Cans C (2012) Epilepsy and cerebral palsy: characteristics and trends in children born in 1976-1998. Eur J Paediatr Neurol 16(1):48–55. https://doi.org/10.1016/j.ejpn.2011.10.003

Stewart K, Harvey A, Johnston LM (2017) A systematic review of scales to measure dystonia and choreoathetosis in children with dyskinetic cerebral palsy. Dev Med Child Neurol 59:786–795. https://doi.org/10.1111/dmcn.13452

Sun D, Wang Q, Hou M, Li Y, Yu R, Zhao J, Wang K (2018) Clinical characteristics and functional status of children with different subtypes of dyskinetic cerebral palsy. Medicine (Baltimore) 97(21):e10817. https://doi.org/10.1097/md.0000000000010817

Twitchell TE (1961) The nature of the motor deficit in double athetosis. Arch Phys Med Rehabil 42:63–67

Weir FW, Hatch JL, McRackan TR, Wallace SA, Meyer TA (2018) Hearing loss in Pediatric Patients with Cerebral Palsy. Otology & Neurotology, Jan 2018, Vol 39, Issue 1, p 59–64. https://doi.org/10.1097/MAO.0000000000001610

Ataxia in Cerebral Palsy

5

Psiche Giannoni and Liliana Zerbino

The form of cerebral palsy (CP) formerly labelled "ataxia" is now referred to as non-progressive congenital ataxia (NPCA) and concerns about 10% of children with CP. The current advanced diagnostic technologies have made it possible to give broader, etiological explanations on this type of CP and to focus on the growing genetic components of the pathology. Many infantile ataxic forms can have additional and/or different prenatal causes than those highlighted in the past, such as stroke and hypoxic-ischemic encephalopathy, and many studies report at least 50% of ataxic CP is inherited as an autosomal recessive trait (Lee et al. 2014; Parolin Schnekenberg et al. 2015; Bertini et al. 2018; Burgeln 2018). This is the case, for example, of ataxia-telangiectasia or Joubert syndrome, in which cerebellar hypoplasia or hereditary chromosome mutations are mainly responsible for the pathology.

However, considering the basic characteristic of a cerebellar disorder, the NPCA form analysed here shows muscle hypotonia, motor delay and other associated dysfunctions such as oculomotor and speech disorder and sometimes some cognitive impairment. Recent studies report how the cerebellum also affects sensory behaviour (Bastian 2011).

Ataxia, a term meaning "lack of order" in Greek etymology, is defined as a disturbance of coordination and statics and as a disorder of the integration of normal movement patterns in time and space, which manifests with the involvement of the cerebellar pathways, in the absence of lesions of the direct corticospinal motor pathways. This means that there is no impairment of movement but a disturbance in its execution. For this reason, an early diagnosis of ataxia is not easy. Superficially, an infant with ataxia may seem just a little awkward and clumsy and often is considered a quiet child, perhaps with only a motor delay.

P. Giannoni (✉)
DIBRIS, University of Genoa, Genoa, Italy

L. Zerbino
DSS, University of Florence, Florence, Italy

Frequently family members (often a grandmother) are the first to have doubts about this child's development when it appears that they are struggling with some usual developmental milestones. Typically, the child needs to exaggerate motor control patterns to maintain postures with a high centre of mass (CoM), which require adequate antigravity tonic reactions and greater body stability.

The characteristic features of ataxia can only be observed during movement since the neural impairment does not affect the overall organisation of the motor patterns but the detailed spatiotemporal aspects of its execution. Milani-Comparetti and Gidoni (1971) underlines how the child with ataxia cannot be identified if observed in a photograph, which "freezes" the movement, and thus the static evidence of the photograph does not reveal the defect of this pathology.

The cerebellum is a very sophisticated part of the nervous system. It is not primarily responsible for generating movement but for its coordination, timing and precision. In fact, all the efferent pathways from Purkinje cells, which constitute the sole output of all motor coordination in the cerebellar cortex, exert inhibitory effects on their functional targets.

Despite its relatively small size, the cerebellum has three times more neurons than the cerebrum and many more topographic maps that highlight its important functional role and its far-reaching connectivity with the other parts of the brain (Thivierge and Marcus 2007; Schlerf et al. 2010; Manto and Oulad Ben Taid 2010; Guell and Schmahmann 2020).

The first experimental studies of the cerebellum (Bolk 1904; Edinger 1910; Comolli 1910) led to a classification according to anatomical-functional criteria. An anatomical division distinguishes the cerebellum in the vermis, the intermediate zone, the lateral hemisphere and the flocculonodular lobe, and another functional division differentiates (a) vestibulocerebellum, mainly regulating balance and eye movements; (b) spinocerebellum, more involved in the regulation of postural tone; and (c) cerebrocerebellum linked, albeit indirectly, with the cortex. All of these parts have distinct afferent inputs and efferent outputs through their deep nuclei.

Further studies have focused on the existence of a distinctive and wide somatotopia of the cerebellum, different for afferent and efferent information and with many fragmented homunculi.

Currently, the functional anatomy of the cerebellum, based on the division of Larsell into ten lobules (Larsell 1947), is differentiated into three domains:

1. The vestibulo-cerebellar syndrome (VCS), related to oculomotor deficits and imbalance
2. The cerebellar motor syndrome (CMS), with postural deficits, motor incoordination and dysarthria
3. The cerebellar cognitive affective syndrome (CCAS), with impairments of executive functions, verbal memory and visuospatial deficits (Schmahmann and Schmahmann 1998; Steilin et al. 1999; Koziol et al. 2014; Manto and Mariën 2015; Popa and Ebner 2019; Manto et al. 2020)

The "cognitive cerebellum" linked to the CCAS, due to its connectivity with the cortex, has a very important role in motor learning. According to the Marr and Albus theory (Marr 1969; Albus 1971), revisited by Ito (Ito et al. 2014), the cerebellum receives two different types of sensory-motor information from the periphery: (1) signals that specifically encode the expected interaction with the environment, through mossy fibres, and (2) error or alarm signals, coming from the olive nucleus through the climbing fibres, which specifically encode unexpected environmental occurrences, capable to induce a long-lasting acquisition of the relevant information. This organisation in two parallel routes promotes the cerebellum as an efficient novelty or error detector and a refined learning device. It is particularly important to keep this theory well in mind, as it also provides the basis of the clinical reasoning and guides the correct rehabilitation intervention required for these children. In this light, treatment aims to promote the learning of new skills, and treatment proposals need to be significant and meaningful. Therapy is based on activating the nervous system through a variety of creative, captivating inputs, which stimulate the attention and interest of the child. The therapists need to help and support the children to accept learning through a trial and error and problem-solving approach to the new problems that come along in their functional development, improving their generalization process.

The feedforward processing of the input of the array of motor and sensory information is a peculiar aspect of the cerebellum for learning, which allows the nervous system to anticipate how to act quickly for the best motor control or the best sensory perception (Eccles et al. 1967). Ataxic disorders make it difficult for the child to exploit these predictive sequences and consequently to store them in a solid learned experiences. For this reason, according to the Schmidt theory on motor control (Schmidt 1975; Schmidt and Lee 2005), children with ataxia need much more practice to acquire motor skills with a long repetitive training that includes elements of variability from trial to trial.

5.1   Main Features of the Child with Ataxia

The cerebellum is a tuning device, not a prime mover, as underlined above. Therefore, the child with ataxia, although capable of voluntary movement, will show the specific manifestations of the impairment in the function of the cerebellar affected areas or the pathways linked with them. Many areas can be involved together.

As far as treatment is concerned, there are so many distinctive aspects to consider, such as movement, vision, speech and cognition, that a very collaborative multidisciplinary approach between all practitioners is mandatory. However, it is possible to make a broad distinction between two basic problematic areas of motor function in ataxia that imply the particular involvement of specific therapists: the first is related to antigravity postural control, including balance and gait (physiotherapist), and the other to the fine movements of the upper limbs (occupational therapist and physiotherapist).

The practitioner needs to distinguish and make an accurate evaluation of these aspects because they should be handled differently, even if both impairments are observed in the same child.

The child with ataxia often suffers also from dysarthria, which is closely related to the lack of vocal coordination, making their speech performance sometimes incomprehensible and impaired by aprosodia. Articulatory inaccuracy causes frequent, marked breakdowns of speech, with slow movements of the vocal apparatus and errors of range of articulatory movements and direction. Moreover, prosodic abnormalities show slowness, monoloudness, monotone and prolonged syllables (Brown et al. 1970; Yorkston and Beukelman 1981; Ackermann and Ziegler 1992). There is a close relationship between speech performance and hypotonia of the thoracic and phonatory muscles, and therefore physiotherapists and speech therapists should work in unison to train the child to achieve more powerful and greater respiratory coordination during the emission of the voice. Collaboration with the speech therapist is indicated to deal with problems of dysphagia and drooling caused by hypotonia of the orbicular muscles (see Chap. 10). The developmental vision therapist will be part of the rehabilitation team for the child's needs concerning oculomotor coordination (see Chap. 11).

5.1.1   Child with Relevant Ataxic Postural Impairment

This child usually shows hypotonia, asthenia and balance problems. The decreased discharge of the fusimotor fibres and the consequent reduced proprioceptive inflow limit the muscle ability to maintain a constant tonic activation level. There is also a delay in initiating movement which invokes slowness because the phasic component activity of the agonist muscle is weaker. When they are attempting to get up, the child stabilises by using a wider base of support (BoS) and uses their hands to support on something to move around (Figs. 5.1 and 5.2).

Difficulty in balance is another characteristic feature in ataxia. Gait disturbances can be caused by direct involvement of the vestibular-cerebellar tract and/or by problems related to muscle contraction and therefore by a disturbed control of the upright position, together with incoordination of the multi-joint movements (Fig. 5.3).

Both vestibular deficit and ataxic gaits show spatiotemporal instability on the sagittal and frontal planes, a wide BoS, reduced step length and trunk oscillation. However, Schniepp et al. (2017) have shown that the walking features of these two impairments include specific defects in the speed of the gait: the vestibular deficit makes gait more difficult at low speed, while in most cases of ataxia, problems occur at both low and high speeds due to the deficiency in sensory integration and feedforward coordination.

To manage these problems in standing and to move with less effort, the child with ataxia spontaneously adopts the following postural adjustments:

(a) Slight bending of the knees to lower the CoM and so reduce body sway
(b) Increase in the width of the step to increase the BoS and keep the projection of the CoM inside it
(c) Outward stretching of the upper limbs to increase the moment of inertia of the body around the front/rear axis

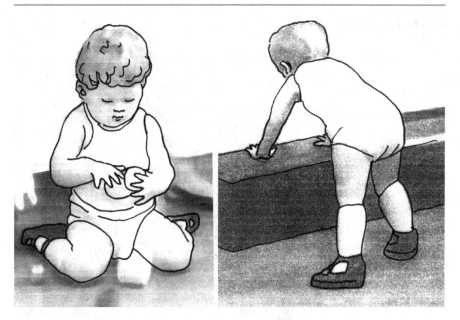

Figs. 5.1 and 5.2   The typical wide BoS organised by the child with ataxia

These are smart strategies that the child can use whenever they are in difficulty, but the goal of the treatment is precisely to train basic abilities to reduce the need for them to resort to these compensation strategies. For this reason, the treatment plan should include the increase of muscle tone through the different techniques of tapping and joint compression and the improvement of balance through dynamic motor tasks.

5.1.2   Child with Difficulties in Manual Dexterity

With regard to arm movements, the child with ataxia has difficulty to reach a manual target with smooth arm movements and must continually adjust their trajectory and/or zigzagging movements before succeeding to touch and grasp the target. These problems are related to the concept of "dysmetria", which ultimately results in the lack of accuracy of voluntary movement (Manto 2009).

This inaccuracy can be observed when the child overshoots or undershoots a manual target, due to an incorrect judgement of distance (hyper-/hypometria). An attempt to correct the amplitude of the previous ballistic motion may then follow, thereby triggering a kind of kinetic tremor of the arm around the target.

These errors occur both at the proximal and distal joint level and are more evident when the child is engaged in fine purposeful movements. The amplitude of the curvature of the trajectories to reach the target may be exaggerated with respect to that necessary and the acceleration/deceleration profile is asymmetrical, with a shorter deceleration time.

Fig. 5.3 Gait stance in
ataxia

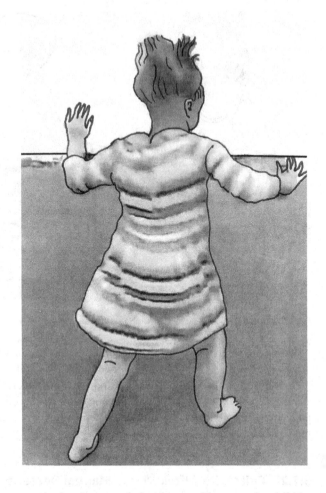

Motor performance worsens in the absence of visual control because the child is more dependent upon visual guidance, although the overuse of this compensation is not optimal because of the visual feedback delay.

The way the child deals with the task of drawing or writing is quite particular. They are unable to grade the amount of strength to hold the pen and draw a smooth line. Efficient handwriting requires in-hand manipulation, fine motor skills, proprioception and visual perception, which are not the best capabilities of a child with ataxia. When they are a toddler, they have distal primitive grasp patterns, but, unlike the problem-free child, they are unable to control the proximal joints at the same time as well. Handwriting is a challenging task for them, due also to their proprioceptive problems: the child is unable to lightly rest their wrist on the paper to stabilise the upper limb, while they move their hand to draw a line with a dynamic grasp of the pen. Instead they place their wrist heavily on the paper, hold the pen with a very tight grip and press down hard, reducing the range of movement (RoM) of the wrist joint. The writing ends up with very heavy, frequently interrupted, lines and

Fig. 5.4 Handwritten scribbles traced by a child with ataxia before and after a treatment session

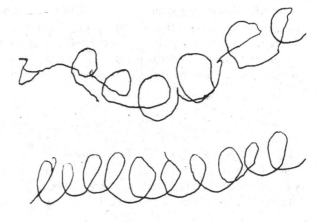

Fig. 5.5 A drawing done a child with ataxia before and after a treatment session

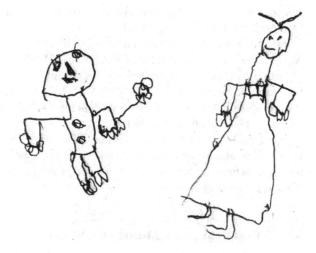

with many jerky peaks. Figure 5.4 shows two examples of a handwritten scribble traced by a child, the first before and the second after a treatment session.

The same difficulties can be noted for hand-drawing (Fig. 5.5). Before the treatment session, the child drew a small-sized figure with heavy lines, due to the excessive pressure on the paper and the consequent limited RoM at the wrist. After the treatment, the figure is larger and the lines are lighter and smoother.

5.1.2.1 Assessment of Ataxia

The most frequently used scales to evaluate ataxia are the Scale for Assessment and Rating of Ataxia (SARA) (Schmitz-Hubsch et al. 2006) and the older International Cooperative Ataxia Rating Scale (ICARS) (Trouillas et al. 1997). Regarding ICARS, there is also a modified version (MICARS) and a short version (BARS) (Schmahmann et al. 2009).

MICARS divides the symptomatology into four compartments which fit very well with the areas to consider during treatment: (1) posture and gait disturbances; (2) kinetic functions; (3) speech disorders; and (4) oculomotor disorders.

Some practical treatment suggestions on the first two aspects of ataxia will be provided below, while the problems relating to oculomotor disorders are described in Chap. 11.

Regarding postural control and balance, it is useful to assess children from 6 years up also with other tests that are usually used to evaluate adults: for example, the Trunk Impairment Scale (TIS) (Verheyden et al. 2004, 2007) and the Balance Evaluation Systems Test (BESTest) (Horak et al. 2009) or Mini-BESTest (Franchignoni et al. 2010) which includes many interesting items to keep in mind for the treatment plan: functional reaching, position transitions (e.g. Timed Up and Go) (Podsiadlo and Richardson 1991), balance (e.g. Berg Balance Test) (Berg et al. 1992), gait (e.g. Dynamic Gait Index) (Shumway-Cook and Woollacott 1995; Herdman 2000), the orientation of the sensory response with either open or closed eyes and many other evaluations. The tests hosted in the BESTest could also be used partially, according to specific needs.

Regarding manual dexterity and coordination, the Box and Block Test (BBT) (Mathiowetz et al. 1985; Jongbloed-Pereboom et al. 2014) is a simple and enjoyable evaluation tool, as well as the Functional Dexterity Test (FDT) (Aaron and Jansen 2003) and the Strength-Dexterity (SD) test (Dayanidhi et al. 2013).

To evaluate cognitive and affective deficits, the Schmahmann syndrome scale was developed (Hoche et al. 2018).

The multi-modal Nottingham Sensory Assessment (NSA) is an evaluation tool designed for adults with stroke, which nevertheless examines some very important aspects of sensation such as kinesthesia and stereognosis which are also valid for children (Lincoln et al. 1998).

5.2   Practical Suggestions

As the main characteristics of NPCA are deficits in postural and motor control and in sensory-motor coordination, the following therapy aims are focused here on these two aspects.

Different aims of intervention of the therapist:
- *For the child (autonomy and quality of life)*
  - Increase anti-gravity postural stability to facilitate interaction with the environment
  - Enhance the use of perception to better exploit the feedback and feedforward mechanisms
  - Improve the child's ability to deal with problems related to activities of daily life (ADL)
  - Provide useful functional equipment as necessary

> • *For the parents and caregivers (child management)*
>   – Help parents and caregivers to understand the particular characteristics of the child and to respect their execution times
>   – Provide advice to promote independence in the ADLs, such as washing, eating, un-/dressing, etc., suggesting minimal effort, functional modalities
>   – Provide aids for easier and more functional mobility of the child
>   – Enhance augmentative communication strategies (e.g. gaze, gestures) to ease problems of vocal communication
> • *For the treatment session*
>   – Improve postural tone and the recruitment of more motor units (MU) to obtain greater antigravity stability and endurance
>   – Improve both dynamic and quiet stance balance reactions
>   – Train fine movement coordination
>   – Propose practice of in-/variant tasks, to improve the feedforward strategy
>   – Improve visual coordination
>   – Improve coordination between respiration and voice production
>   – Investigate and provide aids to facilitate the child's functioning

5.2.1   Tasks for Stability

5.2.1.1 On All Fours

The child with NPCA, compared to the one with bilateral spastic CP, has many advantages in moving on the floor due to their low tone. The task is easier for them as the CoM is lower, with a wider BoS and more support points—their four limbs—compared to when they are standing.

For this reason, proposals to move in situations with lower antigravity level can signify offering occasions for the child to increase their confidence in moving. The proposal of moving on all fours has the advantage of (1) supporting on a large, four-point base; (2) recruiting more tone; (3) allowing the experience of different, easy transfers from that position to others; and (4) improving endurance.

Suggestion
• Promote stability and postural control in the all-four position:
  1. *With the child on all fours, align their trunk and limbs.*
  2. *Take care that the upper limbs have good support with open hands.*
  3. *Verify that the shoulders are not internally rotated, that there is active adduction of the shoulder blades and that arm support is with straight elbows.*
  4. *If the tone of the* rhomboideus, trapezius *and other external rotator muscles is insufficient for a good shoulder girdle stability, apply the tapping technique over the area* (for more details on tapping, see Chap. 4).
  5. *To facilitate effective weight-bearing on the four limbs, exert some joint compression through the long axes of the arm and forearm and from the thigh to the knee.*

Fig. 5.6 Toddler on all
fours, raising one arm

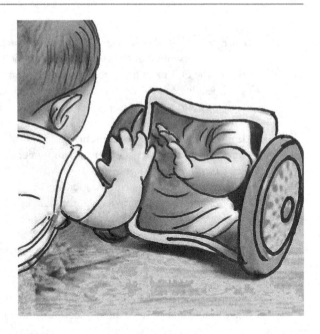

- Motivate the child to move from the starting position:
  - *Attract the interest of the toddler with suitable toy to reach, and ask them to raise a limb so that they need to actively stabilise their balance* (Fig. 5.6).
  - *Challenge a skilled child to lift an arm and then the contralateral leg as well.*
  - *From the position on all fours, induce the child to transfer into other positions like side-sitting and kneeling, and move crawling on hands and knees.*

5.2.1.2 Sitting Position

As specified before, the child with ataxic impairment prefers being and moving in positions with a large BoS and when the projection of their CoM is low. To transfer into higher positions, they lean on furniture or other types of support. For this reason, the child should also be treated in different higher position than those on the floor, to provide experiences offering a variety of sensory information (proprioceptive, vestibular and visual) and to solicit antigravity reactions at all levels of the body. If the child's spontaneous recruitment of muscle tone is not enough to stabilise adequately, the therapist can help by applying tapping on the hypotonic muscle groups or joint compression along the body axis.

Suggestion
- Choose a starting position, and verify the correct alignment in prevision of the activity to be carried out:
  (a) *Possibilities for a small child:*
    - *The toddler in long-sitting on the floor with their arms extended to the sides and slightly externally rotated to enhance the extension of the trunk; open hands will provide valid support on the floor.*

- *The child sitting on your lap, their feet supported on the floor, their upper limbs in extension supporting on an anterior surface* (Fig. 5.7), *preferably slightly inclined.*
- *The infant sitting astride the corner of a small bench with arms and legs as above.*

(b) *Possibilities for an older child:*
  - *The child sitting astride a bench or stool, without back support, feet on the floor, upper limbs straight against a support surface placed in front, at a lower level than the height of their shoulders*

• Work to increase MU recruitment and muscle tone and improve the activation of antigravity postural control:

1. *Stay behind the child, apply the most appropriate techniques (tapping or joint compression) to induce a prolonged upright reaction in extension of the head and trunk, and improve the perception of weight-bearing on the four limbs. Examples:*
   - *Place your hands on each side of the infant/child's head, hold the head and make a gentle but firm compression from top to bottom along the spine to obtain a sustained righting reaction of the trunk.*
   - *With your hands on both sides of the child's head, apply gentle, firm intermittent compressions through the head down the spine to sustain the trunk righting reaction* (see also Fig. 4.17 in Chap. 4). *This facilitation can help the child to feel more stable, and facilitate the visual scanning towards different targets.*
   - *Raise the child's arms straight up along the sides of their head, and apply joint compression through the arms down the spine, as done previously from the head* (Fig. 5.8). *The same technique can be applied directly from the shoulders.*
   - *Position the child with their arms extended and open hands along their sides or supporting on a surface, and then apply tapping to increase the*

Fig. 5.7 Support on straight arms, with closed kinetic chain

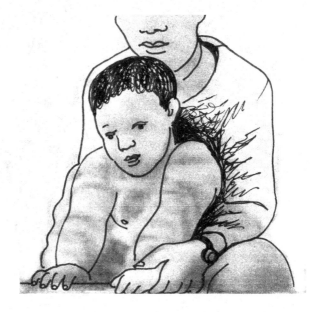

activity of the rotator cuff, trapezius, latissimus dorsi *and* erector spinae *muscles. The tapping needs to go from top to bottom along the direction of the muscle fibres. Obviously, care needs to be taken when using this manoeuvre with a young and/or frail infant.*

2. *After obtaining a more active and stable upright posture, ask the child to perform simple actions (e.g. chatting with their parent, looking at something of interest) or a more complex request (e.g. reaching with an upper limb for an object and giving it to their parent and then playing together) without losing their balance and the support achieved previously on the other upper limb.*

3. *Through your manual contact, remain aware, and anticipate when the child begins to lose their antigravity control, so they can "recharge" the muscle spindles in time through application of tapping or compression once again.*

- Work for an upright straight trunk together with active support on the upper limbs:
    1. *Verify the correct position of trunk and shoulder girdle and then the correct orientation of arms and forearms.*
    2. *Guide the child to dorsiflex their wrists and open hands; this facilitates the child to place their upper limbs on a surface in front, with extended elbows.*

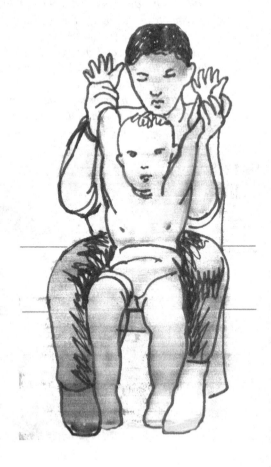

Fig. 5.8 Joint compression technique from top to bottom

3. *Induce more tonic recruitment, if necessary, and therefore active support on the upper limbs, applying a certain compression from the elbows towards the hands and then from the shoulders along the whole axis of the arms.*

4. *Gradually propose more complex skills, such as keeping the child's hands open and the upper limbs extended on a vertical surface, with a 90° flexion of the shoulders. In this case, compression is given from the back of the shoulder along the arms; the use of a mirror as a vertical surface is very useful because vision plays an important role in reinforcing the postural stability* (Fig. 5.9).

5. *If the child has a stable back support (e.g. the therapist's body), it is possible to keep the child's hands and direct compression from the distal to proximal joints.*

5.2.2 Tasks for Stability and Coordination

5.2.2.1 Upper Limb Functional Activities

The child needs to learn to have a steady balance when they move because this ability is essential for their independence not only at home but also at school. To challenge the child in achieving this function, it is necessary to gradually introduce dynamic tasks, which require precise motor control in conditions with upper limbs in closed kinetic chain (e.g. holding a movable object with both hands) and an efficient core stability in action.

Suggestion
- Propose play and/or functional activities that require control of the upper body:
  - *Ask the child to hold a stick, a hoop, or a big ball in front with both hands, and move it forwards, sideways and a little higher and lower, to give it to someone or put it somewhere* (Fig. 5.10a).

Fig. 5.9 Forward upper limb support on an anterior mirror

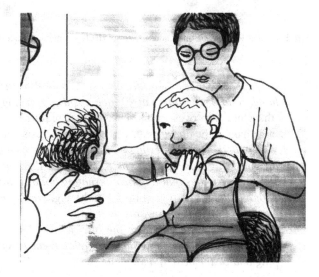

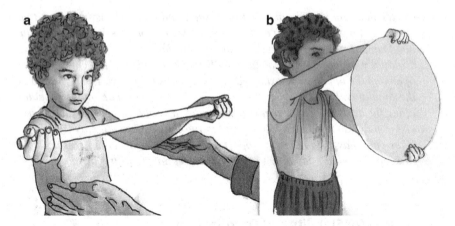

Fig. 5.10 (**a, b**) Activities with kinetic chain closed at the arms and core stability at the trunk

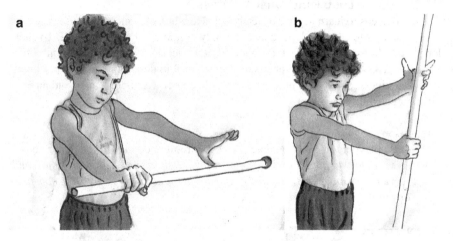

Fig. 5.11 (**a**) Release of one hand at a time. (**b**) Dynamic sequence with alternating upper limb movements

- *Propose activities where the child is required to hold the object with both hands, and then rotate it at 90° and upside down* (Fig. 5.10b).
- As the child improves, propose tasks that require the partial opening of the kinetic chain at the upper limbs and diadochokinesis abilities:
  - *With both their hands resting on a surface, ask the child to move one, and pick up something close,* e.g. *a cookie, to bring to their mouth and eat.*
  - *Propose activities that require alternating holding and letting go of an object with one hand at a time* (Fig. 5.11a, b), e.g. *turning a hoop or a toy steering wheel, pulling a rope towards their body.*
  - *Propose games that require the alternating movements of the hands in a dynamic sequence, adding auditory reinforcement such as voice, hand clapping and/or the beat of a tambourine.*

Fig. 5.12 Fixing part of the body to improve the accuracy of a distal movement

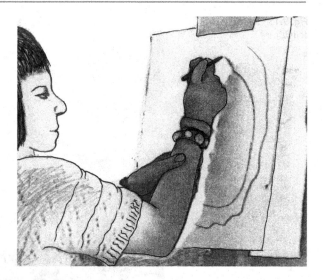

5.2.3   Tasks for Coordination

5.2.3.1 Bimanual/Manual Activities

To play with objects and toys and later to cope with drawing and handwriting tasks, the child should acquire fine and coordinated unilateral and bimanual skills that include the use of tools, such as a pencil and the management of spatial limitations like a page of a notebook. The basic motor patterns are already present in ataxic impairment, and the difficulty is the spatiotemporal incoordination in the execution of the movement.

Furthermore, imprecise proprioceptive information does not allow the child to correctly dose the force to be used both to hold the instrument and to carry out the task.

This child has great difficulty to coordinate multi-joint movements, in particular to stabilise proximal joints when performing fine distal movements. For this, they often adopt functional compensations to facilitate their manual skills, such as fixing the forearm and/or wrist for improving the accuracy of the end-point control (Fig. 5.12). The practitioner and the school teacher can accept these stratagems and even propose them since they do not alter the execution of the gesture, but, on the contrary, they often facilitate it. For writing and drawing, the adults can help the child reduce the number of joints to be controlled, by getting them to wear a light gym wrist weight or by using strips of Velcro,[1] one attached to their wrist and the other to the table surface.

Suggestion
- Involve the child in upper arm activities of reaching, grasping and bimanual manipulation:
  - *Give the child a roll of kitchen paper or similar, and play the game of trapping small objects inside the hole* (Fig. 5.13).

---

[1] Velcro Ltd., Knutsford (UK), www.velcro.uk

Fig. 5.13 Bimanual
activities

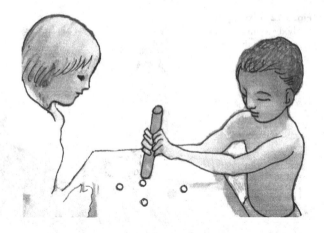

Fig. 5.14 Heavy graphic
trace

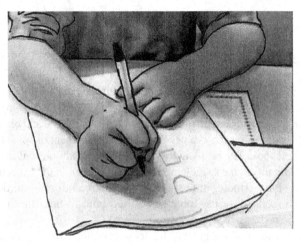

- *Propose activity with play dough to improve fine motor skills; encourage the
  child to squeeze, stretch, roll, pinch and pat the dough to make shapes and
  objects like animals, pretend to make cookies and so on.*
- *Propose activities with children's scissors like cutting out paper figures, such
  as paper dolls and their clothes.*
- *Practise manual feeding skills by introducing a "cookie break" during the
  therapy session inviting them to take some cookies from a box and eat them
  and have a drink.*
- ......
- Depending on the age of the child, propose manual activities with different levels
  of difficulty, such as drawing and pre-/writing.
  1. *Observe the strategies adopted by the child to manage their upper limb insta-
     bility while using a pen/pencil, referring to those described in the short sec-
     tion above. Here below the graphic trace is not fine and light but heavy, due
     to excessive force applied on the medial side of the wrist* (Fig. 5.14).

Fig. 5.15 Piercing
activities

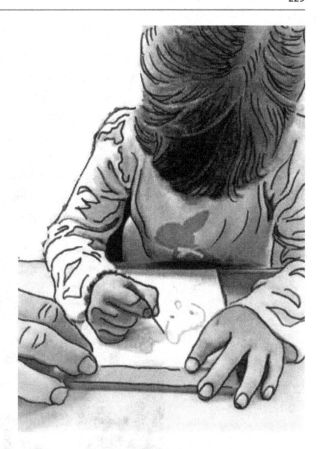

2. *Train the child with activities to improve their control of the execution of distal fine movements:*
   - *Place some cards with figures drawn with dotted lines on a semi-soft board, and ask the child to pierce the points calibrating the force of the pressure with an awl: too much pressure would damage the paper (Fig. 5.15).*
   - *Facilitate selective hand movements by investigating with the child which part of the arm they would like to have stabilised and which part to leave free to perform. For example, the forearm can be stabilised by applying a small gym weight around it and leaving the wrist free to move.*
   - *Ask the child to follow as smoothly as possible some pre-writing lines or a graphic track traced on paper or wood with their index finger or a pen (Fig. 5.16). It is particularly challenging for a schoolchild to trace the line of an Archimedes spiral, as proposed in a MICARS item.*
   - *Today's schoolchildren will be more challenged and have more fun interacting with technological devices that require similar computer-based tasks, e.g. follow a spiral path with a manipulandum, and play video games which have not only rewards for success but also penalties for mistakes (Fig. 5.17).*

Fig. 5.16 Finger tracing

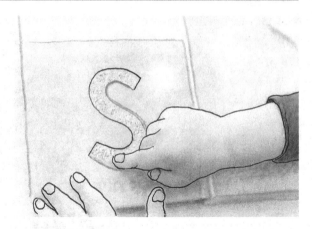

Fig. 5.17 Computer-based tracking tasks

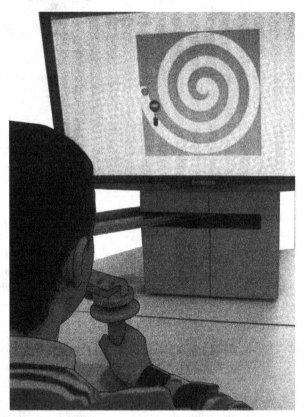

Note

- Interactive videogames, the so-called exergames, including those requiring the use of simple low-cost platforms, can be very enjoyable for the children and, at the same time, a complement to the physiotherapy treatment. Although there is currently little scientific evidence on this sector, home training can incorporate video games with full-body activities that entertain the children and, at the same time, involve them in balance control and multi-joint coordination (Salem et al. 2012; Synofzik and Ilg 2013; Synofzik et al. 2013).

5.2.4 Tasks for Mobility

5.2.4.1 Transfers into Standing

If hypotonia is not a major problem for the individual child with NPCA, they will succeed in walking independently, even though with greater expenditure of energy than other children.

To achieve full independence, it is important to train the child to deal with all transfers from ground level to standing, including all the variabilities that they will encounter in the various phases of moving from one position to the other.

Suggestion
- Propose many transfers from one position to another, varying the levels of antigravity forces:
  - *Guide the child through all transfers to the standing position, including passing through kneeling and half-kneeling*
  - *Remember that, for an ataxic child, moving towards gravity is extremely demanding but also very necessary and therefore it needs to be worked on (Fig. 5.18)*
  - *When the child has poor antigravity stability, in particular in standing, tapping and compression techniques can be useful to recruit and sustain muscle activity and co-contraction (Fig. 5.19a, b)*
- Facilitate a cadenced and paced gait:
  - *Improve the cadence of the gait by adding auditory input like giving vocal timing, beating a tambourine or inviting the child themself to sing a good-rhythm song together while walking*
- Propose more demanding, complex and varied walking experiences:
  - *Walk when pushing a cart and/or person, so that the child is moving against graded resistance, a very efficient and simple facilitation to increase muscle activity*
  - *Practise walking in lifelike environments with a variety of paths and unexpected obstacles: very open areas, uphill and downhill, climb over obstacles, narrow corridors (Fig. 5.20a, b)*
  - *Step in and out and move between different forms with intense perceptual contrasts (Fig. 5.21)*
  - *Walking on surfaces with different perceptual characteristics: sand, pebbles, water, grass, foam, etc.*
  - *Play walking games that require the control of foot placing, for example, without making a noise with their feet, with long "giant" steps or small ant-like steps*
  - *.....*

Fig. 5.18 The half-kneeling position in the transfer to standing

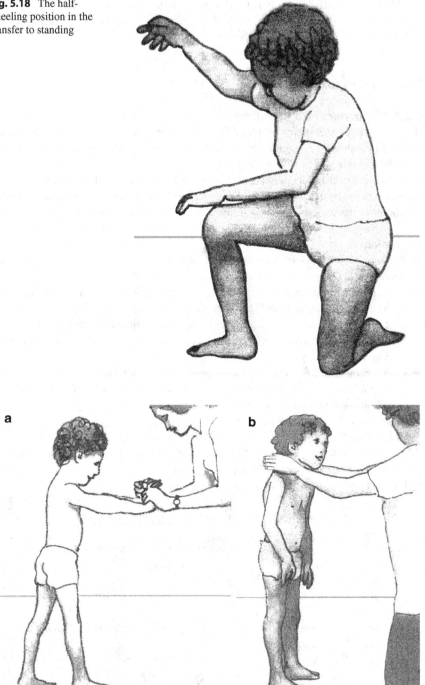

Fig. 5.19 (**a**, **b**) Joint compression techniques in standing

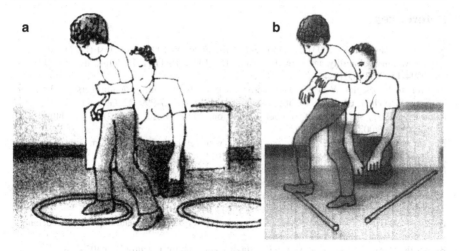

Fig. 5.20   (a) Walking on a narrow path. (b) Stepping over obstacles

Fig. 5.21 Stepping
between blocks

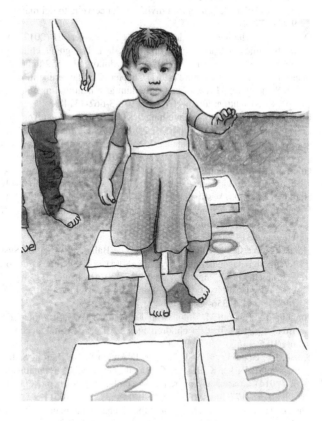

References

Aaron DH, Jansen CW (2003) Development of the Functional Dexterity Test (FDT): construction, validity, reliability, and normative data. J Hand Ther 16(1):12–21. https://doi.org/10.1016/s0894-1130(03)80019-4

Ackermann H, Ziegler W (1992) Die zerebelläre Dysarthrie—eine Literaturübersicht. Fortschr Neurol Psychiatr 60(1):28–40. https://doi.org/10.1055/s-2007-999122. German

Albus JS (1971) A theory of cerebellar function. Math Biosci 10(1–2):25–61. https://doi.org/10.1016/0025-5564(71)90051-4

Bastian AJ (2011) Moving, sensing and learning with cerebellar damage. Curr Opin Neurobiol 21(4):596–601. https://doi.org/10.1016/j.conb.2011.06.007

Berg KO, Wood-Dauphinee SL, Williams JI, Maki B (1992) Measuring balance in the elderly: validation of an instrument. Can J Public Health 83(Suppl 2):S7–S11

Bertini E, Zanni G, Boltshauser E (2018) Nonprogressive congenital ataxias. Handb Clin Neurol 155:91–103. https://doi.org/10.1016/B978-0-444-64189-2.00006-8

Bolk L (1904) Das Cerebellum der Säugetiere: Eine vergleichend anatomische Untersuchung. Nederl Bydragen Anat 3:1–136

Brown JR, Darley FL, Aronson AE (1970) Ataxic dysarhria. Int J Neurol 7(2):302–318

Burgeln N (2018) Atassie congenite. EMC—Neurologia 18(3):1–8. https://doi.org/10.1016/S1634-7072(18)91372-3

Comolli A (1910) Per una nuova divisione del cervelletto dei mammiferi. Arch Ital Anat Embriol 9:247–273

Dayanidhi S, Hedberg A, Valero-Cuevas FJ, Forssberg H (2013) Developmental improvements in dynamic control of fingertip forces last throughout childhood and into adolescence. J Neurophysiol 110(7):1583–1592. https://doi.org/10.1152/jn.00320.2013

Eccles J, Ito M, Szentágothai J (1967) Chapter XV: The cerebellum as a computer? In: Eccles J, Ito M, Szentágothai J (eds) The cerebellum as a neuronal machine. Springer, Berlin Heidelberg, pp 300–315. https://doi.org/10.1007/978-3-662-13147-3

Edinger L (1910) Über die Einteilung des Cerebellums. Anat Anz 35:319–323

Franchignoni F, Horak F, Godi M, Nardone A, Giordano A (2010) Using psychometric techniques to improve the Balance Evaluation Systems Test: the mini-BESTest. J Rehabil Med 42:323–331. https://doi.org/10.2340/16501977-0537

Guell X, Schmahmann J (2020) Cerebellar functional anatomy: a didactic summary based on human fMRI evidence. Cerebellum 19(1):1–5. https://doi.org/10.1007/s12311-019-01083-9

Herdman SJ (2000) Vestibular rehabilitation, 2nd edn. F. A. Davis Co. Publ., Philadelphia

Hoche F, Guell X, Vangel MG, Sherman JC, Schmahmann JD (2018) The cerebellar cognitive affective/Schmahmann syndrome scale. Brain 141(1):248–270. https://doi.org/10.1093/brain/awx317

Horak FB, Wrisley DM, Frank J (2009) The Balance Evaluation Systems Test (BESTest) to differentiate balance deficits. Phys Ther 89(5):484–498. https://doi.org/10.2522/ptj.20080071

Ito M, Yamaguchi K, Nagao S, Yamazaki T (2014) Chapter 1: Long-term depression as a model of cerebellar plasticity. In: Progress in brain research, vol 210, pp 1–30. https://doi.org/10.1016/B978-0-444-63356-9.00001-7

Jongbloed-Pereboom M, Nijhuis-van der Sanden MWG, Steenbergen B (2014) Norm scores of the Box and Block Test for children ages 3–10 years. Am J Occup Ther 67:312–318. https://doi.org/10.5014/ajot.2013.006643

Koziol LF, Budding D, Andreasen N, D'Arrigo S, Bulgheroni S, Imamizu H, Ito M, Manto M, Marvel C, Parker K, Pezzulo G, Ramnani N, Riva D, Schmahmann J, Vandervert L, Yamazaki T (2014) Consensus paper: the cerebellum's role in movement and cognition. Cerebellum 13(1):151–177. https://doi.org/10.1007/s12311-013-0511-x

Larsell O (1947) The development of the cerebellum in man in relation to its comparative anatomy. J Comp Neurol 87(2):85–129. https://doi.org/10.1002/cne.900870203

Lee RW, Poretti A, Cohen JS, Levey E, Gwynn H, Johnston MV, Hoon AH, Fatemi A (2014) A diagnostic approach for cerebral palsy in the genomic era. Neuromol Med 16(4):821–844. https://doi.org/10.1007/s12017-014-8331-9

Lincoln NB, Jackson JM, Adams SA (1998) Reliability and revision of the Nottingham Sensory Assessment for stroke patients. Physiotherapy 84(8):358–365. https://doi.org/10.1016/S0031-9406(05)61454-X

Manto M (2009) Mechanisms of human cerebellar dysmetria: experimental evidence and current conceptual bases. J Neuroeng Rehabil 6:10. https://doi.org/10.1186/1743-0003-6-10

Manto M, Oulad Ben Taib N (2010) Cerebellar nuclei: key roles for strategically located structures. Cerebellum 9(1):17–21. https://doi.org/10.1007/s12311-010-0159-8

Manto M, Mariën P (2015) Schmahmann's syndrome - identification of the third cornerstone of clinical ataxiology. Cerebellum Ataxias. 2015 Feb 27;2:2. https://doi.org/10.1186/s40673-015-0023-1

Manto M, Gandini J, Feil K, Strupp M (2020) Cerebellar ataxias: an update. Curr Opin Neurol. 2020 Feb;33(1):150–160. https://doi.org/10.1097/WCO.0000000000000774

Marr D (1969) A theory of cerebellar cortex. J Physiol 202(2):437–470. https://doi.org/10.1113/jphysiol.1969.sp008820

Mathiowetz V, Federman S, Wiemer D (1985) Box and Block Test of manual dexterity: norms for 6-19 year olds. Can J Occup Ther 52:241–245. https://doi.org/10.1177/000841748505200505

Milani-Comparetti A, Gidoni EA (1971) Significato della semeiotica reflessologica per la diagnosi neuroevolutiva. Neuropsichiatr Infantile 121:252–271

Parolin Schnekenberg R, Perkins EM, Miller JW, Davies WI, D'Adamo MC, Pessia M, Fawcett KA, Sims D, Gillard E, Hudspith K, Skehel P, Williams J, O'Regan M, Jayawant S, Jefferson R, Hughes S, Lustenberger A, Ragoussis J, Jackson M, Tucker SJ, Németh AH (2015) De novo point mutations in patients diagnosed with ataxic cerebral palsy. Brain 138(Pt 7):1817–1832. https://doi.org/10.1093/brain/awv117

Podsiadlo D, Richardson S (1991) The timed "Up & Go": a test of basic functional mobility for frail elderly persons. J Am Geriatr Soc 39(2):142–148. https://doi.org/10.1111/j.1532-5415.1991.tb01616.x

Popa LS, Ebner TJ (2019) Cerebellum, predictions and errors. Front Cell Neurosci 12:524. https://doi.org/10.3389/fncel.2018.00524

Salem Y, Gropack SJ, Coffin D, Godwinc EM (2012) Effectiveness of a low-cost virtual reality system for children with developmental delay: a preliminary randomised single-blind controlled trial. Physiotherapy 98:189–195. https://doi.org/10.1016/j.physio.2012.06.003

Schlerf JE, Verstynen TD, Ivry RB, Spencer RM (2010) Evidence of a novel somatopic map in the human neocerebellum during complex actions. J Neurophysiol 103(6):3330–3336. https://doi.org/10.1152/jn.01117.2009

Schmahmann JD, Schmahmann JC (1998) The cerebellar cognitive affective syndrome. Brain 121:561–579. https://doi.org/10.1093/brain/121.4.561

Schmahmann JD, Gardner R, MacMore J, Vangel MG (2009) Development of a brief ataxia rating scale (BARS) based on a modified form of the ICARS. Mov Disord 24(12):1820–1828. https://doi.org/10.1002/mds.22681

Schmidt RA (1975) A schema theory of discrete motor skill learning. Psychol Rev 82(4):225–260. https://doi.org/10.1037/h0076770

Schmidt RA, Lee TD (2005) Motor control and learning: a behavioral emphasis, 4th edn. Human Kinetic, Champaign

Schmitz-Hubsch T, du Montcel ST, Baliko L, Berciano J, Boesch S, Depondt C, Giunti P, Globas C, Infante J, Kang JS, Kremer B, Mariotti C, Melegh B, Pandolfo M, Rakowicz M, Ribai P, Rola R, Schöls L, Szymanski S, van de Warrenburg BP, Dürr A, Klockgether T, Fancellu R (2006) Scale for the assessment and rating of ataxia: development of a new clinical scale. Neurology 66:1717–1720. https://doi.org/10.1212/01.wnl.0000219042.60538.92

Schniepp R, Möhwald K, Wuehr M (2017) Gait ataxia in humans: vestibular and cerebellar control of dynamic stability. J Neurol 264(Suppl 1):S87–S92. https://doi.org/10.1007/s00415-017-8482-3

Shumway-Cook A, Woollacott M (1995) Motor control theory and applications. Williams and Wilkins Baltimore, pp 323–324

Steinlin M, Styger M, Boltshauser E (1999) Cognitive impairments in patients with congenital nonprogressive cerebellar ataxia. Neurology 53(5):966–973

Synofzik M, Ilg W (2013) Motor training in degenerative spinocerebellar disease: ataxia-specific improvements by intensive physiotherapy and exergames. Biomed Res Int 583507, 11 p. https://doi.org/10.1155/2014/583507

Synofzik M, Schatton C, Giese M, Wolf J, Schöls L, Ilg W (2013) Videogame-based coordinative training can improve advanced, multisystemic early-onset ataxia. J Neurol 260:2656–2658. https://doi.org/10.1007/s00415-013-7087-8

Thivierge JP, Marcus GF (2007) The topographic brain: from neural connectivity to cognition. Trends Neurosci 30(6):251–259. https://doi.org/10.1016/j.tins.2007.04.004

Trouillas P, Takayanagi T, Hallett M, Currier RD, Subramony SH, Wessel K, Bryer A, Diener HC, Massaquoi S, Gomez CM, Coutinho P, Ben Hamida M, Campanella G, Filla A, Schut L, Timann D, Honnorat J, Nighoghossian N, Manyam B (1997) International Cooperative Ataxia Rating Scale for pharmacological assessment of the cerebellar syndrome. J Neurol Sci 145:205–211. https://doi.org/10.1016/s0022-510x(96)00231-6

Verheyden G, Nieuwboer A, Mertin J, Preger R, Kiekens C, De Weerdt W (2004) The Trunk Impairment Scale: a new tool to measure motor impairment of the trunk after stroke. Clin Rehabil 18(3):326–334. https://doi.org/10.1191/0269215504cr733oa

Verheyden G, Nieuwboer A, Van de Winckel A, De Weerdt W (2007) Clinical tools to measure trunk performance after stroke: a systematic review of the literature. Clin Rehabil 21(5):387–394. https://doi.org/10.1177/0269215507074055

Yorkston KM, Beukelman DR (1981) Ataxic dysarthria: treatment sequences based on intelligibility and prosodic considerations. J Speech Hear Disord 46(4):398–404. https://doi.org/10.1044/jshd.4604.398

Sensory-Motor and Perceptual Problems in Cerebral Palsy

6

Psiche Giannoni

Sensation and perception are closely related, but they have different roles in the organization of purposeful functional behaviour and the interpretation of the interaction of the person with the environment. Sensation is the process of acquisition of information and the detection of events through multiple, parallel channels that initiate in the specific peripheral sensory organs (tactile, visual, vestibular, proprioceptive, auditory, olfactory and gustative) and reach specific cortical areas through the thalamus. To a large extent, this continuous and parallel flow of information occurs with little subjective awareness. In contrast, perception is a typically conscious process that extracts "abstract" information from multimodal sensory information, with the aid of acquired cognitive expectations. Examples of this are the perception of shape, discriminating a spherical from a cubic object and the recognition of an apple compared to an orange. To carry out such perceptual-cognitive functions, the brain must learn to "filter" out only the relevant components from the sensory flow, ignoring all the rest, and match the filtered information with learned expectations. Therefore, all sensory inputs and their processing are fundamental requirements for a correct representation of the internal body schema, for postural control and for movement.

In the 1970s, the occupational therapist Jean Ayres developed an approach to address functional disorders of sensory integration processing in children with different disabilities, including cerebral palsy (CP), and she finally designed the Sensory Integration and Praxis Test (SIPT) (Ayres 1973, 1989; Parham et al. 2018) to evaluate these problems. Numerous review articles have investigated the effectiveness of interventions based on sensory integration therapy (SIT). Some are strongly in favour of the approach (May-Benson and Koomar 2010; Kim et al. 2012), and others are positive but with some criticisms because of limited, well-controlled studies (Polatajko and Cantin 2010; Davies and Tucker 2010; Schaaf et al. 2018).

P. Giannoni (✉)
DIBRIS, University of Genoa, Genoa, Italy

© The Author(s), under exclusive license to Springer Nature Switzerland AG 2022
P. Giannoni, L. Zerbino (eds.), *Cerebral Palsy*,
https://doi.org/10.1007/978-3-030-85619-9_6

237

Ayers' assessment addresses a broad category of children with sensory disturbances or minimal brain dysfunctions, but it can also be considered for children with CP (Blanche et al. 1995). CP strokes can also primarily affect the sensorimotor network linked to the cortical and thalamic regions. Evidence confirms that many preterm babies who subsequently develop a spastic or dyskinetic form of CP may exhibit reduced or even increased sensory processing. These deficits further contribute to disturbing their psychomotor development and their relationship with the environment, with a percentage close to 90% in children with USCP being affected (Cooper et al. 1995; Hoon et al. 2009; Tao et al. 2014; Wickremasinghe et al. 2013; Papadelis et al. 2014; Myoung-Ok 2017).

Dunn's model of sensory processing selects four styles of perceptual processing in children, with different neurological thresholds regarding stimulation (high-low) and self-regulation (active-passive) strategies. Children with CP can also react differently to stimulation. For example, they can be hypo-responsive to tactile and proprioceptive inputs and therefore have a low level of arousal and attention to the environment and consequently a more difficult development of body schema and praxis. These children can benefit from sensory input facilitations, such as deep pressure or tapping. Conversely, dyskinetic children can feel disturbed by very "noisy" environments and need an environment filtered from unnecessary stimuli.

Dunn has developed numerous sensory profile tests to evaluate all paediatric age groups and even adults. She also prepared a Sensory Profile Questionnaire for Caregivers to help them better understand the child's perceptual style (Dunn 1997, 2001; Dunn and Daniels 2002).

6.1 Sensory Channels

Although no sensory channel should be excluded a priori, there is clear evidence that some types of sensory information—vestibular, visual and proprioceptive—are more crucial for motor control. The vestibular system is linked to the geocentric frame of reference and allows the body and head to remain aligned with the gravitational environment. Vision, referring to exocentric frames, allows the person to realize their position with respect to the environment, and proprioception provides an egocentric reference of the relationship between different parts of the body. These sensory systems interact closely with each other, as well documented by the studies of Nashner, who developed the Sensory Organization Test (SOT) (Nashner et al. 1982).

Considering SOT, it is interesting to note that, in a play environment, it is also possible to deduce which sensory channels the child use most—and which are problematic—for their interaction with the environment. This is done by momentarily removing an important sensory information to the child (e.g. in sitting or standing with closed eyes) and observing their resulting behaviour.

6.1.1   Dynamic Touch

There is no doubt that all the sensory channels of a normal subject must be integrated to allow them to experience the real world and the shape of their body image through action, with multimodal sensory cooperation (Maravita et al. 2003). Through muscle spindles, Golgi tendon organs and joint receptors, and also with not only passive but also active touch, a child can simultaneously receive both cutaneous and propriocep-tive information, thus having a wider and global haptic experience.

What Is a Haptic Experience
The word "haptic" comes from the Greek *haptikós* that means "suitable for touch" and could be intended as the ability "to grasp something".

Haptic experience is the main vehicle of sensorimotor learning and has the following features:

- It is related to touch but is not the same as touch: it is active, not passive.
- It integrates multimodal sensory information: tactile, kinesthetic, force, sense of effort, sensorimotor expectations and many others.
- Haptic exploration extracts the properties of persons and objects through (1) lateral motion; (2) pressure; (3) static contact; (4) unsupported holding; (5) enclosure; and (6) contour following (Lederman and Klatzky 1987, 2009).
- Haptic experiences are in all activities of daily life: grasping, hitting, pat-ting, squeezing, raking, pinching, weighing, cutting, etc.

In dyadic physical interactions between practitioner and child and parent and child, the haptic experience has multiple benefits and functions:

- Evaluating the haptic features of the child (generally speaking "of the partner")
- Understanding the motor intentions of the child
- Learning the haptic effects on the child of the actions of the adult (parent/ practitioner)
- Evaluating the status of the child, their functional level, their compensation strategies, …
- Providing haptic stimuli to promote active learning
- Optimizing the interaction paradigm in a "personalized" manner (Avila Mireles et al. 2017)

Infants explore and encode the actionable properties of persons and objects and the affordance, i.e. what the environment offers the individual (Gibson 1979), mainly through vision and active touch. However, the capacity to integrate visual and haptic information develops slowly in able-bodied children. Most studies indicate that only children over the age of 8–10 years seem to be able to integrate different sensory inputs with the accuracy of adults. They mostly use vision for orientation discrimination, while haptic strategies are mainly used to determine the size and detailed characteristics of persons and things. Through visual perception, young children usually underestimate the size of the object but become more precise when the object is inside their peri-personal space, in such a way to allow rich haptic interaction (Gori et al. 2008, 2012; Broadbent et al. 2019).

Furthermore, other studies (Purpura et al. 2017, 2019) report that 4-year-olds are already able to recognize common objects through multimodal information processing and even children with BSCP follow the same age-related development, although their performance is generally worse than that of able-bodied children and their preference is always for visual sensory processing over haptics.

It has been shown that children with CP are less able to accurately perceive the property of an object through purposive exploration based on active touch. This is undoubtedly due to the motor problems of these children which limit their interaction with the environment and therefore do not favour significant perceptual experiences (Eliasson et al. 2007; Ocarino et al. 2014). Furthermore, they cannot benefit from previous experiences of manipulation, as can adults after a stroke, who have past experiences of skilled interaction with the environment.

In everyday clinical practice, it often emerges that even the performance of the unaffected arm of the child with unilateral CP shows perceptual problems during active touch, presumably due to their unbalanced sensorial experiences, similar to those reported in studies on adult subjects with stroke (Brasil-Neto and de Lima 2008; Zhang et al. 2014).

These considerations suggest how important it is for the child with motor disabilities to have rich, varied and significant tactile experiences and so plenty of opportunities to touch, be touched and interact tactilely with the environment, while always maintaining attention to their postural alignment, particularly in infants and toddlers.

Concerning the above, it is useful to evaluate children with CP with the Manual Ability Classification System (MACS) or with the Mini-MACS (Eliasson et al. 2007, 2017) for children under the age of 4 years and, consequently, plan intervention based on the outcome of the adopted assessment system.

As for stereognosis, which excludes the use of vision, most evaluations are carried out following the scheme proposed by the tests for adults, although proposing the recognition of objects that the youngster already knows. Since children with difficulty in performing selective movements consequently have less ability in manipulating objects (Wingert et al. 2008; Kinnucan et al. 2010), the practitioner can move the object around in the child's hand and only afterwards ask them to recognize it. Although this may be the only practical solution for an individual child, the therapist should be aware of the difference: an assisted sensory experience is not the same as independent active exploration. Considering the example described, it is the object that is moved in the child's hand, and the child's experience is conditioned by both the way the person has moved the object in their hand and by the child's limited perceptual abilities which allow them to perceive only generic and non-functional characteristics of the object, such as "cold", "hard" and/ or "long".

Some suggestions on how to improve manipulation abilities in the child with CP are discussed in Chap. 9.

6.1.2 Passive Touch

Passive touch occurs when cutaneous mechanoreceptors are stimulated by contact with external persons and things without a voluntary movement related to the object touched. It is a sensory modality that is worth assessing because the cutaneous mechanoreceptors are essential tools for manipulation and the haptic experience of the whole body with the environment. Most of the studies on sensory deficits in CP concern the unilateral form, also involving the unaffected side, and there is much less reported in the other forms (Krumlinde-Sundholm and Eliasson 2007; Sanger and Kukke 2007).

Specific tests concerning tactile sensation are the following:

(a) Light touch, intended here as passive touch and not an active one-finger touch to enhance stability (see below)
(b) Pressure, measured more precisely with Semmes-Weinstein monofilaments
(c) Pinprick
(d) Temperature, using two identical containers filled with hot and cold water
(e) Two-point discrimination, using a calliper or other standardized tools
(f) Tactile localisation and bilateral simultaneous touch

Also for the tactile localisation, it is better to consider the side of the body that is assumed to be not involved or less involved.

Obviously, during the test, the child has to be blindfolded or not be able to use their vision in another way. The assessment should not be limited to the area of the hand but also proposed to other parts of the body.

Another concept to keep in mind is that mechanoreceptors respond differently to the contact modalities and the examiner can voluntarily vary the intensity and/or duration of the stimulus and also vary the time interval between the stimulus and the recognition request. Whatever protocol is chosen, it is implied that the same procedure must always be followed carefully.

Moreover, since this kind of assessment is performed manually, it should only be considered an indicative, qualitative characterization.

6.1.3 Proprioception

Proprioception is a somatosensory modality that allows the appreciation of the position of the joints, the movements of the limbs and the relationship between them.

This information, provided by many sensory channels including muscles, tendons, joints and skin receptors, has a fundamental role in the construction and maintenance of the body schema (Paillard 1980; Schwoebel and Coslett 2005; Pitron et al. 2018).

It is assumed that even the foetus has some primitive perception of its own body. The sense of touch is the first to develop during human gestation. By 8 weeks of gestational age, the foetus responds to touch around lips and cheeks, and, by 11 weeks, they have begun exploring their own face and body and the intra-uterine cavity with their mouth, hands and feet. The motor system develops early too so; from the second trimester, movement and touch together become the baby's two earliest tools for learning about the world around them. The foetus is busy kicking, changing position and practising respiratory movements and non-nutritive thumb-sucking. In the limited space, they experience continual contact of all parts of body with each other and with the uterine wall which defines the spatial boundaries. Studies report that body awareness is already present in newborns and infants (Rochat and Striano 2000; Filippetti et al. 2013).

A crucial functional ability for the baby is the maturation of eye-hand coordination from 3 to 4 months of age, together with the progressive development of movement and relationships with people and the environment, which continues throughout childhood and adolescence. The proprioceptive maturation of fine and selective hand movements takes many years. A study using robot-assisted assessment interestingly reports that wrist movements reach the adult-like level of performance at about the age of 12 years (Marini et al. 2017).

Most studies on impairment in CP are focused mainly on children with a diagnosis of hemiplegia (Hohman et al. 1958; Opila-Lehman et al. 1985; Cooper et al. 1995; Auld et al. 2012; Pavão et al. 2015; Pavão and Rocha 2017), and unfortunately instrumental evaluations, as discussed in Chap. 13 Sect. 13.2.5, are not common (Wingert et al. 2009).

When evaluating the kinaesthetic sense, it is important to distinguish different levels of perceptive competence, as proposed in the Nottingham Sensory Assessment (NSA) (Lincoln et al. 1998), arranged as follows:

0. The child does not detect any movement.
1. The child appreciates movement but not the correct direction.
2. The child can detect the direction of movement.
3. The child reproduces or refers to the position of the joint.

Due to the many levels of impairment of the child, it may be difficult to accurately evaluate their kinaesthesia and joint-position sense. It is implied that, during the assessment, the child should not use their sight and that the adult should first move the less able part when the verification requires the involvement of the opposite side. If motor impairment hinders movement reproduction, a verbal response can be requested, using alternative communication systems if necessary. Furthermore, in these subjective evaluations, close co-operation between the adult and child is necessary, first with a clear formulation of the request by the therapist and then with a valid response by the child. Only a good degree of repeatability of the results can guarantee the accuracy and feasibility of the assessment.

The Affolter-Modell
The Affolter-Modell is based on the concept that a child's development is influenced by their interaction with the environment, a concept that fits in with Bronfenbrenner's ecological development theory (1981). It is therefore particularly important how and how much the child perceives and uses the tactile-kinesthetic information coming from the environment during their daily life. Several authors describe the therapeutic approach aimed at supporting children (and adults) with perceptual difficulties to overcome them (Affolter 1981; Hofer 2009; Affolter and Bischofberger 2016).

The therapeutic guidance by the therapist and child's caregiver is very physical, in the sense that it involves very close, body-body contact. Together, the child and the adult plan an action that should be concluded with the effective functional use of what has been planned and carried out. During the training session, the therapist transmits and underlines tactile and proprioceptive information, such as pressure, weight, weight shifts, active response to hand contact (see CHOR below), rotations, etc., needed to perform and end the planned action. No verbal suggestions are given, only the facilitation of being and acting in close contact with the child.

6.1.4 Vision

Visual problems in CP and suggestions for rehabilitation are discussed in Chap. 11. However, having considered the role of proprioceptive information here, it is interesting to reflect on how and how much vision and proprioception interact with each other and if one prevails over the other.

The area of the head houses two important sensory systems: vision and balance. Antigravity head control develops immediately after birth being the first part of the body that responds to gravity. This early head stability in space allows visual function, already functioning from 36 weeks of gestational age, to be used immediately after and mature in the first months.

Foveal and peripheral vision together play an important role in the detection of objects and motion (Gibson 1966, 1979). When a person moves, they perceive an optic flow that gradually moves around them and expands in the opposite direction, due to the relative movement between them and the environment.

The speed of the flow perceived depends on the speed of the person, on the distance of the destination and therefore of the focus of expansion as well as on the many possible layouts of the environment that expand with different speeds. This happens when moving in a linear direction, but if a transfer requires a combination of translational and rotational movement, the coordinated eye-head movements must intervene and contribute to the rotation.

Another function of vision is to distinguish between self-motion and externally generated motion. If an object moves when the head and eyes are tracking it, the object image remains fixed in the fovea. But, at the same time, the brain knows that the object is moving. Furthermore, when a person looks around to explore the environment and possibly search for objects and persons of interest, they must reconcile the shifting images over the retina with the fact that probably the viewed objects are fixed in the environment.

All these abilities are possible not only due to vision but also with the contribution of the vestibular system and proprioception, the latter provided through the muscle receptors in the neck and the cognitive system. All these systems provide information on the movement of the head and ensure proper eye-head coordination.

There may certainly be primary impairments underlying the sensory problems of the child with CP. However, considering that there are also the pathological deficits of movement in the environment which characterizes all the different forms of CP, it is easily understandable the difficulty the children have in coordinating simultaneously the functions of the different sensorimotor systems.

Abercrombie (1964) pointed out how a motor disability can limit the child's development of spatial awareness and navigation skills. A study by Pavlova et al. (2007) confirmed that teenagers with CP motor impairments caused by perinatal periventricular leukomalacia have more difficulties in visual navigation than other healthy teenagers. A similar conclusion is reported in the research conducted by Ritterband-Rosenbaum et al. (2011, 2012), where improvements in the sense of agency of children with CP were observed after a computer training program in which they had to detect if the track that appeared on the monitor was caused by their movement or by the computer program.

These various sources of knowledge indicate the importance of early experiences in head verticalization and movement in different contexts for the infant and toddler with motor impairment. Many youngsters will need guidance and facilitations to support the maturation of active antigravity control at various levels and to experience being moved and moving independently, all integrated with paying attention to the surrounding environment. Moreover, the young child can practise different modalities of moving in the environment from independent walking, with the use of aids and/or transferring in a chair on wheels with the broader intent of improving spatial awareness and so motor awareness and skills.

6.1.5 Vestibular System

Vestibular dysfunctions in children with CP are often not considered because the motor problems seem more important. However, the vestibular system is critical for effective postural control and visual stabilization. A study of Akbarfahimi et al. in 2016 indicates that 48.4% of children with BSCP have vestibular dysfunction. This is most likely related to the characteristics of the CP pathology, including white matter lesions and/or deficits in the transmission of the vestibulospinal axons and probably also to the reduced use of the vestibular end organs not involved in significant and constant movement training (Rine and Wiener-Vacher 2013; Ghai et al. 2019).

Recent studies are reporting good results for the practice of vestibular stimulation with children with CP or other balance dysfunctions, adapting the traditional vestibular rehabilitation therapy (VRT) with the specifically tailored "pediatric balance therapy (PBT)" training (Lotfi et al. 2016). The main goals of the VRT and PBT programmes are to improve gaze competences and postural stability and so achieve more efficient and richer participation in daily life.

Proposals to enhance gaze stability include head and head-trunk rotation exercises while maintaining visual fixation on a target. Other exercises aim at improving eye movements and imagery pursuit with open and closed eyes (Han et al. 2011).

As for postural stability, exercises require the control of the body position by adopting postural recovery strategies while moving (e.g. on a treadmill) or being moved (sitting in a chair on wheels) and the integration of different somatosensory inputs, such as recognizing one's own position in space and the distance to a target.

Tramontano et al. (2017) report significant improvements in the Goal Attainment Scale in children with BSCP, USCP and ataxia, who received neurodevelopmental treatment and vestibular training over 10 weeks. Positive results are also reported in other studies on the effects of vestibular stimulation on balance in CP children (Hosseini et al. 2015; Shahanawaz et al. 2015).

6.1.6 Vibration

The sensation of vibration, or pallesthesia, is generated by mechanoreceptors that send their inputs to the brain through connective tissue and bones. It is usually tested by placing a low-frequency (usually 128 Hz) long-lasting tuning fork on a bony prominence, as bone tissue is a good vibration resonator.

In recent decades there is a growing interest in vibratory therapy (VT) and its effects on children with CP. In particular, there are two modalities to use VT: (a) focal vibration, applied directly to a muscle belly or a tendon; and (b) whole-body vibration (WBV), which is transmitted through the whole body, usually by asking a subject to stand on a vibrating platform.

The short-term aims of VT are mainly to reduce spinal excitability and hypertonicity and so improve competitive muscle activity, strength and mobility. The long-term aim is to maintain a reduction in spasticity.

There are not many studies reporting the focal application of vibration. Repeated muscle vibrations produced a satisfactory reduction of spasticity when applied on the Achilles tendons of eight children with CP (Celletti and Camerota 2011) and the triceps surae of one 5-year-old child with diplegia (Camerota et al. 2011). One particular study reports the positive effects of muscle vibrations on oro-motor control in 22 children with CP with drooling and swallowing problems (Russo et al. 2019).

Whole-body vibration has been applied and tested on a more significant number of CP cases. Most studies report immediate effects such as improved gait speed, reduced spasticity in knee extensors and a higher score in the Timed Up and Go (TUG) test (Ahlborg et al. 2006; Ruck et al. 2010; Lee and Chon 2013; El-Shamy 2014; Dudoniene et al. 2017; Park et al. 2017). Other trainings with WBV have had positive effects on the upright posture with increased abdominal muscle activity (Unger et al. 2013; Ali et al. 2019).

Some reviews (Sá-Caputo et al. 2016; Ritzmann et al. 2018) and an analysis of the WBV protocol (Pin et al. 2019) conclude that, despite the heterogeneity of the application parameters reported in scientific studies and the strong need for data on long-term outcome, VT is feasible and well tolerated by children with moderate form of CP.

6.2 Pain

Accurate review (van der Slot et al. 2020) and studies (Schwartz et al. 1999; Jahnsen et al. 2004; Opheim et al. 2009; Penner et al. 2013; Poirot et al. 2017; Eriksson et al. 2020) report that 55–70% of adults with CP experience pain, much higher than in general individuals or with other acquired neurological diseases. The prevalence of pain problems is still significant at the average age of 34.3 years, particularly in subjects with CP with Gross Motor Function Classification System (GMFCS) level II and IV, the latter due to the difficulties in managing their daily life with musculo-skeletal problems and joint contractures. Subjects with GMFCS III refer to pain mainly in the legs, perhaps because of the effort to walk with misalignments and progressive patterns in flexion or because they have been using walking aids for a long time. Neck and arm pain also occurs with ageing.

Many features in CP can cause pain including, first of all, the altered sensory and autonomic functioning due to the pathology, spasticity, joint dislocations, soft tissue changes and constipation. Another source of pain could be inappropriate handling during procedures that involve passive movement like dressing and transfers (Parkinson et al. 2013; Bourseul et al. 2016). Pain is often experienced more by highly emotional individuals.

Suggestions for parents to help them understand the signals used by children to communicate discomfort and pain are illustrated in Chap. 1. The presence of pain can limit the social life of the child and cause them to be more aggressive, lose interest in actively participating in therapy sessions and give up trying to be independent.

A fundamental part of the therapist's intervention is to prevent the onset of serious and non-functional body misalignments, which can produce increased muscle tone, secondary contractures and retractions with a consequent reduction of joint range of movement (RoM) and joint subluxations: all this can cause pain.

Pain prevention is also dealt with in Chap. 7 dedicated to soft tissue care where interventions to manage the problem of soft tissue modifications are discussed, both as prevention and as treatment to improve already altered conditions.

Gate Control Theory (GCT)

Melzack and Wall (1965) formulated a model regarding the perception and transmission of pain. They explained that touch, pressure and vibration receptors have a large diameter size and do not transmit pain stimuli, unlike the nociceptive receptors that carry quick and intense pain through the thin myelinated A-δ fibres and chronic pain through the unmyelinated C ones. If a nociceptive and a non-nociceptive stimulus occurs simultaneously, all these fibres behave differently towards the inhibitory interneurons of the spinal cord while sending their signals to the brain. The large fibres excite the interneurons and therefore modulate the pain intensity, while the thin ones do not, bypassing the inhibition activity. This can be observed quite simply when a person hits a part of their body and can alleviate the pain they feel by firmly rubbing that part immediately afterwards.

The principles of the GCT can be applied therapeutically. In fact, the aim of transcutaneous electrical stimulation (TENS) is to overcome the pain stimulus by activating the large-diameter afferent fibres (Kandel et al. 2000).

The condition of the tissues seems to be an important base point for correctly conveying tactile and proprioceptive inputs and controlling nociceptive stimuli, and the therapist can influence the excitation of Aβ fibres positively with their careful and sensitive manual ability. Manual release of soft tissues under restricted barrier conditions (see Sect. 7.1 in Chap. 7) will be useful in children who are at risk to experience pain due to soft tissue problems.

6.3 Praxia

Praxia is not a sense, but the ability to perform intentional movements and to use objects appropriately, in the absence of paresis, incoordination, sensory deficits or impaired comprehension. It can be considered a progression of cognitive and physical actions, necessary to execute every intentional activity.

The purpose of bringing this topic into the discussion is precisely to focus on the close link between sensory-motor skills and praxia. Dyspraxia is a dysfunction caused by poor somatosensory processing and the impairments related to CP can increase ideomotor difficulties, e.g. "how" to manipulate objects, just as motor dyspraxia can lead to an impoverishment of sensory information and therefore of action planning. A study by Lust et al. (2016) reports that children with CP are not accustomed to solving tasks using motor imagery strategies and suggest rehabilitation treatments to work on this particular, useful ability.

Referring to the recommendations published by the European Academy of Childhood Disability in 2012, Baxter points out how motor dyspraxia is only a symptom and can be acquired in mild forms of CP, as opposed to the developmental coordination disorder (DCD) which is one of the many possible causes of dyspraxia (Baxter 2012).

Of course, praxic problems can be only identified from the age of 2 years onwards, since symbolic function appears only after that time. The first signs to recognize a praxic disorder may concern the execution of so-called "transitive" gestures (involving the use of an object, e.g. a spoon) or "intransitive" gestures (not aimed at an object, as sending of a kiss).

As for treatment, a task-oriented approach is indicated even more so in the case of praxic dysfunctions, where the therapist should identify specific activities and help the child to practise them by dividing the actions into small steps.

6.4 Perceptual Issues in Treating Different Parts of the Body

Traditionally, postural control is a term referred to the person's ability to achieve, maintain or restore the antigravity positions of the body in both motionless and dynamic conditions. It is an essential functional motor skill achieved through the ability to adequately collect and interpret inputs from the environment.

Berthoz and Weiss (2000) focuses on the way human beings perceive and control body movement. He argues for a rethinking of the traditional separation between action and perception and the division of perception into five senses. In Berthoz's view, perception and cognition are inherently predictive, functioning to allow the individual to anticipate the consequences of current or potential actions. The brain acts like a simulator that is constantly inventing models to project onto the changing world, models that are adjusted by steady, minute feedback. A person moves in the direction they are looking at, anticipates the trajectory of a falling ball, recovers when they stumble and continually updates their physical position, all thanks to this sense of movement. This interpretation of perception and action allows Berthoz to focus on psychological phenomena largely ignored in standard texts: proprioception and kinaesthesis. These two mechanisms maintain balance and coordinate actions—and basic perceptual and memory processes—involved in navigation.

All the senses and parts of the body are involved together in this effort. In rehabilitation, it is unreasonable to be concerned and focused only on one element and ignore the others. However, head, trunk and limbs have their functional peculiarities which—when their contribution is compromised—can be handled separately at the beginning with a specific manual approach. Immediately afterwards, but also simultaneously, they need to be actively linked again with the whole functioning of the body.

For clarity, the parts of the body are discussed separately below, knowing that this is artificial and that they can only be considered together—as one—in function and so in rehabilitation.

6.4.1 The Head

Because the head is the site of the visual and vestibular systems, it has the role of the stable reference framework for the spatial orientation when the child moves. At the same time, the child with spastic CP moves with an evident counterbalancing "bascule" of the whole body on the frontal plane, due to a reduction of the body's joint-related degrees of freedom and consequently with poor rotation between the two girdles and between head and trunk. For these reasons, the head shows greater variability of movements in the frontal plane, as compensation for the difficulty of moving in space (Hsue et al. 2009; Wallard et al. 2012; Bartonek et al. 2019).

In the dyskinetic forms of CP, the head is disturbed by involuntary movements, and therefore the focus on the target is continuously missed. It is easy to understand how disturbing this dysfunction is by noting the benefit that this child has when the therapist manually stabilizes their head. This facilitation allows the child to move with a clearer perception of the destination point and to markedly reduce the "disarray" in their movement.

Similar problems are found in children with ataxia, who display antigravity instability due to the reduced tonic recruitment and poor spatiotemporal coordination.

The stabilization of the head in space, and the consequent better visual acuity, is fundamental for good postural control, for efficient walking and for the future maturation and education of the child when they have to learn to read and write. It also improves control of the mandibular joints and therefore facilitates feeding (Redstone and West 2004).

Saavedra et al. (2010) studied the influence of vision and trunk control on the head stability of 15 children with different forms of CP (GMFCS I-II-II), during quiet sitting. In addition to the fact that the children show greater head instability on the frontal plane, the study reports that children with BSCP have more postural sway, particularly in closed-eye conditions, unlike the children with dyskinesia who, instead, actually benefit from this condition.

The same is found in clinical experience, observing children with CP spasticity who rely heavily on visual feedback to perform accurate movements at the expense of reduced proprioceptive attention. On the other hand, children with dyskinesia have more visual fixation problems due to continuous involuntary movements of the head and the reduced reliability on visual information that results can enhance the perception of the inputs from other sensory channels, including the auditory one.

It must be remembered that head stability is closely related to trunk stability.

6.4.2 The Trunk

Attention to trunk function is often addressed when the child needs to cope with the independent sitting position since the postural task requires that the head-arm-trunk (HAT) complex acts as a short inverted pendulum. However, the initial basis for achieving and maintaining the sitting position begins long before the independent sitting milestone age, when the baby begins to engage the core muscles by moving and kicking their leg in the supine position.

As Massion and Woollacott (1996) wrote, every movement has a postural component responsible for stabilizing the body and a motor component aimed at achieving a functional goal. The trunk, particularly the lower part with its numerous postural muscles, is the segment of the body most involved in providing stability in upright standing and during movement.

As easily understood, the optimal core area for constant control of movement in an antigravity situation is that which corresponds with the centre of mass (CoM) of the body. It is no coincidence that, even in oriental medicine, the lower Tan Tien is in the same place, where the human can accumulate energy through practice.

Core stability depends on the activation of the abdominal muscles, as well as the muscles around the lumbosacral hinge, the diaphragm and the muscles of the pelvic floor. Their activity becomes the internal anchor point of the body which consequently allows all parts of the body to move smoothly and efficiently.

The lower trunk acts as a sort of "meeting point", where two modalities converge and are used for the body to orientate to vertical positions. In the top-down model, the control of the multiple segments of the body first considers the head position and subsequently the trunk, pelvis and legs. This is the physiological sequence model used by the infant to gradually achieve increasing antigravity postures and finally conquer the standing position. As soon as the feet touch the ground for verticalization, and the main task becomes the balance control, the orientation of the verticality of parts of the body first takes the support surface as a reference point, using a bottom-up model, with reference mainly to the involvement of the ankle and hip.

In addition to the main sensory inputs for motor control that come from the labyrinth, vision and proprioceptors including the light touch (see below), there are the graviceptors that also contribute to orientation of verticality. They are mechanoreceptors located in the stomach, intestines and kidneys and the walls of the blood vessels of the trunk, and they belong to a separate, autonomous perception system, whose inputs start from the bowels and reach the posterior parietal cortex allowing the body to be aware of the posture changes (Mittelstaedt 1996, 1998; Vaitl et al. 2002; Sack 2009). Graviceptors are stimulated through the pelvis movements, and therefore they are particularly sensitive when abdominal and multifidus muscles are coactivated, further supporting the importance of paying attention to the trunk during treatment for postural control.

6.4.3 The Feet

The human has two feet, not in the sense of right and left foot, but because the foot has two different functional roles depending on whether it is in contact with the ground or moves in an open kinetic chain situation.

The foot increases its sensory function every time it enters the walking stance phase and touches something, receiving both exteroceptive and proprioceptive inputs. The anatomical shape of the foot is like a large platform, where specific mechanoreceptors are efficiently distributed according to the task to be managed. A bioengineer would say it is a sophisticated precision force platform, exactly like the one used in gait analysis, to record data related to the displacement of CoM and centre of pressure (CoP) of a body positioned and moving on it.

The human body is an inverted pendulum that, in quiet standing, sways imperceptibly back and forth on a sagittal and frontal plane, rotating on the ankle torque. The sway is determined by the difference in the projection of CoM and the point of application of the ground reaction force (CoP) on the ground (Morasso et al. 1999).

In a more dynamic situation, such as walking forwards, the CoP moves at the first contact of the heel on the ground, from the back of the foot to the big toe, preparing the foot for the pushing action. In the transition between these two actions, when there is a full monopodalic load and the body moves forwards, the CoP also displaces sideways, approaching both the transverse and lateral arch of the foot (Winter 1995; Kavounoudias et al. 1998).

This means that, for this shift to take place effectively, the body needs the entire foot area and an appropriate alignment of the three arches of the foot, which is rarely the case in children with CP who often have their feet in equinus and cannot exercise any torque at the tibiotarsal joint.

Furthermore, the characteristics and distribution of the mechanoreceptors on the sole are not by chance but based on the type of stimulus they usually receive for the function. For example, slowly adapting receptors are present more along the borders of the foot, while the toe and heel receptors have a high afferent firing threshold to the traversal arch and metatarsal area, although generally the toes are perceptually more sensitive (Inglis et al. 2002; Strzalkowski et al. 2015).

As for the therapeutic intervention by a practitioner, it is necessary to distinguish the different aims and situations of sensory stimulation:

(a) It is certainly beneficial for the child to have plenty of tactile experiences to the feet and so be barefoot often and take advantage of play, dressing, bathing activities and so on. Therapy sessions can include stimulation to the soles of the feet with objects like sponges, scrubber gloves and soft spiky balls, remembering that it is always fun for youngsters to play with water, in sand and coloured balls pits. The goals are to increase the level of perceptual awareness to the sensory stimulus in the feet when the threshold is too high or to improve perceptual tolerance when it is too low.

(b) When immediate therapeutic goals include transfers such as from sitting to standing and return, or activities like taking steps and walking, training should be primarily focused to modify the tissue tensions in leg and foot, obtain more RoM to the joints and realign the body segments to improve motor control and prepare for the next functional task. The equinus foot can be reduced in the excursion in dorsiflexion at the ankle joint and metatarsophalangeal joints, and the "heel to toe" movement is not performed. This will limit the physiological phases of the gait cycle, and therefore the therapist should prepare the biomechanical conditions to improve the contact of the foot with the ground.

Fig. 6.1 Alignment of the foot before the uprighting of the body

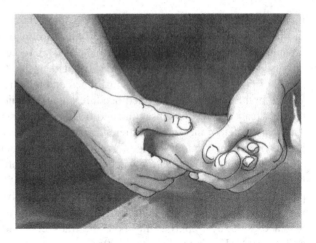

Practical Suggestion
- To promote function in the feet, improve the alignment (Fig. 6.1), and then propose a sit-to-stand transfer or walking, or simply train more efficient pelvis bridging with the child in the supine position:
  - *First, manually elongate the* triceps surae, *and activate concentric contraction of the* tibialis anterior, *to increase RoM of the tibial-tarsal joint.*
  - *Apply the manual distraction-compression technique to the tarsal joints—including those of the cuboid bone—and realign the medial side of the foot to recreate the medial arch that will engage the big toe and be used for the push-off phase.*
  - *As for the lateral side of the foot, manually release* the lumbricalis *and* interossei dorsales *muscles, and activate the* abductor digiti minimi *to gain length and width of the foot with an increased lateral arch.*

Note
- With these premises, the anterior transverse arch is better connected to the other arches, and the foot should be more stable to manage the medial-lateral displacement of the CoM. In the same way, it is more available for the heel-to-toe movement on the sagittal plane. Only after this preparation does it make sense to provide the foot with another type of sensory information that requires greater attention to the contact of the foot with the ground and to the weight-shifting on the sagittal and frontal planes, perceived more with eyes closed.

During the gait stance phase in a child with CP, due to the uneven contact of the foot with the ground, it is difficult to have good integration of the afferent signals coming from the distal part of the leg at the level of the spine, brain stem and cerebellum and those necessary for an efficient antigravity response. Furthermore, the reduced RoM at the ankle and metatarsophalangeal joints limits both the standing still position and dynamic movement.

At the end of the stance phase and in all postural situations where the foot is not in contact with the ground, the foot changes its role and controls its movement in an open chain situation. It is not accurate to no longer consider it a "sensorial foot", because only the influential forces of the different types of inputs are different and the proprioceptive components become more important than the exteroceptive ones.

To support limb movement, the body should be and remain stable posturally so that all muscles can function according to the dynamic task to be performed. It is very important that the therapist is aware of the most likely sequence of the movement in progress and, if necessary, provides in advance the proprioceptive inputs necessary for the child to actively perform it, intervening to improve their body awareness and motor control.

In the chapters concerning the various forms of CP, practical suggestions are provided on how to deal with these functional situations.

Considerations About Orthosis

The prescription of an orthosis to improve the child's anti-gravity posture is a complex decision, which requires a very careful evaluation of the child's characteristics (Brunner et al. 2008).

The purpose of the ankle-foot orthosis (AFO) is to improve the foot alignment, stabilize the ankle and extend the knee. At the same time, it significantly limits the adjustment strategy at the ankle and the heel-to-toe movement of the foot. Nowadays, some orthoses are made of semi-flexible thermoplastic materials, but most of them still allow little or no mobility. From the biomechanical point of view, when the ankle strategy is limited, the mobility needed distally will be compensated elsewhere, normally at the hip joint, as usually happens in the elderly. There is also a close interaction between the ankle, knee and hip, and, in the case of a normal musculoskeletal system and anti-gravity postural adjustment, one joint behaves according to the RoM of the other two.

The strategy at the hip should come into play, but often in the child with CP, the joint is not able to react appropriately due to the poor posterior muscle chain activity. In this case, the most feasible reaction is to over-stabilize the hip with increased concentric activity of the iliopsoas muscles. Being aware of this possibility, the therapist should work to prevent it by strengthening the postural muscles and carefully verifying the RoM of the hip joint, even in a prone position, before the child moves into standing.

There is strong evidence reported in the review article published by Lintanf et al. in 2018 that children with CP benefit greatly from wearing an AFO. Currently there is increased interest in the moulded hinged AFOs and other orthoses that control the ankle while allowing some degree of joint movement and that have a more flexible footplate (Park et al. 2004). These considerations underline the need for close collaboration between therapists and orthotic professionals and a constant, combined interprofessional verification of the effects of the orthosis on the child's posture and movement. They should verify that the planned orthosis meets the real needs of the child and their family, with regard to both the biomechanical aspects and the functional activity, based on the indications of ICF-CY.

6.4.4 The Hand

The way the sensory receptors are distributed in the hand has its particular functional significance, just as in the foot. Their tasks are not only related to the fundamental functions of reaching, grasping and manipulating but also include the stability and orientation of the body in the environment. The hand itself is the principle instrument for dynamic touch, and it represents not only the involvement of the arm but that of the whole body, with the contribution of multiple sensory inputs.

Jeannerod's considerations in 1983 regarding the prehension task accurately described the sequence of the approach of the hand to a target object, distinguishing a fast-velocity initial phase with open hand and fingers stretched and a final phase, at two-thirds of the way, when the velocity slows down and the hand starts to shape its fingers according to the intrinsic-extrinsic characteristics of the object, its position in the environment and the functional use planned for it.

In this sequence, the distal working point is the hand, but the trajectory of the movement takes place within a space that refers to the body as a point of stability. In a prehension task, the hand is the peculiar element that decides to grasp an object, but the movement needs the co-operation of proximal postural stability. Otherwise, the functional movement would be limited and inaccurate.

It is known that objects do not move but that the person approaches them. Every young infant and child with CP should be encouraged to behave in the same way, without the adult automatically transferring things into their hands. Clearly, little real hand function will end up being possible independently in the presence of severe upper arm impairment. To promote and facilitate hand-object behaviour, the therapist should first verify the upright straightening of the child's trunk and the RoM at the shoulder girdle, and, if necessary, work on the soft tissues to obtain more muscle elongation and joint alignment before soliciting the active involvement of the arm. The first phase of the hand approaching a target requires a certain elevation and external rotation at the shoulder, a *biceps-triceps* interaction with the *triceps brachialis* activated for extension and the thumb pointing straight in the direction of the target. Close to the object, the wrist and little finger should maintain a certain extension to prepare the hypothenar side of the hand to make contact with the object and hold it firmly. It is the thenar part of the hand that is most involved in the final phase of grasping.

The function of the hand is not only the interaction with objects but also to approach surfaces to support and push on them in order to increase the core activity and actually take on part of the body weight. The strategies used to perform these tasks are similar to those for grasping, but for these functions the hand must already be open, ready for placement on the surface, to feel and be aware of the surface and be ready to interact with it. For this reason the therapist should selectively strengthen the intrinsic muscles of the hand, before it approaches the surface.

Since the inner side of the forearm and wrist, as well as the hypothenar part of the hand, has a greater stability function than the outer side, it is useful that this side is the first to make contact with the surface in order to promote active placing and perceptual awareness of the whole hand. This "aware" hand can help the child to have more stable reference points and active support, e.g. when rotating the pelvis in the supine position, during bridging and pivoting in sitting.

Raine et al. (2009) reported that the experience of frictional contact of the hand to a surface (contact hand orientation response, CHOR) is transferred to the whole body and allows a person to enhance their midline orientation, balance and weight-bearing on limbs. There do not seem to be many scientific studies on CHOR applied to the treatment of children, but it is successfully applied in adults with motor impairment to improve upright standing and postural transfers, such as sitting to standing (Seo et al. 2018).

Light Touch Contact

Light touch is a particular contribution of the hand to the body's antigravity stability where, if used, it can reduce the postural sway in upright positions (Holden et al. 1994; Jeka and Lackner 1994, 1995; Jeka 1997). Individuals, including children, with sensory-motor impairment can take advantage of this facilitation when standing and walking, for example.

Light touch contact (LTC) is intended as an active touch facilitation. It is the result of cutaneous and kinaesthetic information which is available when a fingertip rests and slides imperceptibly on a stable surface, exerting a load not exceeding 100 gr. or 1 N. This means that, through this light contact, a person can use a stable surface as a reference frame to organize and improve their upright posture. Many studies report how the effect of light touch can be observed when a person touches a surface, even vertical, with a finger or through a stick, both with eyes open and closed (Krishnamoorthy et al. 2002; Baccini et al. 2007; Shima et al. 2013; In et al. 2019; Mitani et al. 2019).

A similar application of LTC has been employed in young adults, using two vibrotactile devices positioned at L5 spinal level as biofeedback, with the aim of improving their postural control and balance. The results reported a significant reduction of the sway amplitude in standing (Ballardini et al. 2020). Shima et al. (2021) obtain similar results applying a wearable light touch system to fingertips.

Few studies report the effects of LTC in infants with traditional development, and one of those was conducted with infants at the beginning of their independent walking experience. A force platform recorded data of their free walking and when holding a floating balloon full of helium, contrived as a possible reference frame. The results showed that body sway decreased when the infants were walking with the balloon (Shimatani et al. 2015a, b; Shima et al. 2017).

There is interesting relevance for daily caregiving and rehabilitation sessions in the analysis of Watanabe and Tani (2020) that investigated the different effects of active and passive light touch and no touch when a person performs a difficult postural task. The experience of passive light touch could reflect the moments when therapists and caregivers touch the person to help them to perceive and maintain their posture, without supporting their body weight. Results showed that the information received passively, even with light touch, is less effective for postural stability than actively performed LT. Moreover, results from the same study report that active LTC is most effective when the person has their eyes closed.

References

Abercrombie MLJ (1964) Perceptual and visuo-motor disorders in cerebral palsy: a review of the literature. Spastics Society, Heinemann, London

Affolter F (1981) Perceptual processes as prerequisites for complex human behaviour. Int Rehabil Med 3(1):3–10. https://doi.org/10.3109/03790798109167107

Affolter F, Bischofberger W (2016) From roots to branches Part III: a contribution to solving problems of everyday life of children, adolescents and adults with disorders of perception—in regular or special schools, in rehabilitation centers and families. Neckar-Verlag

Ahlborg L, Andersson C, Julin P (2006) Whole-body vibration training compared with resistance training: effect on spasticity, muscle strength and motor performance in adults with cerebral palsy. J Rehabil Med 38(5):302–308. https://doi.org/10.1080/16501970600680262

Akbarfahimi N, Hosseini SA, Rassafiani M, Rezazadeh N, Shahshahani S, Tabatabai Ghomsheh F, Karimlou M (2016) Assessment of the saccular function in children with spastic cerebral palsy. Neurophysiology 48(2):141–149. https://doi.org/10.1007/s11062-016-9580-z

Ali MS, Awad AS, Elassal MI (2019) The effect of two therapeutic interventions on balance in children with spastic cerebral palsy: a comparative study. J Taibah Univ Med Sci 14(4):350–356. https://doi.org/10.1016/j.jtumed.2019.05.005

Auld ML, Boyd RN, Moseley GL, Ware RS, Johnston LM (2012) Impact of tactile dysfunction on upper-limb motor performance in children with unilateral cerebral palsy. Arch Phys Med Rehabil 93(4):696–702. https://doi.org/10.1016/j.apmr.2011.10.025

Avila Mireles EJ, Zenzeri J, Squeri V, Morasso P, De Santis D (2017) Skill learning and skill transfer mediated by cooperative haptic interaction. IEEE Trans Neural Syst Rehabil Eng 25(7):832–843. https://doi.org/10.1109/TNSRE.2017.2700839

Ayres AJ (1973) Sensory integration and learning disorders. Western Psychological Services Publ, Los Angeles

Ayres AJ (1989) Sensory integration and praxis test. Western Psychological Services Publ, Los Angeles

Baccini M, Rinaldi LA, Federighi G, Vannucchi L, Paci M, Masotti G (2007) Effectiveness of fingertip light contact in reducing postural sway in older people. Age Ageing 36(1):30–35. https://doi.org/10.1093/ageing/afl072

Ballardini G, Florio V, Canessa A, Carlini G, Morasso P, Casadio M (2020) Vibrotactile feedback for improving standing balance. Front Bioeng Biotechnol 16:137. https://doi.org/10.3389/fbioe.2020.00094

Bartonek A, Lidbeck C, Hellgren K, Gutierrez-Farewik E (2019) Head and trunk movements during turning gait in children with cerebral palsy. J Mot Behav 51(4):362–370. https://doi.org/10.1080/00222895.2018.1485009

Baxter P (2012) Developmental coordination disorder and motor dyspraxia. Dev Med Child Neurol 54(1):3. https://doi.org/10.1111/j.1469-8749.2011.04196.x

Berthoz A, Weiss G (2000) The brain's sense of movement (Perspectives in Cognitive Neuroscience). Harvard University Press, Boston

Blanche EI, Botticelli TM, Hallway MK (1995) Combining neuro-developmental treatment and sensory integration principles: an approach to pediatric therapy. Academic, pp 67–84

Bourseul JS, Brochard S, Houx L, Pons C, Bué M, Manesse I, Ropars J, Guyader D, Le Moine P, Dubois A (2016) Care-related pain and discomfort in children with motor disabilities in rehabilitation centres. Ann Phys Rehabil Med 59(5–6):314–319. https://doi.org/10.1016/j.rehab.2016.04.009

Brasil-Neto JP, de Lima AC (2008) Sensory deficits in the unaffected hand of hemiparetic stroke patients. Cogn Behav Neurol 21(4):202–205. https://doi.org/10.1097/WNN.0b013e3181864a24

Broadbent H, Osborne T, Kirkham N, Mareschal D (2019) Touch and look: the role of visual-haptic cues for categorical learning in primary school children. Inf Child Dev 29:e2168. https://doi.org/10.1002/icd.2168

Bronfenbrenner U (1981) Die Ökologie der menschlichen Entwicklung. Klett, Stuttgart (orig. 1979)

Brunner R, Dreher T, Romkes J, Frigo C (2008) Effects of plantarflexion on pelvis and lower limb kinematics. Gait & Posture, Vol.28, Issue 1, July 2008, pages 150-156. https://doi.org/10.1016/j.gaitpost.2007.11.013

Camerota F, Galli M, Celletti C, Vimercati S, Cimolin V, Tenore N, Filippi GM, Albertini G (2011) Quantitative effects of repeated muscle vibrations on gait pattern in a 5-year-old child with cerebral palsy. Case Rep Med 2011:359126. https://doi.org/10.1155/2011/359126

Celletti C, Camerota F (2011) Preliminary evidence of focal muscle vibration effects on spasticity due to cerebral palsy in a small sample of Italian children. Clin Ter 162(5):e125–e128

Cooper J, Majnemer A, Rosenblatt B, Birnbaum R (1995) The determination of sensory deficits in children with hemiplegic cerebral palsy. J Child Neurol 10(4):300–309. https://doi.org/10.1177/088307389501000412

Davies PL, Tucker R (2010) Evidence review to investigate the support for subtypes of children with difficulty processing and integrating sensory information. Am J Occup Ther 64:391–402. https://doi.org/10.5014/ajot.2010.09070

Dudoniene V, Lendraitiene E, Pozeriene J (2017) Effect of vibration in the treatment of children with spastic diplegic cerebral palsy. J Vibroeng 19(7):5520–5526. https://doi.org/10.21595/jve.2017.18250

Dunn W (1997) The impact of sensory processing abilities on the daily lives of young children and their families: a conceptual model. Infants Young Child 9(4):23–35. https://doi.org/10.1097/00001163-199704000-00005

Dunn W (2001) The sensations of everyday life: empirical, theoretical, and pragmatic considerations. Am J Occup Ther 55(6):608–620. https://doi.org/10.5014/ajot.55.6.608

Dunn W, Daniels DB (2002) Initial development of the infant/toddler sensory profile. J Early Interv 25(1):27–41. https://doi.org/10.1177/105381510202500104

Eliasson AC, Krumlinde-Sundholm L, Rösblad B, Beckung E, Arner M, Öhrvall AM, Rosenbaum P (2007) The Manual Ability Classification System (MACS) for children with cerebral palsy: scale development and evidence of validity and reliability. Dev Med Child Neurol 2006(48):549–554. https://doi.org/10.1111/j.1469-8749.2006.tb01313.x

Eliasson AC, Ullenhag A, Wahlström U, Krumlinde-Sundholm L (2017) Mini-MACS: development of the Manual Ability Classification System for children younger than 4 years of age with signs of cerebral palsy. Dev Med Child Neurol 2017(59):72–78. https://doi.org/10.1111/dmcn.13162

El-Shamy SM (2014) Effect of whole-body vibration on muscle strength and balance in diplegic cerebral palsy: a randomized controlled trial. Am J Phys Med Rehabil 93(2):114–121. https://doi.org/10.1097/PHM.0b013e3182a541a4

Eriksson E, Hägglund G, Alriksson-Schmidt AI (2020) Pain in children and adolescents with cerebral palsy—a cross-sectional register study of 3545 individuals. BMC Neurol 20:15. https://doi.org/10.1186/s12883-019-1597-7

Filippetti ML, Johnson MH, Lloyd-Fox S, Dragovic D, Farroni T (2013) Body perception in newborns. Curr Biol 23(23):2413–2416. https://doi.org/10.1016/j.cub.2013.10.017

Ghai S, Hakim M, Dannenbaum E, Lamontagne A (2019) Prevalence of vestibular dysfunction in children with neurological disabilities: a systematic review. Front Neurol 17(10):1294. https://doi.org/10.3389/fneur.2019.01294

Gibson JJ (1966) The senses considered as perceptual systems. Houghton Mifflin, MA, Boston

Gibson JJ (1979) The ecological approach to visual perception. Houghton Mifflin, MA, Boston

Gori M, Del Viva M, Sandini G, Burr DC (2008) Young children do not integrate visual and haptic form information. Curr Biol 18(9):694–698. https://doi.org/10.1016/j.cub.2008.04.036

Gori M, Giuliana L, Sandini G, Burr D (2012) Visual size perception and haptic calibration during development. Dev Sci 15(6):854–862. https://doi.org/10.1111/j.1467-7687.2012.2012.01183.x

Han BI, Song HS, Kim JS (2011) Vestibular rehabilitation therapy: review of indications, mechanisms, and key exercises. J Clin Neurol 7(4):184–196. https://doi.org/10.3988/jcn.2011.7.4.184

Hofer A (2009) Das Affolter-Modell: Entwicklungsmodell und gespürte Interaktionstherapie. Pflaum, München

Hohman LB, Baker L, Reed R (1958) Sensory disturbances in children with infantile hemiplegia, triplegia, and quadriplegia. Am J Phys Med 37(1):1–6

Holden M, Ventura J, Lackner JR (1994) Stabilization of posture by precision contact of the index finger. J Vest Res 4:285–301

Hoon AH, Stashinko EE, Nagae LM, Lin DDM, Keller J, Bastian A, Campbell ML, Levey E, Mori S, Johnston MV (2009) Sensory and motor deficits in children with cerebral palsy born preterm correlate with diffusion tensor imaging abnormalities in thalamocortical pathways. Dev Med Child Neurol 51(9):697–704. https://doi.org/10.1111/j.1469-8749.2009.03306.x

Hosseini SA, Ghoochani BZ, Talebian S, Pishyare E, Haghgoo HA, Meymand RM, Zeinalzadeh A (2015) Investigating the effects of vestibular stimulation on balance performance in children with cerebral palsy: a randomized clinical trial study. J Rehabil Sci Res 2(2):41–46. https://doi.org/10.30476/JRSR.2015.41073

Hsue BJ, Miller F, Su FC (2009) The dynamic balance of the children with cerebral palsy and typical developing during gait. Part I: spatial relationship between COM and COP trajectories. Gait Posture 29:465–470. https://doi.org/10.1016/j.gaitpost.2008.11.007

In TS, Jung JH, Jang SH, Kim KH, Jung KS, Cho HY (2019) Effects of Light Touch on balance in patients with stroke. Open Med (Wars) 14:259–263. https://doi.org/10.1515/med-2019-0021

Inglis JT, Kennedy PM, Wells C, Chua R (2002) The role of cutaneous receptors in the foot. Adv Exp Med Biol 508:111–117. https://doi.org/10.1007/978-1-4615-0713-0_14

Jahnsen R, Villien L, Aamodt G, Stanghelle JK, Holm I (2004) Musculoskeletal pain in adults with cerebral palsy compared with the general population. J Rehabil Med 36(2):78–84. https://doi.org/10.1080/16501970310018305

Jeannerod M (1983) The timing of natural prehension movements. J Mot Behav 16(3):235–254. https://doi.org/10.1080/00222895.1984.10735319

Jeka JJ (1997) Light touch contact as a balance aid. Phys Ther 77(5):476–487. https://doi.org/10.1093/ptj/77.5.476

Jeka JJ, Lackner JR (1994) Fingertip contact influences human postural control. Exp Brain Res 100(3):495–502. https://doi.org/10.1007/bf02738408

Jeka JJ, Lackner JR (1995) The role of haptic cues from rough and slippery surfaces in human postural control. Exp Brain Res 103(2):267–276. https://doi.org/10.1007/bf00231713

Kandel ER, Schwartz JH, Jessell TM (2000) Principles of neural science, 4th edn. McGraw-Hill, New York, pp 482–486

Kavounoudias A, Roll R, Roll JP (1998) The plantar sole is a 'dynamometric map' for human balance control. Neuroreport 9:3247–3252. https://doi.org/10.1097/00001756-199810050-00021

Kim HH, Hwang-Bo G, Kook Yoo B (2012) The effects of a sensory integration programme with applied interactive metronome training for children with developmental disabilities: a pilot study. Hong Kong J Occup Ther 22(1):25–30. https://doi.org/10.1016/j.hkjot.2012.05.001

Kinnucan E, Van Heest A, Tomhave W (2010) Correlation of motor function and stereognosis impairment in upper limb cerebral palsy. J Hand Surg Am 35(8):1317–1322. https://doi.org/10.1016/j.jhsa.2010.04.019

Krishnamoorthy V, Slijper H, Latash ML (2002) Effects of different types of light touch on postural sway. Exp Brain Res 147(1):71–79. https://doi.org/10.1007/s00221-002-1206-6

Krumlinde-Sundholm L, Eliasson AC (2007) Comparing tests of tactile sensibility: aspects relevant to testing children with spastic hemiplegia. Dev Med Child Neurol 2002(44):604–612. https://doi.org/10.1017/s001216220100264x

Lederman SJ, Klatzky RL (1987) Hand movements: a window into haptic object recognition. Cogn Psychol 19:342–368. https://doi.org/10.1016/0010-0285(87)90008-9

Lederman SJ, Klatzky RL (2009) Haptic perception: a tutorial. Attent Percept Psychophys 71(7):1439–1459. https://doi.org/10.3758/APP.71.7.1439

Lee BK, Chon SC (2013) Effect of whole body vibration training on mobility in children with cerebral palsy: a randomized controlled experimenter-blinded study. Clin Rehabil 27(7):599–607. https://doi.org/10.1177/0269215512470673

Lincoln NB, Jackson JM, Adams SA (1998) Reliability and revision of the Nottingham Sensory Assessment for stroke patients. Physiotherapy 84(8):358–365. https://doi.org/10.1016/S0031-9406(05)61454-X

Lintanf M, Bourseul JS, Houx L, Lempereur M, Brochard S, Pons C (2018) Effect of ankle-foot orthoses on gait, balance and gross motor function in children with cerebral palsy: a systematic review and meta-analysis. Clin Rehabil 32(9):1175–1188. https://doi.org/10.1177/0269215518771824

Lotfi Y, Rezazadeh N, Moossavi A, Haghgoo H, Farokhi Moghadam S, Pishyareh E et al (2016) Introduction of pediatric balance therapy in children with vestibular dysfunction: review of indications, mechanisms, and key exercises. Iran Rehabil J 14(1):5–14. https://doi.org/10.15412/J.IRJ.08140102

Lust JM, Wilson PH, Steenbergen B (2016) Motor Imagery difficulties in children with cerebral palsy: a specific or general deficit? Res Dev Disabil 57:102–111. https://doi.org/10.1016/j.ridd.2016.06.010

Maravita A, Spence C, Driver J (2003) Multisensory integration and the body schema: close to hand and within reach. Curr Biol 13(13):R531–R539. https://doi.org/10.1016/s0960-9822(03)00449-4

Marini F, Squeri V, Morasso P, Campus C, Konczak J, Masia L (2017) Robot-aided developmental assessment of wrist proprioception in children. J Neuroeng Rehabil 14(1):3. https://doi.org/10.1186/s12984-016-0215-9

Massion J, Woollacott MH (1996) Posture and equilibrium. In: Bronstein AM, Brandt T, Woollacoot MH (eds) Clinical disorders of balance, und and gait, 1st edn. Arnold Ed, London

May-Benson T, Koomar J (2010) Systematic review of the research evidence examining the effectiveness of interventions using a sensory integrative approach for children. Am J Occup Ther 64:403–414. https://doi.org/10.5014/ajot.2010.09071

Melzack R, Wall PD (1965) Pain mechanisms: a new theory. Science 150(3699):971–979. https://doi.org/10.1126/science.150.3699.971

Mitani R, Shimatani K, Sakata M, Mukaeda T, Shima K (2019) Effects of somatosensory information provision to fingertips for mitigation of postural sway and promotion of muscle coactivation in an upright posture. In: 2019 41st annual international conference of the IEEE engineering in medicine and biology society (EMBC). https://doi.org/10.1109/EMBC.2019.8856942

Mittelstaedt H (1996) Somatic graviception. Biol Psychol 42(1–2):53–74. https://doi.org/10.1016/0301-0511(95)05146-5

Mittelstaedt H (1998) Origin and processing of postural information. Neurosci Biobehav Rev 22(4):473–478. https://doi.org/10.1016/s0149-7634(97)00032-8

Morasso P, Baratto L, Capra R, Spada G (1999) Internal models in the control of posture. Neural Netw 12(7–8):1173–1180. https://doi.org/10.1016/s0893-6080(99)00058-1

Myoung-Ok P (2017) The relationship between sensory processing abilities and gross and fine motor capabilities of children with cerebral palsy. J Korean Soc Phys Med 12(2):67–74. https://doi.org/10.13066/kspm.2017.12.2.67

Nashner LM, Black FO, Wall C (1982) Adaptation to altered support and visual conditions during stance: patients with vestibular deficits. J Neurosci 2(5):536–544. https://doi.org/10.1523/JNEUROSCI.02-05-00536.1982

Ocarino JM, Fonseca ST, Silva PLP, Gonçalves GGP, Souza TR, Mancini MC (2014) Dynamic touch is affected in children with cerebral palsy. Hum Mov Sci 33:85–96. https://doi.org/10.1016/j.humov.201308.007

Opheim A, Jahnsen R, Olsson E, Stanghelle JK (2009) Walking function, pain, and fatigue in adults with cerebral palsy: a 7-year follow-up study. Dev Med Child Neurol 51(5):381–388. https://doi.org/10.1111/j.1469-8749.2008.03250.x

Opila-Lehman J, Short MA, Trombly CA (1985) Kinesthetic recall of children with athetoid and spastic cerebral palsy and of non-handicapped children. Dev Med Child Neurol 27(2):223–230. https://doi.org/10.1111/j.1469-8749.1985.tb03773.x

Paillard J (1980) Le corps situé et le corps identifié. Une approche psychophysiologique de la notion de schéma corporel. Rev Méd Suisse Romande 100:129–141

Papadelis C, Ahtam B, Nazarova M, Nimec D, Snyder B, Grant PE, Okada Y (2014) Cortical somatosensory reorganization in children with spastic cerebral palsy: a multimodal neuroimaging study. Front Hum Neurosci 8:725. https://doi.org/10.3389/fnhum.2014.00725

Parham LD, Smith Roley S, May-Benson TA, Koomar J, Brett-Green B, Burke JP, Cohn ES, Mailloux Z, Miller LJ, Schaaf RC (2018) Development of a fidelity measure for research on the effectiveness of the Ayres Sensory Integration® intervention. Am J Occup Ther 65:133–142. https://doi.org/10.5014/ajot.2011.000745

Park ES, Park CI, Chang HJ, Choi JE, Lee DS (2004) The effect of hinged ankle-foot orthoses on sit-to-stand transfer in children with spastic cerebral palsy. Arch Phys Med Rehabil 85(12):2053–2057. https://doi.org/10.1016/j.apmr.2004.05.008

Park C, Park ES, Choi JY, Cho Y, Rha DW (2017) Immediate effect of a single session of Whole Body Vibration on spasticity in children with cerebral palsy. Ann Rehabil Med 41(2):273–278. https://doi.org/10.5535/arm.2017.41.2.273

Parkinson KN, Dickinson HO, Arnaud C, Lyons A, Colver A, SPARCLE Group (2013) Pain in young people aged 13 to 17 years with cerebral palsy: cross-sectional, multicentre European study. Arch Dis Child 98(6):434–440. https://doi.org/10.1136/archdischild-2012-303482

Pavão SL, Rocha NACF (2017) Sensory processing disorders in children with cerebral palsy. Infant Behav Dev 46:1–6. https://doi.org/10.1016/j.infbeh.2016.10.007

Pavão SL, Silva FP, Savelsbergh GJ, Rocha NA (2015) Use of sensory information during postural control in children with cerebral palsy: systematic review. J Mot Behav 47(4):291–301. https://doi.org/10.1080/00222895.2014.981498

Pavlova M, Sokolov A, Krägeloh-Mann I (2007) Visual navigation in adolescents with early periventricular lesions: knowing where, but not getting there. Cerebral Cortex 17(2):363–369. https://doi.org/10.1093/cercor/bhj153

Penner M, Xie YW, Binepal N, Switzer L, Fehlings D (2013) Characteristics of pain in children and youth with cerebral palsy. Pediatrics 132(2):e407–e413. https://doi.org/10.1542/peds.2013-0224

Pin TW, Butler PB, Purves S (2019) Use of whole body vibration therapy in individuals with moderate severity of cerebral palsy—a feasibility study. BMC Neurol 19(1):80. https://doi.org/10.1186/s12883-019-1307-5

Pitron V, Alsmith A, de Vignemont F (2018) How do the body schema and the body image interact? Conscious Cogn 65:352–358. https://doi.org/10.1016/j.concog.2018.08.007

Poirot I, Laudy V, Rabilloud M, Roche S, Ginhoux T, Kassaï B, Vuillerot C (2017) Prevalence of pain in 240 non-ambulatory children with severe cerebral palsy. Ann Phys Rehabil Med 60(6):371–375. https://doi.org/10.1016/j.rehab.2017.03.011

Polatajko HJ, Cantin N (2010) Exploring the effectiveness of occupational therapy interventions, other than the sensory integration approach, with children and adolescents experiencing difficulty processing and integrating sensory information. Am J Occup Ther 64(3):415–429. https://doi.org/10.5014/ajot.2010.09072

Purpura G, Cioni G, Tinelli F (2017) Development of visuo-haptic transfer for object recognition in typical preschool and school-aged children. Child Neuropsychol 24(5):657–670. https://doi.org/10.1080/09297049.2017.1316974

Purpura G, Perazza S, Cioni G, Tinelli F (2019) Visuo-haptic transfer for object recognition in children with periventricular leukomalacia and bilateral cerebral palsy. Child Neuropsychol 25(8):1084–1097. https://doi.org/10.1080/09297049.2019.1602599

Raine S, Meadows L, Lynch-Ellerington M (2009) Bobath Concept: theory and clinical practice in neurological rehabilitation. Wiley-Blackwell Ltd

Redstone F, West JF (2004) The importance of postural control for feeding. Pediatr Nurs 30(2):97–100. https://doi.org/10.3233/PRM-170435

Rine RM, Wiener-Vacher S (2013) Evaluation and treatment of vestibular dysfunction in children. Neuro Rehabil 32:507–518. https://doi.org/10.3233/NRE-130873

Ritterband-Rosenbaum A, Christensen MS, Kliim-Due M, Petersen LZ, Rasmussen B, Nielsen JB (2011) Altered sense of agency in children with spastic cerebral palsy. BMC Neurol 11:150. https://doi.org/10.1186/1471-2377-11-150

Ritterband-Rosenbaum A, Christensen MS, Nielsen JB (2012) Twenty weeks of computer-training improves sense of agency in children with spastic cerebral palsy. Res Dev Disabil 33(4):1227–1234. https://doi.org/10.1016/j.ridd.2012.02.019

Ritzmann R, Stark C, Krause A (2018) Vibration therapy in patients with cerebral palsy: a systematic review. Neuropsychiatr Dis Treat 14:1607–1625. https://doi.org/10.2147/NDT.S152543

Rochat P, Striano T (2000) Perceived self in infancy. Infant Behav Dev 23(3–4):513–530. https://doi.org/10.1016/S0163-6383(01)00055-8

Ruck J, Chabot G, Rauch F (2010) Vibration treatment in cerebral palsy: a randomized controlled pilot study. J Musculoskelet Neuronal Interact 10(1):77–83

Russo EF, Calabrò RS, Sale P, Vergura F, De Cola MC, Militi A, Bramanti P, Portaro S, Filoni S (2019) Can muscle vibration be the future in the treatment of cerebral palsy-related drooling? A feasibility study. Int J Med Sci 16(11):1447–1452. https://doi.org/10.7150/ijms.34850

Saavedra S, Woollacott M, van Donkelaar P (2010) Head stability during quiet sitting in children with cerebral palsy: effect of vision and trunk support. Exp Brain Res 201(1):13–23. https://doi.org/10.1007/s00221-009-2001-4

Sá-Caputo D, Costa-Cavalcanti R, Carvalho-Lima RP, Arnobio A et al (2016) Systematic review of whole body vibration exercises in the treatment of cerebral palsy: brief report. Dev Neurorehabil 19(5):1–7. https://doi.org/10.3109/17518423.2014.994713

Sack AT (2009) Parietal cortex and spatial cognition. Behav Brain Res 202(2):153–161. https://doi.org/10.1016/j.bbr.2009.03.012

Sanger T, Kukke S (2007) Abnormalities of tactile sensory function in children with dystonic and diplegic cerebral palsy. J Child Neurol 22(3):289–293. https://doi.org/10.1177/0883073807300530

Schaaf RC, Dumont RL, Arbesman M, May-Benson TA (2018 updated) Efficacy of occupational therapy using ayres sensory integration®: a systematic review. Am J Occup Ther 72(1):7201190010p1–7201190010p10. https://doi.org/10.5014/ajot.2018.028431

Schwartz L, Engel JM, Jensen MP (1999) Pain in persons with cerebral palsy. Arch Phys Med Rehabil 80(10):1243–1246. https://doi.org/10.1016/s0003-9993(99)90023-0

Schwoebel J, Coslett HB (2005) Evidence for multiple, distinct representations of the human body. J Cogn Neurosci 17(4):543–553. https://doi.org/10.1162/0898929053467587

Seo T-H, Yang S-E, Lee H-G (2018) The effects of Contact Hand-Orientation Response (CHOR) during Sit-to-stand (STS) in people with stroke. J Korean Soc Neurother 22(3):31–36. https://doi.org/10.17817/2018.10.01.111319

Shahanawaz SD, Palekar TJ, Shah N (2015) Effect of Swiss Ball on balance in children with spastic diplegia: a case study. ARC J Pediatr 1(1):8–11. https://doi.org/10.20431/2455-5711.0101002

Shima K, Shimatani K, Sugie A, Kurita Y, Kohno R, Tsuji T (2013) Virtual Light Touch Contact: a novel concept for mitigation of body sway. In: 7th international symposium on medical information and communication technology (ISMICT), 6–8 Mar 2013. https://doi.org/10.1109/ISMICT.2013.6521710

Shima K, Shimatani K, Sato G, Sakata M, Giannoni P, Morasso P (2017) A fundamental study on how holding a helium-filled balloon affects stability in human standing. In: 2017 IEEE int conf rehabil robot, pp 1061–1066. https://doi.org/10.1109/ICORR.2017.8009390

Shima K, Shimatani K, Sakata M (2021) A wearable light-touch contact device for human balance support. Sci Rep 11(1):7324. https://doi.org/10.1038/s41598-021-85687-4

Shimatani K, Shibanoki T, Shima K, Kurita Y, Otsuka A, Casadio M, Giannoni P, Moretti P, Morasso P, Tsuji T (2015a) Change over time of infants' movements based on motion analysis:

comparison with changes in general movements and the body sway. Physiotherapy 101(Suppl 1):eS1388. https://doi.org/10.1016/j.physio.2015.03.1333

Shimatani K, Shima K, Giannoni P, Moretti P, Morasso P (2015b) The use of a floating balloon as a walking aid for children. Physiotherapy 101(Suppl 1):eS1388. https://doi.org/10.1016/j. physio.2015.03.1334

Strzalkowski NDJ, Mildren RL, Bent LR (2015) Thresholds of cutaneous afferents related to perceptual threshold across the human foot sole. J Neurophysiol 114(4):2144–2151. https://doi. org/10.1152/jn.00524.2015

Tao H, Pannek K, Fiori S, Boyd RN, Rose S (2014) Reduced integrity of sensorimotor projections traversing the posterior limb of the internal capsule in children with congenital hemiparesis. Res Dev Disabil 35(2):250–260. https://doi.org/10.1016/j.ridd.2013.11.001

Tramontano M, Medici A, Iosa M, Chiariotti A, Fusillo G, Manzari L, Morelli D (2017) The effect of vestibular stimulation on motor functions of children with cerebral palsy. Mot Control 21(3):299–311. https://doi.org/10.1123/mc.2015-0089

Unger M, Jelsma J, Stark C (2013) Effect of a trunk-targeted intervention using vibration on posture and gait in children with spastic type cerebral palsy: a randomized control trial. Dev Neurorehabil 16(2):79–88. https://doi.org/10.3109/17518423.2012.715313

Vaitl D, Mittelstaedt H, Saborowski R, Stark R, Baisch F (2002) Shifts in blood volume alter the perception of posture: further evidence for somatic graviception. Int J Psychophysiol 44(1):1–11. https://doi.org/10.1016/s0167-8760(01)00184-2

van der Slot WMA, Benner JL, Brunton L, Engel JM, Gallien P, Hilberink SR, Månum G, Morgan P, Opheim A, Riquelme I, Rodby-Bousquet E, Simsek TT, Thorpe DE, Berg-Emons RJVD, Vogtle LK, Papageorgiou G, Roebroeck ME (2020) Pain in adults with cerebral palsy: a systematic review and meta-analysis of individual participant data. Ann Phys Rehabil Med. pii: S1877-0657(20)30034-8. https://doi.org/10.1016/j.rehab.2019.12.011

Wallard L, Bril B, Dietrich G, Kerlirzin Y, Bredin J (2012) The role of head stabilization in locomotion in children with cerebral palsy. Ann Phys Rehabil Med 55(9–10):590–600. https://doi. org/10.1016/j.rehab.2012.10.004

Watanabe M, Tani H (2020) Effects of active and passive light-touch support on postural stability during tandem standing. J Phys Ther Sci 32(1):55–58. https://doi.org/10.1589/jpts.32.55

Wickremasinghe AC, Rogers EE, Johnson BC, Shen A, Barkovich AJ, Marco EJ (2013) Children born prematurely have atypical Sensory Profiles. J Perinatol 33(8):631–635. https://doi. org/10.1038/jp.2013.12

Wingert JR, Burton H, Sinclair RJ, Brunstrom JE, Damiano DL (2008) Tactile sensory abilities in cerebral palsy: deficits in roughness and object discrimination. Dev Med Child Neurol 50(11):832–838. https://doi.org/10.1111/j.1469-8749.2008.03105.x

Wingert JR, Burton H, Sinclair RJ, Brunstrom JE, Damiano DL (2009) Joint-position sense and kinesthesia in cerebral palsy. Arch Phys Med Rehabil 90(3):447–453. https://doi.org/10.1016/j. apmr.2008.08.217

Winter DA (1995) Human balance and posture control during standing and walking. Gait Posture 3(4):193–214. https://doi.org/10.1016/0966-6362(96)82849-9

Zhang L, Li P, Mao Z, Qi X, Zou J, Yu Z (2014) Changes in motor function in the unaffected hand of stroke patients should not be ignored. Neural Regen Res 9(13):1323–1328. https://doi. org/10.4103/1673-5374.137581

Therapeutic Approaches for the Soft Tissues

7

Psiche Giannoni

The vast family of body tissues includes epithelial, connective, muscle, and neural tissues (Fig. 7.1), often referred to by the broad term *soft tissues*, without considering the bones that are hard tissue.

These tissues are the components of structures that allow the body's systems to function. Each system makes its separate contribution to movement, but every one of them must work together to provide the complete support framework.

In cerebral palsy, the care of muscle tissue is fundamental to improve the work of weak muscles or, on the other hand, to counteract excessive muscle recruitment due to poor core stability of the body, for example, that, in a short time, can cause postural misalignment.

Since the muscles and the nervous system are so closely related, children with CP also benefit greatly from the mobilization of the CNS, particularly those children who have very poor movements and remain in the same position for a long time.

At the same time, the care of connective tissue is particularly important because this tissue gives shape and support to every part of the body, including muscles and nerves, connects and protects the internal organs, moves fluids like blood and lymph, and stores energy. Lack of care to this tissue means compromising its general functioning and that of the connected parts of the body.

The connective tissue is present in the dermis, fasciae, tendons, ligaments, entheses, and aponeurosis. Unlike epithelial, muscle, and neural tissues, which mainly depend on their cellular elements, the properties of the connective tissue that forms these structures mainly depend on the amount, type, and arrangement of the extracellular protein fibers and characterize their function (Fig. 7.2).

For example, fasciae have a different consistency depending on their function: the superficial fascia, composed of loose connective tissue, allows the layers of dermis to slide through them, and the fascia profunda or deep fascia, characterized

P. Giannoni (✉)
DIBRIS, University of Genoa, Genoa, Italy

© The Author(s), under exclusive license to Springer Nature Switzerland AG 2022   263
P. Giannoni, L. Zerbino (eds.), *Cerebral Palsy*,
https://doi.org/10.1007/978-3-030-85619-9_7

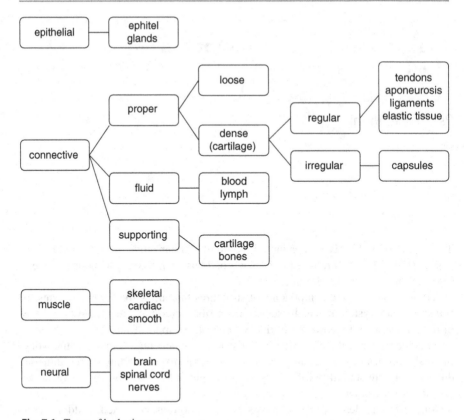

Fig. 7.1 Types of body tissues

Location	Main cell type	Dominant fiber	Mechanical properties
dermis	fibroblasts	collagen / elastin	resistance to tension, moderate compression and stretching
tendon	tenocytes	collagen	resistance to tension forces
joint cartilage	condrocytes	collagen	resistance to compression forces
bone	osteoblasts/osteocytes	collagen	resistance to tension, compression and torsion

Fig. 7.2 Summary of properties of the major types of connective tissue

by a dense connective, allows the more internal organs to slide but in particular surrounds the blood vessels and the three layers of each muscle and nerve so that they can move and function properly (Schleip et al. 2012).

Fasciae are often considered passive structures that transmit the mechanical tension generated by muscle activity or external forces throughout the body. Yet some research suggests that they can contract independently and actively influence muscle dynamics and therefore play an important role as force transmitters in human posture and movement regulation (Schleip et al. 2005). The interconnections of the fascia with muscles, joints, and ligaments create a very strong network of interacting, interrelated, and interdependent tissues that, in all respects, can be considered a "fascial system" (Stecco and Schleip 2016; Adstrum et al. 2017; Schleip et al. 2019).

That also means that, when manipulating a tissue, at the same time the therapist is influencing the condition of all the surrounding tissues that are part of the other organs.

The child's well-being will benefit from both active physical treatment intended to promote movement and coordination through alignment between the parts of the body and enhancement of muscle strength as well as the only apparently "passive" treatment intended as manual treatment of the body tissues. Weakness, as well as spasticity, spasms, and misalignment, leads to excessive stiffness in the body segments, causing a change in the intrinsic qualities of specific tissues and long-term joint and muscle pain (Jahnsen et al. 2004; Opheim et al. 2009; Alriksson-Schmidt and Hägglund 2016; Eriksson et al. 2020).

7.1 The Connective Tissue

The dermis, immediately beneath the epithelial tissue, has two tasks: (1) it provides information about the nearby environment through its tactile receptors, and (2) it protects the underlying internal organs.

The processing of tactile information, which develops much earlier than other sensory modalities, not only allows the child to differentiate and protect their body from the external world but also provides a powerful means of physical and social interaction with other people (Gallace and Spence 2014).

It is very important that the child with motor impairments can touch and be touched to enhance their understanding of the environment. Sometimes these touching experiences are infrequent because often the adults are worried and distressed by the child's limitations. To overcome this impasse, it is of great advantage for parents and caregivers to interact with the child not only through correct handling but also through the practice of infant massage (Vickers et al. 2000; McClure 2017; Pados and McGlothen-Bell 2019).

The benefit received from sensory experiences is undoubtedly important, as will be explained in Chap. 6 of this book.

As suggested by the family care approach (see Chap. 1), it is important to involve and empower the family in a collaborative intervention process (Novak 2011; Novak and Berry 2014; An et al. 2019). The therapist can ask the parent or caregiver for collaboration not only for what concerns the postural care of the child during daily life but also for the well-being of their soft tissue. Simple play motor activities with the child, as a "small gymnastic interaction," improve the empathic linkage with the adult and also favor the maintenance of the important metabolic functions of the connective tissue (Fig. 7.3).

Fig. 7.3 "Small gymnastic
interaction"

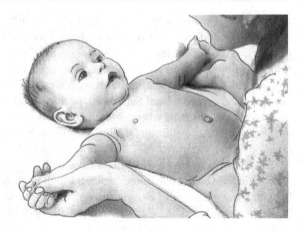

To understand how to influence the connective tissue, it is necessary to consider its three main specific mechanical properties: viscoelasticity, thixotropy, and piezoelectricity.

Viscoelasticity is given by the macromolecular structure of the tissue, composed mainly of fibroblast cells and a matrix that incorporates a viscous fluid called "ground substance" and the specific fibers of the tissue.

Thixotropy refers to the ability of some fluids as the ground substance, which is thick or viscous under static conditions, to become less viscous when shaken or subjected to shear stress. Thixotropy is a time-dependent property and therefore requires a fixed time to return to a more viscous state.

Furthermore, collagen, which is the most dominant fiber of the connective tissue, exhibits piezoelectric properties (Curie and Curie 1880) in response to a gradual and prolonged pressure and latent heat. That means that collagen can accumulate electric charge and therefore modulate its tissue structure and function (Fukada and Yasuda 1964; Shamos and Lavine 1967). This can happen, for example, during a manual release technique when the therapist exerts pressure on the dermis, and consequently, their hands transmit a certain amount of heat.

Soft tissue-releasing techniques had their first applications in osteopathic medicine but were soon applied to physiotherapy as well when studies focused on the contribution of the fascial system in the physiological equilibrium of the body (Barnes 2004; Davis 2009; Stecco and Schleip 2016).

Currently, there are several approaches to soft tissue treatment, and often the related manual techniques work in a similar fashion. Many studies report positive results when treating soft tissue dysfunctions, most of the time in favor of adults but also of children. The application of these techniques is useful in CP both for prevention in toddlers and young children and in particular in adolescents or adults with CP for an effective release of tight tissues, and particularly of the myofascia (Macgregor et al. 2007; Whisler et al. 2012; Hansen et al. 2014; Kumar and Vaidya 2014; Loi et al. 2015).

Anyway, the purpose of this chapter is not to choose one manual technique over another but to report which kind of interventions is best suited to be applied to a child, and to argue that the purpose of these techniques is not to relax but to change the state of the compromised tissue and so improve its functioning: a therapeutic approach that involves a combination of pressure and movement can have a positive effect on the connective tissue (Juhan 1987; Lederman 1997).

In particular, connective tissue massage (CTM) (Dicke 1953; Shiffer and Harms 2014) is a specific method addressed to the connective tissue that is often applied together with soft tissue release (STR). Manipulation with CTM can produce both local effects, favoring the restoring of the intrinsic properties of the tissue, and general effects, influencing the autonomic functions (Barr and Taslitz 1970; Goats and Keir 1991). To better understand the manipulative technique of CTM, it is fundamental to refer to the concept of "barrier" and to realize the amount of pressure that the therapist must exert on the tight tissue.

The "Barrier" Concept

Practitioners of osteopathy adopted first the term "barrier," which originally referred to joints, but it can also refer to elasticity and mobility of soft tissues and muscles.

Kuchera (1997) defined the barrier as the limit of active motion, but, according to Lewit (1999), it is more appropriate to define the barrier as the limit of maximum passive motion, having a greater range of motion than the active one.

The practitioner investigating movement restriction of a person can identify different kinds of barrier:

1. Anatomical barrier: limit of motion or of the extreme passive range of movement (RoM) due to the anatomical structure of the joints, ligaments, muscles, and fasciae. If, for some event, this barrier is overcome, there will be disruption in the tissue.
2. Physiological barrier: limit of active RoM, less than passive RoM. It is the point where the examiner feels the first resistance that warns the tension present in the muscle fibers and in the fascia.
3. Elastic barrier: range between the physiological and anatomical barrier of motion. In this range the barrier yields slightly with a sense of "springing," defining a potential workspace.
4. Pathological or restricted barrier: RoM limit, less than physiological, present in pathological situations and felt as an abrupt stop, with lack of the sense of springing. This limitation can change the neutral resting position of a segment, provoking, for example, asymmetry.

In the case of dysfunction or pathology, the practitioner can work on a restriction of mobility not only observing the active RoM but also examining the condition of the tissues through palpation. The goal of their treatment is to find the restricted barrier and then, with the application of their fingers to the surface of the tissue, move it as close as possible to the physiological one. They must be always aware of what they sense under their hands and fingers: initially they will encounter the resistance of the restricted barrier, which they can "engage" with a gentle but firm thrust to obtain some release and springing of the tissue and reach a new possible elastic barrier (Fig. 7.4).

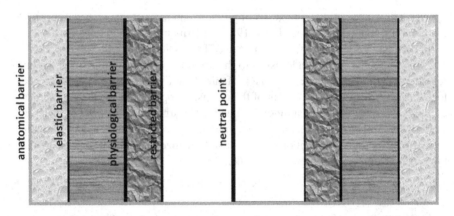

Fig. 7.4 The barriers

Key Points for the Evaluation and Treatment of the Connective Tissue
- The final aim of a manual release technique is to restore elasticity and mobility of the tissue in order to improve motion and function.
- Manual contact is for the evaluation and treatment of soft tissue restriction, and both are intertwined.
- The release technique must not be forced and the child must not feel any pain.
- Evaluation through palpation is not a matter of visual inspection as it could also be done with closed eyes. The hands and fingers have receptors not only for touch but also for motion, texture, and many other sensations, and only light pressure allows the therapist's hands to have a better perception of the modification of the underlying tissue.
- Palpation and engagement of the barrier must be done with light pressure. Minimal, light stimuli help to feel the reaction in the tissue, while deep pressure stimuli do the opposite.
- The resolution of the pathological barrier is always associated with the disappearance of painful symptoms.
- Early interruption of the releasing manipulation does not allow to achieve the desired goal.
- Tendons, ligaments, entheses, and aponeuroses are also composed of dense connective tissue, but their intrinsic properties sometimes require to be manipulated with specific techniques, as will be seen later.
- The release technique is not a massage, but a preparation for functional activity. The use of oils and creams would not allow the therapist to feel the modifications in the tissue under their hands.
- **Steps to "Engage" and Overcome a Barrier** (Lewit 1999)
  1. Engagement of the barrier through palpation
  2. Slight pressure or stretching the tissue, as indicated by manual release techniques
  3. No/minimal pressure or variation in stretching during the manipulation

4. Perception of the tissue release (normally after 90–120 s. or longer in more critical situations)
5. Repeat palpation in a nearby area to find any other areas with the same characteristics of tension or pain

7.1.1 Practical Suggestions

As said before, the purpose of taking care of connective and other tissues is not relaxation, because that would induce passivity in the person or the child and not help them to move more actively. It is another matter to release a tissue because it is too tight or because an underlying tender point hinders the efficiency of a functional motor pattern.

The main and fundamental aim is to prepare the child for better motor function, and therefore, immediately after the tissue release, the therapist will have to propose new active, functional problem-solving activities.

Different aims of soft tissue therapy:

- *For the child (independence and quality of life)*
  - Prevent infants from developing contractures caused by a limited variety of movement patterns or body segment misalignments
  - Let the child or adult with CP to feel less tense and therefore more confident of solving a functional problem
  - Help the child deal with the fear of a possibly painful event and reduce the stiffening up caused by the anticipation of feeling discomfort
  - Give the child the opportunity, after the release technique therapy, to improve their sensory experience and increase their functional motor repertoire
  - Improve their autonomic system
- *For the parents/caregivers (child management)*
  - Help their understanding of the problems related to compromised tissue
  - Make them feel more confident to touch the child (infant massage, care of swelling, scars, sweat, etc.)
  - Improve communication between parents and child through good touch
- *For treatment planning*
  - Reduce the tightness in the soft tissues that cause limitation in ARoM and/or pain in children, adolescents, and adults with CP
  - Improve the intrinsic properties of the fascia and consequently of the muscles and tendons and so improve the RoM at the joints, alignment, and muscle activity
  - Improve functional movement

Some basic techniques can be applied to release soft tissues and in particular myofascia, to recover to some extent their specific intrinsic properties and restore their mechanical functions, contributing to the execution of sequences of movement that are not only smoother but even more effective (Lewit 1999; Sanderson 2021).

7.1.1.1 Stretching of the Skin

This technique is performed with one or two fingers and is particularly useful for working on small parts of the body. Stretching reaches the first layers of the dermis and aponeurosis and should be applied in a soft but determined way (Fig. 7.5).

Suggestions

- *Gently stretch the child's cheeks and the area around the mouth, following the shape of the underlying* orbicular oris *muscle, or if necessary, stretch the inner cheek with a finger, to help the child, e.g., to control their drooling and to improve the closure of the lip during feeding or mimic.*
- *If a child shows a flexor synergy or hunching shoulders has tension at the superior part of* trapezius, *release it stretching the tissue with one or two fingers.*
- *A child with a flexor synergy most likely sits with a poking chin to keep the center of mass (CoM) inside the base of support (BoS) and prevent losing balance. It is useful in this case to take the* sternocleidomastoid *muscle with two fingers and exert a slight transversal stretching, to realign the head to the shoulders, and then work for a straightening of the trunk.*
- *A diaphragm release can help children with poor diaphragmatic mobility and a fixed open ribcage to improve the pulmonary function and diaphragmatic motion* (Diwan et al. 2014; Rocha et al. 2015; Rutka et al. 2021).
- *Stay behind the child, and gently press with both hands and two or more fingers under the costal arches, following the child's breathing.*
- *Treat a scar tissue holding the part between thumb and forefinger, and then impress a slight shear stretch until a springing of the barrier is felt.*

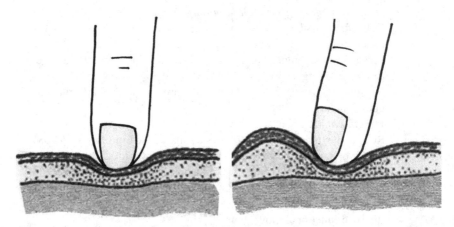

Fig. 7.5 Skin stretching (modified from Sanderson 2021)

7.1.1.2 Pressure

With this technique, it is possible to reach different layers of tissue, depending on the amount of pressure exerted, but manipulation with a light hand is always mandatory. Figure 7.6 shows the different amount of hand pressure in these two first techniques. After feeling the first barrier, the finger exerts further slight pressure to feel the springing that leads to the new physiological barrier.

Suggestions

- *A flexed shoulder girdle and an internally rotated humerus mean reduced passive RoM and a too stiff pectoral major, which can be released with this technique using two fingers or with the hand fully open, depending on the size of the child. Besides, a warm open hand transmits some heat, in favor of the piezoelectric properties of the connective tissue (Fig. 7.7).*

Fig. 7.6 Pressure (modified from Sanderson 2021)

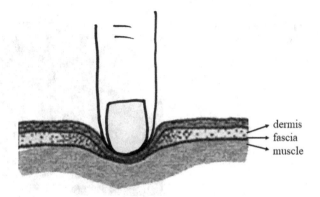

dermis
fascia
muscle

Fig. 7.7 Release of the connective components of *pectoral major*

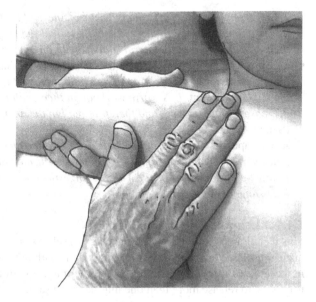

Fig. 7.8 Stretching of the palmar fascia

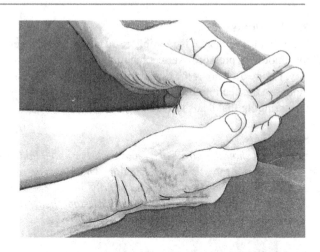

Fig. 7.9 Release of the *subscapularis* muscle

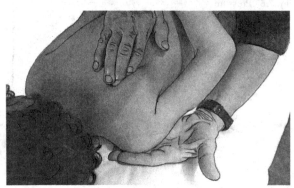

- *Transversely stretch the palmar fascia of the child's fisted hand, to obtain a larger palmar surface to allow the child to feel the surfaces, touch themself or their parent, or maintain lateral support with an open hand* (Fig. 7.8).
- *Many painful tight bands in the* soleus *muscle, the* medial gastrocnemius, *and the* tibialis posterior *can be found through palpation when a difficult dorsiflexion of the ankle is present. It is worth working on them with the pressure technique, to decrease muscle stiffness and therefore realign the ankle joint to a certain extent* (Sanderson 2021).
- *A* subscapularis *muscle tightened due to a fixed protraction of the scapula can be reached from the lateral edge of the scapula or its medial edge. In the latter case, it may be easier to press not with the fingertips but with the lateral side of the index finger* (Fig. 7.9).

7.1.1.3 Lengthening of the Deep Fascia

This technique is used to release the deep muscle fascia or when a chain of synergistic muscles is involved. It is often applied in combination with stretching because in these cases it is not possible to reach the muscle with the fingers or when it is necessary to release more than one muscle at the same time.

Fig. 7.10 Manual lengthening of the deep fascia

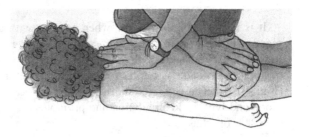

Suggestion

- *An evident misalignment of the trunk also means an unbalanced muscle activity and therefore a suffering fascial system. Working on a large area of the body, it is necessary to manipulate the part with open and warm hands. In this case, it may be important to work on the* latissimus dorsi *muscle, with one hand on an iliac crest and the other on the scapula of the same side, and both hands move gently in opposite directions* (Fig. 7.10).

Note

- *Latissimus dorsi* muscle has two important actions: the scapular segment rotates the humerus into the glenoid, and the vertebral segment assists the movements of the lower trunk. According to the functional problem to be solved, the therapist can emphasize movement and stretch one part with one hand while holding the other.
- Remember that after the first release of a muscle group, it is important to engage the child in functional and play activities in which the same muscles group is involved (Fig. 7.11).
- An equinus foot with inversion is often associated with a stretching of the *tibialis anterior* muscle, and a friction massage with transverse action on its tendon (Cyriax 1982; Chamberlain 1982) can allow a certain decreasing of muscle tension and a certain realignment of the ankle joint for a more efficient weight-bearing on the foot (Fig. 7.12).

Taping Technique

Nowadays elastic therapeutic taping is often applied to children with CP as part of a multimodal therapy program. Many reviews have reported that this technique is a useful addition to physiotherapy (Ortiz Ramírez and Pérez de la Cruz 2017; Cunha et al. 2018; Unger et al. 2018) although there is still moderate evidence supporting its efficacy. Children with better developmental and motor levels, e.g., GMF test level I or II, seem to obtain greater benefits from this technique.

At first, taping was used mainly for athletes, with the aim of facilitating muscle contraction and increasing the strength of specific muscles. This is not the aim in CP, although the application of taping with a mixed compression technique is sometimes used in rehabilitation practice to improve, for example, the activity of *transversus abdominis* muscle.

It is a much more effective when applied with a decompressive technique, with any tension of the tape and the muscle initially held in elongation (da Costa et al. 2013; Shamsoddini et al. 2016). The action of this type of application is quite similar to the manual one on the dermis and fascia (Fig. 7.13) because it lifts and moves the tissues and therefore promotes blood and lymphatic circulation and promotes the maintenance of intrinsic muscle properties.

Fig. 7.11 Active stretching of the deep fascia

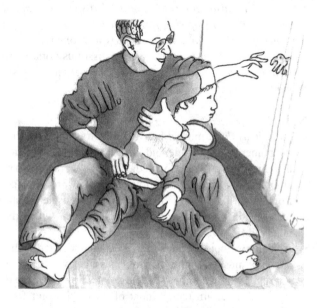

Fig. 7.12 Release of the *tibialis anterior* tendon

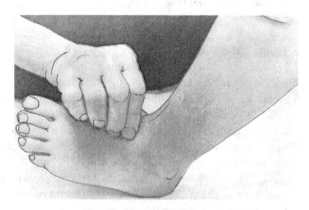

Fig. 7.13 Action of taping applied with decompression technique

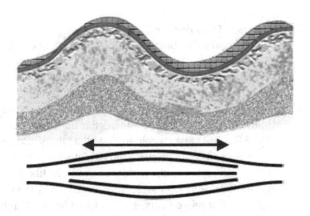

7.2 The Muscle Tissue

It is necessary to remember that connective, muscle, and neural tissues are closely connected. All bundles of muscle fibers are separated from each other by layers of connective tissue (Turrina et al. 2013). However, compared with other tissues, the muscle has its specific behavior, which is to convert chemical energy into mechanical work and heat.

Children with CP initially have muscle weakness due to a lack of motor unit recruitment caused by the affected neural fibers of the descending tract. This weakness is part of the negative features observed after a lesion of the upper motor neuron (Rose and McGill 2005; Barnes and Johnson 2008). As positive features, there is spasticity, the definition of which has been widely revised concerning Lance's restricted statement (1980). The definition referred to now is that reported by the SPASM consortium in 2005, which revised and redefined the concept of spasticity as "disordered sensory-motor control, resulting from an upper motor neuron lesion, presenting as intermittent or sustained involuntary activation of muscles" (Pandyan et al. 2005; Burridge et al. 2005).

Muscle weakness, although limited to only some body segments, leads to a general imbalance of all muscle groups. This muscle imbalance is a determining factor in worsening the development of abnormal postural control and limitations of full joint RoM and the shortening of many muscle groups (Downing et al. 2009; Barrett and Lichtwark 2010; Mockford and Caulton 2010; Barber et al. 2011; Shortland 2011; Gough and Shortland 2012, 2014).

Therefore, rehabilitation treatment should focus on the problem of this basic weakness and involve the child's muscles through active and adequate functional training, through intelligent proposals of play, which the child will find enjoyable.

Henneman's Size Principle
It is well known that there are three types of muscle fibers:

- Type I: (S) slow-twitch, low threshold, small diameter, high fatigue resistance, high oxidative capacity, reduced force generation. This means that they can function for a long time with little fatigue and are mainly used to maintain posture and produce small movements that do not require large amounts of energy.
- Type IIa: (FR) fast-twitch, intermediate threshold, medium diameter, moderate resistance to fatigue, high oxidative capacity, moderate force generation. The motor units with these muscle fibers are mainly recruited to perform movements that require more energy than postural control but not for very fast movements, such as throwing something.
- Type IIb: (FF) very fast-twitch, high threshold, large diameter, small resistance to fatigue, low oxidative capacity, very high force generation. They tire quickly, so they are used for quick and powerful movements.

According to Henneman's size principle, motor neurons with small cell bodies tend to innervate small-sized muscle fibers, while motor neurons with large cell bodies tend to innervate larger muscle fibers. In most cases the order of activation of the motor units is fixed during a muscle contraction: first, the type I fibers are activated, capable of a lower contractile force, and then the larger type II fibers, if necessary (Henneman 1957; Henneman et al. 1965).

To improve strength, it is necessary to recruit an increasing number of motor units, as the able-bodied child does during their first year of life, and even later to achieve an increasingly high level of antigravity competence.

The child with CP cannot follow this path due to the primary damage to the motor system, and therefore their neural system can activate the type I fibers but has difficulties going beyond and engaging type II fibers.

One possible strategy to counteract motor unit poor fire is to recruit additional motor units through co-contraction (Chae et al. 2002a, b). That is the way the child with CP often uses when attempting to stand against gravity: they recruit all the muscles of the lower limbs to avoid collapsing, but consequently, they are then unable to move freely.

The child can adopt similar extreme strategies even when seated to cope with poor balance because their trunk muscles are not strong enough for a good core stability. The same can occur when they attempt functional reaching and use the trunk and arm as a whole to achieve the goal.

This restricted repertoire quickly leads to a secondary and often progressive dysfunction with modification of the intrinsic qualities of the connective tissue and of the morphological and mechanical characteristics of the muscle. The limited use of few and stereotyped patterns leads to an increase in the activity of stretch reflex in the shortened muscles (Gracies 2005a, b), hindering the interplay with the antagonist muscles that remain silent (Nielsen et al. 2007).

Several studies also report changes in muscles of children with constant spasticity, with a variability of the extracellular matrix (Booth et al. 2001) and an increased percentage of type I fibers (Marbini et al. 2002).

Therefore, it is necessary to introduce in the therapeutic play and functional proposal variations to involve the child in repetitive but variable activities, in agreement with the Schmidt's schema theory (1975) already explained in Chap. 2. Repetition may induce learning and strengthening of those specific muscles that do not work properly for a function (Sheperd 2014) and increasing endurance. In the scientific literature, this strength-training is often proposed to achieve effective and efficient walking (Yang et al. 2006; Clutterbuck et al. 2019; Hegarty et al. 2019), but it can also be proposed for other activities like moving from sitting to standing and vice versa and going up and down stairs or for functional reaching while keeping an active steady trunk.

The therapist should take into account that the main steps and characteristics of the able-bodied child's sensorimotor development might not be followed in the child with motor impairment: one possibility is to use personalized "shortcuts" that take advantages of the individual characteristics of the child.

Furthermore, following the Henneman's size principle, the therapist should work to engage first the postural muscles before the phasic ones, to sustain the motor activity, and, during the execution of a task, guide the concentric or eccentric muscle activity according to the sequence necessary for the task, with the exact timing accuracy.

7.2.1 Practical Suggestions

There is such a close link between connective and muscle tissue that many of the aims for connective care are similar to those for muscles. The most substantial differences in the aims mainly concern the planning of the treatment session.

Different aims of therapy:
- *For the child (independence and quality of life)*
  - Prevent infants from developing contractures caused by patterns with few movement variables or by misalignments.
  - Let the child or adult with CP feeling less tight and therefore more confident of solving a functional problem.
  - Allow the child to improve their sensory experience and augment their functional motor repertoire.
- *For the parents/caregivers (child management)*
  - Allow parents and caregivers to handle the child and manage their daily needs more easily and comfortably.
- *For the treatment session*
  - Recruit more motor units and solicit active motor responses to improve strength in weak muscles and endurance.
  - Release the tense muscles to favor the alignment of the body segments.
  - Guide the correct sequence of length-tension muscle activity during a functional task.
  - Prevent or, more realistically, delay the onset of changes in muscle tissue and the loss of their intrinsic properties.

7.2.1.1 Functional Sitting

The aim of improving the child's active motor initiative should be the recurring *Leitmotiv* in the mind of all rehabilitators. The very young child spends a lot of time sitting and playing, and then later sitting at school from about 6 years of age, and their functional strategies in this postural level can be efficient but performed with obvious misalignments.

During a treatment—and it is beneficial during usual daily activities as well—a child with moderate or mild CP should be asked to reach the sitting position by themself, as part of the rehabilitation plan. If this active sequence is not currently possible and the child is put into the sitting position, the therapist should first pay attention to the muscle recruitment and work on that to realign the body segments. Immediately afterward, they should propose a play or functional activity in order to obtain an efficient outcome. An unsupported sitting position engages the child much more than a supported one, and also a small amount of active muscle involvement can give them a greater chance of improving their strength and motor repertoire.

Suggestion
- With the child seated, work for an active foot contact with the floor:
  - *If necessary, manually release the* anterior tibialis *and* extensor hallucis *long tendon to facilitate the foot in touching and maintaining contact with the ground* (as in Fig. 6.1).
  - *Release the fascia of* interosseus *muscles, and then activate the* abductor hallucis *and* abductor digiti minimi *to obtain a "large" foot with active sensory contact with the floor.*
- Align the pelvis on the transverse and sagittal plane:
  - *Work to release the long head of the* rectus femoris *and* psoas major, *and then induce an active anterior pelvic tilt together with the activation of* multifidus, quadratus lumborum *muscle, and the extensors of the spine.*
  - *Induce a small shift of the weight of the child's pelvis toward the contralateral hip joint, to allow the latter to act as a fulcrum, free the opposite joint to come forward, and realign with the contralateral hip.*
  - *With these two steps, prepare the child to co-activate the trunk extensors and the abdominal muscles.*
- Work for the active involvement of all the foot on floor:
  - *Check again the actual contact of the feet on floor: reduce a possible grasp reaction in the toes of the feet, by manually decreasing the activity of the* flexor digitorum *muscles and favoring the involvement of the forefoot* (Fig. 7.14).
- Facilitate the child to move their feet backward on the sagittal plane to ensure that the CoM moves safely on the foot-femur-pelvis BoS. This is fundamental for maintaining the activity of the extensor muscles of the trunk, also when the seated child uses the upper limbs to play, rotate, or transit to standing (Roy et al. 2006):
  - *Release the connective tissue of the* triceps surae, *and then hold with one hand (making an arch between the thumb and forefinger) the dorsal part of the*

Fig. 7.14 Preparation the forefoot to receive weight

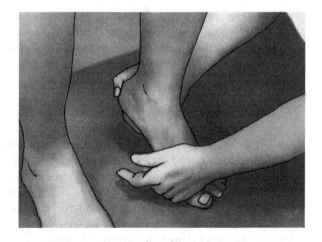

tibiotarsal joint to facilitate an active dorsal flexion of the ankle while maintaining firm heel contact on the supporting surface. This leads to a concentric activation of the tibialis anterior *muscle and a co-activation of the* triceps surae *with lenghthening of the* soleus
- *Before asking the child to move their foot backward, keep the other hand firm on the upper third of their rear leg, to avoid a backward movement of the pelvis while foot moves and knee bends.*
- *Now the child can move forward or rotate the trunk and reach, grasp, or play with objects maintaining their active extension of the spine.*

7.2.1.2 Reaching

Reaching is just one of the many upper limb functions, along with other basics such as support, grasping, and manipulation. From the sensory point of view, the hand can provide important information about the environment, and, for this reason, it should be ready to interact with it. Working to achieve an efficient reaching function requires particular attention, and it does not occur by simply sitting a child and then asking them to move their arm forward but starts beyond that.

Preparation for functional reaching proceeds from the proximal to distal districts. Some basic building blocks are needed: core stability, a linear acceleration for the extension of the trunk, a proper position of the humerus into the glenoid, a good scapulohumeral rhythm, and selective movements of the limb.

It is also important to consider that a reaching task mainly involves fast-twitch muscle fibers, and therefore it is advisable to guide the execution of the reaching at an adequate functional speed and not in slow motion.

Suggestion
- Depending on the starting position—sitting or standing—check the alignment of the pelvis and trunk, to allow a good shoulder dynamic:
  - *Verify the proper position of the pelvis on the three spatial planes: are the postural muscles of the pelvis and lower trunk engaged* (Barr et al. 2005)?

- *Verify the adequate weight-bearing on the lower limbs, based on the position of the target to be reached: is there good foot contact on the floor?*
- *Verify if the trunk can maintain proper control even when it moves:* activate postural muscles as multifidus muscle (Moseley et al. 2002) *and* erector spinae.
- Prepare the shoulder complex (Hess 2000):
  - *Verify the incongruity of the head of the humerus in the glenoid fossa, caused by the misalignment of the scapula.*
  - *Release those overtight muscles that cause the shoulder girdle to flex and the incorrect position of the humerus:* pectoralis major *and* minor *muscles,* latissimus dorsi *(close to its insertion), and* teres major.
  - *Facilitate the correct activity of the muscles of the rotator cuff:* supraspinatus *and* infraspinatus, subscapularis, *and* teres minor, *to obtain the gliding of the humerus and a well-synchronized movement of the scapula.*
- Prepare the limb to lengthen and move forward:
  - *Keeping the position gained at the glenohumeral joint, release the* biceps brachii *and* brachioradialis, *and then activate the* triceps brachii *to improve the RoM at the elbow.*
  - *Release the pronator muscles of the forearm and the carpal flexors.*
  - *Hold the sides of the child's hand, and with your radiocarpal joints, apply some pressure to obtain dorsiflexion of the wrist and abduction of the fingers* (Fig. 7.15).
- Prepare the reaching activity:
  - *Activate and guide the thumb of the child toward the target, to engage the entire posterior muscle chain of the limb, with dorsiflexion of the wrist still present and an open hand that will approach the object to be reached.*
  - *Depending on the height of the target to be reached, it will also be necessary to involve the* deltoid *muscles.*

Fig. 7.15 Dorsiflexion of the child's wrist and abduction of fingers

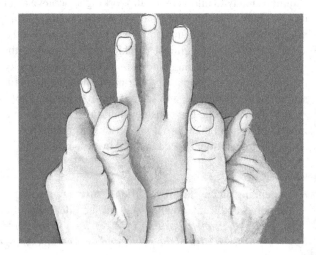

7.2.1.3 Sit Down, Stand Up, and Start Walking

A successful sequence from sitting to stand (STS) and walking requires muscle strength. Therefore, it is necessary to train the child to experience these transfers to activate the muscles that act on the hip, knee, and ankle joints when STS (Yoshioka et al. 2007) and also on the forefoot joints when walking.

It is possible to achieve all this in a play and task-oriented environment, proposing that, during play, the child stands up from sitting to reach a toy, walks to give it to someone, climbs a stair to put it somewhere, or squats down to put it on the floor.

Suggestion
- Prepare the transit from sitting to standing:
  - *Make sure the feet are well placed on the floor, the pelvis is properly anteriorly tilted, and the posterior muscle chain of the trunk is engaged.*
  - *The child should move the trunk forward, transfer the weight on the feet and then lift the pelvis: verify or guide the coordinated lengthening of the* soleus *with the concentric activity of the dorsiflexor muscles, to move the tibial shaft forward.*
  - *The child should now raise the trunk, reduce the anterior tilting of the pelvis, and finally obtain an active extension of hip and knee: engage the child's* glutæi maximi *muscles, and stabilize the hamstrings near the ischial tuberosity and the two* vasti *muscles to support knee extension.*
- Train the reversal activity from standing to sitting as well:
  - *It is not just a matter of rewinding the previous sequence: here there is much more eccentric muscle activity that requires significant control of postural stability toward gravity and with less visual guidance* (Ashford and de Souza 2000).
- Prepare the child to move in a functional context, keeping in mind that it is possible to go in many directions, forward, backward, sideways, and even cross-walking, and each direction requires the activity of different muscles.
- Guide the child to walk forward:
  - *Before the pushing-off phase, it is necessary to stabilize the muscles of the big toe and the* abductor digiti minimi, *to allow the forefoot to receive the weight, and then propel the body forward. The hip flexors are stretched.*
  - *In the pushing off, guide the concentric activity of the* triceps surae (Fig. 7.16) *and immediately after that of the* tibilias anterior *for clearing the foot from the floor. At the hip level, the* tensor fasciae latæ *must work, as well as the* gluteus medius *of the opposite limb, which must receive body weight.*
  - *After the swing phase, efficient heel contact must have the cooperation of a strong tibialis anterior and elongation of the posterior limb muscle chain.*
  - *To gain an efficient weight-bearing on the supporting leg, the* tibialis anterior *continues to work until the foot has full contact on the floor, and at the same time, the* gluteus maximus *and* medius *stabilize the hip joint and the* vasti *stabilize the knee.*

Fig. 7.16 Preparation of the swing phase

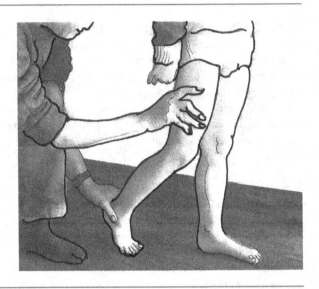

7.3   The Neural Tissue

The neural tissue is the basic component of the brain, spinal cord, and peripheral nerves. This tissue includes neurons that transmit electrical impulses and neuroglia that supports many fundamental functions of the nervous system.

All the components of this system are protected by connective tissue, and therefore the spinal cord and nerves are also sheathed with fasciae, and both tissues move together when a part of the body stretches, bends, or extends. There is close interdependence between them.

The spinal cord and nerves adapt to movement by varying their intraneural pressure and modifying their shape and length, even as much as 9 cm. If they have no or few opportunities to move, they increase in tension, their layers lose elasticity and sliding effects, and the nerve endings suffer from progressive mechanical stress.

There are many tests to evaluate and treat neural tension (Maitland 1985; Elvey 1986; Butler 1991), which consist of a series of multi-joint movements of the limbs and/or trunk that produce mechanical and physiological events in the nervous system.

As written before, there are so many links between neural, connective, and muscle tissue that it is difficult to determine which tissue is most involved during treatment. However, some signs can be distinguished to make a differential diagnosis between muscle and neural tension, adding or subtracting from the basic components of the test the so-called "sensitizing maneuvers" that aim to momentarily modify the tension of the nerve under examination and therefore to highlight its involvement on the previously perceived tensions. One of the most common tests used to distinguish muscle and neural tension is the Slump Test with its sensitizing movements (Butler 1991; White and Pape 1992).

It is difficult to apply these techniques rigorously with a young child who wishes to play. However, with some creativity, some tests may be transformed into a game that involves exactly those test movements. Obviously, it is much easier to apply the technique with a teenager or an adult.

7.3.1   Practical Suggestions

The following aims are very similar to those concerning muscle therapy, with the substantial difference that the intervention is now directed toward the neural tissue which has biomechanical, physiological, and morphological characteristics which are different from the muscle type.
Different aims of therapy for neural tissue:
- *For the child (independence and quality of life)*
  - Allow the child or adult with CP to feel less tension and therefore be more confident in moving and in solving functional problem
  - Overcome a possible painful state arising from neural tension, which causes the child to become anxious and stiffen up in anticipation
  - Give the child the opportunity to increase their functional motor repertoire due to the decrease in the neural tension
- *For the parents/caregivers (child management)*
  - Allow parents and caregivers to handle the child and manage their daily needs more easily and comfortably
- *For the treatment sessions*
  - Reduce the nerve adhesion and facilitation of nerve gliding
  - Improve the physiological functions of the nervous system
  - Facilitate active motor responses and so improve function

Tension tests recommended by Butler can be used by trained therapists not only as an evaluation tool but also as a treatment technique. The therapist can act first on the part of the body with signs of nervous tension by progressively adding the different components required by the test, until the full passive RoM of the interested joints can be achieved without eliciting any pain; thereafter they apply a gentle and continuous mobilization of the affected nerve or spinal cord along with their natural extension. The treatment technique does not require forced stretching but rather a dynamic mobilization with different individual amplitudes, which should always remain below the threshold of pain or tension (Rolf 2001, 2002). After this mobilization, a larger RoM of the interested joints can be appreciated.

Below is described the sequence of the components to be applied in three tests most easily used with children: the therapist should first reach the physiological range of the joints involved and then dynamically mobilize them. This activity can be introduced as a fun during treatment with a child or teenager.

7.3.1.1   Upper Limb Neural Tension Test 1 (ULNTT1)

ULNTT1 is useful to counteract the tension of an upper limb with a synergistic pattern in flexion, as it influences the length and sliding mechanism of the median nerve. The test should be performed following a rigorous sequence and being certain to progressively achieve each of the components indicated in the following steps:

- *Shoulder depression*
- *Shoulder abduction*

- *Shoulder external rotation*
- *Forearm supination*
- *Wrist and finger extension*
- *Elbow extension*
- *Sensitizing movement: lateral cervical flexion toward the opposite side*

Suggestion

- To carry out the test instructions correctly, the child should be lying in a supine position (Fig. 7.17), but if care is taken to maintain the initial depression of the shoulder and all the ranges of movement obtained progressively at the arm joints, it is also possible with the young child in sitting or even standing.
  - *Add all the components required by the test until the limit of RoM at the single joints is perceived.*
  - *Remaining below the threshold of tension, mobilize dynamically the most involved joints, as described before.*
  - *After obtaining a greater RoM, propose activities that include the extension of the upper limb, for example, reaching and grasping a toy and haptically explore it.*

7.3.1.2 Prone Knee Bending (PKB)

This test primarily mobilizes the femoral nerve and is particularly important in prophylactic treatment to counteract the unwanted limited motion at the hip joint, so common in children with CP.

The femoral nerve tension test is performed with the person in the prone position. The therapist places one hand on the child's pelvis to prevent compensatory movements in flexing the hips and then acts as follows:

- *Extension of the hip joint*
- *Flexion of the knee, maintained for 45 s*
- *Main sensitizing movement: flexion of the head*

Fig. 7.17 Upper Limb
Neural Tension Test 1

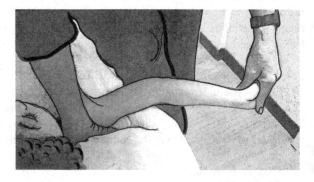

Fig. 7.18 Prone Knee
Bending Test

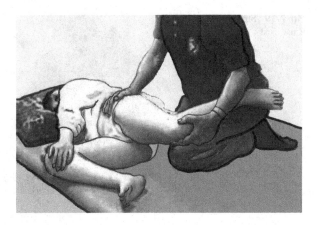

Suggestion

- It is very common to carry out this test with the child side lying. In this case, the therapist should take care of maintaining the correct initial position, with some important precautions:
  - *Ask the child to flex and embrace the lower knee (the one in contact with the surface)*
  - *Stay behind the child, support the femur of the other limb to be treated, and extend the hip joint.*
  - *Counteract with your hand or body any compensatory flexion movement of the hip, and flex the child's knee up to the limit of its passive RoM (Fig. 7.18).*
  - *Hold the position, and then apply a dynamic mobilization of the knee joint below the threshold of tension.*
  - *After this mobilization, do not ask the child to do activities in sitting position, which goes back to a flexed hip, but in kneeling, half-kneeling, or standing.*

7.3.1.3 Straight Leg Raise (SLR)

SLR influences the sciatic nerve but also involves other nerves, such as the tibial or common peroneal nerve, when the ankle moves. It can be applied also on children with CP (Marsico et al. 2016a, b).

The sequence and characteristics of the maneuvers are as follows:

- *Knee extension*
- *Hip flexion*
- *Main sensitizing movements: ankle dorsiflexion or neck flexion*

Suggestion

- The test indicates the child in the supine position (Fig. 7.19), but it is possible to introduce the sequence even if the child is in side lying, paying close attention to reproduce and maintain all the initial positions of the joints:
  - *Lift the leg of the child by the posterior ankle while keeping the knee in a fully extended position.*

Fig. 7.19 Straight Leg
Raise Test

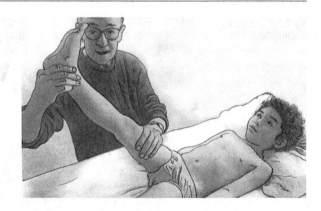

Fig. 7.20 Child
supporting on all fours

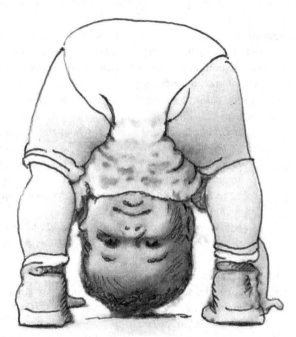

- *Lift the leg until the limit of passive RoM at the hip joint is reached or a tight-*
  ness in the back of the leg is perceived by the child.
- *Remaining below the threshold of tension, mobilize the joint with more lim-*
  ited RoM (hip, knee, or ankle joint).
- *Offer the child some activities that include knee extension with hip flexion and*
  ankle dorsiflexion. For example, a toddler can kick a toy, or support on all
  fours (Fig. 7.20), or a standing child and adolescent can bend their trunk
  forward and touch the floor.

References

Adstrum S, Hedley G, Schleip R, Stecco C, Yucesoy CA (2017) Defining the fascial system. J Bodyw Mov Ther 21(2017):173–177. https://doi.org/10.1016/j.jbmt.2016.11.003

Alriksson-Schmidt A, Hägglund G (2016) Pain in children and adolescents with cerebral palsy: a population-based registry study. Acta Paediatr 105(6):665–670. https://doi.org/10.1111/apa.13368

An M, Palisano RJ, Yi CH, Chiarello LA, Dunst CJ, Gracely EJ (2019) Effects of a collaborative intervention process on parent empowerment and child performance: a randomized controlled trial. Phys Occup Ther Pediatr 39(1):1–15. https://doi.org/10.1080/01942638.2017.1365324

Ashford S, de Souza L (2000) A comparison of the timing of muscle activity during sitting down compared to standing up. Physiother Res Int 5(2):111–118. https://doi.org/10.1002/pri.190

Barber L, Hastings-Ison T, Baker R, Barrett R, Lichtwark G (2011) Medial gastrocnemius muscle volume and fascicle length in children aged 2 to 5 years with cerebral palsy. Dev Med Child Neurol 53(6):543–548. https://doi.org/10.1111/j.1469-8749.2011.03913.x

Barnes JF (2004) Myofascial release—the missing link in traditional treatment. In: Davis CM (ed) Complementary therapies in rehabilitation, 2nd edn. SLACK Inc, Thorofare, pp 59–81

Barnes MP, Johnson GR (2008) Upper motor neurone syndrome and spasticity: clinical management and neurophysiology. Cambridge Univ. Press, Cambridge

Barr JS, Taslitz N (1970) The influence of back massage on autonomic functions. Phys Ther 50(12):1679–1691. https://doi.org/10.1093/ptj/50.12.1679

Barr K, Griggs M, Cadby T (2005) Lumbar stabilization: core concepts and current literature, Part 1. Am J Phys Med Rehabil 84:473–480. https://doi.org/10.1097/01.phm.0000163709.70471.42

Barrett RS, Lichtwark GA (2010) Gross muscle morphology and structure in spastic cerebral palsy: a systematic review. Dev Med Child Neurol 52(9):794–804. https://doi.org/10.1111/j.1469-8749.2010.03686.x

Booth CM, Cortina-Borja MJ, Theologis TN (2001) Collagen accumulation in muscles of children with cerebral palsy and correlation with severity of spasticity. Dev Med Child Neurol 43(5):314–320. https://doi.org/10.1017/s0012162201000597

Burridge JH, Wood DE, Hermens HJ, Voerman GE, Johnson GR, Wijck F, Platz T, Gregoric M, Hitchcock R, Pandyan AD (2005) Theoretical and methodological considerations in the measurement of spasticity. J Disabil Rehabil 27(1–2):69–80. https://doi.org/10.1080/09638280400014592

Butler DS (1991) Mobilisation of the nervous system. Churchill Livingstone, Elsevier Publ.

Chae J, Yang G, Park BK, Labatia I (2002a) Delay in initiation and termination of muscle contraction, motor impairment, and physical disability in upper limb hemiparesis. Muscle Nerve 25(4):568–575. https://doi.org/10.1002/mus.10061

Chae J, Yang G, Park BK, Labatia I (2002b) Muscle weakness and cocontraction in upper limb hemiparesis: relationship to motor impairment and physical disability. Neurorehabil Neural Repair 16(3):241–248. https://doi.org/10.1177/154596830201600303

Chamberlain GJ (1982) Cyriax's friction massage: a review. J Orthop Sports Phys Ther 4(1):16–22. https://doi.org/10.2519/jospt.1982.4.1.16

Clutterbuck G, Megan A, Johnston L (2019) Active exercise interventions improve gross motor function of ambulant/semi-ambulant children with cerebral palsy: a systematic review. Disabil Rehabil 41(10):1131–1151. https://doi.org/10.1080/09638288.2017.1422035

Cunha AB, Lima-Alvarez CD, Rocha ACP, Tudella E (2018) Effects of elastic therapeutic taping on motor function in children with motor impairments: a systematic review. Disabil Rehabil 40(14):1609–1617. https://doi.org/10.1080/09638288.2017.1304581

Curie P, Curie J (1880) Développement, par pression, de l'électricité polaire dans les cristaux hémièdres à faces inclinées—Comptes Rendus des séances de l'Académie des Sciences, Tome XCI, Parigi, pagg. 294–295

Cyriax J (1982) Textbook of orthopaedic medicine, 11th edn. Bailliere Tindall, London

da Costa CS, Rodrigues FS, Leal FM, Rocha NA (2013) Pilot study: investigating the effects of Kinesio Taping® on functional activities in children with cerebral palsy. Dev Neurorehabil 16(2):121–128. https://doi.org/10.3109/17518423.2012.727106

Davis CM (2009) Complementary therapies in rehabilitation—evidence for efficacy in therapy. In: Prevention and wellness. SLACK, Inc., Thorofare

Dicke E (1953) Meine Bindegewebsmassage. Marquardt, Stuttgart

Diwan SJ, Bansal AB, Chovatiya H, Kotak D, Vyas N (2014) Effect of anterior chest wall myofascial release on thoracic expansion in children with spastic cerebral palsy. Int J Contemp Pediatr 1(2):94–99

Downing AL, Ganley KJ, Fay DR, Abbas JJ (2009) Temporal characteristics of lower extremity moment generation in children with cerebral palsy. Muscle Nerve 39(6):800–809. https://doi.org/10.1002/mus.21231

Elvey RL (1986) Treatment of arm pain associated with abnormal brachial plexus tension. Aust J Physiother 32(4):225–230. https://doi.org/10.1016/S0004-9514(14)60655-3

Eriksson E, Hägglund G, Alriksson-Schmidt AI (2020) Pain in children and adolescents with cerebral palsy—a cross-sectional register study of 3545 individuals. BMC Neurol 20(1):15. https://doi.org/10.1186/s12883-019-1597-7

Fukada E, Yasuda I (1964) Piezoelectric effects in collagen. J Appl Phys 3:117

Gallace A, Spence C (2014) In Touch with the Future: The Sense of touch from cognitive neuroscience to virtual reality. Publ. Oxford Scholarship Online, Apr. 2014, https://doi.org/10.1093/acpro:oso/9780199644469.001.0001

Goats GC, Keir KA (1991) Connective tissue massage. Br J Sports Med 25(3):131–133. https://doi.org/10.1136/bjsm.25.3.131

Gough M, Shortland AP (2012) Could muscle deformity in children with spastic cerebral palsy be related to an impairment of muscle growth and altered adaptation? Dev Med Child Neurol 54(6):495–499. https://doi.org/10.1111/j.1469-8749.2012.04229.x

Gough M, Shortland AP (2014) Early muscle development in children with cerebral palsy: the consequences for further muscle growth, muscle function, and long-term mobility. In: Sheperd R (ed) Cerebral palsy in infancy, 1st edn. Churchill Livingstone, Elsevier Publ., pp 157–173

Gracies JM (2005a) Pathophysiology of spastic paresis. I: paresis and soft tissue changes. Muscle Nerve 31(5):535–551. https://doi.org/10.1002/mus.20284

Gracies JM (2005b) Pathophysiology of spastic paresis. II: emergence of muscle overactivity. Muscle Nerve 31(5):552–571. https://doi.org/10.1002/mus.20285

Hansen AB, Price KS, Feldman HM (2014) Myofascial structural integration: a promising complementary therapy for young children with spastic cerebral palsy. J Evid Based Complement Altern Med 17(2):131–135. https://doi.org/10.1177/2156587211430833

Hegarty A, Kurz MJ, Stuberg W, Silverman AK (2019) Strength training effects on muscle forces and contributions to whole-body movement in cerebral palsy. J Mot Behav 51(5):496–510. https://doi.org/10.1080/00222895.2018.1519691

Henneman E (1957) Relation between size of neurons and their susceptibility to discharge. Science 126(3287):1345–1347. https://doi.org/10.1126/science.126.3287.1345

Henneman E, Somjen G, Carpenter DO (1965) Excitability and inhibitability of motoneurons of different sizes. J Neurophysiol 28:599–620. https://doi.org/10.1152/jn.1965.28.3.599

Hess SA (2000) Functional stability of the glenohumeral joint. Man Ther 5(2):63–71. https://doi.org/10.1054/math.2000.0241

Jahnsen R, Villien L, Aamodt G, Stanghelle JK, Holm I (2004) Musculoskeletal pain in adults with cerebral palsy compared with the general population. J Rehabil Med 36:78–84. https://doi.org/10.1080/16501970310018305

Juhan D (1987) Job's Body: a handbook for bodywork. Station Hill Press, Barrytown

Kuchera WA (1997) Glossary of osteopathic terminology. In: Foundations of osteopathic terminology. Williams and Wilkins, Baltimore

Kumar C, Vaidya SN (2014) Effectiveness of myofascial release on spasticity and lower extremity function in diplegic cerebral palsy: randomized controlled trial. Int J Phys Med Rehabil 3:1. https://doi.org/10.4172/2329-9096.1000253

Lance JW (1980) Symposium synopsis. In: Feldman RG, Young RR, Koella WP (eds) Spasticity: disordered motor control. Symposia Specialists. Year Book Medical Publishers, Chicago

Lederman E (1997) Fundamentals of manual therapy: physiology, neurology and psychology. Churchill Livingstone, Edinburgh

Lewit K (1999) Manipulative therapy in rehabilitation of the locomotor system, 3rd edn. Butterworth-Heinemann Publ.

Loi EC, Buysse CA, Price KS, Jaramillo TM, Pico EL, Hansen AB, Feldman HM (2015) Myofascial structural integration therapy on gross motor function and gait of young children with spastic cerebral palsy: a randomized controlled trial. Front Pediatr 3:74. https://doi. org/10.3389/fped.2015.00074

Macgregor R, Campbell R, Gladden MH, Tennant N, Young D (2007) Effects of massage on the mechanical behaviour of muscles in adolescents with spastic diplegia: a pilot study. Dev Med Child Neurol 49(3):187–191. https://doi.org/10.1111/j.1469-8749.2007.00187.x

Maitland GD (1985) The Slump Test: an examination and treatment. Aust J Physiother 31:215–219. https://doi.org/10.1016/S0004-9514(14)60634-6

Marbini A, Ferrari A, Cioni G, Bellanova MF, Fusco C, Gemignani F (2002) Immunohistochemical study of muscle biopsy in children with cerebral palsy. Brain Dev. 24:63–66. https://doi. org/10.1016/s0387-7604(01)00394-1

Marsico P, Tal-Akabi A, Van Hedel HJ (2016a) Reliability and practicability of the straight leg raise test in children with cerebral palsy. Dev Med Child Neurol 58(2):173–179. https://doi. org/10.1111/dmcn.12797

Marsico P, Tal-Akabi A, van Hedel HJA (2016b) The relevance of nerve mobility on function and activity in children with Cerebral Palsy. BMC Neurol 16:194. https://doi.org/10.1186/ s12883-016-0715-z

McClure V (2017) Infant massage: a handbook for loving parents, 4th edn. Bantam Pub.

Mockford M, Caulton JM (2010) The pathophysiological basis of weakness in children with cerebral palsy. Pediatr Phys Ther 22(2):222–233. https://doi.org/10.1097/PEP.0b013e3181dbaf96

Moseley GL, Hodges PW, Gandevia SC (2002) Deep and superficial fibers of the lumbar multifidus muscle are differentially active during voluntary arm movements. Spine 27:E29–E36. https://doi.org/10.1097/00007632-200201150-00013

Nielsen JB, Crone C, Hultborn H (2007) The spinal pathophysiology of spasticity—from a basic science point of view. Acta Physiol (Oxf) 189(2):171–180. https://doi. org/10.1111/j.1748-1716.2006.01652.x

Novak I (2011) Parent experience of implementing effective home programs. Phys Occup Ther Pediatr 31(2):198–213. https://doi.org/10.3109/01942638.2010.533746

Novak I, Berry J (2014) Home program intervention effectiveness evidence. Phys Occup Ther Pediatr 34(4):384–389. https://doi.org/10.3109/01942638.2014.964020

Opheim A, Jahnsen R, Olsson E, Stanghelle JK (2009) Walking function, pain, and fatigue in adults with cerebral palsy: a 7-year follow-up study. Dev Med Child Neurol 51(5):381–388. https://doi.org/10.1111/j.1469-8749.2008.03250.x

Ortiz Ramírez J, Pérez de la Cruz S (2017) Therapeutic effects of kinesio taping in children with cerebral palsy: a systematic review. Arch Argent Pediatr 115(6):e356–e361. https://doi. org/10.5546/aap.2017.eng.e356

Pados BF, McGlothen-Bell K (2019) Benefits of infant massage for infants and parents in the NICU. Nurs Womens Health 23(3):265–271. https://doi.org/10.1016/j.nwh.2019.03.004

Pandyan AD, Gregoric M, Barnes MP, Wood D, Van Wijck F, Burridge J, Hermens H, Johnson GR (2005) Spasticity: clinical perceptions, neurological realities and meaningful measurement. Disabil Rehabil 27(1–2):2–6. https://doi.org/10.1080/09638280400014576

Rocha T, Souza H, Brandão DC, Rattes C, Ribeiro L, Campos SL, Aliverti A, de Andrade AD (2015) The Manual Diaphragm Release Technique improves diaphragmatic mobility, inspiratory capacity and exercise capacity in people with chronic obstructive pulmonary disease: a randomised trial. J Physiother 61(4):182–189. https://doi.org/10.1016/j.jphys.2015.08.009

Rolf G (2001) Unpublished lectures given during the post-graduate course: patho-neurodynamics following lesions of the central nervous system. ART Educational and Rehabilitation Centre, Genova, Italy, 9–13 Oct 2000, pp 22–27

Rolf G (2002) The puzzle of pain, loss of mobility, evasive movements and the self-management; 25th March 2002. http://fysio1.inforce.dk/graphics/PDF/PDFJob.p65.PDF

Rose J, McGill KC (2005) Neuromuscular activation and motor-unit firing characteristics in cerebral palsy. Dev Med Child Neurol 47(5):329–336. https://doi.org/10.1017/s0012162205000629

Roy G, Nadeau S, Gravel D, Malouin F, McFadyen BJ (2006) The effect of foot position and chair height on the asymmetry of vertical forces during sit-to-stand and stand-to-sit tasks in individual with hemiparesis. Clin Biomech 21(6):585–593. https://doi.org/10.1016/j.clinbiomech.2006.01.007

Rutka M, Myśliwiec A, Wolny T, Gogola A, Linek P (2021) Influence of chest and diaphragm manual therapy on the spirometry parameters in patients with cerebral palsy: a pilot study. Biomed Res Int 2021:6263973. https://doi.org/10.1155/2021/6263973

Sanderson M (2021) Soft Tissue Release: a practical handbook for physical therapists, 4th edn. Lotus Publ., Chichester

Schleip R, Klingler W, Lehmann-Horn F (2005) Active fascial contractility: fascia may be able to contract in a smooth muscle-like manner and thereby influence musculoskeletal dynamics. Med Hypotheses 65(2):273–277. https://doi.org/10.1016/j.mehy.2005.03.005

Schleip R, Jäger H, Klingler W (2012) What is 'fascia'? A review of different nomenclatures. J Bodyw Mov Ther 16:496–502. https://doi.org/10.1016/j.jbmt.2012.08.001

Schleip R, Hedley G, Yucesoy CA (2019) Fascial nomenclature: update on related consensus process. Clin Anat 32(7):929–933. https://doi.org/10.1002/ca.23423

Schmidt RA (1975) A schema theory of discrete motor skill learning. Psychol Rev 82(4):225–260. https://doi.org/10.1037/h0076770

Shamos MH, Lavine LS (1967) Piezoelectricity as a fundamental property of biological tissues. Nature 213:267–269. https://doi.org/10.1038/213267a0

Shamsoddini A, Rasti Z, Kalantari M, Hollisaz MT, Sobhani V, Dalvand H, Kazem Bakhshandeh-Bali M (2016) The impact of Kinesio taping technique on children with cerebral palsy. Iran J Neurol 15(4):219–227

Sheperd RB (2014) Cerebral palsy in infancy, 1st edn. Churchill Livingstone, Elsevier Publ.

Shiffer R, Harms E (2014) Connective tissue massage: Bindegewebsmassage according to Dicke (English Edition). Georg Thieme Verlag KG

Shortland A (2011) Muscle volume and motor development in spastic cerebral palsy. Dev Med Child Neurol 2011(53):482–489. https://doi.org/10.1111/j.1469-8749.2011.03926.x

Stecco C, Schleip R (2016) A fascia and the fascial system. J Bodyw Mov Ther 20(1):139–140. https://doi.org/10.1016/j.jbmt.2015.11.012

Turrina A, Martínez-González MA, Stecco C (2013) The muscular force transmission system: role of the intramuscular connective tissue. J Bodyw Mov Ther 17:95–102. https://doi.org/10.1016/j.jbmt.2012.06.001

Unger M, Carstens JP, Fernandes N, Pretorius R, Pronk S, Robinson AC, Scheepers K (2018) The efficacy of kinesiology taping for improving gross motor function in children with cerebral palsy: a systematic review. S Afr J Physiother 74(1):459. https://doi.org/10.4102/sajp.v74i1.459

Vickers A, Ohlsson A, Lacy JB, Horsley A (2000) Massage for promoting growth and development of preterm and/or low birth-weight infants. Cochrane Database Syst Rev. https://doi.org/10.1002/14651858.CD000390.pub2

Whisler SL, Lang DM, Armstrong M, Vickers J, Qualls C, Feldman JS (2012) Effects of myofascial release and other advanced myofascial therapies on children with cerebral palsy: six case reports. Explore (NY) 8(3):199–205. https://doi.org/10.1016/j.explore.2012.02.003

White MA, Pape KE (1992) The Slump Test. Am J Occup Ther 46:271–274. https://doi.org/10.5014/ajot.46.3.271

Yang YR, Wang RY, Lin KH, Chu MY, Chan RC (2006) Task-oriented progressive resistance strength training improves muscle strength and functional performance in individuals with stroke. Clin Rehabil 20(10):860–870. https://doi.org/10.1177/0269215506070701

Yoshioka S, Nagano A, Himeno R, Fukashiro S (2007) Computation of the kinematics and the minimum peak joint moments of sit-to-stand movements. Biomed Eng Online 6:26. https://doi.org/10.1186/1475-925X-6-26

Guidelines for Upper Limb Rehabilitation

8

Gabriella Veruggio

8.1 The Upper Limb Functional Development

The development of increasingly refined and complex upper limb motor and perceptual skills is of critical importance. These skills are needed for play, touch, explore, caress and indicate and to carry out all activities of daily life including self-help tasks, such as feeding, toileting, dressing, drawing and writing (Fig. 8.1).

The hand can sense and act at the same time and therefore has an essential relevance in the neuropsychological development of the child and in the achievement of skills that will lead to autonomy.

8.1.1 The Physiological Development of Function in the Upper Limb

In the first years of life, the basic patterns of reaching, prehension and release evolve rapidly into increasingly efficient manipulative patterns. The child gradually acquires the ability to control reaching with increasing accuracy and to voluntarily grasp and release all kinds of objects (Fig. 8.2) (Koupernik and Dailly 1968; Twitchell 1970; Rosembloom and Horton 1971; Erhardt 1974, 1981; Jeannerod 1990, 1994; Henderson and Pehoski 2006; O'Brien and Kuhaneck 2019).

Later, during the child's development, it is possible to observe an increasing differentiation and modulation of the use of the upper limb (UL) segments and the acquisition of intrinsic movements for in-hand manipulation (Fig. 8.3) (Exner 1990a, b, 1992, 2005; Pehoski et al. 1997), together with a more differentiated and coordinated bilateral hands activity (Elliott and Connolly 1974; Henderson and Pehoski 2006).

G. Veruggio (✉)
AAC Service of Benedetta d'Intino Centre, Milan, Italy

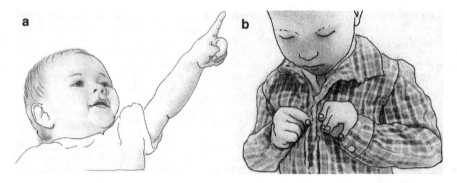

Fig. 8.1 Hands used to point

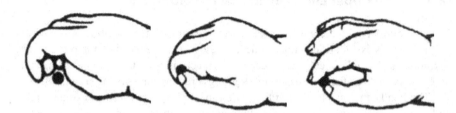

Fig. 8.2 Primarily voluntary movements (grasp of the pellet) (from EDPA by R.P. Erhardt 1994, reprinted by permission)

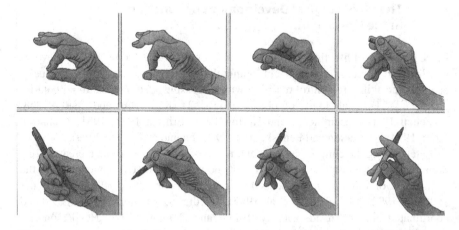

Fig. 8.3 Some in-hand manipulation movements (Modified from Elliott and Connolly 1984)

These acquired skills will allow the child to achieve increasingly complex motor skills and efficient use of different tools (Napier 1956; Denckla 1974; Kamakura et al. 1980; Elliott and Connolly 1984; Connolly and Dalgleish 1989; Humphry et al. 1995) (Fig. 8.4), which are essential abilities for all the daily occupations of

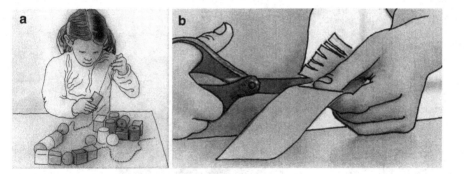

Fig. 8.4 Differentiated and coordinated bilateral hand use

childhood, e.g. play, activities of daily life (ADL), instrumental ADL (IADL) and handwriting.

After the second year of life, the quality of the gesture improves and shows more fluency, harmony, speed, adaptability and efficacy.

It is essential to have a thorough knowledge in the physiological development of the UL and hand control to better understand the functional problems of the child with cerebral palsy (CP), even though the therapist can only rarely translate the exact developmental sequences into treatment.

In the literature, there are many interesting studies, useful for a better knowledge of the natural functional development of the UL of the child (Halverson 1940; Piaget 1952; Bruner 1970; Connolly 1970; Kopp 1974; Touwen 1975; Sheridan 1977; Holstein 1982; Fedrizzi et al. 1994; Forssberg 1998; Henderson and Pehoski 2006).

8.1.2 The Upper Limb Functional Development in Cerebral Palsy

In the child with CP, the most basic hand function achievements, such as reaching, prehension and release, are often delayed in time and often limited or completely absent in children with severe motor impairment. Almost 50% of children with CP present an arm-hand dysfunction (Uvebrant 1988; Fedrizzi et al. 2003; Arnould et al. 2007).

Abnormal stiffness, the persistence of primitive reflexes, motor coordination problems and perceptual disorders are the most common features that limit the child's development of hand skills (Twitchell 1965; Gilfoyle et al. 1981; Mark Carter 1983; Pratt and Allen 1989; Erhardt 1995; Henderson and Pehoski 2006; Arnould et al. 2007, 2014; Eliasson et al. 1991, 2006a; Himmelmann et al. 2006). Significant impairments in most basic hand functions affect or preclude the more complex and mature manipulative abilities achievement, such as the more differentiated and coordinated in-hand manipulation and bilateral hand use.

The impact of CP on a child's hand functioning may be formalized through the theoretical framework of the children and youth version of the International Classification of Functioning (WHO 2007), which considers three separate but

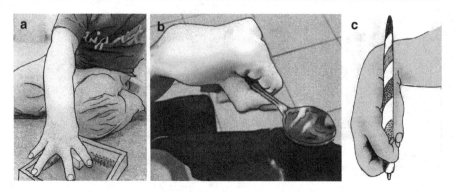

Fig. 8.5 Prehension dysfunctions in the child with cerebral palsy

Fig. 8.6 Dysfunction in the coordinated and differentiated use of both upper limbs

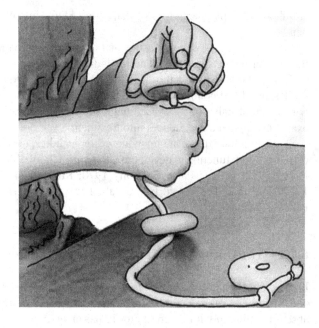

related functioning domains, referring to body functions and structures, activities and participation (Beckung and Hagberg 2002; Rosenbaum and Stewart 2004; Arnould et al. 2014) (Fig. 8.5).

The quality of gestures is also compromised. Even mild CP children are clumsy, slow and poorly efficient in performing finer and complex tasks, such as assembling constructions, using pens and pencils, buttoning, using scissors, etc. (Fig. 8.6).

Problems of control of upper limbs and fine motor skill achievement result from the combination of several factors:

– Many children with CP have difficulties using UL depending on trunk control disorders. Therefore, they often need to use one or both upper extremities to support themself and stabilize their sitting/standing position, and cannot use their arms and hands for functional tasks.

– The lack of ability to maintain a stable position or even an abnormal posture in sitting limits bilateral hand use and fine motor skill development.

– The child, in the effort to play or perform various ADLs, learns to use compensatory patterns, such as the lateral trunk flexion for reaching, the trunk and head extension for moving the UL on the sagittal plane or even the wrist flexion for opening their hand.

– Disorders in complementary two-hand use (symmetrical and asymmetrical) are common. Some children may find it difficult to place both hands on the midline when performing a defined task; others fail due to a severe functional deficit of a limb, using it only in simpler locking tasks, e.g. blocking a paper sheet on the desk to scribble with the more able hand, or in simple holding, the task to easily manage objects. Furthermore, some children, although able to work in the midline and with good grasping patterns at both upper extremities, are unable to dissociate the movements of the two hands and have difficulty in performing tasks that require their use in a finest, differentiated and complementary manner.

– The child with CP also has difficulty in grading upper limb movements. They perform movements of amplitude, speed and strength often inappropriately for the task, showing the difficulty in coordinating the various segments of the upper limbs and in controlling their intermediate movements. Often, to overcome such difficulties, the child learns to "lock" one or more joints to facilitate the upper limb's functional use, such as taking advantage of shoulder protraction, elbow extension, forearm pronation and flexion wrist with extended fingers.

– Another problem, particularly in mildly impaired children, is the difficulty of isolating the movements required for a specific task. The child tends to move arm and hand in synergistic patterns and, in the case of fine motor activities, is lacking the ability to isolate distal movements, to differentiate the hand's radial side use from the ulnar side, for example, and to isolate a single finger to type on a keyboard, etc.

– To overcome these problems, the child learns to use different compensatory strategies. These strategies may be effective initially, but, in the long term, they can restrict the acquisition of more complex movements or cause contractures, reduction in joint excursion and, in some cases, more severe skeletal deformities.

– Perceptual, sensory and cognitive disorders, which have significant interrelationship, can affect upper limb use and will need to be properly assessed in order to define a realistic, functional prognosis and to set up an appropriate rehabilitation project (Henderson and Pehoski 2006; Odding et al. 2006; Himmelmann et al. 2006; Sigurdardottir and Vik 2011; Case-Smith 2019).

– Finally, the upper limbs functional use and, more generally, the participation of children with CP in all daily occupations of childhood, can also be affected by environmental factors (physical environments, caregiver attitudes, culture, etc.) (Law et al. 1999; Ostensjo et al. 2003; Rosenbaum and Stewart 2004; Mihaylov et al. 2004; Arnould et al. 2014), that will need to be carefully analysed.

8.2 General Guidelines for Intervention

The intervention, aimed at improving the UL functional use in all-day activities of the child, as stressed by ICF (Beckung and Hagberg 2002; Rosenbaum and Stewart 2004), is implemented with a "mixed"-type approach.

Through play and specific activity proposals (Fig. 8.7) rehabilitation intervention is aimed at optimizing the UL performance to reach specific, realistic and achievable functional goals, in agreement with the child and/or their family (Gordon 1992; Missiuna and Pollock 2000; Case-Smith 2019).

However, the rehabilitation intervention is also aimed at providing the child with CP with real opportunities for play, communication and movement, using various compensatory strategies, (bypass strategies). For example, simplifications of tasks could be the application of straps (Fig. 8.7) or the use of gloves with Velcro,[1] environmental adaptations or the use of assistive technology (AT) to overcome the UL problems (Pratt and Allen 1989; Ostensjo et al. 2003; Eliasson and Burtner 2008; Henderson et al. 2008; Sadao and Robinson 2010; Case-Smith 2019).

To set up an appropriate project, it is necessary to carry out a careful and prolonged observation and assessment of the UL functionality, after collecting information about the child's strong points, interests, their goals and the characteristics of the environment. This assessment should be repeated over time to record any modification in the UL performances and to update the functional prognosis and consequent short- and long-term goals (Gordon 1992; Missiuna and Pollock 2000; Case-Smith 2019).

8.3 Upper Limb Assessment

First of all, the therapist carries out a general observation of the use of UL, both in the clinical setting and in the different environments of the child's life (home, school, etc.), recording how the upper limbs are used in the natural contexts of play, communication and ADL, also considering the environmental constraints.

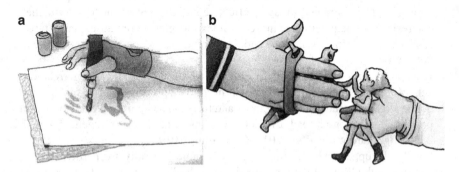

Fig. 8.7 Bypass strategies

---

[1] Velcro Co., https://www.velcro.com

Table 8.1 Methodological framework for UL observation and assessment (Veruggio 2000)

(A)	**Postural control/positioning**
1.	Assessment of the sitting position and the child's pathological patterns which affect the ability to maintain it, e.g. flexion/extension synergies, involuntary movements, primitive reflexes
2.	Identification of a better positioning system which facilitates the maintenance of the posture, the functional use of the ULs and eye-gaze control, taking into consideration, for example, the chair/wheelchair, table/lap tray with a recess or other postural system components, stabilizations and anchoring systems
3.	Assessment of UL control in other positions (side-lying, standing, on standing frame, etc.)
(B)	**Spontaneous upper limb use/possible functional performances/reaching control/ most proficient upper limb identification**
1.	Overall observation of spontaneous use of ULs and their functionality, during play, the ADL activities and communication
2.	Reaching control assessment and, particularly, identification of the most proficient UL
3.	Use of specific assessment scales to highlight possible problems related to unestablished handedness
4.	Evaluation of the potential of other segments of the child's body or gaze, for functional activities and/or for alternative access to AT
5.	Early formulation of hypotheses on sensory, perceptual and cognitive factors that can influence the performance of the ULs, with an in-depth analysis of these factors
(C)	**Prehension/manipulation**
1.	(a) Under 36 months: observation/assessment of the basic hand skill development (reaching, prehension, release)
	(b) Assessment of prehension patterns of both ULs, through the use of standardized clinical scales
2.	Assessment of in-hand manipulation movements, strength and precision grip and bilateral hand use (according to UL performances emerged in b) and the chronological age of the child)
3.	Observation and critical evaluation of any involuntary movements and their influence on the use of ULs and postural control, in addition to the compensatory strategies used to overcome the involuntary movements

Usually, when the child is three, a further, more precise assessment of the ULs is suggested, as reported in the methodological framework of Table 8.1.

- In the first phase of the assessment, the therapist looks for the best positioning system that optimizes the voluntary and functional UL use and visual control (Ward 1984; Pratt and Allen 1989; Myhr and von Wendt 1991; Myhr et al. 1993, 1995; Trefler et al. 1993; Sahinoğlu et al. 2017; Case-Smith 2019). For this, it is necessary to position the child sitting in a chair of adequate size, with their feet resting on the ground, in front of a table, preferably with recess and at a height allowing forearm support (Fig. 8.8). If the child is unable to sit alone, because of postural control difficulties, special chairs or posture systems can be used, even adopting additional components, such as pelvic belt, armrest, lateral hip pad, headrest, footplates, etc. Some clinical scales assessing the sitting posture can also be used (Myhr et al. 1993; Field and Roxborough 2011; Field and Livingstone 2013).

Fig. 8.8 Appropriate
positioning system to
optimize the UL use and
eye-gaze control

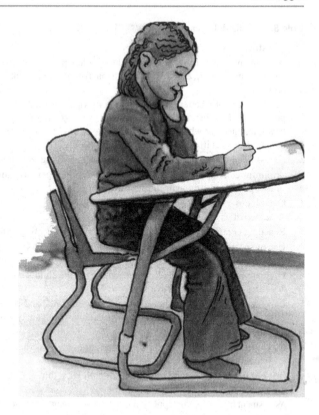

- Later, it is necessary to evaluate the UL reaching control, through play proposals, meaningful for the child but also adequate to their functional level, assessing the child's abilities to control their UL movements on the three different planes (Fig. 8.9). Regarding this aspect, the therapist can also use specific standardized clinical scales for functional assessment of the UL, as suggested in Table 8.2. Based on this assessment, it is often possible to identify the most proficient upper limb to be used for functional activities and the overall potential use of the "assisting" arm.
- Sometimes, in children with mild and moderate impairment, it may be necessary to extend the investigation of the problems related to unestablished handedness, here again using a specific assessment scale (Auzias 1984; Henderson and Pehoski 2006; Erhardt 2012).
- Furthermore, the therapist should evaluate other impairments (e.g. sensory, perceptual, cognitive) conditioning the UL use, particularly hand-eye coordination.
- In children with severe disabilities, if even limited use of the upper limbs is not possible or extremely difficult, it is necessary to evaluate other parts of the child's body (head, lower limbs, etc.) or the use of other controlled movements (e.g. fixed gaze) (Henderson et al. 2008; Borgestig et al. 2015). Appropriate alternative access and aids can also be adapted (Fig. 8.10).

Fig. 8.9 Reaching
assessment

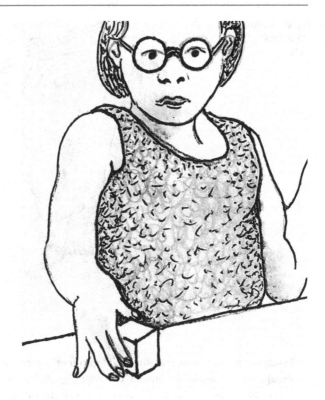

Table 8.2 Standardized clinical scales for the evaluation of UL function in CP

Body function domain

- The Gross Motor Function Classification System (GMFCS, Palisano et al. 1997)
- The Quality of Upper Extremity Skills Test (QUEST, De Matteo et al. 1992)
- The Melbourne Assessment of Unilateral Upper Limb Function (MUUL, Randall et al. 1999)

Activity domain

- Assisting Hand Assessment (AHA, Krumlinde-Sunddholm and Eliasson 2003)
- Manual Ability Classification System (MACS, Eliasson et al. 2006b)
- Mini-MACS (Eliasson et al. 2017)
- Jebsen-Taylor Test of Hand Function (JTHFT, Jebsen et al. 1969)
- Besta Scale (Rosa-Rizzotto et al. 2014)

Participation domain

- Pediatric Evaluation of Disability Inventory (PEDI, Haley et al. 1992)
- ABILHAND-Kids (Arnould et al. 2004).
- Canadian Occupational Performance Measure (COPM, Law et al. 1994)

Fig. 8.10 Possible use of
other parts of the
child's body

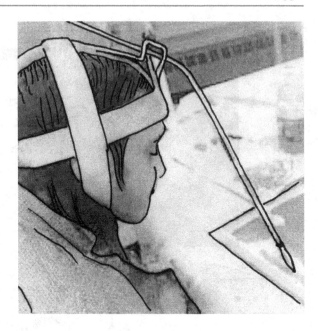

- In children with moderate/mild impairment, both hand prehension patterns should be assessed. In younger children, the prehension assessment is mainly based on the observation of prehension patterns during playing and ADLs, for example using the Erhardt Developmental Prehension Assessment (EDPA) (Erhardt 1994) which proposes a series of objects that requires basic reaching, prehension and release patterns (Fig. 8.11).
- After the age of three, concerning the UL function previously observed (see Table 8.1(B)) and the child's chronological age, the therapist should also evaluate the in-hand manipulation movements, the bilateral hand activity as well as the strength and precision grip.
- Some standardized scales for the evaluation of the UL function in CP are suggested below (see in Table 8.2). The application of the ICF helps considerably in the selection of those evaluation tools useful for defining aims and decision-making processes and also for measuring the outcomes (Coster 1998; Rosenbaum and Stewart 2004; Majnemer 2006; Gilmore et al. 2010; Klingels et al. 2010; Hoare et al. 2011; Lemmens et al. 2012; Santos et al. 2015; Wallen and Stewart 2015).
- Finally, the therapist observes any involuntary movements caused by UL use, their effect on functional activities and the compensatory strategies that the child adopts to control these movements, to overcome their interference and to play and to perform the ADLs.

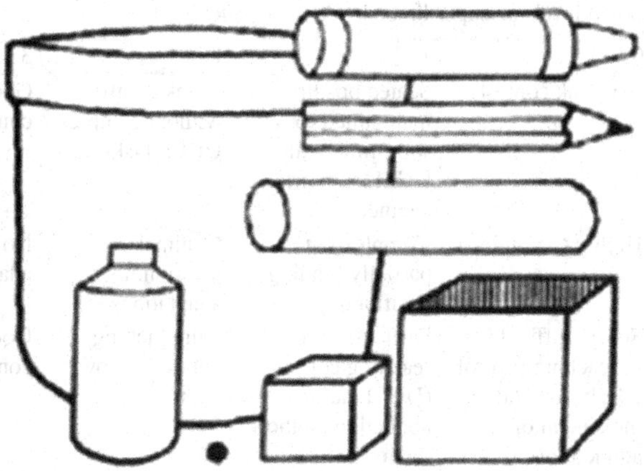

Fig. 8.11 Materials used for prehension assessment in younger children (from EDPA scale, by R.P. Erhardt 1994, reprinted by permission). Graduated set of large containers (5–8 cm wide). Graduated set of small bottles (opening from diam. 1–3 cm). Graduated series of wood dowels (diam. 1–2 ½ cm). Graduated series of wood or foam cubes (from 3 to 6 cm). Graduated series of three edible or Play Dough pellets (diam. from 5 mm to 1 ½ cm). Crayon (diam. 1 ½ cm). Pencil (diam. 7 mm)

8.4 Planning a Functional Treatment

Based on the UL assessment of the child, it is possible to determine an initial prognosis on the achievable functional level, to be continuously verified and updated during the treatment and following evaluations.

Factors influencing the functional prognosis of the upper limbs include also sensation, perception, cognition, relationship and environment.

Clinical evaluation data concerning sitting posture control, reaching, grasping and manipulation patterns create a "picture" of the child's UL function (excluding unilateral forms), defining three levels of score from 0 to 3 (Table 8.3).

The functional level 0 and 1 means a severe impairment, a limitation in body function and all the child's activities (i.e. play, ADLs, mobility, education and communication). Children with this score require continuous support from caregivers, with important adaptations for feasible tasks, using bypass strategies.

Children with functional levels 2 and 3 have a better prognosis with greater autonomy in daily life, based on the tasks required in the environment.

Based on this evaluation, a therapeutic plan is then formulated, identifying the short-/medium-/long-term goals, which should be continuously updated over time (Law et al. 1999). The rehabilitation project is aimed at improving specific arm/hand performances and ADL/IADL autonomy; with level 0 or 1, the goal is to identify bypass solutions that provide for real participation of the child in social life (Rosenbaum and Stewart 2004).

Table 8.3 Functional levels of upper limbs in CP (Veruggio 2000)

	0	1	2	3
Postural control	No trunk control	Seated posture maintained for a short time with UULL support/ balance	Trunk control, without complex UULL tasks	Good head/trunk control
Positioning	Highly customized	Complex but partially binding positioning	Minimal positioning adaptations	No positioning adaptations
Possible functional performance Reaching control	Severe difficulties in reaching control (UL horizontal movement of adduction/ abduction)	Difficulties in reaching control (UULL adduction/ abduction—elbow flexion/extension)	Fair reaching control (elbow use)	Good reaching control
More proficient upper limb	Single UL use only (if possible)	Use of only most proficient hand/ arm or alternative use of a single UL	Limited bilateral hands use (one in assisting function)	Bilateral hands use
Prehension/ manipulation	No prehension and manipulation	Sometimes possible palmar grasp and lateral pinch	Palmar or three-point pinch grasp	Power and precision grip (various type of two-point pinch)
	Sometimes possible simple contact of the object or shifting or switch activation	Severely limited manipulation Possible simple contact of object or shifting or switch activation	Limited bilateral hands use (one in assisting function)	Bilateral hands use (possible simultaneous and cooperative hands use)
		Sometimes possible single finger use	Possible single finger use	In-hand manipulation

8.5   Practical Suggestions

Here below are indicated some possible planning paths for the rehabilitation treatment, the first concerning CP children with severe impairment (level 0–1) and the second one regarding moderate/mild impaired children (level 2–3).

Level 0–1
– Good positioning that allows the best voluntary functional use of the UL, with particular attention to head and trunk control, visual control
– Analytical intervention on the upper limbs, through play activities, aimed mainly at achieving voluntarily controlled movements, essential for access to play, to AAC systems, to AT tools (e.g. writing access, system environmental control, power supply for wheelchair mobility); search for the simplest patterns to reach, grasp and release; one finger/pointing control; activation/release of special switches, electric wheelchair control device)

- Identification of any other part of the child's body to replace the use of the upper limbs, subsequently implementing a specific rehabilitation treatment
- Facilitation of access to play as independent as possible, through placement for the toys, their adaption, selected strategies; caregiver training is recommended to educate them on how to modify toys and how to use them
- Support for access to Augmentative and Alternative Communication (AAC) systems (face-to-face, written and remote communication, e.g. access to mobile technologies, the Internet, etc.) in children with communication problems, identifying and developing the "natural resources" available for unaided and assisted communication (e.g. communication cards, eye-transfer boards (ETRAN), speech-generating device (SGD)) (see also Chap. 12)
- Direct intervention in favour of the child to achieve partial autonomy, or indirect intervention in favour of caregivers, aimed at facilitating their care assistance
- Improvement of sensory/perceptual and cognitive development
- Support for access to school activities by identifying appropriate adaptations of learning tools: from simple solutions for access to learning to technologically advanced ones, such as training on the use of the keyboard, special switches or use of the eye-tracking, scanning software, etc. (see also Chap. 13)
- Suggest transfer modes during ADL and support access to electric wheelchair mobility if possible

Level 2–3
- Identification of different positionings to facilitate different ADLs, as in the child with traditional development
- Analytical intervention on upper limbs and fine motor skills, e.g. reaching control in the three spatial plans, prehension and release of objects with radial and terminal pincer, in-hand manipulation and bilateral hand activities, as differentiated as possible
- Support to play development, through toys, play and environmental adaptations
- Facilitation to school activities access, e.g. environmental adaptations, intervention on the executive aspects of writing for access to pen-and-paper writing, computer writing and other school device access
- Direct/indirect rehabilitation intervention on the ADL/IADLs, e.g. environmental and self-care technique adaptations, as for dressing, hygiene, etc.
- Intervention on mobility with or without aids, with focus on daily transfers, outdoor mobility or public transport access, if feasible
- Longitudinal support to AAC systems access, e.g. face-to-face, written and remote communication, such as access to the Internet with mobile technologies, if needed (see also Chap. 12)

Finally, to set up a rehabilitation plan, it is necessary to know more details about the general UL problems in the different forms of CP, as described in the next chapter.

References

Arnould C, Penta M, Renders A et al (2004) ABILHAND-Kids: a measure of manual ability in children with cerebral palsy. Neurology 2004(63):1045–1052. https://doi.org/10.1212/01. wnl.0000138423.77640.37

Arnould C, Penta M, Thonnard JL (2007) Hand impairments and their relationship with manual ability in children with cerebral palsy. J Rehabil Med 2007(39):708–714. https://doi.org/10.234 0/16501977-0111

Arnould C, Bleyenheuft Y, Thonnard JL (2014) Hand functioning in children with cerebral palsy. Front Neurol 2014(5):48. https://doi.org/10.3389/fneur.2014.00048

Auzias M (1984) Enfants gauchers, enfants droitiers. Delachaux et Niestlé, Neuchatel

Beckung E, Hagberg G (2002) Neuroimpairments, activity limitations, and participation restrictions in children with cerebral palsy. Dev Med Child Neurol 2002(44):309–316. https://doi. org/10.1017/S0012162201002134

Borgestig M, Sandqvist J, Parsons R, Falkmer T, Hemmingsson H (2015) Eye gaze performance for children with severe physical impairments using gaze-based assistive technology—a longitudinal study. Assist Technol 2015(28):93–102. https://doi.org/10.3109/17518423.2015.1132281

Bruner JS (1970) The growth and structure of skills. In: Connolly K (ed) Mechanism of motor skill development. Academic, London

Case-Smith J (2019) Occupational therapy for children and adolescents. Elsevier

Connolly K (1970) Mechanism of motor skill development. Academic, London

Connolly K, Dalgleish M (1989) The emergence of a tool-using skill in infancy. Dev Psychol 25(6):894–912. https://doi.org/10.1037/0012-1649.25.6.894

Coster W (1998) Occupation-centered assessment of children. Am J Occup Ther 52:337–344. https://doi.org/10.5014/ajot.52.5.337

De Matteo C, Law M, Russell D, Pollock N, Rosenbaum P, Walter S (1992) Quality of upper extremity skills test manual. McMaster University, CanChild, McMaster University, Hamilton, Ontario, Hamilton

Denckla MD (1974) Development of motor coordination in normal children. Dev Med Child Neurol 1974(15):635–645. https://doi.org/10.1111/j.1469-8749.1974.tb03393.x

Eliasson AC, Burtner PA (2008) Improving hand function in children with cerebral palsy: theory, evidence and intervention. Mac Keith Press, Cambridge

Eliasson AC, Gordon AM, Forssberg H (1991) Basic co-ordination of manipulative forces of children with cerebral palsy. Dev Med Child Neurol 33:661–670. https://doi.org/10.1111/j.1469-8749.1991.tb14943.x

Eliasson AC, Forssberg H, Hung YC, Gordon AM (2006a) Development of hand function and precision grip control in individuals with cerebral palsy: a 13-year follow-up study. Pediatrics 118:1226–1236. https://doi.org/10.1542/peds.2005-2768

Eliasson AC, Krumlinde-Sundholm L, Rösblad B, Beckung E, Arner M, Ohrvall AM, Rosenbaum P (2006b) The Manual Ability Classification System (MACS) for children with cerebral palsy: scale development and evidence of validity and reliability. Dev Med Child Neurol 2006(48):549–554. https://doi.org/10.1017/S0012162206001162

Eliasson AC, Ullenhag A, Wahlström U, Lena Krumlinde-Sundholm L (2017) Mini-MACS: development of the Manual Ability Classification System for children younger than 4 years of age with signs of cerebral palsy. Dev Med Child Neurol 2017(59):72–78. https://doi.org/10.1111/ dmcn.13162

Elliott JM, Connolly KJ (1974) Hierarchical structure in skill development. In: Connoly KJ, Bruner JS (eds) The growth of competence. Academic, London, pp 135–168

Elliott JM, Connolly KJ (1984) A classification of manipulative hand movements. Dev Med Child Neurol 1984(26):283–296. https://doi.org/10.1111/j.1469-8749.1984.tb04445.x

Erhardt RP (1974) Sequential level in developmental prehension. Am J Occup Ther 28(10):592–596

Erhardt RP (1994) The Erhardt Developmental Prehension Assessment (EDPA). Erhardt Developmental Products, Maplewood. www.ErhardtProducts.com

Erhardt RP (1995) Developmental Hand Dysfunction: theory, assessment, treatment, 2nd edn. Communication Skills Builders, Tucson

Erhardt RP (2012) Hand preference: theory, assessment and implication for function. Erhardt Developmental Product

Erhardt RP, Beatty PA, Hertsgaard DM (1981) A development prehension assessment for handicapped children. Am J Occup Ther 1981(4):237–242. https://doi.org/10.5014/ajot.35.4.237

Exner CE (1990a) In-hand manipulation skills in normal young children: a pilot study. Occup Ther Pract 1(4):63–72

Exner CE (1990b) The zone of proximal development. In: In-hand manipulation skills of non-dysfunctional 3 and 4 year-old children. Am J Occup Ther 44:884–891. https://doi.org/10.5014/ajot.44.10.884

Exner CE (1992) In-hand manipulation skills. In: Case-Smith J, Pehoski C (eds) Development of hand skills in the child. The Am. Occup. Ther. Association Inc., Rockville, pp 35–45

Exner CE (2005) The development of hand skills. In: Case-Smith J (ed) Occupational therapy for children, 5th edn. Mosby, St Louis, pp 304–355

Fedrizzi E, Avanzini G, Crenna P (1994) Motor development in children. John Libbey & Company, London

Fedrizzi E, Pagliano E, Andreucci E, Oleari G (2003) Hand function in children with hemiplegic cerebral palsy: prospective follow-up and functional outcome in adolescence. Dev Med Child Neurol 2003(45):85–91. https://doi.org/10.1111/j.1469-8749.2003.tb00910.x

Field DA, Livingstone R (2013) Clinical tools that measure sitting posture, seated postural control or functional abilities in children with motor impairments: a systematic review. Clin Rehabil 2013(27):994–1004. https://doi.org/10.1177/0269215513488122

Field DA, Roxborough LA (2011) Responsiveness of the seated postural control measure and the level of sitting scale in children with neuromotor disorders. J Disabil Rehabil Assist Technol 6:473–482. https://doi.org/10.3109/17483107.2010.532255

Forssberg H (1998) The neurophysiology of manual skills development. In: Connolly KJ (ed) The psychobiology of the hand. Cambridge University Press, Cambridge

Gilfoyle EM, Grady AP, Moore JC (1981) Children adapt. Slack Inc., Thorofare

Gilmore R, Sakzewski L, Boyd R (2010) Upper limb activity measures for 5- to 16-year-old children with congenital hemiplegia: a systematic review. Dev Med Child Neurol 2010(52):14–22. https://doi.org/10.1111/j.1469-8749.2009.03369.x

Gordon N (1992) Independence for the physically disabled. Child Care Health Dev 18:97–105. https://doi.org/10.1111/j.1365-2214.1992.tb00344.x

Haley SM, Coster WJ, Ludlow LH et al (1992) Pediatric Evaluation of Disability Inventory (PEDI). New England Medical Center Hospitals, Boston

Halverson HM (1940) Prehension and manipulation. In: Gesell A (ed) The first five years of life New York. Harper & Brothers

Henderson A, Pehoski C (2006) Hand function in the child: foundations for remediation. Elsevier Health Sciences. https://doi.org/10.1016/B978-0-323-03186-8.X5001-1

Henderson S, Skelton H, Rosenbaum P (2008) Assistive devices for children with functional impairments: impact on child and caregiver function. Dev Med Child Neurol 50(2):89–98. https://doi.org/10.1111/j.1469-8749.2007.02021.x

Himmelmann K, Beckung E, Hagberg G, Uvebrant P (2006) Gross and fine motor function and accompanying impairments in cerebral palsy. Dev Med Child Neurol 2006(48):417–423. https://doi.org/10.1017/S0012162206000922

Hoare B, Imms C, Randall M, Carey L (2011) Linking cerebral palsy upper limb measures to the international classification of functioning, disability and health. J Rehabil Med 2011(43):987–996. https://doi.org/10.2340/16501977-0886

Holstein R (1982) The development of prehension in normal infants. Am J Occup Ther 1982(3):170–176. https://doi.org/10.5014/ajot.36.3.170

Humphry R, Jewell K, Rosenberger RC (1995) Development of in-hand manipulation and relationship with activities. Am J Occup Ther 49(8):763–771. https://doi.org/10.5014/ajot.49.8.763

Jeannerod M (1990) The neural and behavioural organisation of goal-directed movements. Oxford University Press, new ed.

Jeannerod M (1994) Chapter 3: Development of reaching and grasping. In: Fedrizzi E, Avanzini G, Crenna P (eds) Motor development in children. John Libbey & Co. Ltd, London, pp 25–32

Jebsen RH, Yaylor N, Trieshmann RB, Trotter MJ, Howard LA (1969) An objective and standardized test of hand function. Arch Phys Med Rehabil 1969(50):311–319

Kamakura N, Matsuo M, Ishii H, Misuboshi F, Miura Y (1980) Patterns of static prehension in normal hands. Dev Med Child Neurol 7:437–445. https://doi.org/10.5014/ajot.34.7.437

Klingels K, Jaspers E, Van de Winckel A, De Cock P, Molenaers G, Feys H (2010) A systematic review of arm activity measures for children with hemiplegic cerebral palsy. Clin Rehabil 2010(24):887–900. https://doi.org/10.1177/0269215510367994

Kopp CB (1974) Fine motor abilities of infants. Dev Med Child Neurol 16:629–636. https://doi.org/10.1111/j.1469-8749.1974.tb04181.x

Koupernik C, Dailly R (1968) Le développement neuro-psychique du nourrisson (Sémiologie normale et pathologique). Press Universitare de France, Paris

Krumlinde-Sunddholm L, Eliasson AC (2003) Development of the Assisting Hand Assessment, a Rash built measure intended for children with unilateral upper limb impairments. Scand J Occup Ther 2003(10):16–26. https://doi.org/10.1080/11038120310004529

Law M, Polatajko H, Pollock N, McColl MA, Carswell A, Baptiste S (1994) Pilot testing of the Canadian Occupational Performance Measure: clinical and measurement issues. Can J Occup Ther 61(4):191–197. https://doi.org/10.1177/000841749406100403

Law M, Haight M, Milroy B, Willms D, Stewart D, Rosenbaum P (1999) Environmental factors affecting the occupations of children with physical disabilities. J Occup Sci 6:102–110. https://doi.org/10.1080/14427591.1999.9686455

Lemmens RJ, Timmermans AA, Janssen-Potten YJ, Smeets RJ, Seelen HA (2012) Valid and reliable instruments for arm-hand assessment at ICF activity level in persons with hemiplegia: a systematic review. BMC Neurol 12:21. https://doi.org/10.1186/1471-2377-12-21

Majnemer A (2006) Assessment tools for cerebral palsy. Future Neurol 1:755–763. https://doi.org/10.2217/14796708.1.6.755

Mark Carter B (1983) Reflex development and the prehensile deficit in cerebral palsy. Aust Occup Ther J 30:3–13. https://doi.org/10.1111/j.1440-1630.1983.tb01412.x

Mihaylov SI, Jarvis SN, Colver AF, Beresford B (2004) Identification and description of environmental factors that influence participation of children with cerebral palsy. Dev Med Child Neurol 46:299–304. https://doi.org/10.1017/s0012162204000490

Missiuna C, Pollock N (2000) Perceived efficacy and goal setting in young children. Can J Occup Ther 67:101–109. https://doi.org/10.1177/000841740006700303

Myhr U, von Wendt L (1991) Improvement of functional sitting position for children with cerebral palsy. Dev Med Child Neurol 33:246–256. https://doi.org/10.1111/j.1469-8749.1991.tb05114.x

Myhr U, von Wendt L, Sandberg KW (1993) Assessment of sitting in children with cerebral palsy from videofilm. Phys Occup Ther Pediatr 12(4):21–35. https://doi.org/10.1080/J006v12n04_03

Myhr U, von Wendt L, Norrlin S, Radell U (1995) Five-year follow-up of functional sitting position in children with cerebral palsy. Dev Med Child Neurol 37:587–596. https://doi.org/10.1111/j.1469-8749.1995.tb12047.x

Napier J (1956) The prehensile movements of the human hand. J Bone Joint Surg 38:902–913. https://doi.org/10.1302/0301-620x.38b4.902

O'Brien JC, Kuhaneck H (2019) Case-Smith's Occupational therapy for children and adolescent, 8th edn. Elsevier-Mosby

Odding E, Roebroeck ME, Stam HJ (2006) The epidemiology of cerebral palsy: incidence, impairments and risk factors. Disabil Rehabil 2006(28):183–191. https://doi.org/10.1080/09638280500158422

Ostensjo S, Carlberg EB, Vollestad NK (2003) Everyday functioning in young children with cerebral palsy: functional skills, caregiver assistance and modifications of the environment. Dev Med Child Neurol 45:603–612. https://doi.org/10.1017/S0012162203001105

Palisano R, Rosenbaum P, Walter S, Russel D, Wood E, Galuppi B (1997) Development and reliability of a system to classify gross motor function in children with cerebral palsy. Dev Med Child Neurol 39:214–223. https://doi.org/10.1111/j.1469-8749.1997.tb07414.x

Pehoski C, Henderson A, Tickle-Degnen L (1997) In-hand manipulation in young children: rotation of an object in the fingers. Am J Occup Ther 51:544–552. https://doi.org/10.5014/ajot.51.7.544

Piaget J (1952) The origins of intelligence in children. WW Norton & Co. https://doi.org/10.1037/11494-000

Pratt PN, Allen AS (1989) Occupational Therapy for children. Mosby Co.

Randall M, Johnson L, Reddihough D (1999) The Melbourne Assessment of Unilateral Upper Limb Function: test administration manual. Royal Children's Hospital, Melbourne, Melbourne

Rosa-Rizzotto M, Visonà Dalla Pozza L, Corlatti A, Luparia A, Marchi A, Molteni F, Facchin P, Pagliano E, Fedrizzi E, GIPCI Study Group (2014) A new scale for the assessment of performance and capacity of hand function in children with hemiplegic cerebral palsy: reliability and validity studies. Eur J Phys Rehabil Med 50(5):543–556

Rosembloom L, Horton ME (1971) The maturation of fine prehension in young children. Dev Med Child Neurol 1971(13):3–8. https://doi.org/10.1111/j.1469-8749.1971.tb03025.x

Rosenbaum P, Stewart D (2004) The World Health Organization International Classification of Functioning, Disability, and Health: a model to guide clinical thinking, practice and research in the field of cerebral palsy. Semin Pediatr Neurol 11:5–10. https://doi.org/10.1016/j.spen.2004.01.002

Sadao CK, Robinson NB (2010) Assistive Technology for young children. Paul Brookes Publishing Co.

Sahinoğlu D, Coskun G, Bek N (2017) Effects of different seating equipment on postural control and upper extremity function in children with cerebral palsy. Prosthetics Orthot Int 41(1):85–94. https://doi.org/10.1177/0309364616637490

Santos CA, Franco de Moura RC, Lazzari RD, Dumont AJ, Braun LA, Oliveira CS (2015) Upper limb function evaluation scales for individuals with cerebral palsy: a systematic review. J Phys Ther Sci 2015(27):1617–1620. https://doi.org/10.1589/jpts.27.1617

Sheridan MD (1977) Children's developmental progress from birth to five years. NFER Publishing Company

Sigurdardottir S, Vik T (2011) Speech, expressive language, and verbal cognition of preschool children with cerebral palsy in Iceland. Dev Med Child Neurol 53(1):74–80. https://doi.org/10.1111/j.1469-8749.2010.03790.x

Touwen BCL (1975) Neurological development in infancy. Spastic International Medical Publishers

Trefler E, Hobson DA, Johnson Taylor S, Monahan LC, Shaw CG (1993) Seating and mobility for persons with physical disability. Therapy Skill Builders, AU

Twitchell TE (1965) The automatic grasping responses of infants. Neuropsychologia 3:247–259. https://doi.org/10.1016/0028-3932(65)90027-8

Twitchell TE (1970) Reflex mechanism and the development of prehension. In: Connolly K (ed) Mechanism of motor skill development. Academic, London

Uvebrant P (1988) Hemiplegic cerebral palsy: etiology and outcome. Acta Paediatr Scand 345:1–100. https://doi.org/10.1111/j.1651-2227.1988.tb14939.x

Veruggio G (2000) Linee generali di intervento abilitativo sugli arti superiori. In: Giannoni P, Zerbino L (eds) Fuori schema, 1st edn. Springer, Italia, Milano, pp 272–286

WHO (World Health Organization) (2007) The International Classification of Functioning, Disability and Health; children and youth version (ICF CY), Geneva, World Health Organization.

Wallen M, Stewart K (2015) Upper limb function in everyday life of children with cerebral palsy: description and review of parent report measures. Disabil Rehabil 37(15):1353–1361. https://doi.org/10.3109/09638288.2014.963704

Ward D (1984) Positioning the handicapped child for functions. St. Louis Mosby

Upper Limbs Functional Problems in Different Forms of Cerebral Palsy

9

Gabriella Veruggio

9.1 The Child with Bilateral Spastic Cerebral Palsy

In bilateral spastic forms of cerebral palsy (BSCP), different levels of upper limb performances can be observed, as indicated in Table 8.3 of Chap. 8.

Children with moderate/mild impairment (functional levels 2–3, Table 8.3) can acquire basic reaching, prehension, and release patterns. However, it is possible to notice delays and difficulties in acquiring more advanced and mature prehension patterns (e.g., superior pincer grasp with extended wrist), release, in-hand manipulation movements, and bilateral hand use, which may be even more or less limited by the presence of unintended movements in the nonperforming hand (Kuhtz-Buschbeck et al. 2000; Kim et al. 2020).

Generally, these children can access the daily activities of childhood. However, it may be necessary to use the equipment and environmental adaptations, aids, and strategies allowing access to activities of daily life, handwriting, and other school tasks.

In these children with moderate/mild motor impairment, disorders in perceptual-cognitive development and educational achievements may also be present (Yin Foo et al. 2013). Perceptual, visual, and cognitive disorders can affect upper limb use and need to be properly assessed to carry out a realistic functional prognosis and to set up an appropriate rehabilitation project (Henderson and Pehoski 2005; Sigurdardottir et al. 2008; Case-Smith and O'Brien 2019).

On the other hand, in children with severe motor impairment (functional levels 0–1, Table 8.3), the upper limb use is extremely limited or completely impossible. They often tend to use primitive and synergistic patterns of flexion or extension, which can severely limit the functions of daily life.

G. Veruggio (✉)
AAC Service of Benedetta d'Intino Centre, Milan, Italy

Even though access to the daily occupations of childhood will require ongoing support from caregivers, the therapist should highlight and value the child's available
functional resources—accepting their deficits—by identifying one or more voluntarily
controlled movements, which the child could use functionally. Consequently, it is possible to modify and/or adapt some of the child's daily life activities (ADL), which they
can manage to carry out through bypass strategies. In some cases, the therapist can
evaluate the use of other parts of the child's body (head, foot, etc.) or of their eye-gaze
(Borgestig et al. 2015, 2016) to make them achieve some functional goals.

These children pose significant problems in daily care. They have difficulties in
feeding (severe oral control dysfunction), in toileting, in performing their physiological functions (frequent constipation problems), in bathing, in dressing, etc.
Therefore, through direct observation in natural contexts and interviews, it is necessary to evaluate the environmental factors (supports and barriers) that can affect
daily care. Subsequently, the therapist can set up a rehabilitation project directed to
ADL, aimed at supporting the caregivers, identifying and negotiating appropriate
handling procedures, e.g., how to dress and undress the child. Often equipment
adaptations, ADL aids, and environmental adaptations are needed, to lighten the
burden of daily care (Fig. 9.1) (French et al. 1991; Korpela et al. 1992; Hammel
1996; Finnie 2009; Dormans and Pellegrino 1998; Østensjø et al. 2003, 2009;
Henderson and Pehoski 2005; Pirila et al. 2018; Case-Smith and O'Brien 2019).

Very often children with severe motor impairment also have communication difficulties, and therefore, it is important to identify communication strategies and support that allow them to guide the adult's care, for example, by communicating their
likings and choosing food preferences, clothes, or hairstyles (Fig. 9.2) (Morris and
Klein 1987; Millar and Aitken 2003; Beukelman and Mirenda 2013).

> *"When I look up with my eyes, I am telling you to stop tipping the cup.*
> *When I shake my head and say 'uh-uh', I don't want any more"*
> *(Message added in the Personal Communication Passport, to guide care while drinking,*
> Morris and Klein 1987)

Fig. 9.1 Environmental
adaptations and aids,
facilitating daily care

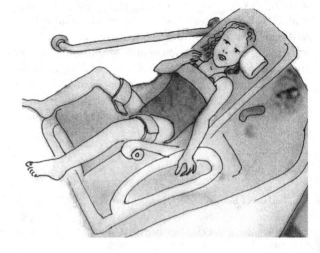

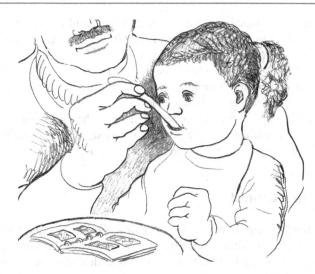

Fig. 9.2 Exploiting a communication strategy based on iconic indication with finger or eye-gaze (redrawn from Morris and Klein 1987)

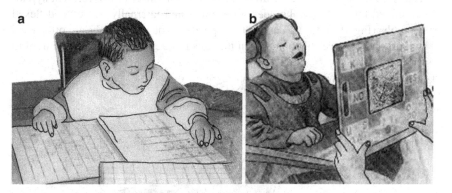

Fig. 9.3 Use of a communication board (**a**) and an Etran board (**b**)

They also have evident limitations in playing. Opportunities to enjoy and progress through the various stages of independent and cooperative play development depend greatly on the support of the caregiver as well as on the adaptation of toys (Pratt and Allen 1989; Case-Smith and O'Brien 2019).

Authors report that between 33 and 88% of children with severe CP impairment have speech and language disorders, such as decreased speech production, poor articulation, and reduced speech intelligibility (Yorkston et al. 2010; Beukelman and Mirenda 2013). These problems require a specific and earl intervention of augmentative and alternative communication (AAC) (see also Chap. 12) (Fig. 9.3a, b).

In severe bilateral spastic forms, there are often perceptual disorders, especially regarding stereognosis and two-point discrimination (Bolanos et al. 1989; Odding et al. 2006; Arnould et al. 2008, 2014; Auld et al. 2011; Ferrari et al. 2014).

Disorders in visual function, such as acuity deficit, oculomotor problems, etc., are common, and the literature shows that from 60 to 70% of children with severe BSCP manifest cerebral visual impairment (CVI), as also described in Chap. 11 (Fazzi et al. 2007, 2009, 2012; Dufresne et al. 2014).

Moreover, many children have an intellectual impairment (Bottcher 2010; Yin Foo et al. 2013; Stadskleiv et al. 2018; Batorowicz et al. 2018).

In children with BSCP, functional performance in the upper limbs is strongly determined by the combination of limitations in various factors, including postural control, reaching, and prehension/manipulation.

9.1.1 Postural Control

The child with BSCP will be more or less able to achieve and maintain independent sitting, the position they will use most frequently for play and during ADL.

The seated posture can be affected by synergistic flexion or extension patterns, by symmetrical tonic neck reflex (STNR), asymmetrical tonic neck reflex (ATNR), and startle reaction.

The child sits with a posterior tilt of the pelvis, with more or less relevant kyphosis, extended lower limbs, shoulder protraction, and internally rotated and flexed upper limbs (Fig. 9.4). In such an unstable position, the upper limbs are often used in support and balance function. When the upper extremities are fixed and used to

Fig. 9.4 Common sitting position of the child with BSCP

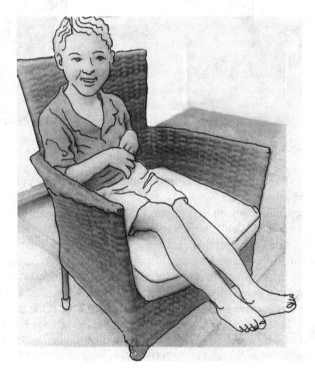

help stabilize and control the sitting posture, arms and hands are unavailable to be used for functional tasks.

Therefore, the choice of a personalized positioning system is essential to obtain better alignment and more stable shoulder girdle and to allow for better use of the upper limbs for the various ADLs.

The identification of a positioning system is essential in children with severe motor disabilities because it can improve interpersonal relationship and functional activities, prevent or delay deformities, increase comfort, and, if possible, permit powered mobility (Myhr et al. 1995; Furusamu 1997; Bottos et al. 2001; Stavness 2006; Ryan 2012; Case-Smith and O'Brien 2019) (Fig. 9.5).

Many of these children fail to adapt their body to the seat system because they cannot anchor the pelvis to the chair or cannot dissociate the trunk movements from those of the pelvis. Sometimes they do not even tolerate the sitting system itself for a long time. Therefore, it is important to evaluate the structural features of all components of the system (frame, texture, consistency, etc.) in case of possible perceptual interference.

Multidisciplinary teamwork, together with the caregivers, allows the identification of a positioning system that adapts to the needs of the child. Time is needed together with the caregivers to verify its effects on the child's posture and their functional abilities. In the case of severe impairment, custom-molded systems are often needed (Ward 1983; Noronha et al. 1989; Costigan and Light 2011; Ju et al. 2012; Sahinoğlu et al. 2017).

Fig. 9.5 Seating system

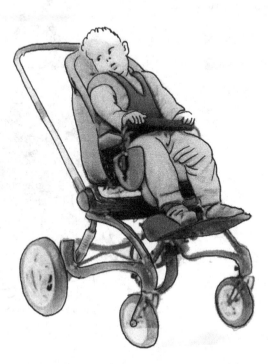

Trunk stability and performances in upper limbs and other parts of the body can also be enhanced through the use of a lap tray with recess, in particular when the lap tray cutout follows the contour of the child's thorax. The lap tray or school desk should be of the appropriate size for the child and adjustable in height and inclination (Fig. 9.6).

Sometimes, it is necessary to set up customized workstations, i.e., sitting posture aid and other positioning components, together with assistive technology (AT) devices. This requires the mounting of these alternative access systems also to allow access to AT systems for communication, playing, and writing to optimize the upper limbs or other body parts performances (Fig. 9.7) (see also Chap. 13).

Children with severe BSCP, especially those with speech impairments or a lack of speech, often tend to trigger total synergistic patterns to communicate, e.g., to express emotions and to declare YES/NO. The positioning system should be designed to minimize these effects, if the main goal is also to let the child acquire early or timely communication strategies through effective tools adapted to their needs (Fig. 9.8) (see Chap. 12).

In younger children, the performance of the upper limb can initially be enhanced also in the prone position or in side-lying (as described in Chap. 2), using various positioning aids, or even sitting the child on a parent's lap or playing in front of a table with a recess (Fig. 9.9).

Fig. 9.6 School desk with a recessed lap tray

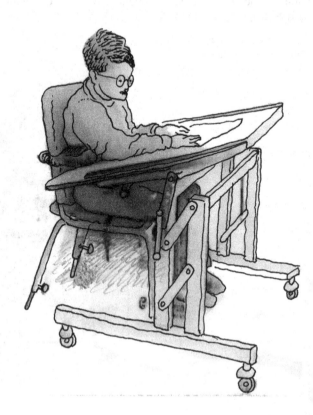

Fig. 9.7 Customized workstation with switches activated by a movement of the thigh

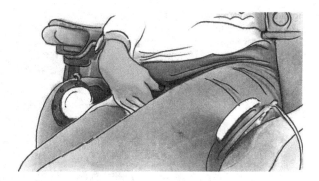

Fig. 9.8 Extensor synergy used to communicate

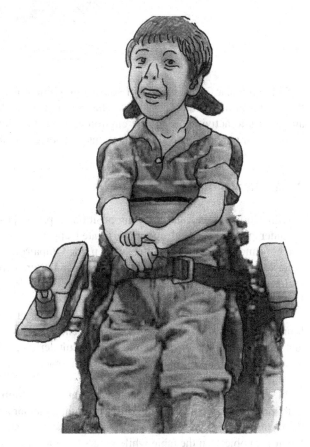

To improve stability, trunk extension, and upper limb performance in children with mild/moderate motor impairment, less complex solutions can be adopted, such as standard wheelchairs and special chairs, sometimes by adapting existing equipment at home or in the classroom. Examples of these adaptions include anti-slip pads applied to the seat, special cushions that abduct the lower limbs, and a pelvic belt to improve the upright posture of the trunk. Even these children can benefit from the use of a desk with recess.

Fig. 9.9 Alternative positioning device to enhance upper limb functioning

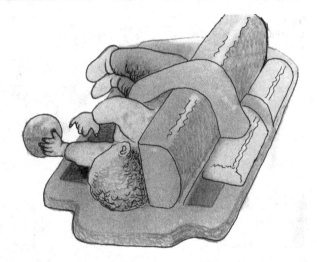

In the mildest forms, the use of adapted equipment may be essential to enhance the child's participation in all ADLs. This equipment should also facilitate transfers and access to activities in all the environments of the child's life, e.g., accessible furniture for playing, bedroom adaptations, or choice of table/desk for accessing PC.

9.1.2 Reaching

Inability to maintain a stable sitting position, kyphotic posture, misalignment with shoulder protraction, and internally rotated upper limbs can all negatively affect reaching movements. In children with milder impairment, a predominantly parabolic approach to the target can be observed, and often there are difficulties in bilateral hand use (Koupernik and Dailly 1968; Erhardt 1995; Pratt and Allen 1989; Henderson and Pehoski 2005) (Fig. 9.10).

Reaching movements are possible mainly in front of the child, in a more or less limited area close to their body. They are generally slow and limited in amplitude and require a lot of effort. The child has difficulty crossing the midline, elevating the upper limbs, and accessing the lateral or rear spaces, e.g., to perform many ADLs, such as dressing and toilet hygiene.

In children who show greater impairment in one limb, reaching is carried out with the more efficient arm with different complementary use of the other. Some of them can only rest the less functional limb on the work surface; others can use it for locking an object on the table while others for grasping it with a massive grip.

Sometimes, stabilization and anchoring systems of the "secondary" upper limb can also be proposed to improve trunk and head postural control and promote a better use of the dominant working arm (Fig. 9.11).

In children with severe motor impairment, the persistence of primitive or atypical reactions, and disorders in muscle tone, all have a relevant negative impact on reaching. In these children, this movement is extremely laborious, reduced in

Fig. 9.10 Difficult bilateral hand use

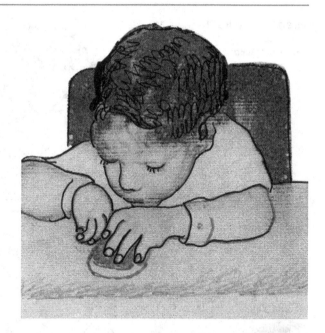

Fig. 9.11 Anchoring system of the "secondary" arm

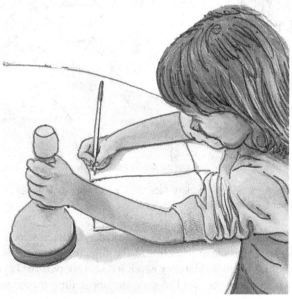

amplitude, and limited to certain areas of the work surface within a flexion or extension synergistic pattern (Fig. 9.12).

Often only imprecise, limited adduction/abduction horizontal movements and/or flexion/extension of the upper limbs is possible, which greatly restricts access to daily occupations of childhood.

Fig. 9.12 Difficult and
limited reaching, with
synergistic pattern

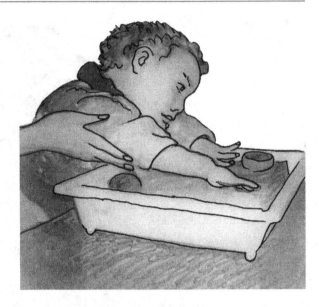

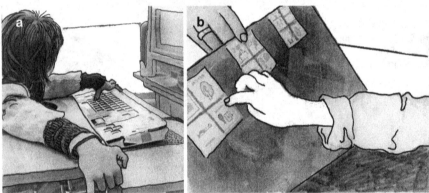

Fig. 9.13 Special work surface to enhance upper limb movements: (**a**) two-tiered desk and key-guard; (**b**) angled lap tray easel

Sometimes, besides special seated systems, a selection of a customed work surfaces is indicated to optimize the functional use of these limited abilities. These include an angled lap tray easel, forearm supports or keyguard, or a two-tiered desk, which allow the child to slide the upper limb on the work surface and play (e.g., move a car or activate a battery-operated toy) or access AT (e.g., computer writing) and AAC system (Fig. 9.13).

It is also extremely important to pay attention to the adequate positioning of the caregiver with respect to the child (e.g., the adult's face at the child's eye level) and the position of all the objects and screens surrounding them (Goossens' and Crain 1992).

Furthermore, it is very important that the child achieves all possible elbow control for a more direct and accurate pointing, as well as the isolation of one finger for

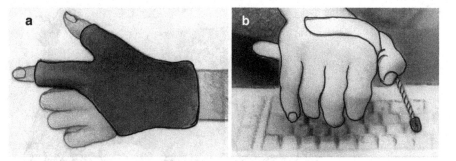

Fig. 9.14 Keyboard access tools: (**a**) special mitten and (**b**) typing aids

direct selection on a communication board, a speech-generating device (SGD) or for typing on the keyboard.

To isolate a finger and to allow typing, keyboard access tools can also be used (Fig. 9.14).

However, when reaching and pointing control are impossible or extremely tiring for the child, it is necessary to consider the use of other parts of the child's body and/ or eye gaze (Borgestig et al. 2015, 2016), as alternative access to playing, writing, education, and AAC systems (Pratt and Allen 1989; Henderson et al. 2008; Sadao and Robinson 2010; Case-Smith and O'Brien 2019) (see also Chap. 11). For this, it is necessary to set up an adequate rehabilitation plan, selecting positioning and mounting systems.

9.1.3 Prehension and Manipulation

Prehension difficulties are linked to various factors, such as the child's postural control, reaching modalities, the persistence of primitive or atypical reactions, perceptual disorders, stiffness, contractures, and deformities (Twitchell 1965; Erhardt 1995; Mark Carter 1983; Henderson and Pehoski 2005; Eliasson et al. 2006).

In children with severe motor impairment, prehension is extremely difficult, limited to some objects and using only primitive grasp patterns. Sometimes, it is completely impossible. These youngsters can have considerable difficulty even in hand opening control, due to the grasping reflex, perceptual disorders and limited haptic experiences. Often the opening and closing of the hand are carried out using synergistic patterns.

The child could be able to only hold an object placed in their hand and for a limited time, also needing the objects to have particular features (in texture, weight, dimension, and ease to grip).

Manipulation is not present, and sometimes the child can only use a fisted hand, for example, to make contact with or move objects, press a large key, or a switch linked to a battery-operated toy or a large button in a music box (Fig. 9.15).

Fig. 9.15 Child operating
a large key

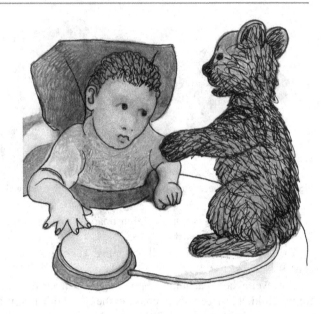

Fig. 9.16 Adapted
equipment or orthoses to
improve the functioning

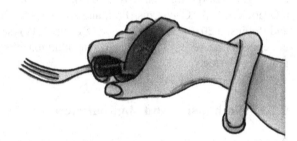

Limited use of upper limbs can cause muscle contractures, increasing fore-arm pronation and wrist flexion, which may over time turn into deformities. It is therefore important to consider more global functional goals and other sup-porting solutions, such as adaptations of the workstation, adapted equipment, medical-pharmacological interventions, and orthoses, to improve function and limit deformity (Wilton 2003; Morris et al. 2011; Case-Smith and O'Brien 2019) (Fig. 9.16).

Children with moderate impairment can grasp and release objects with different modalities to control the pronation and supination of the forearm and wrist and fingers extension. They can usually grasp large objects using the surface of all finger pads and small objects with three-point or radial pinch, with little differentiation between radial and ulnar fingers (Fig. 9.17).

Manipulation is possible but there are difficulties in dissociating the two upper limb movements.

A milder impaired child can achieve more upper limb function: direct reaching with pre-shaping of the hand, adequate strength and precision of grip, in-hand

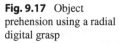

Fig. 9.17 Object prehension using a radial digital grasp

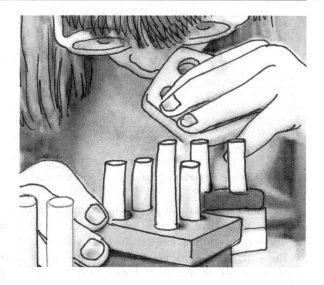

manipulation movements, and coordinated and more differentiated bilateral hand use (Koupernik and Dailly 1968). The therapist should work on the differentiation between radial and ulnar fingers and complex in-hand manipulation movements, e.g. combine translation with rotation and use tools and objects with varied shapes and sizes during ADL.

In the case of moderate/mild disabilities, the need for caregiver engagement is less, as the children can achieve greater autonomy in ADLs, although they often have limitations in more complex activities like fastening of smaller buttons, use of scissors, cutting, and lacing of shoes.

Mastery of the ADL tasks leads to increased self-esteem, self-confidence, and self-determination and gives the child a sense of autonomy. The acquisition of self-care skills in childhood is not only strictly involved in the development of motor skills but also conditioned by perceptual, cognitive, cultural, and environmental factors. Knowledge of the sequences in which typical children become self-reliant in ADLs is invaluable for the understanding of the possible milestones that the child with impairment can achieve (Henderson and Pehoski 2005; Case-Smith and O'Brien 2019).

To set up an appropriate ADL rehabilitation plan, a general and client-focused analysis is required, aimed at examining the essential components and physical requirements to carry out that specific activity and to identify possible intervention opportunities for the child with impairment (Coley and Procter 1989; Spitzer 2019). Based on this analysis, on the previous evaluation of the upper limbs and, if possible, on the observation of the child in their everyday environments, the therapist should use standardized assessment tools to define the goals of intervention for ADL, shared with the child and their family (Gordon 1992; Missiuna and Pollock 2000; Shepard 2019) (see Chap. 8).

In children with functional level 2–3 (see Table 8.3), it is sometimes necessary to propose alternative strategies that allow a more independent life, introducing

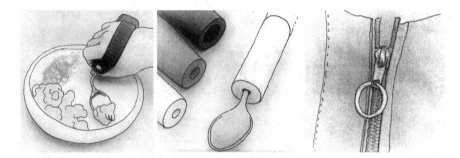

Fig. 9.18 Aids and adaptations to enhance independence in ADL

environmental changes and proposing alternative postures and aids that facilitate function: e.g., self-undressing in a sitting position instead of standing or using handles for toileting. To improve the child's self-feeding, the therapist can select more functional glasses, cutlery, and dishes, and, as support to dressing, they can suggest easy-to-tie shoes or modified clothes to overcome the difficulties in buttoning (Fig. 9.18).

It may also be necessary to identify the most suitable ADL teaching techniques for the child, such as gradually increasing the number of steps to complete an activity or using only verbal instructions, involving and educating their caregivers in these modalities (Klein 1983; Morris and Klein 1987; Shepard 2019).

In adolescents and adults, the aim is to support them to achieve everything essential for independent living and community participation, where necessary with the help of feasible instrumental ADLs (IADL) for the use of public transport, shopping, meal preparation, home management, and employment activities.

The child with mild bilateral spastic CP (level 3) can achieve handwriting. They can have handwriting movements that are slow, tiring, and of limited amplitude. They often hold the writing tools with unorthodox and contracted grips and put considerable pressure on the paper. The handwriting layout appears irregular, slanting, creased, and not fluid (Fig. 9.19).

Some children may need a specific intervention for handwriting, and/or the use of different bypass solutions (see Chap. 8, Sect. 8.3), such as a special pencil holder to enhance the tripod grasp, special notebooks with clearly marked margins, and colored guidelines to facilitate writing in rows, an anti-slip pad (Ajuriaguerra et al. 1964; Klein 1982; Edwards et al. 2002; Henderson and Pehoski 2005; Kim 2016; Case-Smith and O'Brien 2019) (Fig. 9.20).

To promote body stability and better upper limb use on the work surface, it may be advisable to extend the support of the forearms on the surface of the recessed desk.

In the presence of fatigue, excessive slowness, poor readability, and/or numerous written assignments, handwriting can be replaced or supplemented by computer writing or other advanced devices (see also Chap. 13).

In some milder children, the problem of unestablished handedness may emerge, which may affect the development of fine motor skills, particularly handwriting performances (Henderson and Pehoski 2005). Therefore, the therapist should carry out a prolonged evaluation with careful observation of the functional performance

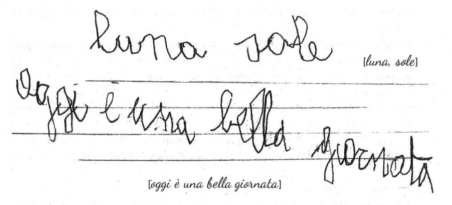

[luna, sole]

[oggi è una bella giornata]

Fig. 9.19 Handwriting layout of two children with mild BSCP

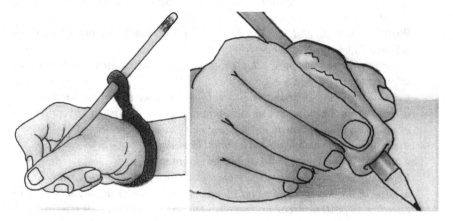

Fig. 9.20 Adaptive handwriting tools

of the two upper limbs and then propose the most efficient hand for writing (Auzias 1975) (see Chap. 8).

9.1.4 Aims of Functional Treatment of the Upper Limb in Children with BSCP

Based on the upper limb functional levels described in Table 8.3, the following aims and treatment modalities are proposed for children with severe (level 0–1) or moderate/mild (level 2–3) impairment. Aims for children with moderate/mild impairment can also be suitable in the rehabilitation plan for children with diplegia.

- **The child with severe motor impairment**
  - *Reaching control: from adduction/abduction horizontal movement control to elbow control. Particularly, enhancing wide-ranging movements toward the*

preferred working area and proximal movements toward the most difficult area to reach

- *Hand use: from hand opening to maintaining/releasing contact with an object (e.g., switch contact and releasing); from only moving objects on a surface to palmar grasp use and, if feasible, to three-point palmar or lateral pinch achievement*
- *Isolation of at least one finger for direct selection on AAC systems or for typing on the keyboard*
- *Bilateral hand use: from the simple maintenance of both upper limbs on the work surface to initial use of a more involved arm to stabilize objects, without grasping*
- *Eye/hand coordination*
- *Functional use of other parts of the body, particularly in severe upper limb impairment*
- *ADLs: caregiver training for positioning, handling strategies, and in the use of ADLs aids*
- *Writing: selection and training of alternative access to computer writing or advanced technology (AT) devices*
- *Play: positioning for play, adapted environment, alternative strategies, and adapted toy use; selecting AT for play*
- *Contractures and deformities prevention/containment, in association with general rehabilitation plan: positioning improvement, task modification, use of orthoses, eventual medical-pharmacological intervention*
- *Assessment and treatment of perceptual disorders*
- **The child with moderate/mild motor impairment**
  - *Reaching and pointing control: control of more precise trajectories, implemented in different postures and planes, with particular attention to midline crossing, to posterior reaching patterns (required for many ADLs, as in dressing and hygiene), prone/supination of the forearm, and the extension of the wrist*
  - *Prehension: from radial pinch to superior pinch with thumb opposition; gradual reduction of ulnar fingers use, in favor of the radial finger one; prehension of objects with various features (e.g., flat, heavy); anticipatory control of the hand*
  - *Release: from control of hand opening with extended fingers to the precise and controlled release, with the increase of wrist extension—on a surface or in space or a small container—of objects of various sizes and features*
  - *In-hand manipulation: from isolated finger movements to the differentiation between radial and ulnar fingers; from finger to palm translation to complex intrinsic movements, combining, e.g., translation with rotation; parallel intervention on tactile and proprioceptive awareness/discrimination*
  - *Bilateral hand use: from less proficient hand use in stabilizing (without or with grasp) function to bilateral simultaneous and differentiated hand use, even with smaller objects*

- *Handedness: investigate any problem of unestablished handedness, particularly in choosing hand for handwriting; related intervention, if necessary*
- *Handwriting: handwriting rehabilitation intervention, if necessary; training in computer writing*
- *ADLs: facilitation of functional strategies; environmental and equipment adaptations (e.g., bathroom, classroom), ADL aids choice; caregiver training; IADL aids for adolescents/adults*
- *Assessment and intervention on perceptual disorders, if needed*

9.2 The Child with Unilateral Spastic Cerebral Palsy

In the hemiplegic child, the effective use of the arm and hand to reach, grasp, release, and manipulate objects is often compromised. The upper extremity is usually affected more than the lower extremity, in 40% of cases according to Uvebrant (1988) and in 30% of cases according to Beckung and Hagberg (2002).

Hand impairment depends on several factors, including the severity of paresis, the extent of sensory loss, the degree of stiffness or spasticity, and in some cases on cognitive disorders (Twitchell 1958; Uvebrant 1988; Cioni et al. 1999; Brown and Walsh 2001; Niemann 2001; Hoare et al. 2018). Different levels of hand impairment and different levels of bilateral hand use can be observed, which can differently affect functional independence and quality of life (Beckung and Hagberg 2002; Eliasson et al. 2006; Rosa-Rizzotto et al. 2014).

In children with unilateral spastic cerebral palsy (USCP), and particularly in severe cases, there are often upper limb perceptual disorders, especially concerning stereognosis and two-point discrimination (Bolanos et al. 1989; Yekutiel et al. 1994; Gordon and Duff 1999; Brown and Walsh 2001; Krumlinde-Sunddholm and Eliasson 2002; Fedrizzi et al. 2003; Odding et al. 2006; Kinnucan et al. 2010; Auld et al. 2011). Some authors also report sensory impairment in the unaffected hand (Lesny et al. 1993; Cooper et al. 1995).

Many studies report problems, such as hemianopia, visual hemiagnosia, hemiasomatognosia, and visual hemi-inattention, that need careful evaluation and sometimes a specific intervention (Fazzi et al. 2012; Dufresne et al. 2014; Philip et al. 2020).

The incidence of intellectual disability is lower than in BSCP and to a different extent (Cioni et al. 1999; Niemann 2001; Hoare et al. 2018). It is related to other features, such as epilepsy and language and visual problems (Cohen Levine et al. 1987; Vargha-Khadem et al. 1994; Bates et al. 1999; Salam et al. 2016; Stadskleiv et al. 2018; Blair et al. 2018).

Generally, these children can access the daily occupations of childhood, and, as adults, many are fully integrated into society after regular academic education and vocational training. Therefore, according to the suggestions of the International

Classification Functioning (ICF), the most general rehabilitation goal is promoting functional activity and the person's full participation in all aspects of life (Rosenbaum and Stewart 2004; WHO 2007).

9.2.1 Assessment of the Upper Limbs in USCP

To set up an adequate rehabilitation plan, it is necessary to assess both the prehension skills of the child and the spontaneous use of the affected limb in playing and in ADLs. Several standardized tools for functional assessment of prehension, manipulation, and daily life activities can be used (Gilmore et al. 2010; Klingels et al. 2010; Lemmens et al. 2012) (see Chap. 8) to assess the extent of spontaneous use of the affected hand and its involvement with the other hand.

Clinical experience suggests the use of the Besta scale (Rosa-Rizzotto et al. 2014), which was developed in 1985 to assess the quality of grasp (hand function on request) and spontaneous hand use (bilateral manipulation) in the child with USCP.

In the rehabilitation setting, this tool is a reliable method to follow-up and monitor the clinical evolution of unimanual and bimanual manipulation, to distinguish capacity from performance as suggested by ICF, and to identify the appropriate interventions in the short and long term (Fedrizzi et al. 1994, 2003; Rosa-Rizzotto et al. 2014).

The Besta scale considers three domains: (a) assessment of the grasp function of the impaired hand, (b) assessment of spontaneous use in bimanual manipulatory activities, and (c) assessment of spontaneous use of the impaired hand in ADL. A score from 0 to 3 is assigned for each domain, defined as follows:

(a) Grasp assessment:
    0: grasp absent
    1: palmar grasp
    2: whole-hand, radial, or three-finger grasp
    3: pincer grasp
(b) and (c) Spontaneous use in bimanual activities:
    0: no use of impaired limb
    1: use of an impaired limb (not hand) in a stereotyped pattern (wrist support) for holding
    2: cooperation of the impaired hand by holding with a restricted number of stereotyped patterns
    3: cooperation of the impaired hand by holding and manipulation, using a varied repertoire of patterns

Grasp function on request is assessed by using three cubes of different sizes (side measurements 4, 2.5, and 1 cm) and a marble. The unaffected hand is evaluated before the impaired one because it could often have subtle deficits as well (Gordon et al. 1999).

Spontaneous hand use in bimanual activities during playing and ADL is then assessed. The play and the ADL proposals have been standardized to age range (four tasks for each age group) and to play material that necessarily involves both hands use.

Based on the assessment of the grasp function on request, children with lower scores (score 0–1) show a severe upper limb motor deficit. Those with high scores can grasp objects with different grip patterns, from radial pinch to three-point pinch (score 2) and superior pinch (score 3).

Based on the assessment of the impaired hand spontaneous use, children with lower scores (score 0–1) have absent or severely limited impaired hand use in bilateral manipulatory activities. Those with high scores (score 2–3) spontaneously use the impaired hand in bilateral manipulatory activities with a more or less stereotyped pattern.

However, in younger children, more informal observation of possible perceptual disorders may be carried out, as suggested below.

Tips for an Informal Observation
- How does the child spontaneously use their affected hand? (Do they try to use it, to bring it to the mouth, suck finger, or leave it unused, against the body, or under the table?)
- Does the child look at their affected hand?
- Does the child turn their head and explore all the space around them or focus only on the unaffected side?
- Does the child accept that you put an object in their palm and that you touch their impaired hand?
- Does the child forget small objects inside the hand while playing, like bits of paper or crumbs, for example?
- How does the child react to caresses, tickles, or touches; to flowing water or to a blow on their hand; to a "sting" made for fun with the tip of a pencil; and to a toy car moved for fun on their affected side?
- Are there differences in the various parts of the arm and hand?
- Does the child use their affected hand in bimanual activities and in bimanual gestures (e.g., stretches their arms toward parent or claps their hands)?

9.2.2 Stereognosis

The evaluation of the upper limbs should therefore be completed by the evaluation of perceptual disorders, particularly stereognosis, as well as visual functions, muscle retractions, and RoM limitations.

Stereognosis is assessed first in the unaffected hand and then in the affected one and usually at the age of 5 because younger children often do not cooperate or lack the necessary attention. The literature agrees on the characteristics of the objects, which should be familiar and of different shapes and materials, but the type of objects is not specified. Some studies use different objects, like a small ball, money, combs, toothbrushes, keys, etc. (Tyler 1972; Van Heest et al. 1993; Yekutiel et al. 1994), and other studies assess stereognosis by identifying shapes (Bolanos et al. 1989) or a combination of familiar objects and shapes (Cooper et al. 1995).

Examples of Different Sets of Objects Used to Assess Stereognosis
- Tyler (1972): two-inch diameter rubber ball, five-inch plastic spoon, two-inch metal car with movable wheels, three-inch plush stuffed dog, one-inch toy plastic chair, penny, one-inch plastic button with four holes, ticker than the penny
- Van Heest et al. (1993): block, pencil, little spoon, paper clip, safety pin, penny, button, pill, glove, string, marble, key
- Krumlinde-Sunddholm and Eliasson (2002): a LEGO[1] brick and an eraser, a wooden bead and a paper pellet, a coin and a shirt-button

The worsening of hand function in some children after the age of 11 years might be attributed to limb growth and to increased retraction of wrist tendons.

Further differences emerge between the methods used because, in some assessments, children are allowed to look at and touch objects before the test, and in others they are not. Other times, the task is to match the object with a corresponding visible object or with a photograph; others ask the child to verbally describe or name the object (Bolanos et al. 1989; Yekutiel et al. 1994; Fedrizzi et al. 2003).

For the assessment of stereognosis, each object is placed separately into the child's hand, shielded from vision behind a screen or a piece of cardboard, helping the child to manipulate and explore them if necessary. In Fig. 9.21, there is an example of a commercially available tool.[2]

Stereognosis was assessed in 25 of the 31 children at a mean age of 4 years 4 months. The other six children did not cooper ate sufficiently at this age to perform the test. All 25 children recognized the 5 objects with the unaffected hand: 13 were able to identify all the objects with the affected hand, and the other 12 children had astereognosis. Stereognosis in relation to the affected hand function is shown in Table I. Of the 13 children who identified all objects in the stereognosis test, none had a score of 0 or 1 on grip and use assessment; furthermore, all used the affected hand in bilateral manipulation activities: five used it to hold (score 2) and eight used the fingers to manipulate (score 3). By contrast, none of the 12 children with astereognosis scored 3 on either grip or spontaneous use.

---

[1] LEGO System A/S, Billund (DK), https://www.lego.com
[2] Officina Ortopedica Ferrero Srl, Venaria Reale (IT), http://ferreromed.it

Fig. 9.21 Device for the
stereognosis assessment

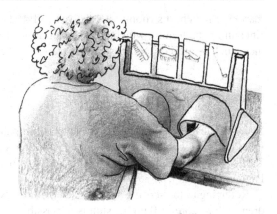

9.2.3   Postural Control

Regardless of the level of impairment in the lower limbs, the child achieves autonomous independent walking, with a lot of variability in their motor behavior depending on the task to be achieved. The therapist should observe the child in their daily life environments and evaluate their behavior, as well as the characteristics of the equipment used (chairs, tables, etc.), suggesting to the family any changes, if necessary.

For infants, commercially available seats or postural systems can be suggested, to facilitate a better postural alignment and allow more involvement of the affected limb in the midline, within their visual field, for example placing a little cushion behind the child's scapula. The supported sitting position is useful to facilitate eye-hand-mouth coordination and the integration of the two sides of the body to favor the development of the interior mental body image.

The child with USCP can have the advantage of sitting in stable chairs of adequate height already in use in the home and school environments. Adaptations can be added, such as small anti-slip wedges applied to the seat to improve the distribution of weight-bearing. In preschool and school children, particularly those with severe upper limb deficits, a recessed table is very useful to favor forearm support on the work surface and allow better visual control and bimanual hand use (Kavak and Bumin 2009).

During the training to achieve some selective activities, such as self-feeding or writing, the therapist could also propose the use of anchoring systems of the affected arm, to promote a better postural alignment.

Moreover, to facilitate the affected arm function in playing and in ADLs, it may be necessary to reorganize the environments of child's daily life, for example, to rearrange the child's room with shelves and desks of adequate height or selecting sinks in the bathroom, which allow better arm support, or utilizing adaptive equipment such as soap or toothpaste dispensers (Fig. 9.22).

9.2.4 Prehension

Many studies focus on the different levels of impairment regarding prehension ability in children with USCP (Uvebrant 1988; Eliasson et al. 1991; Sugden and Utley 1995; Kuhtz-Buschbeck et al. 2000; Fedrizzi et al. 2003; Holmefur et al. 2009; Pagliano et al. 2001).

Referring to the scoring system used by the previously cited Besta scale, in children with a score of 0 prehension is impossible. However, in some cases, the child will try on request to grasp the proposed items between the side surface of the thumb and index finger. Other children try to grasp with a half-opened hand and extended fingers. There is no thumb opposition, the forearm is generally semipronated, the elbow is flexed, the wrist is flexed in ulnar deviation, and the hand is closed.

During assessment of grasp on request, children with score 1 can use a digital palm grip, blocking the object with thumb adduction against the palm, or use a multi-digital grip with extended fingers, i.e., blocking a small object between the fingers. This object should be "easy to grip," be placed near the child's body, and has particular features, like be lightweighted, soft, and medium-sized. The prehension and release of the object is usually carried out using synergistic upper limb flexion and extension patterns. Furthermore, many authors report that children with scores 0–1 not only have hand impairments but also significant perceptual disorders (Van Heest et al. 1993; Cooper et al. 1995; Kinnucan et al. 2010).

Children with moderate motor impairment, i.e., with a score of 2, can grasp objects with radial (Fig. 9.23) or three-point grip. The thumb is usually adducted or in some cases in opposition with the middle finger; the wrist may have different

Fig. 9.22 Sink with large forearm support

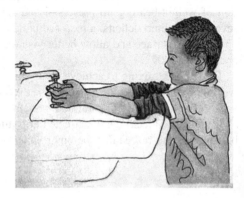

Fig. 9.23 Radial grip with wrist flexion (redrawn from Erhardt 1995)

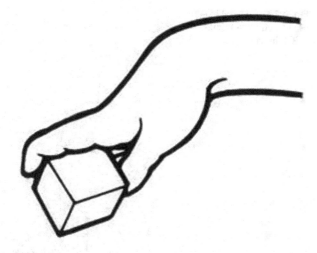

RoM of flexion and ulnar deviation, with some simpler in-hand manipulation movements, e.g., simple rotations. The resulting lack of experience can possibly lead to stereognosis disorders.

Children with mild impairment, i.e., with a score of 3, can use various power and precision grips, such as lateral and superior pinch, and their thumb can be opposed. The child can pre-shape the hand in relation to the features of the objects and accurately release them on both on a surface and into a small container (Eliasson and Gordon 2000; Gordon et al. 2003). Pronation-supination of the forearm is possible, and the wrist can be in a neutral position or extended. More complex in-hand manipulation movements are possible, and therefore these children do not have major stereognosis disorders (Fedrizzi et al. 2003; Kinnucan et al. 2010.)

9.2.5 Bilateral Hand Use

Already in the first months of life of a child with USCP, it is possible to observe asymmetry in postural organization and active movements of the upper limbs (see also Chap. 3). Difficulties are noted when the child brings both hands to the mouth to explore them when fingering or reaching for objects on the midline (Fig. 9.24). Very often, parents or grandparents are the first to notice these postural and functional asymmetries.

In children with moderate/mild impairment, symmetric reaching can be observed early on, but as soon as the unaffected hand reaches the object faster and more effectively, there is a progressive reduction in the use of the affected hand.

Over time there is a continuous maturation in the functional use of the unaffected hand to the detriment of the impaired one, and a reduced spontaneous use of the affected arm and hand can be observed during bimanual activities (Kuhtz-Buschbeck

Fig. 9.24 Bilateral hand
use in a child with mild
USCP impairment

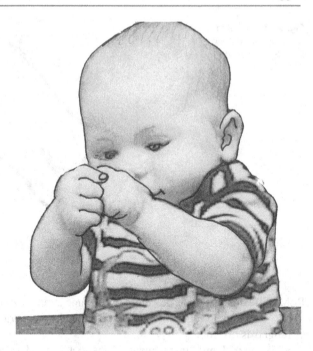

et al. 2000; Beckung and Hagberg 2002; Eliasson et al. 2006; Rosa-Rizzotto et al. 2014).

Children with severe unilateral impairment have extremely limited or no use of the affected arm and become increasingly skilled at performing bimanual tasks, such as drinking, using a fork, combing, etc., by using more and more the most efficient hand. This is the beginning of neglect of the affected arm (Taub et al. 2004, 2006; Aarts et al. 2010; Fedrizzi et al. 2013).

Seated in front of a table, the child with 0 score often leaves the affected arm under the table and does not use it for simple tasks, like blocking/holding objects, even when the limb is in their visual field.

In other cases, i.e., in children with a score of 1, the affected upper limb is used in a synergistic pattern with the aim of carrying out simple tasks, like moving a toy car on the table or blocking an object by bringing the upper limb to the chest or mouth.

The child with moderate impairment and a score of 2, even only with a limited number of stereotyped patterns, can spontaneously use their upper limb particularly in bimanual tasks, such as blocking an object on the work surface or holding medium-sized objects (Fig. 9.25). The bimanual activity can also be affected by the presence of involuntary movements in the unaffected hand (Kim et al. 2020; Kuhtz-Buschbeck et al. 2000). Difficulties in stereognosis recognition tasks can be observed also if with a limited number of stereotyped patterns.

The child with mild impairment and score 3 spontaneously involves the affected hand in bimanual activities using a varied repertoire of patterns, and in-hand manipulation movements of medium complexity are possible. The child can manipulate

Fig. 9.25 Spontaneous use of the affected hand to hold an "easy to grip" object

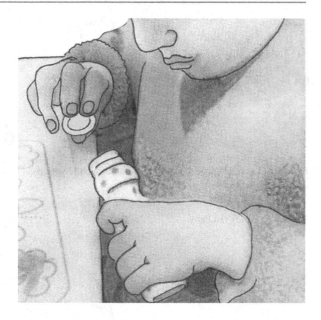

small objects, such as medium-sized and small beads, with both hands and can switch them from one hand to the other even without visual control. Generally bimanual activity is not disturbed by involuntary movements of the unaffected hand, and no stereognosis disturbances have been reported (Fedrizzi et al. 2003; Kinnucan et al. 2010).

The main goal of upper extremity rehabilitation in the child with USCP is to reach functional independence in ADLs by improving bimanual skills.

Intervention should start early from the first months of life and be implemented continuously and intensively until school age, because the greatest improvements are obtained during this period, and they generally last over time. Several studies have reported that the intensity of treatment and coaching to parents are the most important factors to facilitate the learning of new strategies and to improve the quality of the hand use (Hanna et al. 2003; Charles and Gordon 2006; Holmefur et al. 2009; Gordon 2011; Akhbari Ziegler et al. 2019).

During daily handling, the caregiver can promote early sensory experiences for both "hemi-sides" of the child's body, to improve the reception of visual, tactile, and proprioceptive inputs of the affected limb and to seek its integration into the body schema (Nuara et al. 2019).

To encourage the child's visual contact toward space on their impaired side, therapists and caregivers should pay attention to where toys and other interesting objects are positioned with respect to the child. For the same reason, adults should also remember to enter the child's visual field from their most problematic side. Another possible suggestion to the family is to rearrange the child's bedroom, for example, orienting the cot/bed in such a way the child is attracted to look at interesting toys or light from windows (Finnie 2009) (Fig. 9.26).

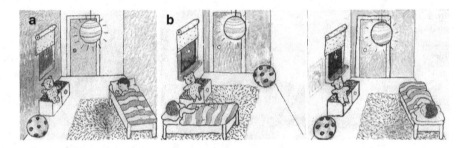

Fig. 9.26 (**a**) Inadequate sleeping position for a child with right hemiplegia; (**b**) Adequate sleeping position (redrawn from Finnie 2009)

Fig. 9.27 Handwrist baby rattle

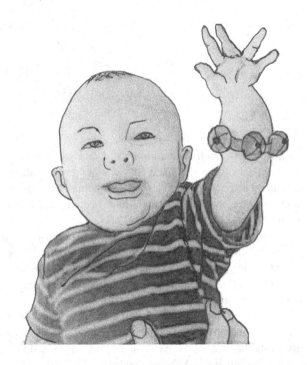

To promote the child's interest in the affected arm, as well as eye-hand-mouth coordination, it is useful to offer toys with different properties (tactile, visual, auditory) or use a handwrist baby rattle, equipped with bells, pets, and even lights (Fig. 9.27). It is also important to encourage exploration of the face, facilitating the child's hand to reach and touch their mouth, nose, and head. With a toddler, caregivers can propose play with the finger colors, water, sand, and beans.

Involvement of the affected arm/hand in their daily routine activities is also important, for example, during feeding, toileting, and hygiene, even using commercially available adapted equipment (Finnie 2009; Case-Smith and O'Brien 2019). During bathing, the toddler can be washed with different kinds of sponges and can play with water or with floating objects to stimulate them to use both hands (Fig. 9.28).

Fig. 9.28 Floating toys in the tub, during bathing

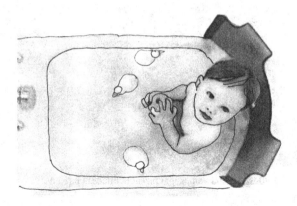

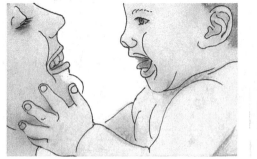

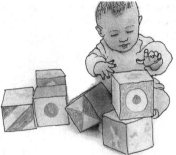

Fig. 9.29 Baby games and toys that promote bilateral hand use

It should be remembered that, during un/dressing of the child with USCP, there is a specific procedure to follow where the impaired arm (or leg) is always the first to be involved in the functional sequence: during dressing, the first arm to be brought forward is the impaired one, and vice-versa during undressing.

Parents offer to the infant baby games and toys of different sizes and tactile properties, proposing play activities to promote bilateral hand use (Fig. 9.29).

These games and toys have to gradually adapt to changes in the child's interests, to play development, and to their acquisition of functional abilities, e.g., by selecting toys suitable for the size and other features that enhance bimanual use (Fig. 9.30).

Already from the first year of the child's life, the presence of parents and caregivers at the rehabilitation treatment is important because they need to be able to understand the child's difficulties and therefore pay attention to their postural orientation, the criteria for choosing toys, and the modalities to propose them.

In preschoolers with moderate/mild impairment, two of the main goals are fine motor skills development and the use of the affected hand in more complex and differentiated bimanual activities. Through play activities, related to the child's mental development, the therapist can promote, where possible, the pre-shaping of the hand, according to the object's features, the differentiated power and precision

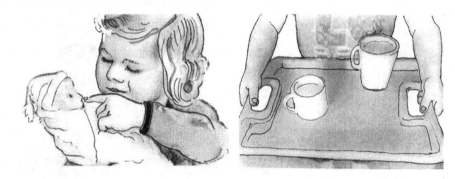

Fig. 9.30 Toys and games that promote bilateral hand use

Fig. 9.31 Play activity for
fine motor skill
development

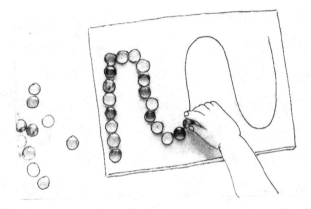

grips, the release, the finger singularization, the distinction of use of the radial and ulnar fingers, and the in-hand manipulation movements, while simultaneously refining various tactile discriminatory skill.

These goals can also be achieved by using commercially available toys that require fine motor skills but also crafted toys, created with everyday objects that can be easily found in the family environment (Fig. 9.31).

In children with severe motor difficulties, the main goal is to involve the impaired hand as an auxiliary to the unaffected one during ADLs: for example, involving the affected hand in blocking a sheet or in a holding function, such as to unscrew the lid of a jar or holding the play dough to break into small pieces with the unaffected hand.

To promote a more functional bimanual activity, adults can suggest to the child alternative ways of fixing objects, e.g., locking objects against the trunk or inserting them between the fingers. If possible, they can also try to improve the involvement of the affected limb, promoting horizontal adduction/abduction movements in some play activities, such as coloring with finger colors, or the palmar/interdigital grip use, identifying, also together with the child, feasible ways to open their hand.

In some cases, it could be necessary to consider, the prescription of orthoses and/ or medical-pharmacological interventions within the rehabilitation plan in order to

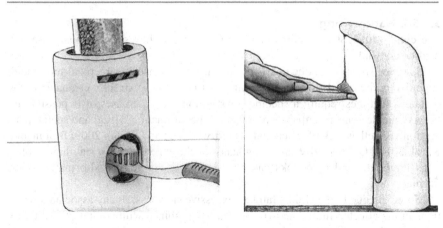

Fig. 9.32 Adapted equipment for one-hand use

improve function and prevent or reduce deformities (Wilton 2003; Burtner et al. 2008; Morris et al. 2011; Case-Smith and O'Brien 2019).

9.2.5.1 ADLs
Based on the functional ability level of the child, the therapist should carry out a further evaluation regarding the ADLs, focusing on goals shared with the child and/or their family, and feasible both in the short and long term (Shepard 2019; Spitzer 2019). Depending on the age and level of impairment, they can also identify and agree on possible compensations, using bypass strategies or modifying equipment to allow one-hand use, e.g., folded toilet paper, toothpaste, and soap dispenser (Fig. 9.32) (Klein 1983; Morris and Klein 1987; Pratt and Allen 1989; Finnie 2009; Missiuna and Pollock 2000; Spitzer 2019; Case-Smith and O'Brien 2019).

As in the BSCP form, the therapist should suggest step-by-step facilitation techniques for ADL not only to the child but also techniques which involve parents and caregivers (Klein 1983; Morris and Klein 1987; Shepard 2019).

Adolescents and adults may need periodic reassessment to evaluate not only ADLs but also IADLs, because sometimes previous functional strategies need to be updated, such as, for example, to address the needs of a new job.

Adolescents with USCP can often be stressed out by attending rehabilitation services for a long time, especially if the rehabilitation goals are not constantly verified and updated. Because of this, they *be quite upset,* and so, for this reason, many authors underline the importance of adapting therapy to life rather than having the young person's life adapt to therapy (Scrutton 2001; Goodman and Yude 2001; Fedrizzi et al. 2003; Skold et al. 2004; Blank et al. 2012).

From the early years of life, these youngsters can be encouraged to engage in sports and play activities, such as swimming, volleyball, horseback riding, canoeing, or skiing, to promote not only motor skills but also social interaction.

9.2.5.2 Handwriting

The child with USCP acquires handwriting because they spontaneously use the unaffected hand.

However, sometimes, due to arm dominance or to sensory-perceptual-motor and cognitive problems, there may be writing that need to be carefully evaluated early on and sometimes require a specific intervention. In these cases, it is possible to observe tactile-sensory impairment, bilateral incoordination, visual and spatial perception, as well as lack of speed and dexterity (Kavak and Bumin 2009; Bumin and Kavak 2010). Occasionally "assisting hand" anchoring systems or stabilizing solutions for books and notebooks can be used, for example, anti-slip materials or magnets.

Moreover, due to the child's fatigue, excessive slowness, or any associated reactions in the affected limb, handwriting can be combined with computer writing to overcome these difficulties.

9.2.6 Aims of Functional Treatment of the Upper Limb in Children with USCP

– *Intervention for perceptual aspects: early sensory experiences during play and daily handling, to integrate visual, tactile, and proprioceptive inputs between all parts of the body and improve the body schema and later on, if possible, enhance the tactile discrimination in the impaired limb*
– *Prehension: from hand opening/closing control to three-point pinch and, if possible, to superior pinch use; hand pre-shaping depending on the object features; improving wrist control and thumb opposition; differentiation between radial and ulnar fingers*
– *Release: from whole hand opening to precise release control, with previous wrist extension, of objects of various sizes and features on a surface or in space or small containers*
– *In-hand manipulation: from the differentiation between radial and ulnar fingers to more complex intrinsic movements; parallel intervention on tactile and proprioceptive awareness/discrimination*
– *Bilateral hand use: early experiences of bilateral hand use, stimulating the spontaneous use of the affected hand in more complex bimanual play activities; parent and caregiver training, sharing postural care, toy choice criteria and modalities to propose games and toys*
– *ADLs: selecting compensatory strategies; teaching standard and adapted techniques; environmental and equipment adaptations; use of ADL aids; caregiver training; IADL intervention in adolescents*
– *Orthoses: possible use to improve function and/or to prevent or reduce deformities, in association with eventual medical-pharmacological intervention, if needed*

9.3 The Child with Dyskinesia

The child with dyskinesia shows more difficulties in the upper limb use compared to the child with spastic CP, related to several factors such as postural control disorders, primitive reflexes persistence, tone fluctuations, involuntary movements, and perceptual disorders. These difficulties also greatly affect participation in daily occupations of childhood.

In children with moderate/mild impairment (functional levels 2 and 3 of the Table 8.3), there is a significant delay and sometimes limitations in some strength and precision grip achievements (e.g., superior pinch), in more complex in-hand manipulation movements and bilateral, coordinated, and differentiated hand use. Generally, these children can access the daily activities, but it will often be necessary to adapt or modify the task features.

Children with severe motor impairment (functional levels 0 and 1) have a significant limitation in the most basic hand functions, such as reaching, grasping, and releasing. The use of the upper limbs for even simple tasks can be extremely difficult and sometimes completely impossible (Kyllerman et al. 1982; Monbaliu et al. 2016, 2017b).

Access to ADLs is greatly limited and requires continuous support from caregivers. Therefore, for the child with dyskinesia, it is important to rely on all the functional resources available, identifying one or more voluntarily controlled movements, which can be used functionally, and modifying and/or adapting the daily activities through bypass strategies (see Chap. 8, Sect. 8.3). For some functional goals in more complex cases, other parts of the body, such as head, foot, or eye-gaze use can be evaluated (Borgestig et al. 2015, 2016).

These children have significant limitations in achieving autonomy in many ADLs, as in toileting, bathing, dressing, and feeding, the latter due to dysfunction in oral control and upper limb use (Monbaliu et al. 2017a). It is also necessary to evaluate environmental factors, such as types of assistance and barriers, that may affect day-to-day care, as well as interviewing and supporting the caregivers regarding the handling procedures for the child. Equipment adaptations, ADL aids and environmental adjustments are often needed to lighten the burden of care (Finnie 2009; French et al. 1991; Korpela et al. 1992; Dormans and Pellegrino 1998; Østensjø et al. 2003, 2009; Henderson and Pehoski 2005; Pirila et al. 2018; Case-Smith and O'Brien 2019).

It is also important to identify communication strategies and supports (Millar and Aitken 2003; Beukelman and Mirenda 2013) that allow the child to guide their caregivers in taking care of them.

Limitations in play are considerable, especially in children with severe impairment. For most of them, the opportunity to enjoy and progress through the various stages of play development, independent or cooperative, depends greatly on caregiver support and play adaptations. The therapist can suggest some simple play aids: if the child does not have a functional grip, a Velcro[3] glove can lock a small toy, or

---

[3] Velcro Ltd., Knutsford (UK), www.velcro.uk

Fig. 9.33 Play adaptation: battery-operated toy with a customed switch

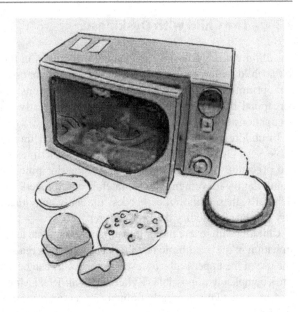

the child can activate a battery-operated toy with a customed switch (Fig. 9.33) (Pratt and Allen 2009; Case-Smith and O'Brien 2019).

The child with communication difficulties can also use AAC boards to guide a partner, for example, to play with them (see also Chap. 12).

If manipulation of play materials is impossible, other parts of the body could become involved for play, for example, for using a head pointer with a brush to paint, a head switch as an alternative access to special computer games, or eye pointing to play a memory game (Fig. 9.34).

Bypass strategies are also needed for children with moderate/mild dyskinesia to access many ADLS, enhance autonomy, and guarantee safety. For example, in washing, toileting, and grooming, they can use compensatory strategies, environmental adaptations, and/or simpler aids, sometimes also adopting bathing and commercially available toileting equipment for kids (Fig. 9.35).

Regarding self-feeding, there may be difficulties related to oral control, perceptual disorders, and upper limbs use, especially in more complex tasks, like cutting with a knife, eating with a fork, using a spoon, and pouring water.

Disorders in fine motor skills often limit physical access to more complex toys and games, and it is necessary to select among commercially available products toys that are easy to handle and appropriate to the interests and performance capacities of the child, with characteristics like easy-to-grip, of medium size, magnetic, or Velcro-fitted objects (Fig. 9.36).

Another problem for the child is that, due to their involuntary movements, their toys tend to move when they attempt to manipulate them. Therefore, it is advisable to adopt a wide table or lap-tray with edges or to propose toys to put into socket

Fig. 9.34 Play with other
parts of the body: head
pointer with a paintbrush

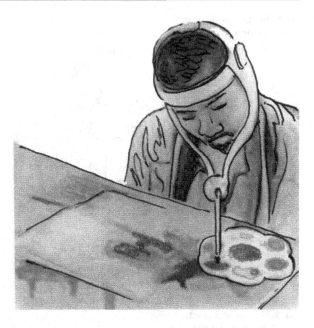

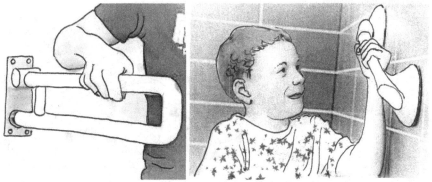

Fig. 9.35   Equipment commercially available for toileting and bathing

frames or that are stabilized on the work surface with a non-slip mat, suction cups, or c-clamps or strapped to the child hand (Fig. 9.37).

The child usually has dysphonia and dysarthria. These problems make it difficult to understand their speech, more than in the child with BSCP, and they often require a specific and early intervention of AAC (Yorkston et al. 1998; Himmelmann et al. 2013; Beukelman and Mirenda 2013) (see further details in Chap. 12).

Perceptual disorders are very frequent mainly related to the selection, suppression, and calibration of the various sensory inputs (Odding et al. 2006; Sanger and Kukke 2007; Himmelmann et al. 2009; Monbaliu et al. 2017b).

Especially in the most severe children, there are often auditory impairment (Shevell et al. 2009) and visual disorders (Jan et al. 2001; Fazzi et al. 2007; Ghasia et al. 2008; Dufresne et al. 2014; Ego et al. 2015).

Fig. 9.36 Easy-to-handle
and magnetic toys

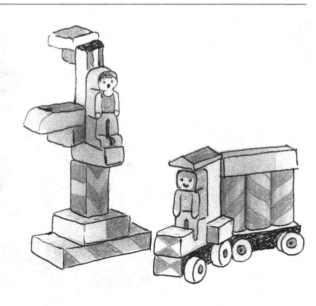

Fig. 9.37 Toy socket set
placed on a non-slip mat

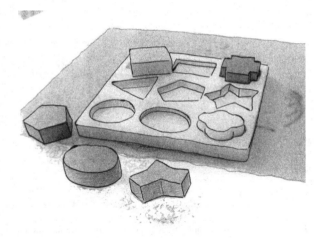

Also, again mainly in the severe motor challenged children, there may be relevant cognitive impairment (Kyllerman et al. 1982; Sigurdardottir et al. 2008; Himmelmann et al. 2009; Yin Foo et al. 2013; Stadskleiv et al. 2018; Batorowicz et al. 2018; Ballester-Plané et al. 2018; Laporta-Hoyos et al. 2019).

Perceptual, visual, and cognitive disorders, which are significantly interrelated, can affect the use of the upper limbs and need to be properly assessed to define a realistic functional prognosis and to set up an appropriate rehabilitation project (Beckung and Hagberg 2002; Henderson and Pehoski 2005; Case-Smith and O'Brien 2019).

In dyskinetic forms of CP, the use of the upper limbs is influenced by a combination of several different factors. It can even be impossible in cases of severe motor impairment.

9.3.1 Postural Control

The child with dyskinesia has considerable difficulties in maintaining the sitting posture, which is the most used during play and ADLs. Sitting can be affected by various factors, such as synergistic flexion or extension patterns, involuntary movements, atypical or abnormal primitive reflex persistence (e.g., ATNR, Galant. etc.), tone fluctuations, and perceptual disorders (see also Chap. 4).

Seated on a chair, this child tends to be dominated by synergistic patterns, which force their lower limbs to extend or to go into flexion under the seat, making it difficult to keep their feet on the ground (Fig. 9.38).

The problems above make it difficult to use the upper limbs for support. If the child manages to stabilize their posture with their arms, then they cannot use their hands for other functional tasks.

To improve the use of the upper limbs and visual control and to provide greater stability and alignment, the therapist should choose positioning aids that can contain the child without preventing them from moving. Different aids may be needed for the various ADLs, when the child needs different positioning for self-feeding, un/dressing, playing, or writing.

Sometimes, in moderate/mild forms, commercially available stable chairs can be adopted, using soft or anti-slip pads, modifying existing equipment, or adding the simplest sitting aids, such as foot support with a back edge to promote better control of the lower limbs.

Children with severe motor impairment greatly benefit from a seating system, often customized, which will allow them - as seated - to enhance their relationships with people, feasible functional activities and facilitate caregiving (Costigan and Light 2011; Ryan 2012; Sahinoğlu et al. 2017). Here, teamwork between different

Fig. 9.38 Inappropriate posture with synergistic pattern in extension

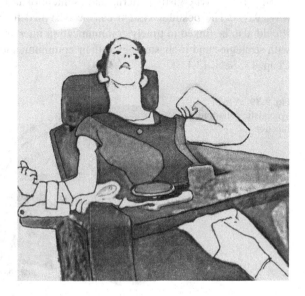

rehabilitation professionals is highly recommended because together they need to evaluate and verify the effects of the proposed system on the child's posture and functional abilities.

For a long time, many of these children cannot even tolerate the separation from caregivers and the seating system itself, and they only accept to sit on their parents' and other known adults' lap.

Due to the child's perceptual disorders, it is important to consider the features (texture, consistency, measures) of all components of the positioning system and identify the most suitable strategies to help the child gradually accept the posture system.

Depending on the extent of the motor impairment, additional components for hips, lower limbs, and the head as well as any anchoring system can be considered.

To improve stability in sitting, this child benefit from a recessed table that facilitates arm support and functional activities. It is typical for them to organize compensatory strategies when seated, such as anchoring one foot to the chair's leg. These strategies should be carefully evaluated because sometimes they are functional, but in other cases, they could cause future contractures and deformities.

Sometimes, it is necessary to set up customized workstations, including some alternative access to AT on the seating system to facilitate communication, play, writing, etc. The same problem can arise about mobility with a wheelchair when the arms are dysfunctional. In these cases, the therapist evaluates and proposes the use of control interfaces managed by other parts of the body (e.g., head or foot) or scanning methods (Furusamu 1997; Bottos et al. 2001; Case-Smith and O'Brien 2019). For further information on AT for mobility aids, read Chap. 13, Sect. 13.1.5.

Children with dyskinesia, especially those with impaired or absent speech, tend to trigger total synergistic patterns and unintentional movements, to communicate (Fig. 9.39). The postural system can be designed to minimize these effects and should also be linked to timely communication intervention that provides the child with strategies and tools suitable to their communication needs (see Chap. 12 and Chap. 13, Sect. 13.1.3).

Fig. 9.39 A total synergistic pattern for function

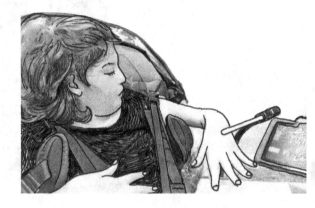

9.3.2   Reaching in the Child with Dyskinesia

Here reaching is greatly affected by various factors, which include postural control problems, persistence of abnormal primitive reflex (mostly by ATNR and avoiding reactions) involuntary movements, tone fluctuations, and perceptual disorders.

Children with severe disabilities have considerable difficulties in maintaining postural alignment and the upper limbs on the work surface, under visual control. They can therefore functionally engage only one upper limb, often exploiting the extension of the facial arm of the ATNR, which allows the use of the hand to perform sweeping movements. Despite this, intervention might be aimed at optimizing the use of these even limited movements for some functional activities, for example, to operate a toy with a switch (Fig. 9.40).

To enhance participation in ADLs using AT, it is important to identify a functional work area for the child, within which to place objects, toys, or switches. However, when reaching and other upper limb use is impossible or extremely tiring, it is necessary to evaluate the use of other parts of child's body, eye gaze, or voice, as alternative accesses to play, writing, and education. The therapist can propose the use of AT or AAC systems, planning adequate rehabilitation training for a better positioning and functional use of the alternative parts of the body and/or eye gaze (Henderson et al. 2008; Pratt and Allen 2009; Sadao and Robinson 2010; Borgestig et al. 2015, 2016; Case-Smith and O'Brien 2019) (Fig. 9.41).

Children who are moderately impaired show better postural alignment and visual control over their actions than those with severe impairment, even if using various compensatory strategies. They often alternate the use of the two upper limbs, depending on the task and the localization of the target, even when the more functional arm is in extension when ATNR is present. For tasks which require more precision, such as for pointing to symbols on a communication board or typing on a computer keyboard, they usually isolate one finger exploiting the wrist flexion

Fig. 9.40 Operating a toy with a switch, despite the influence of ATNR

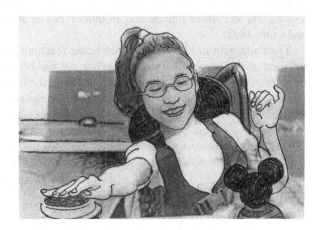

Fig. 9.41 Using
eye-tracking to access
computer game

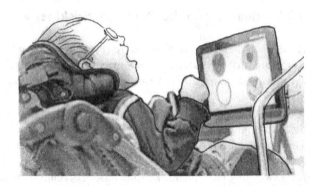

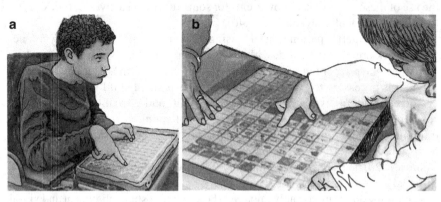

Fig. 9.42 Isolation of index finger exploiting the wrist flexion

(Fig. 9.42). In other tasks requiring wide movements in a large working area (e.g., painting), they carry out the task moving the extended arm in adduction/abduction.

Sometimes, to promote better postural alignment and improve functional use of the more competent arm, the therapist may introduce "no-accessing" arm anchoring systems or apply boundary bumpers to improve the postural stability of the child (Fig. 9.43). It is also important to pay attention to the position of people in relation to the child and where objects and all other types of inputs are placed (Goossens' and Crain 1992).

The child with mild dyskinesia has better reaching control; more coordinated, differentiated bilateral hand use; and better eye-hand coordination. They also have more postural and forearms alignment, allowing them to move both upper limbs closer to the midline, sometimes even crossing it, and have better control of elbow flexion/extension movements. They may also have a supination range between full pronation and neutral position, which allows for more direct reaching and functional hand orientation toward objects.

As previously stated, it is fundamental to the use of a desk or lap-tray with recess, which allows the child to firmly rest their forearms on a surface and has supination and wrist extension for an easier use of the hand.

Fig. 9.43 Boundary bumpers for promoting a functional use of arms in midline

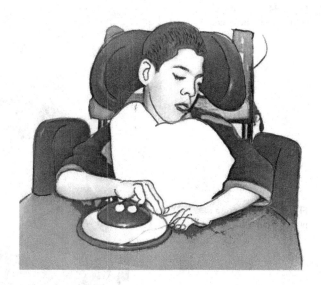

9.3.3   Prehension and Manipulation

In the child with dyskinesia, the prehension and manipulation difficulties are considerable, even in the mildest form and are related to several factors, such as those described regarding reaching problems (Sanger et al. 2010; Monbaliu et al. 2016).

In the case of severe impairment, the child is unable to handle objects and is greatly limited in performing even simple actions. Hand use is possible only with an extended arm. The hand is brought to the object in various ways, for example, with flexion of the wrist and extended fingers or with pronation of the forearm and ulnar deviation of the fisted hand. At the first contact with an object, the hand often closes or moves away from the object due to the avoiding reaction, together with the associated gaze avoiding. Bimanual manipulative activity is not possible.

Hand use can also be disturbed by hand-eye coordination disorders. To have visual control over their actions, this child sometimes uses peripheral vision or dissociates gaze and action (first looks and then touches).

The main goal of intervention for these children is to let help them achieve some voluntary hand opening (Fig. 9.44) and, if feasible, to facilitate a palmar grasp pattern when a change in arm position is required, for example, to manipulate a joystick and drive a power chair (Fig. 9.45).

In the case of moderate impairment, the child handles a limited selection of easily manageable objects in an adapted situation. If well seated, the child with dyskinesia can have better reaching and a better range of supination control, which allows them to grasp with palmar or three-point grip objects with particular features, such as a drinking cup with wide handles or "easy-to-grip" pencil, brushes, etc. (Figs. 9.20 and 9.49).

Fig. 9.44 Pressing a
device with open hand

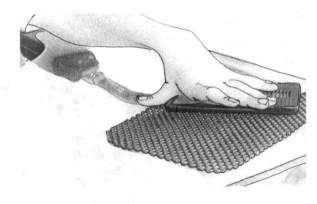

Fig. 9.45 Operating a
power chair with a joystick

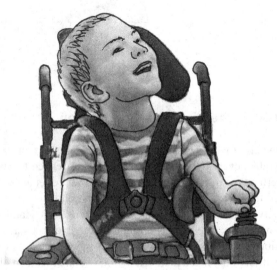

Prehension and release of objects can also be facilitated by the use of anchoring systems on the not-accessing arm and by stabilization of these objects on non-slippering surfaces, as in Fig. 9.44.

These children can usually achieve one finger isolation, often by flexing the wrist, for typing on the keyboard or for direct selection on a communication board or speech-generating device (SGD).

A child with a moderate motor disability can achieve manipulation and the more basic skills for bilateral use of the hand, even if influenced by the ATNR. They usually hold objects still with one hand, for example, to hold a piece of paper on the desk, while the other hand has manipulative tasks, such as coloring.

To manipulate easy objects and enhance visual control over their actions, the child with dyskinesia often uses compensatory strategies, e.g., leaning forward on the table or even using shoulder protraction to block the upper limbs against their body.

These children can access some ADLs, even if it is often necessary to modify or adapt to the characteristics of the environment.

Children with mild impairment can achieve some power and precision grip, more complex in-hand manipulation movements, and coordinated and differentiated bilateral hand use, even when arms are in an open kinetic chain. The acquisition of better fine motor skills depends on reaching control, on the influence of the unintentional movements (which often become more evident over time), and on the child's ability to adopt compensatory strategies. It is important to evaluate the functionality of such compensatory strategies, sometimes helping the child to organize those that are easier to use, less strenuous, and more effective for performing various tasks, e.g., holding a pencil with a "cross-thumb" grip, to control unintentional distal movements when writing (Fig. 9.46).

9.3.3.1 ADLs

Usually, children with moderate/mild impairment can achieve greater autonomy, but with some limitations in more complex ADLs (e.g., buttoning, scissors using, lacing shoes, hair combing). Adolescents and adults may also have difficulties in achieving some IADLs, for example, public transportation use, home management, jobs, and leisure time.

To set up a good functional rehabilitation project, it is always necessary to periodically evaluate the child's potential and difficulties, first making an assessment of the upper limbs and then observing them in their everyday environments (Law et al. 1999). The use of standardized assessment tools allows the therapist to define more precisely the short-/medium-/long-term aims of the project, sharing them with the youngster (child and adolescent) and the family (Gordon 1992; Missiuna and Pollock 2000; Shepard 2019; Spitzer 2019).

Fig. 9.46 Cross-thumb pencil grip

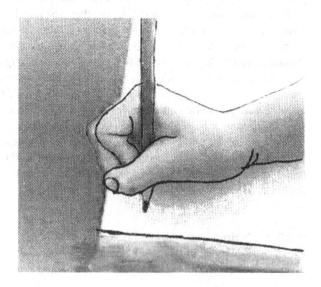

Fig. 9.47 Self-feeding: strategy to bring food to the mouth

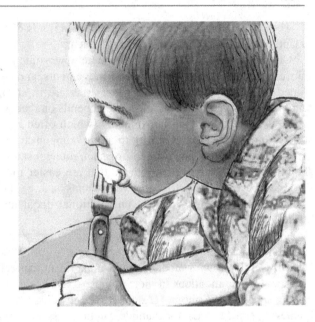

In the case of dyskinesia, it is often necessary to modify the environment or/and adapt tasks (with bypass strategies) to allow them to achieve more autonomy in ADL. For example, in self-feeding, professionals can reduce sensory inputs from the environment, facilitate better positioning with suitable chair and table, and/or select ADL aids, such as easy-to-hold cutlery or drinking devices with big handles (Morris and Klein 1987). The therapist could also accept compensatory strategies, if necessary, for function.

The child with dyskinesia can have many difficulties with self-feeding, for example, in bringing a bowl or food in the mouth using cutlery (Fig. 9.47).

Positioning also requires attention: the therapist may have to adapt the chair with a recessed tray or table, to provide greater stability to the trunk and shoulders or propose adaptive equipment, such as rubber strips to secure the cutlery to the hand or suction cup with a raised edge to facilitate the scooping of food (Fig. 9.48).

To facilitate self-drinking, it is possible to select a suitable device according to the child's prehension patterns, such as a mug with a wide handle (Fig. 9.49). Some children with good oral control prefer cups with flexible straws, but in severe cases, special drinking aids, which do not require upper limb use, can be proposed.

As in BSCP, the child with dyskinesia also needs to learn step-by-step strategies to best perform ADLs, and the family and caregivers need to be involved and trained to help the child achieve these goals. In adolescents and young adults, intervention should be aimed not only at independence but also at positive participation in the community.

9.3.3.2 Writing

Children with moderate/mild impairment may be able to draw and paint, usually using easy-to-hold tools such as large markers and brushes, faceting pencils, or a

Fig. 9.48 Adaptive equipment: rubber strip fixing the fork

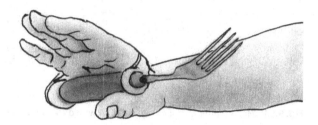

Fig. 9.49 Adaptations for self-drinking

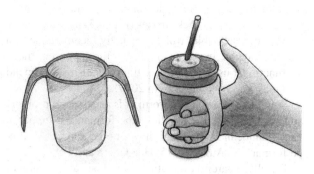

Fig. 9.50 Adaptive tools for writing

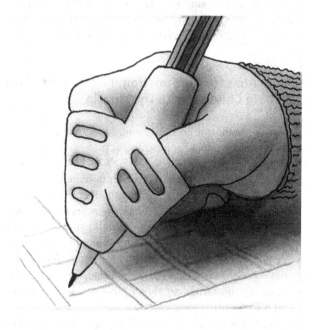

special pencil/brush holder (Klein 1982). It may also be necessary to facilitate such activities by using anti-slip materials on which to place the paper or notebooks (Fig. 9.50).

Children with moderate dyskinesia can only do—and with great effort—a limited amount of handwritten work. Generally, they write a few single words to take

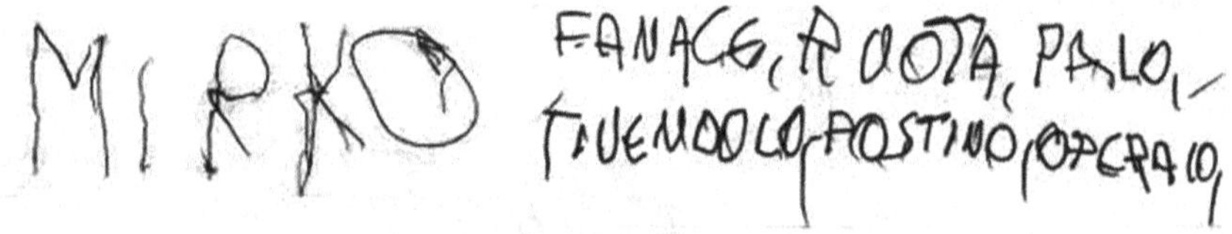

Fig. 9.51 Handwriting layout of two children with dyskinesia

notes or to make a simplified signature and prefer to write in capital letters that require only short, quick strokes (Fig. 9.51).

The recessed table, which is usually recommended for all children with CP and severe/moderate impairment to favor the support of the forearms and therefore better functional use of the upper limbs, is also recommended for children with mild dyskinesia (Kavak and Bumin 2009).

Sometimes, in this mild form, it is necessary a prolonged and careful observation and assessment of the functional performance of upper limbs, because the unestablished handedness problem may emerge and could affect the child's handwriting performances (Auzias 1975; Henderson and Pehoski 2005).

Equally, a careful evaluation should be carried out with the moderate/mild child, if they access computer writing to meet educational needs, identifying also the most functional positioning and/or adaptive equipment for the computer access, e.g., type of keyboard, keyguard, and/or alternatives mouse use (Fig. 9.52).

9.3.4 Aims for the Functional Treatment of the Upper Limb in Children with Dyskinesia

According to the child's upper limb functional level, as indicated in Table 8.3, suggestions for the upper limb treatment plan are presented below.

For Children with Severe Motor Impairment
- *Reaching control: from adduction/abduction horizontal movement control to elbow control. Particularly: improve movement's range of at least one arm, moving closer to the midline, more visual control on the action*
- *Hand use: from voluntary hand opening to maintaining/releasing contact with an object (e.g., switch) and, if feasible, initiating and sustaining a palmar grasp pattern with changes in the arm positions (e.g., to operate a joystick to drive a power chair)*
- *Isolation of at least one finger for direct selection on AAC systems or for typing on a keyboard*
- *Bilateral hand use: from the simple maintenance of both upper limbs on the work surface to initial use of a more involved arm to stabilize object, without grasp*
- *Assessment and intervention on perceptual disorders*
- *Eye/hand coordination*
- *Rehabilitation intervention for the functional use of other parts of the body (if upper limbs are severely impaired)*

Fig. 9.52 Alternative keyboard with keyguard, for computer writing

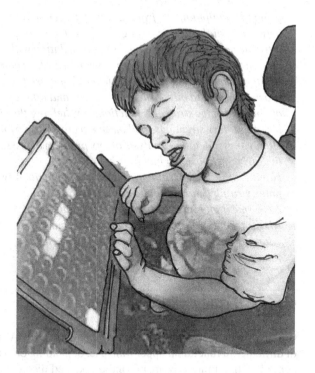

– *ADLs: caregiver training for positioning, handling strategies and ADLs aids use, etc.*
– *Writing: selection of alternative access to computer writing (hardware and software selection and training)*
– *Play: positioning for play, adapted environment, alternative strategies and adapted toys use; selecting AT for play*

For Children with Moderate/Mild Motor Impairment

– *Reaching and pointing control: control of more precise trajectories, implemented in different postures and planes, with particular attention to midline crossing and posterior reaching patterns required for many ADLs (e.g., in dressing, hygiene, etc.), pronation/supination of the forearm, extension of the wrist, etc.*
– *Prehension: from three-point pinch to superior pinch with thumb opposition; gradual inhibition of ulnar fingers, using only the radial fingers; prehension of objects with various features (e.g., flat, heavy, etc.)*
– *Release: from the control of hand opening with extended fingers and neutral wrist to the precise and controlled release—on a surface or in space or a small container—of objects of various sizes and features*
– *Isolation of at least one finger for direct selection on AAC systems or for typing on a keyboard*

- *In-hand manipulation: from isolated finger movements to the differentiation between radial and ulnar fingers; from finger to palm translation to complex intrinsic movements, e.g., combining translation with rotation; parallel intervention on tactile and proprioceptive awareness/discrimination*
- *Bilateral hand use: from less proficient hand use for stabilizing (without or with grasp) function to bilateral simultaneous and differentiated hand use; evaluation of compensatory strategies functionality, helping the child to organize those easier to use, less strenuous, and more effective for performing various tasks*
- *Handedness: detailed analysis of any problem of unestablished handedness, particularly to choose the hand for handwriting*
- *Handwriting: handwriting training, when functionally possible; training of computer writing (hardware and software selection)*
- *Assessment and intervention on perceptual disorders, if needed*
- *ADLs: teaching standard and adapted techniques; environmental and equipment adaptations (e.g., bathroom), ADL aids selection; caregiver training; IADLs rehabilitation intervention in adolescents*

9.4   The Child with Ataxia

Children with nonprogressive congenital ataxia (NPCA) may have varying degrees of difficulty in functional upper limb use, depending on whether antigravity postural control or fine limb movements and associated disorders are more involved. Their performance is characterized by a lack of muscle coordination, and therefore movements are performed with abnormal strength, rhythm, and precision. Also, slow tremor and low pitch are observed. However, albeit with very long learning times, these children can reach good levels of autonomy in playing and in the ADLs, with difficulties in some more complex and coordinated activities, such as self-feeding, writing, buttoning, and other fine motor skills.

Many authors report a high incidence of associated problems in NPCA (Hagberg et al. 1993; Esscher et al. 1996; Steinlin et al. 1998). They are related to (a) cognitive function (2/3 of children have learning problems, half of which are quite severe); (b) visual problems, detected in more than 50% of children (Black 1982; Dufresne et al. 2014; Kozeis and Jain 2018); (c) perception and language disorders; and (d) epilepsy (Bertini et al. 2018).

It is essential to evaluate all these aspects in order to plan an adequate upper limb rehabilitation project, following the guidelines suggested in Chap. 8.

9.4.1   Postural Control

Postural instability is the main problem that conditions the maintenance of the sitting posture, the position most frequently used by the child while playing and performing ADLs.

The use of the upper limbs together with the visual control of the environment is essential to provide greater stability to the child, choosing suitable positioning

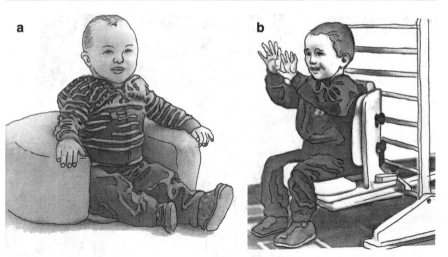

Fig. 9.53 Positioning for children with ataxia

sitting systems to improve writing, self-feeding, and more complex and coordinated play activities.

For this purpose, it is also possible to use commercially available, very stable chairs or other equipment already existing at home or in the classroom. In some cases, it is necessary to use non-slip mats applied to the seat surface or special cushions that improve stability.

To facilitate and enhance the functions of the upper limbs, the child with ataxia also needs to be seated with a recess in front, to facilitate the support of the forearms, and, in some cases, with a non-slip pad under their buttocks or feet, to increase stability. The same measures are also proposed in the infant/toddler to facilitate play, even while sitting on the ground (Fig. 9.53).

As in all other forms of CP, here again it is necessary to evaluate the characteristics of the environment in which the child lives and consequently adapt it to their needs. To improve the child's transfers and their participation in all ADLs, it may be useful to reorganize the bathroom, bedroom, etc. and allow furniture to be accessible for feeding, play, or pc use, sometimes applying adaptive equipment, e.g., grab bars in the bathroom (Fig. 9.35).

9.4.2 Upper Limb Use

Children with ataxia usually have a normal repertoire of the basic patterns of the upper limbs, but their functional acquisitions can be delayed in time and their use is affected by dysmetria (hyper/hypometria). Poor temporal coordination of the motor sequences causes acceleration, braking, and sudden adjustments of the gesture (asynergy). Another typical feature is past-pointing, i.e., the over-/undershooting of goal-directed movement. This means that children with ataxia may have a "plan" for how to achieve a goal but fail to execute it with accuracy. Further details about these features can be found in Chap. 5, Sect. 5.1.2.

Fig. 9.54 Using the trunk to transfer weight to arms

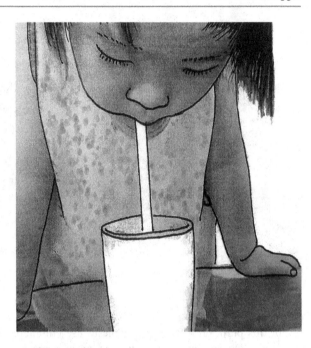

Typical "ataxic" behaviors can be observed frequently in these children. For example, during self-feeding, they bring the spoon to their mouth and the movement is adequate but starts with a rapid, uncontrolled movement, and they risk hurting themselves. Particularly when the infant is not too stiff, they could begin to feed by themselves without apparent problems, but as feeding progresses, their posture becomes more unstable and movements less controlled. In this case, the therapist should facilitate the task by providing more support to arms and trunk, with specific equipment to reduce fatigue and effort.

Concerning visual-motor behavior, it is frequently observed that, during tasks that require to coordinate the movements of the eyes with arm-hand, these children exhibit peculiar patterns. For example, in order to fixate a target, they break down the task in two phases: first they rotate the head to an extreme opposite position and thereafter they turn the eyes to the target.

In the case of mild/moderate ataxia, the child can generally improve over time their strength, precision grip, simple in-hand manipulation movements (e.g., rotation, translational movement), and coordinated or differentiated bilateral use of the hand. The acquisition of these fine motor skills depends on postural and manual control, on the incidence of movement incoordination and on the child's ability to adopt compensatory strategies.

Indeed, this child may be very able and imaginative in discovering compensatory patterns to succeed in the task. Examples of the most common compensatory strategies include keeping the arms close to the body, fixing the elbows on a surface, and using the trunk to support weight on the arms (Fig. 9.54).

These compensatory strategies reduce the task of managing multiple joints, thus facilitating the functional performance of only a few joints, with the benefit of controlling dysmetria and allowing for more efficient manipulation.

However, families and therapists should pay attention to avoid the use of too many abnormal compensatory patterns in the infant/toddler while encouraging the habitual use of normal functional patterns. Nonetheless, when the child begins to be more independent, it is equally important to evaluate the functionality of such compensatory strategies, sometimes helping the child to organize those that are easier to use, less tiring, and more effective for performing various tasks.

To allow this child to achieve the greatest autonomy in ADL, it is often necessary to adapt tasks introducing bypass strategies. For example, with regard to self-feeding, professionals can implement positioning adaptations, e.g., suitable chair and table, also commercially available, and/or use ADL aids, e.g., easy-to-hold cutlery (Morris and Klein 1987; Case-Smith and O'Brien 2019).

Bimanuality can also be facilitated by proposing objects of adequate weight, size, texture, and friction and stable, robust, and easy-to-handle magnetized toys. Sometimes, it is enough to make some simple adaptations, like stiffen the end of the thread used to make a necklace with wooden beads.

Manipulation can also be facilitated by encouraging greater use of visual control to verify, guide, and adapt the gesture to the task. It is also important to propose more complex and fine activities to induce an accurate perception of auditory, visual, and tactile inputs regarding the task, supporting their intermodal integration.

In infants and toddlers, rehabilitation intervention to improve fine motor skills should start early and be integrated into all daily activities. As with other age groups, careful evaluation by the rehabilitation team is needed as well as precise indications for home activities and, in particular, for kindergarten time, where many creative manipulation experiences can be proposed to promote hand and arm development (Novak et al. 2009).

9.4.2.1 ADLs

Impairments of gestures and postures greatly influence the acquisition of some ADLs and subsequently of IADLs. The ADL assessment generally highlights clumsiness and major difficulties evident in some finer and more coordinated activities, such as picking up small items, dressing up, and self-feeding. Also, handwriting problems are often encountered, as described below.

9.4.2.2 Self-Feeding

In self-feeding, the child may have difficulty performing all or most of the necessary bowl-to-mouth tasks, for example, managing cutlery and coordinating simultaneously the movements necessary to bring the food to the mouth. To partially overcome these problems, it could be wise to fix the cutlery with rubber strips to the child's hand or to use a plate with borders to facilitate food collection (Fig. 9.55).

With regard to positioning during self-feeding, a regular chair with a recessed tray or table can provide greater trunk and shoulder stability and reduce the tendency of the trunk to slump forward.

Together with an oral control intervention, it may be necessary to identify first of all useful bypass strategies for the simplification of the task and to promote the gradual acquisition of self-feeding.

Fig. 9.55 Plate with borders and sucker

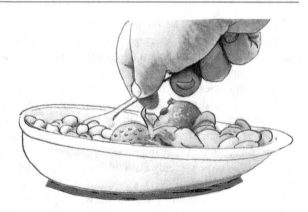

Particular care should be taken to facilitate the independent drinking, evaluating the most suitable drinking device for the child's current abilities, proposing, for example, a stable plastic cup with or without handle/s. For some children with significant motor function disorders, the therapist can suggest the strategy of "mouth to drinking device" by using, for example, a tilting cup fixed to a stable support, or a stable tumbler with a straw, with or without a straw holder (Fig. 9.49).

As in all other forms of CP, the rehab team should propose a gradual increase in the number of steps to complete every functional task, involving and training family and caregivers at home and school. In young adults, the aims are focused mainly on the most realistic IADLs, for work and leisure activities and community participation.

Practical Suggestions
- It is always useful to suggest a few simple basic tips to caregivers to improve self-feeding in the child with ataxia:
- *Ask the child to place their elbow firmly on the table to stabilize the upper limb and to steady their hand*
- *Choose finger foods and textures such as mashed potatoes and so on which make self-feeding easier*
- *Use a non-slip placemat, to stabilize bowls and plates, or a bowl with a suction cup to stop them moving around*

9.4.2.3 Bathing and Toileting

Placing bars and rails near the tub and/or toilet (Fig. 9.35) can increase safety and independence in the bathroom. It is important to foresee the problems that will arise when the child grows up and therefore to also plan the use of a bath chair or a shower to decrease the effort involved and increase independence. A further useful tip is the use of a washcloth with soap or "soap on a string" to avoid the soap slipping around and being dropped (Fig. 9.56).

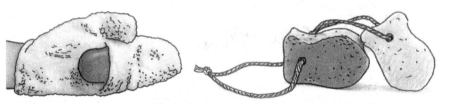

Fig. 9.56   Washcloth with soap and "soaps on a string"

9.4.2.4 Handwriting

Generally, children with ataxia can achieve the task of handwriting, first in capital letters, which requires only single-stroke movements, and then in cursive letters, with significant interpersonal differences in acquisition time and regarding speed, fatigue, and legibility. The child may have difficulty in adjusting and coordinating the upper hand/arm movements of progression and inscription, especially when prolonged for a long time (Ajuriaguerra et al. 1964). Especially in the dynamic phase of handwriting, they can maintain childlike and sometimes bizarre grips of the writing tool.

To facilitate handwriting, the child can adopt compensatory strategies such as leaning the trunk and upper limbs heavily on the work surface to give stability to the forearm and wrist. Particularly, they can press the ulnar side heavily on the table to allow the radial side to move more freely, but this behavior, together with the need to control involuntary movements, causes the child to put excessive hand pressure on the graphic instrument and indirectly also on the sheet of paper.

The handwriting trace appears broken, trembling, imprecise, and sometimes too light but other times too heavy, with variations in the size and orientation of signs and letters that will make the handwriting often unreadable (Fig. 9.57).

The therapist needs first to evaluate the child's drawing ability when they are at the prewriting stage between 2 and 3 years old. Later, between 5 and 5 years, handwriting can be assessed, if the development of handwriting looks promising and special handwriting tools and other adaptive equipment may be indicated.

The therapist can also propose easy-to-hold tools, such as large markers and brushes, faceting pencils for drawing and painting activities, suggesting the use of anti-slip pads on which the child can place paper or notebooks (Klein 1982). Furthermore, a writing board inclined at 45° may provide more stability for the forearm and make it easier for the child to look at the task (Fig. 9.58).

Commercially available writing tools are often suitable for the handwriting of the child with ataxia. Of course, it is necessary to evaluate the different characteristics of the tools regarding their smoothness, size, and shape, e.g., hexagonal pens can be more functional than cylindrical ones. In some cases, the child can take advantage of adaptive handwriting tools such as a weighted pen or a magnetic cuff that facilitates the maintenance of their forearm and wrist on the work surface or special notebooks with clearly marked margin lines and colored guidelines as a reference for writing in rows (Fig. 9.59).

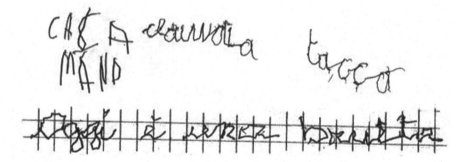

Fig. 9.57 Handwriting layout of two children with ataxia

Fig. 9.58 Adapted
equipment for handwriting

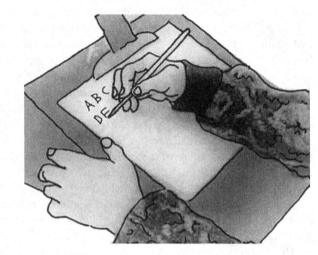

Fig. 9.59 A magnetic cuff
to facilitate handwriting

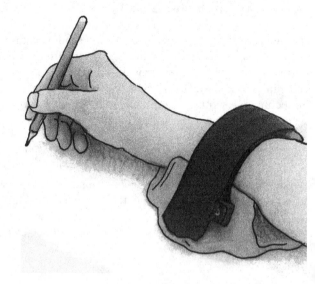

As well as during feeding time, the child can sit with a recessed table in front for handwriting, drawing, or activities using different writing devices (Kavak and Bumin 2009).

Often due to fatigue, excessive slowness, poor readability, and/or the great amount of written work requirements, handwriting can be replaced or complemented by computer writing ("mixed writing") and other educational devices.

However, computer writing may pose other access difficulties for the child, e.g., a finger singularization, and accurate typing may be problematic like activating a selected key or two keys at the same time.

Once more, careful assessment of the functional resources of the upper limbs is necessary, to identify the most functional positioning and/or adaptive equipment for computer access and the type of keyboard, keyguard, touchscreen, and/or alternative mouse use followed by an appropriate rehabilitation intervention.

In the child with ataxia, it can also be necessary to define which is the dominant hand for fine skill development and handwriting. This requires an accurate observation and specific assessment of the functional performance of both upper limbs and, if indicated, specific training (Auzias 1975).

9.4.3 Aims for the Functional Treatment of the Upper Limb in Children with Ataxia

- *Support for perceptual development (active tactile, visual, etc.) and intermodal integration*
- *Support for the acquisition of more advanced prehension and manipulation patterns (with a particular focus on bimanual hand use and in-hand manipulation) through the proposal of gradually more complex play and everyday activities, carried out first with the child seated "at the table" and then in different positions*
- *Continuous monitoring of compensatory strategies, spontaneously adopted by the child and, if necessary, proposals of more functional solutions (with a focus on positioning equipment selection in some activities such as writing and feeding)*
- *Play: toys selection, fixation systems use*
- *ADLs: teaching standard and adapted techniques; environmental and equipment adaptations, if needed (e.g., bathroom), ADL aids choice; caregiver training; IADL intervention in adolescents*
- *Handedness: study in detail of unestablished handedness problems, particularly for choosing hand for handwriting; related intervention, if necessary*
- *Handwriting: handwriting rehabilitation intervention, if needed and if it is predicted that the child should be able to develop a usable handwriting; training to computer writing*

9.5 Play Activities for Children with Cerebral Palsy: Some Suggestions

The games and toy proposals suggested here need to be selected and adapted to the child's interests, functional abilities, level of development, as well as the rehabilitation goals.

- **Reaching**
- Activities to improve adduction/abduction horizontal movements, elbow flexion/extension, and progressive hand opening control:
  - *Touch and hold, if possible, objects, toys, and materials to explore/activate them (e.g., put a hand in a water bowl and play with water, activate a battery-operated toy with one large switch and then with two switches)*
  - *Push objects (in relation to play developmental level) from one side of the work surface to the other and closer and further (e.g., push a toy dog near peers, push toy cars into the parking lot, or slide objects, classifying them by color or shape)*
  - *As above, but requiring the object to be introduced into a toy house (e.g., put a toy dog into a large and then smaller kennel)*
  - *As above, but requiring the child to do "multiple stops" with toys (e.g., the toy car runs on petrol and then goes to the car wash and then to the garage)*
  - *Paint with finger colors and then with sponges or easy-to-hold brushes, within larger (or smaller) spaces, gradually reaching areas where the use of the upper limbs becomes more difficult*
  - *Wash a doll, iron, brush, or dust (fixing/stabilizing objects on the table, if needed)*
  - *Play musical instruments with large buttons*
  - *....*
- **Prehension/Release**
  - *Grasp easy-to-hold items in two or more containers (e.g., arrange the goods in various baskets to prepare the shop game, etc.)*
  - *Build large ring towers; play with large and magnetic constructions with easy-grip items: animals, car, brand puzzles with large knobs, etc. (elements arranged on stable planks, if needed)*
  - *Play with a LEGO DUPLO[4] construction games, pegboards, etc.*
  - *....*
- **In-hand manipulation**
- Looking for translation, shift, and rotation patterns:
  - *Getting a coin out of a purse (e.g., in a shop pretending to pay)*
  - *Getting a coin in a box with holes in different positions*
  - *Crumpling paper*

---

[4]LEGO System A/S, Billund (DK), https://www.lego.com

- *Moving a magnetic piece—from palm to finger—to put it on a magnetic panel (e.g., two-dimensional magnetic game)*
- *Separating playing cards*
- *Putting on/removing or rotating little characters in/out a toy car*
- *Turning pages in a book*
- *Buttoning (e.g., playing with doll)*
- *Playing with the stickers*
- *Holding pen and pushing its top off with the same hand*
- *....*

- **Bilateral Hand Use**
- Aim: from less efficient hand use (in stabilizing function, with/without grasp) to bilateral simultaneous and differentiated hand use, even with smaller objects:
  - *Hold a paper with one hand while coloring/drawing on the paper with the other hand*
  - *Blocking a puzzle base*
  - *Uncap and cap markers for coloring; disassemble necklaces with large plastic pieces*
  - *Pouring water or sand in a large container, using two hands*
  - *Use play dough, squeeze, roll, and squish it with two hands*
  - *Play musical instruments that require two hands: cymbals, drums, xylophone*
  - *Pulling interlocking blocks apart or putting interlocking blocks together*
  - *Make necklaces with medium-sized pearls*
  - *Scissoring*
  - *Make origami*
  - *....*

References

Aarts PB, Jongerius PH, Geerdink YA et al (2010) Effectiveness of modified constraint-induced movement therapy in children with unilateral spastic cerebral palsy: a randomized controlled trial. Neurorehabil Neural Repair 24:509–518. https://doi.org/10.1177/1545968309359767

Ajuriaguerra J, De Auzias M, Denner A, Coumes F, Denner A, Lavondes Monod V, Perron R, Stamback M (1964) L'écriture de l'enfant. Delachaux et Niestlé Ed., Neuchâtel

Akhbari Ziegler S, Dirks T, Hadders-Algra M (2019) Coaching in early physical therapy intervention: the COPCA program as an example of translation of theory into practice. Disabil Rehabil 41(15):1846–1854. https://doi.org/10.1080/09638288.2018.1448468

Arnould C, Penta M, Thonnard JL (2008) Hand impairments and their relationship with manual ability in children with cerebral palsy. J Rehabil Med 2007(39):708–714. https://doi.org/10.2340/16501977-0111

Arnould C, Bleyenheuft Y, Thonnard JL (2014) Hand functioning in children with cerebral palsy. Front Neurol 5:48. https://doi.org/10.3389/fneur.2014.00048

Auld ML, Boyd RN, Moseley GL, Johnston LM (2011) Tactile assessment in children with cerebral palsy: a clinimetric review. Phys Occup Ther Pediatr 31:413–439. https://doi.org/10.3109/01942638.2011.572150

Auzias M (1975) Enfants gauchers, enfants droitiers. Delachaux et Niestlé Ed., Neuchatel

Ballester-Plané J, Laporta-Hoyos O, Macaya A, Narberhaus A, Segarra D, Pueyo R (2018) Cognitive functioning in dyskinetic cerebral palsy: its relation to motor function, communication and epilepsy. Eur J Pediatr Neurol 22:102–112. https://doi.org/10.1016/j.ejpn.2017.10.006

Bates E, Vicari S, Trauner D (1999) Neural mediation of language development: perspectives from lesion studies of infants and children. In: Tager-Flusberg H (ed) Neurodevelopmental disorders. MIT Press

Batorowicz B, Stadskleiv K, Renner G, Dahlgren Sandberg A, von Tetzchner S (2018) Assessment of aided language comprehension and use in children and adolescents with severe speech and motor impairments. Augment Altern Commun 34(1):54–67. https://doi.org/10.1080/0743461 8.2017.1420689

Beckung E, Hagberg G (2002) Neuroimpairments, activity limitations, and participation restrictions in children with cerebral palsy. Dev Med Child Neurol 44:309–316. https://doi.org/10.1017/S0012162201002134

Bertini E, Zanni G, Boltshauser E (2018) Non progressive congenital ataxias. Handb Clin Neurol 155:91–103. https://doi.org/10.1016/B978-0-444-64189-2.00006-8

Beukelman DR, Mirenda P (2013) Augmentative and Alternative Communication; supporting children and adults with Complex Communication Needs, 4th edn. Paul H. Brookes, Baltimore

Black P (1982) Visual disorders associated with cerebral palsy. Br J Ophthalmol 66:46–52. https://doi.org/10.1136/bjo.66.1.46

Blair E, Cans C, Sellier E (2018) Epidemiology of the cerebral palsies. In: Panteliadis CP (ed) Cerebral palsy, a multidisciplinary approach. Springer Int Publ, pp 19–28. https://doi.org/10.1007/978-3-319-67858-0

Blank R, Smits-Engelsman B, Polatajko H, Wilson P, European Academy for Childhood Disability (2012) European Academy for Childhood Disability (EACD): recommendations on the definition, diagnosis and intervention of developmental coordination disorder (long version). Dev Med Child Neurol 54(1):54–93. https://doi.org/10.1111/j.1469-8749.2011.04171.x

Bolanos AA, Bleck EE, Firestone P, Young L (1989) Comparison of stereognosis and two-point discrimination testing of the hands of children with cerebral palsy. Dev Med Child Neurol 31:371–376. https://doi.org/10.1111/j.1469-8749.1989.tb04006.x

Borgestig M, Sandqvist J, Parsons R, Falkmer T, Hemmingsson H (2015) Eye gaze performance for children with severe physical impairments using gaze-based assistive technology—a longitudinal study. Assist Technol 28(2):93–102. https://doi.org/10.3109/17518423.2015.1132281

Borgestig M, Sandqvist J, Ahlsten G, Falkmer T, Hemmingsson H (2016) Gaze-based assistive technology in daily activities in children with severe physical impairments—an intervention study. Dev Neurorehabil 20(3):129–141. https://doi.org/10.3109/17518423.2015.1132281

Bottcher L (2010) Children with spastic cerebral palsy, their cognitive functioning, and social participation: a review. Child Neuropsychol 16:209–222. https://doi.org/10.1080/09297040903559630

Bottos M, Bolcati C, Sciuto L, Ruggeri C, Feliciangeli A (2001) Powered wheelchairs and independence in young children with tetraplegia. Dev Med Child Neurol 43:769–777. https://doi.org/10.1111/j.1469-8749.2001.tb00159.x

Brown JK, Walsh EG (2001) Neurology of the upper limb. In: Neville B, Goodman R (eds) Congenital hemiplegia. Clinics in developmental medicine, No. 150. Mac Keith Press, London

Bumin G, Kavak ST (2010) An investigation of the factors affecting handwriting skill in children with hemiplegic cerebral palsy. Disabil Rehabil 32:692–703. https://doi.org/10.3109/09638288100365478

Burtner P, Poole J, Torres T, Medora AM, Abeyta R, Keene J, Qualls C (2008) Effect of wrist hand splints on grip, pinch, manual dexterity and muscle activation in children with spastic hemiplegia: a preliminary study. J Hand Ther 21:36–42. https://doi.org/10.1197/j.jht.2007.08.018

Case-Smith J, O'Brien JC (2019) Occupational therapy for children and adolescents, 7th edn. Elsevier Mosby, St. Louis

Charles J, Gordon AM (2006) Development of hand–arm bimanual intensive training (HABIT) for improving bimanual coordination in children with hemiplegic cerebral palsy. Dev Med Child Neurol 48:931–936. https://doi.org/10.1017/S0012162206002039

Cioni G, Sales B, Paolicelli PB et al (1999) MRI and clinical characteristics of children with hemiplegic cerebral palsy. Neuropediatrics 30:249–255. https://doi.org/10.1055/s-2007-973499

Cohen Levine S, Huttenlocher P, Banich MT, Duda E (1987) Factors affecting cognitive functioning of hemiplegic children. Dev Med Child Neurol 29:27–35. https://doi.org/10.1111/j.1469-8749.1987.tb02104.x

Coley IL, Procter S (1989) Self-maintenance activities. In: Pratt PN, Allen AS (eds) Occupational therapy for children, 2nd edn. Mosby, St Louis

Cooper J, Majnemer A, Rosenblatt B (1995) The determination of sensory deficits in children with hemiplegic cerebral palsy. J Child Neurol 22:289–293. https://doi.org/10.1177/088307389501000412

Costigan FA, Light J (2011) Functional seating for school-age children with cerebral palsy: an evidence-based tutorial. Lang Speech Hear Serv Sch 42(2):223–236. https://doi.org/10.1044/0161-1461(2010/10-0001)

Dormans JP, Pellegrino L (1998) Caring for children with cerebral palsy. A team approach. Paul Brookes Publishing Co.

Dufresne D, Dagenais L, Shevell MI, REPACQ Consortium (2014) Spectrum of visual disorders in a population-based cerebral palsy cohort. Pediatr Neurol 50(4):324–328. https://doi.org/10.1016/j.pediatrneurol.2013.11.022

Edwards SJ, Buckland DJ, McCoy-Powlen JD (2002) Developmental & functional hand grasping. Slack Inc., Thorofare

Ego A, Lidzba K, Brovedani P, Belmonti V, Gonzalez-Monge S, Boudia B, Ritz A, Cans C (2015) Visual–perceptual impairment in children with cerebral palsy: a systematic review. Dev Med Child Neurol 57:46–51. https://doi.org/10.1111/dmcn.12687

Eliasson AC, Gordon AM (2000) Impaired force coordination during object release in children with hemiplegic cerebral palsy. Dev Med Child Neurol 42:228–234. https://doi.org/10.1017/s0012162200000396

Eliasson AC, Gordon AM, Forssberg H (1991) Basic co-ordination of manipulative forces of children with cerebral palsy. Dev Med Child Neurol 33:661–670. https://doi.org/10.1111/j.1469-8749.1991.tb14943.x

Eliasson AC, Forssberg H, Hung YC, Gordon AM (2006) Development of hand function and precision grip control in individuals with cerebral palsy: a 13-year follow-up study. Pediatrics 118:1226–1236. https://doi.org/10.1542/peds.2005-2768

Erhardt RP (1995) Developmental Hand Dysfunction: theory, assessment, treatment, 2nd edn. Communication Skills Builders, Tucson

Esscher E, Flodmark O, Hagberg G, Hagberg B (1996) Non-progressive ataxia: origins, brain pathology and impairments in 78 Swedish children. Dev Med Child Neurol 38:285–296. https://doi.org/10.1111/j.1469-8749.1996.tb12095.x

Fazzi E, Signorini SG, Bova SM, La Piana R, Ondei P, Bertone C, Misefari W, Bianchi PE (2007) Spectrum of visual disorders in children with cerebral visual impairment. J Child Neurol 22:294–301. https://doi.org/10.1177/08830738070220030801

Fazzi E, Bova S, Giovenzana A, Signorini S, Uggetti C, Bianchi P (2009) Cognitive visual dysfunctions in preterm children with periventricular leukomalacia. Dev Med Child Neurol 51:974–981. https://doi.org/10.1111/j.1469-8749.2009.03272.x

Fazzi E, Signorini SG, La Piana R, Bertone C, Misefari W, Galli J, Bianchi PE (2012) Neuro-ophthalmological disorders in cerebral palsy: ophthalmological, oculomotor, and visual aspects. Dev Med Child Neurol 54:730–736. https://doi.org/10.1111/j.1469-8749.2012.04324.x

Fedrizzi E, Avanzini G, Crenna P (1994) Motor development in children. John Libbey & Co., London

Fedrizzi E, Pagliano E, Andreucci E, Oleari G (2003) Hand function in children with hemiplegic cerebral palsy: prospective follow-up and functional outcome in adolescence. Dev Med Child Neurol 45:85–91. https://doi.org/10.1111/j.1469-8749.2003.tb00910.x

Fedrizzi E, Rosa-Rizzotto M, Turconi AC, Pagliano E, Fazzi E, Pozza LV, Facchin P, GIPCI Study Group (2013) Unimanual and bimanual intensive training in children with hemiplegic cerebral palsy and persistence in time of hand function improvement: 6-month follow-up results of a multisite clinical trial. J Child Neurol 28(2):161–175. https://doi.org/10.1177/0883073812443004

Ferrari A, Sghedoni A, Alboresi S, Pedroni E, Lombardi F (2014) New definitions of 6 clinical signs of perceptual disorder in children with cerebral palsy: an observational study through reliability measures. Eur J Phys Rehabil Med 50:709–716

Finnie N (2009) Handling the young cerebral palsy child at home, 4th edn. Butterworth-Heinemann, Oxford

French C, Tapp Gonzales R, Trinson-Simpson J (1991) Caring for people with multiple disabilities. An interdisciplinary guide for caregivers. Therapy Skill Builders

Furusamu J (1997) Pediatric powered mobility: developmental perspectives, technical issues, clinical approaches. RESNA, Arlington

Ghasia F, Brunstrom J, Gordon M, Tychsen L (2008) Frequency and severity of visual sensory and motor deficits in children with cerebral palsy: Gross Motor Function Classification Scale. Invest Ophthalmol Vis Sci 49:572–580. https://doi.org/10.1167/iovs.07-0525

Gilmore R, Sakzewski L, Boyd R (2010) Upper limb activity measures for 5- to 16-year-old children with congenital hemiplegia: a systematic review. Dev Med Child Neurol 52:14–22. https://doi.org/10.1111/j.1469-8749.2009.03369.x

Goodman R, Yude C (2001) Emotional, behavioural and social consequence. In: Neville B, Goodman R (eds) Congenital hemiplegia. Clinics in developmental medicine No. 150. Mac Keith Press, London

Goossens' C, Crain S (1992) Utilizing switch interfaces with children who are severely physically challenged. Pro-Ed Inc.

Gordon N (1992) Independence for the physically disabled. Child Care Health Dev 18:97–105. https://doi.org/10.1111/j.1365-2214.1992.tb00344.x

Gordon AM (2011) To constrain or not to constrain, and other stories of intensive upper extremity training for children with unilateral cerebral palsy. Dev Med Child Neurol 53:56–61. https://doi.org/10.1111/j.1469-8749.2011.04066.x

Gordon AM, Duff SV (1999) Relation between clinical measures and fine manipulative control in children with hemiplegic cerebral palsy. Dev Med Child Neurol 41:586–591. https://doi.org/10.1017/s0012162299001231

Gordon AM, Charles J, Duff SV (1999) Fingertip forces during object manipulation in children with hemiplegic cerebral palsy. II: bilateral coordination. Dev Med Child Neurol 41:176–185. https://doi.org/10.1017/s0012162299000365

Gordon AM, Lewis SR, Eliasson AC, Duff SV (2003) Object release under varying task constraints in children with hemiplegic cerebral palsy. Dev Med Child Neurol 45(4):240–248. https://doi.org/10.1017/s0012162203000471

Hagberg B, Hagberg G, Olow I (1993) The changing panorama of cerebral palsy in Sweden. VI. Prevalence and origin during the birth year period 1983–1986. Acta Paediatr 82(4):387–393. https://doi.org/10.1111/j.1651-2227.1993.tb12704.x

Hammel J (1996) What's the outcome? Multiple variables complicate the measurement of assistive technology outcomes. Rehabil Manag 2(3):97–99. https://doi.org/10.1055/s-2007-970586

Hanna S, Law M, Rosenbaum P et al (2003) Development of hand function among children with cerebral palsy: growth curve analysis for ages 16 to 70 months. Dev Med Child Neurol 45:448–455. https://doi.org/10.1017/S0012162203000847

Henderson A, Pehoski C (2005) Hand function in the child: foundations for remediation. Elsevier Health Sciences. https://doi.org/10.1016/B978-0-323-03186-8.X5001-1

Henderson S, Skelton H, Rosenbaum P (2008) Assistive devices for children with functional impairments: impact on child and caregiver function. Dev Med Child Neurol 50:89–98. https://doi.org/10.1111/j.1469-8749.2007.02021.x

Himmelmann K, McManus V, Hagberg G, Uvebrant P et al (2009) Dyskinetic cerebral palsy in Europe. Arch Dis Child 94:921–926. https://doi.org/10.1136/adc.2008.144014

Himmelmann K, Lindk K, Hidecker MJC (2013) Communication ability in cerebral palsy: a study from the CP register of western Sweden. Eur J Paediatr Neurol 17:568–574. https://doi.org/10.1016/j.ejpn.2013.04.005

Hoare B, Ditchfield M, Thorley M, Wallen M et al (2018) Cognition and bimanual performance in children with unilateral cerebral palsy: protocol for a multicentre, cross-sectional study. BMC Neurol 18:63. https://doi.org/10.1186/s12883-018-1070-z

Holmefur M, Krumlinde-Sundholm L, Bergström J, Eliasson AC (2009) Longitudinal development of hand function in children with unilateral cerebral palsy. Dev Med Child Neurol 2010(52):352–357. https://doi.org/10.1111/j.1469-8749.2009.03364.x

Jan JE, Lyons CL, Heaven R, Matsuba C (2001) Visual impairment due to a dyskinetic eye movement disorder in children with dyskinetic cerebral palsy. Dev Med Child Neurol 43:108–112. https://doi.org/10.1017/S0012162201000184

Ju YH, Hwang IS, Cherng RJ (2012) Postural adjustment of children with spastic diplegic cerebral palsy during seated hand reaching in different directions. Arch Phys Med Rehabil 93:471–479. https://doi.org/10.1016/j.apmr.2011.10.004

Kavak ST, Bumin G (2009) The effects of pencil grip posture and different desk designs on handwriting performance in children with hemiplegic cerebral palsy. J Pediatr (Rio J) 85:346–352. https://doi.org/10.2223/JPED.1914

Kim HY (2016) An investigation of the factors affecting handwriting articulation of school aged children with cerebral palsy based on the international classification of functioning, disability and health. J Phys Ther Sci 28:347–350. https://doi.org/10.1589/jpts.28.347

Kim KS, Park HK, Park ES (2020) Contra-lateral unintended upper arm movement during unimanual tasks in children with cerebral palsy. Yonsei Med J 6:235–242. https://doi.org/10.3349/ymj.2020.61.3.235

Kinnucan E, Van Heest A, Tomhave W (2010) Correlation of motor function and stereognosis impairment in upper limb cerebral palsy. J Hand Surg Am 35:1317–1322. https://doi.org/10.1016/j.jhsa.2010.04.019

Klein DM (1982) Pre-writing skills. Communication Skill Builder, Tucson

Klein DM (1983) Pre-dressing skill. Communication Skill Builder, Tucson

Klingels K, Jaspers E, Van de Winckel A, De Cock P, Molenaers G, Feys H (2010) A systematic review of arm activity measures for children with hemiplegic cerebral palsy. Clin Rehabil 24:887–900. https://doi.org/10.1177/0269215510367994

Korpela R, Seppänen RV, Koivikko M (1992) Technical aids for daily activities: a regional survey of 204 disabled children. Dev Med Child Neurol 34:985–998. https://doi.org/10.1111/j.1469-8749.1992.tb11404.x

Koupernik C, Dailly R (1968) Le développement neuro-psychique du nourisson. Press Universitare de France

Kozeis N, Jain S (2018) Visual impairment. In: Panteliadis CP (ed) Cerebral palsy: a multidisciplinary approach. Springer ed.

Krumlinde-Sunddholm L, Eliasson AC (2002) Comparing test of tactile sensitivity: aspects relevant to testing children with spastic hemiplegia. Dev Med Child Neurol 44:604–612. https://doi.org/10.1017/s001216220100264x

Kuhtz-Buschbeck JP, Sundholm LK, Eliasson AC, Forssberg H (2000) Quantitative assessment of mirror movements in children and adolescents with cerebral palsy. Dev Med Child Neurol 42:728–736. https://doi.org/10.1017/s0012162200001353

Kyllerman M, Bager B, Bensch J, Bille B, Olow I, Voss H (1982) Dyskinetic cerebral palsy: clinical categories, associated neurological abnormalities and incidences. Acta Prediatr Scand 71:543–550. https://doi.org/10.1111/j.1651-2227.1982.tb09472.x

Laporta-Hoyos O, Ballester-Plané J, Leiva D, Ribas T, Miralbell J et al (2019) Executive function and general intellectual functioning in dyskinetic cerebral palsy: comparison with spastic cerebral palsy and typically developing controls. Eur J Paediatr Neurol 2019:546–559. https://doi.org/10.1016/j.ejpn.2019.05.010

Lemmens RJ, Timmermans AA, Janssen-Potten YJ, Smeets RJ, Seelen HA (2012) Valid and reliable instruments for arm-hand assessment at ICF activity level in persons with hemiplegia: a systematic review. BMC Neurol 12:21. https://doi.org/10.1186/1471-2377-12-21

Lesny I, Stehlik A, Tomásek J, Tománková A, Havlicek I (1993) Sensory disorders in cerebral palsy: two-point discrimination. Dev Med Child Neurol 35:402–405. https://doi.org/10.1111/j.1469-8749.1993.tb11661.x

Mark Carter B (1983) Reflex development and the prehensile deficit in cerebral palsy. Aust Occup Ther J 1982(30):3–13. https://doi.org/10.1111/j.1440-1630.1983.tb01412.x

Millar S, Aitken S (2003) Personal communication passports. Guidelines for good practice. Call Centre, Edinburgh

Missiuna C, Pollock N (2000) Perceived efficacy and goal setting in young children. Can J Occup Ther 67:101–109. https://doi.org/10.1177/000841740006700303

Monbaliu E, De Cock P, Ortibus E, Heyrman L, Klingels K, Feys H (2016) Clinical patterns of dystonia and choreoathetosis in participants with dyskinetic cerebral palsy. Dev Med Child Neurol 58:138–144. https://doi.org/10.1111/dmcn.12846

Monbaliu E, De Cock P, Mailleux L, Dan B, Feys H (2017a) The relationship of dystonia and choreoathetosis with activity, participation and quality of life in children and youth with dyskinetic cerebral palsy. Eur J Paediatr Neurol 21:327–335. https://doi.org/10.1016/j.ejpn.2016.09.003

Monbaliu E, Himmelmann K, Lin JP, Ortibus E, Bonouvrié L, Feys H, Vermeulen RJ, Dan B (2017b) Clinical presentation and management of dyskinetic cerebral palsy. Lancet Neurol 16:741–749. https://doi.org/10.1016/S1474-4422(17)30252-1

Morris SE, Klein MD (1987) Pre-feeding skills, 1st edn. Therapy Skills Builders

Morris C, Bowers R, Ross K, Stevens P, Phillips D (2011) Orthotic management of cerebral palsy: recommendations from a consensus conference. NeuroRehabilitation 28:37–46. https://doi.org/10.3233/NRE-2011-0630

Myhr U, von Wendt L, Norlin S et al (1995) Five-year follow-up functional sitting position in children with cerebral palsy. Dev Med Child Neurol 37:587–596. https://doi.org/10.1111/j.1469-8749.1995.tb12047.x

Niemann GA (2001) New MRI-based classification. In: Neville B, Goodman R (eds) Congenital hemiplegia. Clinics in developmental medicine No. 150. Mac Keith Press, London

Noronha J, Anita Bundy A, Groll J (1989) The effect of positioning on the hand function of boys with cerebral palsy. Am J Occup Ther 43:501–512. https://doi.org/10.5014/ajot.43.8.507

Novak I, Cusick A, Lannin N (2009) Occupational therapy home programs for cerebral palsy: double-blind, randomized, controlled trial. Pediatrics 124(4):e606–e614. https://doi.org/10.1542/peds.2009-0288

Nuara A, Papangelo P, Avanzini P, Fabbri-Destro M (2019) Body representation in children with unilateral cerebral palsy. Front Psychol 10:354. https://doi.org/10.3389/fpsyg.2019.00354

Odding E, Roebroeck ME, Stam HJ (2006) The epidemiology of cerebral palsy: incidence, impairments and risk factors. Disabil Rehabil 28:183–191. https://doi.org/10.1080/09638280500158422

Østensjø S, Carlberg EB, Vøllestad NK (2003) Everyday functioning in young children with cerebral palsy: functional skills, caregiver assistance and modifications of the environment. Dev Med Child Neurol 45:603–612. https://doi.org/10.1017/S0012162203001105

Østensjø S, Eva Brogren E, Carlberg EB, Vøllestad NK (2009) The use and impact of assistive devices and other environmental modifications on everyday activities and care in young children with cerebral palsy. Disabil Rehabil 27:849–861. https://doi.org/10.1080/09638280400018619

Pagliano E, Andreucci E, Bono R, Semorile C, Brollo L, Fedrizzi E (2001) Evolution of upper limb function in children with congenital hemiplegia. Neurol Sci 22:371–375. https://doi.org/10.1007/s100720100067

Philip SS, Guzzetta A, Chorna O, Gole G, Boyd RN (2020) Relationship between brain structure and Cerebral Visual Impairment in children with Cerebral Palsy: a systematic review. Res Dev Disabil 99:103580. https://doi.org/10.1016/j.ridd.2020.103580

Pirila S, van der Meere J, Seppanen RL, Korpela R, Nieminen P (2018) A pilot study on children with limitations in self-care, mobility, and social functions: effects on family strengths. Fam Soc J Contemp Soc Serv 87:269–276. https://doi.org/10.1606/1044-3894.3520

Pratt PN, Allen AS (1989) Occupational Therapy for children, 2nd edn. C.V. Mosby Co.

Rosa-Rizzotto M, Visonà Dalla Pozza L, Corlatti A, Luparia A, Marchi A, Molteni F, Facchin P, Pagliano E, Fedrizzi E, GIPCI Study Group (2014) A new scale for the assessment of performance and capacity of hand function in children with hemiplegic cerebral palsy: reliability and validity studies. Eur J Phys Rehabil Med 50:543–556

Rosenbaum P, Stewart D (2004) The World Health Organization International Classification of Functioning, Disability, and Health: a model to guide clinical thinking, practice and research in the field of cerebral palsy. Semin Pediatr Neurol 11:5–10. https://doi.org/10.1016/j.spen.2004.01.002

Ryan SE (2012) An overview of systematic reviews of adaptive seating interventions for children with cerebral palsy: where do we go from here? Disabil Rehabil Assist Technol 7:104–111. https://doi.org/10.3109/17483107.2011.595044

Sadao KC, Robinson NB (2010) Assistive technology for young children. Paul Brookes Publishing Co.

Sahinoğlu D, Coskun G, Bek N (2017) Effects of different seating equipment on postural control and upper extremity function in children with cerebral palsy. Prosthetics Orthot Int 41(1):85–94. https://doi.org/10.1177/0309364616637490

Salam OA, Esmael A, El-Sherif M (2016) Epilepsy among cerebral palsy children: clinical predictors and frequency. Int Neuropsychiatr Dis J 1–8. https://doi.org/10.9734/INDJ/2016/22785

Sanger TD, Kukke SN (2007) Abnormalities of tactile sensory function in children with dystonic and diplegic cerebral palsy. J Child Neurol 22:289–293. https://doi.org/10.1177/0883073807300530

Sanger TD, Chen D, Fehlings DL et al (2010) Definition and classification of hyperkinetic movements in childhood. Mov Disord 25:1538–1549. https://doi.org/10.1002/mds.23088

Scrutton D (2001) Physical assessment and aims of treatment. In: Neville B, Goodman R (eds) Congenital hemiplegia. Clinics in developmental medicine No. 150. Mac Keith Press, London

Shepard J (2019) Self-care and adaptations for independent living. In: O'Brien J, Kuhaneck (eds) Case-Smith: occupational therapy for children and adolescents, 8th edn. Elsevier Mosby, St. Louis

Shevell MI, Dagenais L, Hall N (2009) Comorbidities in Cerebral palsy and their relationship to neurologic subtype and GMFCS level. Neurology 72:2090–2096. https://doi.org/10.1212/WNL.0b013e3181aa537b

Sigurdardottir S, Eiriksdottir A, Gunnarsdottir E, Meintema M, Arnadottir U, Torstein V (2008) Cognitive profile in young Icelandic children with cerebral palsy. Dev Med Child Neurol 50:357–362. https://doi.org/10.1111/j.1469-8749.2008.02046.x

Skold A, Josephsson S, Eliasson AC (2004) Performing bimanual activities: the experiences of young persons with hemiplegic cerebral palsy. Am J Occup Ther 58:416–425. https://doi.org/10.5014/ajot.58.4.416

Spitzer SL (2019) Observational assessment and activity analysis. In: O'Brien J, Kuhaneck: Case-Smith: occupational therapy for children and adolescents. 8th ed. Elsevier Mosby, St. Louis

Stadskleiv K, Jahnsen R, Andersen GL, von Tetzchner S (2018) Neuropsychological profiles of children with cerebral palsy. Dev Neurorehabil 21:108–120. https://doi.org/10.1080/1751842 3.2017.1282054

Stavness C (2006) The effect of positioning for children with cerebral palsy on upper-extremity function. A review of evidence. J Phys Occup Ther Pediatr 26:39–53. https://doi.org/10.1080/J006v26n03_04

Steinlin M, Zangger B, Boltshauser E (1998) Non-progressive congenital ataxia with or without cerebellar hypoplasia: a review of 34 subjects. Dev Med Child Neurol 40:148–154. https://doi.org/10.1111/j.1469-8749.1998.tb15438.x

Sugden DA, Utley A (1995) Vocabulary of grips in children with hemiplegic cerebral palsy. Physiother Theory Pract 11:67–79. https://doi.org/10.3109/09593989509022403

Taub E, Ramey SL, DeLuca S, Echols K (2004) Efficacy of constraint-induced movement therapy for children with cerebral palsy with asymmetric motor impairment. Pediatrics 113:305–312. https://doi.org/10.1542/peds.113.2.305

Taub E, Uswatte G, Mark VW, Morris DM (2006) The learned nonuse phenomenon: implications for rehabilitation. Eur Medicophys 42:241–256

Twitchell TE (1958) The grasping deficit in spastic hemiparesis. Neurology 8:13–21. https://doi.org/10.1212/wnl.8.1.13

Twitchell TE (1965) Variations and abnormalities of motor development. Phys Ther 45:424–430. https://doi.org/10.1093/ptj/45.5.424

Tyler NB (1972) A stereognostic test for screening tactile sensation. Am J Occup Ther 26(5):256–260

Uvebrant P (1988) Hemiplegic cerebral palsy: etiology and outcome. Acta Paediatr Scand 345:1–100. https://doi.org/10.1111/j.1651-2227.1988.tb14939.x

Van Heest AE, House J, Putnam M (1993) Sensibility deficiencies in the hands of children with spastic hemiplegia. J Hand Surg Am 18:278–281. https://doi.org/10.1016/0363-5023(93)90361-6

Vargha-Khadem F, Isaacs E, Muter V (1994) Review of cognitive outcome after unilateral lesions sustained during childhood. J Child Neurol 9:2867–2873. https://doi.org/10.1177/088307389400900210I

Ward D (1983) Positioning the handicapped child for functions. Phoenix, St. Louis

Wilton J (2003) Casting, splinting, and physical and occupational therapy of hand deformity and dysfunction in cerebral palsy. Hand Clin 19:573–584. https://doi.org/10.1016/s0749-0712(03)00044-1

WHO (World Health Organization) (2007) The International Classification of Functioning, Disability and Health; children and youth version (ICF CY). World Health Organization, Geneva

Yekutiel M, Jariwala M, Stretch P (1994) Sensory deficits in the hands of children with cerebral palsy: a new look at assessment and prevalence. Dev Med Child Neurol 36:619–624. https://doi.org/10.1111/j.1469-8749.1994.tb11899.x

Yin Foo R, Guppy M, Johnston LM (2013) Intelligence assessments for children with cerebral palsy: a systematic review. Dev Med Child Neurol 55:911–918. https://doi.org/10.1111/dmcn.12157

Yorkston KM, Beukelman DR, Strand EA (2010) Management of motor speech disorders in children and adult, 3rd edn. Pro-Ed.

Feeding and Dysphagia in Children with Cerebral Palsy

10

Monica Panella

Every child is unique, as are those affected with cerebral palsy (CP), where each youngster is different from any other presenting with the same pathology. The same principle applies to their oro-motor function, which will be one of a kind in all its characteristics. Some children will have difficulty producing sounds, and others will have problems with drooling, managing solid food, and/or controlling liquids. However, appropriate, careful and early intervention based on, personalized, and specific rehabilitation plan improves oral function and the mouth's ability to be a receptor of the sensory inputs, including flavors, aromas, and colors, keeping in mind that meals and food should be a source of joy and pleasure.

When dedicating attention to the function of the oral cavity in these children, it is important to keep in mind that the persistent disorders of posture and movement that characterize CP are accompanied by sensory, perceptual, cognitive, communication, and/or behavioral disturbances. These need to be considered in oro-motor rehabilitation.

Breathing, sucking, and swallowing are activities which involve the mouth, and, from birth onward, all three actions are essential for survival, ensuring the necessary supply of nutrition and the passage of air in support of nasal respiration.

From the first months after birth, the infant perceives, explores, and satisfies their primary nutritional needs by sucking, chewing, and coordinating their respiration with their alimentation.

Infants with feeding disorders benefit greatly from very early therapeutic intervention. Nowadays, in the neonatal intensive care unit (NICU), even before a precise diagnosis, it is a common clinical practice that rehabilitation therapists support the nursing staff and parents in the care of babies presenting with pathological feeding problems. This specialized intervention is particularly indicated for infants with CP, and it needs to continue after dismission, in each stage of development.

M. Panella (✉)
Rehabilitation Department, Degli Infermi Hospital, Ponderano (Biella), Italy
e-mail: monica.panella@aslbi.piemonte.it

© The Author(s), under exclusive license to Springer Nature Switzerland AG 2022   371
P. Giannoni, L. Zerbino (eds.), *Cerebral Palsy*,
https://doi.org/10.1007/978-3-030-85619-9_10

10.1   The Oral Cavity Functioning of the Child

Physiological Swallowing

Swallowing is primarily an alimentary ability, in which a system of forces allows the passage of a bolus from the outside (oral cavity) to the inside (stomach) of the organism through the coordinated contraction of muscles of the mouth, tongue, pharynx, larynx, and esophagus.

Deglutition, a complex and dynamic function, is a highly integrated neuro-muscular act regulated by a bulbar center. This function is synchronous with breathing, and controlled by cortical and subcortical centers and by the sensitivity that comes from the effectors. It is neurophysiologically related to respiration and phonation. *"Neuromuscular coordination must engage the central nervous system, afferent sensory input, motor responses of voluntary and involuntary muscles, the brain stem, and the enteric nervous system. Hormonal factors also play a critical, although poorly understood role"* (Arvedson et al. 2020).

It has various functions according to age, starting from neonatal nutritive sucking to stages of middle and late adulthood.

Phase 0: Extraoral preparation of the substances. This occurs through cooking, crushing, preservation, and the association between different substances. Foods that otherwise would not be edible are prepared for consummation, taking into consideration different ages and preferences and particular circumstances, including illness or disability. It involves attention for taste, sight, smell, temperature, and consistency.

Phase 1: Preparation of the bolus. This is the moment in which the bolus enters the mouth and is explored and prepared to be swallowed. It is the phase of cleansing with possible buccal expulsion of food. The infant up to 4–6 months of age takes liquid food, from the breast or bottle, through sucking; the infant's lips adhere to the areola; and the tongue, the gums, and the jaw rest under the nipple, and, using the upper gums, they begin the activity of squeezing the milk. The baby's intake of liquids is not complex because the consistency of the food allows it to slide quickly and smoothly into the oral cavity. A period of gradual weaning follows, during which foods evolve in consistency, and in the way they are introduced into the oral cavity. The biting and chewing functions appear later.

Phase 2: Oral stage. Food is channeled to the posterior oral cavity, functioning as a trigger for this to occur involuntarily. The oral phase coincides with the beginning of swallowing: the food is ready to be ingested, and the tongue implements a retropulsion and transports the bolus backward, toward the pharynx, where swallowing is triggered (involuntary act). In the infant, retropulsion occurs due to the opening and closing of the jaw, combined with an anteroposterior movement of the tongue.

Phase 3: Pharyngeal stage. This is a place for anatomical and functional crossing between the respiratory and swallowing route (crossroads area), where tongue thrust and sucking for negative pressure, created by the hypopharynx and pharyngeal contraction, allow the passage of the bolus. *"The pharyngeal phase begins with the elevation of the soft palate to close off the nasopharynx. Pharyngeal constrictors contract to propel the bolus through the pharynx. Simultaneously, the larynx is closed to protect the airway"* (Arvedson et al. 2020).

Phase 4: Esophageal phase. This is an automatic peristaltic wave that carries the bolus to the stomach. Compared to the smooth muscle, the skeletal muscle in the cervical esophagus propels the food more quickly into the thoracic esophagus. The primary wave goes from the upper to the lower esophageal sphincter in a single contraction. The secondary wave tends to start at the mid-esophagus and extends to the stomach. Regurgitation and reflux are frequently found during this stage in the presence of abnormal peristalsis.

Phase 5: Gastric stage. This includes the whole time in which the food passes through the lower esophageal sphincter and remains inside the stomach until it is emptied into the duodenum. Stomach functioning is influenced by myenteric neural and hormonal factors. Food volume, texture, consistency (solid or liquid) and specific food content all affect gastric emptying (Arvedson et al. 2020).

Reference Concepts

Feeding: It concerns the nature of foods, their quality and safety, the most convenient preparation methods, and how they are used.

Nutrition: The branch of science and the process of providing and obtaining the food necessary for the health and growth of the individual. It concerns the ways and measures in which the nutrients contained in food are used, the satisfaction of specific nutritional needs, and their consequent balance and imbalances.

Malnutrition: The state of functional and structural alteration, resulting from the discrepancy between the body's needs and its nutritional intake. In the child with similar clinical conditions to those of adults, nutritional needs are necessary for growth, and food intake influences the steady increase of body weight, the functional maturation of organs and systems, and the cognitive and psychomotor development. Furthermore, these needs are closely related to immunological alterations (Rempel 2015; Leal-Martínez et al. 2020).

Dysphagia: From the Greek words *"dis"* (problematic) and *"phagia"* (swallowing). This is the difficulty, or inability, to implement an autonomous and safe oral diet. It is related to the difficulty in swallowing food of any consistency (solid, liquid, gaseous, or mixed) and its passage from the mouth to the stomach.

The presence of aspiration, meaning the passage of foreign material into the airways, can influence the general, pulmonary, and oral health of the individual.

Children with CP often present both sensory and motor deficits in the functions of the mouth. International data estimates an incidence of oro-motor dysfunction in a range of 27–99%, of the children, depending on the study population and the measures adopted for assessing eating and drinking abilities (Parkes et al. 2010; Van Hulst 2019). The sensorial function is involved because of the innervation, both sensory and motor, of all the cranial nerves (with the exception of the XII) involved in swallowing from the perioral phase to the pharyngeal one. As a consequence, this causes not only dysphagia problems, i.e., episodes of mistaken pathway, implying possible risks for the respiratory tract, but also problems involving feeding and its correlated sensorial integration, through which the brain receives and organizes information coming from the sense organs.

Savoring food means perceiving its taste, seeing its colors, smelling its odors and aromas, recognizing through touch how it feels, and manipulating and handling it in the appropriate, socially accepted manner (it is sufficient to think of how cutlery is used), integrated into the individual mealtime setting. These considerations explain the importance of approaching the topic of "feeding" as a combination of functions that are inseparable from each other.

The therapeutic approach for the child with dysphagia should be holistic (Arvedson et al. 2020). In addition to evaluating the organs and functions, it needs to include the assessment of the levels of limitation in activity (individual execution of tasks and actions) and participation (involvement in everyday social situations) of the young person, according to the International Classification of Functioning and Disability (WHO 2007; Arvedson 2008; Grosso et al. 2011).

A rehabilitation project, shared between professionals, family members, and caregivers, allows to increase the child's developmental potential and guarantees the achievement of the highest possible level of functionality and autonomy (Setaro and Fedrizzi 2016). Early intervention for dysphagia integrates easily into the general therapy plan and will contribute to not only improving the maturation of the child's feeding competences but also preventing collateral medical complications.

10.2   Evaluation of the Child

It is well-known that a diagnosis is a static phase and that it is not a sufficient indicator of the rehabilitation needs of the individual, which, instead, are based on dynamic criteria deriving from the understanding of ongoing processes and, in the pediatric age group, the evaluation of the potential of development. For these reasons, it is essential to investigate how the impairments caused by the pathology impact on the child's functioning and then move on to outlining a targeted and personalized rehabilitation plan, which is continually updated and which remains attuned to the context of the child's activity and participation level (WHO 2007). Clinical reasoning considers the profile of the child as a whole, applying scientific evidence and a holistic, child-centered approach.

The assessment of the functions of swallowing is closely connected to the child's everyday environment. The professional observes and evaluates the ways the child organizes their oro-motor skills and their general postural and motor abilities. The speech and language therapist (SLT) identifies the main feeding problems and formulates the aims of treatment.

They propose the appropriate methods of feeding and the types and consistencies of food that the child can manage, all within the criteria of maximum safety, which guarantees adequate nutrition and hydration, together with good respiratory function. The presence of dysphagia is determined, and its nature and causes are established.

10.2.1 Collecting the Child's History

The SLT gathers the physiological and pathological anamnesis and all the information which makes up the child's past and present history. The specific SLT information includes the perinatal period, the stages of neuromotor development, and the history of feeding from breastfeeding and/or bottle-feeding to weaning as well as the first solid meals on to the current eating habits, which provides an understanding of the functional situation of the infant. A specific history of the previous feeding experiences, obtainable through interviews with the family and videotaped documentation, provides important indications on how to deal with the nutrition problems and plan the rehabilitation intervention.

The clinical evaluation (Grosso et al. 2011; Ramella and Panella 2011; Arvedson et al. 2020) includes a pre-feeding baseline check and functional and instrumental assessments.

To obtain the pre-feeding baseline, the following vital parameters are needed:

- Oxygen saturation (greater than 85%)
- Heart rate (80–220 beats/min)
- Respiratory rate (30–80 acts/min)
- Surveillance status
- Reactivity status (Neonatal Behavioral Observation, Brazelton and Nugent 2011)

Functional evaluation:

- Oral functions related to nutrition
- Bucco-facial neuromotor balance (observation of automatic responses and oral reflexes)
- Observation of respiratory components and characteristics during food-related and nonfood-related activities
- Observation and analysis of drooling

Instrumental evaluation:

- Cervical auscultation (Frakking et al. 2016)
- Fiber-optic endoscopic evaluation of swallowing (Sitton et al. 2011)
- Videofluoroscopy (Galván and Mendoza 2020)

(Sellers et al. 2014) developed the classification system Eating and Drinking Ability Classification System (EDACS) for use by parents and/or professionals, for evaluating the feeding abilities of the child with CP. More recently, the tested Mini-EDACS has been proposed for infants between 18 and 36 months (Sellers et al. 2019).

10.2.2 Evaluation Through Observation

The program for the management of swallowing difficulties needs to be an ongoing process in continual evolution. It changes and is updated as the child matures and moves from one stage of development to the next. The therapeutic plan is based on observation and evaluation through the following actions:

- Interviews with the parents to share information on the newborn period, the baby's behavior and the feeding problems and aims of intervention that have been identified (Molinaro et al. 2017)
- Research of the modalities and facilitations to improve the child's feeding abilities and to share with the parents and other caregivers
- Support to the activities of the infant and caregiver, according to the goals to be achieved
- Care of the interaction between the child, the family, and multidisciplinary team
- Support to the active participation of the child in their daily life activities

In dealing with dysphagia and feeding problems in children, the specialized SLT should involve all members of the rehabilitation team and the child's family, helping them to understand all the most important details of the SLT assessment and intervention, which will contribute to everyone intervening with safety.

When educating in the most appropriate ways to feed the child, the SLT needs to be very supportive of the caregivers. Indeed, they have not only the responsibility of nourishing the child with the adequate quantities and types of food and liquids, but often, in the case of CP and dysphagia, this task can be very difficult and exhausting, becoming a source of tension and anxiety, instead of calm and enjoyment. Helping the caregivers to be—and to feel—competent in feeding the child means transforming everyday meals into experiences that can promote enriching relationships, health, and development.

10.3 The Development of Feeding

Swallowing can be observed in the fetus starting from the 10th to the 11th week of gestational age (Arvedson et al. 2020). From the 18th week, sucking is observed more and more, in preparation of the nutritive sucking ability of the newborn (Schindler et al. 2011). The neurophysiological mechanism of swallowing consists in a precise succession of motor actions coordinated at timed intervals by the bulbar center. This distinct rhythmic activity takes place at three different levels:

- The cortical level (voluntary trigger: anterior end of Rolando's cleft).
- The level of the bulbar lateral reticulum (through specific stimulation, the muscular response should not be conditioned or controlled by reflexes).
- The adaptive level in which the features of food and liquid, such as consistency, temperature, and volume, stimulate different actions (e.g., tongue activity that triggers the swallowing action through the hypoglossal-trigeminal, without the intervention of the XII pair of the cephalic nerves) (Schindler et al. 2011).

Throughout the first year of life, the baby learns new feeding mechanisms and adapts to new foods. All this new knowledge and these new skills mature in attunement with general psychomotor development.

10.3.1 The Development of Feeding in Children with Neurological Impairments

10.3.1.1 Preterm Infant

In preterm babies with neurological impairment, feeding difficulties can include the inability to seal the lips properly and produce a propulsive force of the tongue, as well as physiological peristalsis. They can present with incoordination between sucking, swallowing, and breathing, weak and ineffective cough, and irritability. Nowadays, nutrition is included in personalized, family-centered developmental care through programs, such as the Neonatal Individualized Developmental Care and Assessment Program (NIDCAP) of Heidelise Als, which are applied in most NICUs. These programs involve the parents and the multiprofessional team (neonatologist, nurse, child neuropsychiatrist, physiotherapist, SLT, psychologist) who have both transdisciplinary and specialized roles in supporting the physiological development of the baby and managing neonatal functional impairments (Hilditch et al. 2019). The SLT has an important role in the nutrition program supporting the team, particularly the nurses and parents, in the management of feeding and the promotion of feeding skills (Ericson and Palmér 2019; Maastrup et al. 2021; Majoli et al. 2021a, b).

Practical Suggestions
- *Evaluate the baby in collaboration with the team and the group of specialists, using validated tools and scales [e.g., Latch, Audible Swallowing, Type of Nipple, Comfort, Hold (LATCH) (Jensen et al. 1994), Premature Infant Behavior Breastfeeding Scale (PIBBS) (Nyqvist et al. 1996), Supporting Oral Feeding in Fragile Infants (SOFFI) (Ross and Philbin 2011), Neonatal Oral Motor Assessment Scale (NOMAS) (da Costa and van der Schans 2008), Preterm Infant Oral Feeding Readiness Assessment Scale (PIOFRAS) (Fujinaga et al. 2013)].*
- *Favor the bonding process through holding and the experience of skin-to-skin kangaroo care, in accordance with the procedures of the NICU (Baley and Committee on Fetus and Newborn 2015).*
- *Support the breastfeeding program of the neonatologists and the nursing staff of the individual NICU.*

- *Propose and share with the nursing staff and parents specific nonnutritive sucking activities, e.g., preterm infant oral motor intervention (PIOMI)* (Lessen Knoll 2012; Ghomi et al. 2019).

Reference Concepts
Gavage feeding: Nutrients are provided through a nasal/orogastric tube, introduced via the nose or mouth until about 2.5 cm of the terminal end in the stomach.

Parenteral nutrition: Partial or total intravenous delivery of nutrition, used only in particular clinical conditions of the infant when enteral and oral feeding are not possible.

Enteral nutrition methods: Tube-feeding is used only when strictly indicated and necessary and when oral feeding is not possible. It is safe and advantageous from a nutritional and growth point of view. The baby passes to oral feeding as soon as possible to promote oro-buccal sensorimotor experiences, fundamental for the development of self-feeding and oral skills.

Family stress and aversion to oral nutrition (food aversion) can delay the maturation of oro-motor skills (e.g., verbal production) at different developmental phases. This can happen in the maturation process of some preterm infants.

10.3.1.2 Infants Up to 6 Months

Nutritive sucking, through both breastfeeding and bottle-feeding, is the physiological oro-motor action to acquire the nutrition required in the first months of life (McFadden et al. 2017; Joffe et al. 2019).

As is well-known, breastfeeding, an intimate action that takes time and practice, should always be encouraged because it has numerous benefits for the infant (including immunological protection in the first months of life) and for the mom, offering that unique and intimate interaction between the mother and the baby. From a sensorial point of view, breast milk is also enriched with the characteristics of individual maternal flavors lacking in formula milk. In complex situations, success with breastfeeding can be supported by specially trained nurses, midwives, pediatricians, SLT, and breastfeeding counselors.

Practical Suggestions to Support Breastfeeding
- *Promote the habit to create an intimate, pleasant, and peaceful setting.*
- *Invite the mother to choose a supported and comfortable position for herself and a suitable hold for the baby, which promotes relaxation and a regular breathing pattern in both. The array of breastfeeding holds include the cradle, the cross-cradle, the laid-back, the rugby ball, the side and inverted side-lying, the upright, etc.*
- *Share baby holding techniques with good head and body stabilization and appropriate handling to use when moving the baby in space and changing their positions.*

- *Encourage the baby to explore the breast and nipple area, facilitating them to grasp both the areola and the nipple within the mouth to suckle.*
- *Suggest manual guidance facilitations to the mother to facilitate the baby's latch to the breast, and more specific oro-motor facilitations as necessary.*

In some circumstances, breastfeeding may not be possible, either for maternal reasons or due to difficulties in the baby. Both situations will be a source of worry and disappointment for the mother, becoming another important stress factor to take into consideration.

Practical Suggestions for Bottle-Feeding
The SLT will work with and share their feeding support plan with the other professionals looking after the mother and the baby (neonatologist, pediatrician, nurse, and/or midwife):

- *Support the mother by promoting tactile experiences with her baby, for example, skin-to-skin kangaroo care, holding and positive touch modalities, and, when possible, infant massage* (McClure 2017).
- *Contribute to the choice of a teat (see characteristics below), and make sure that the bottle is suitable in size and shape, according to the baby's mouth and their sensory features.*
- *Facilitate a forward and backward sucking motion of the teat, as well as placing the tip of the teat on the retro-incisive papilla or in the center of the tongue.*
- *Carefully observe the baby during feeding, and interrupt the sucking sequence in case of breathing-swallowing incoordination.*
- *Introduce manual oral sensorimotor facilitations as necessary.*

Characteristics of the Teat
The teat should be chosen with care to guarantee that the size, material, and number of holes are just right for each individual baby:

- A teat which is too large can prevent the lips from closing or cause a vomiting reflex.
- A teat which is too long can cause not only vomiting but also choking.
- A teat which is too soft can impede a good lip seal, and consequently sucking is not activated or is inefficient.

The number and size of the holes in the teat affect the speed of the flow of the liquid and need to be assessed individually for each baby, according to their ability to coordinate breathing and swallowing.

10.3.1.3 Child from the Age of 6–18 Months
This is the developmental stage when the infant without impairment is engaged in achieving new gross and fine motor abilities. There are important functional conquests at mealtimes too, which include finger feeding and the use of a spoon and a

beaker/cup/tumbler. There is also the capacity to manage different tastes and textures of foods, which pass gradually from only liquid (milk) to a multiplicity of more solid foods, initially blended and mashed to subsequently lumpy and chewable. The finger food phase is important as preparation of self-feeding skills with utensils.

In the small infant with a diagnosis of CP and presenting with dysphagia, sensorimotor development is compromised, along with the maturation of the self-feeding. This group of children usually includes the most severely motor impaired, and feeding and drinking remain caregiver dependent for some time, if not permanently. Because these children are at high risk of malnutrition and are often clinically underweight, their nutrition plan includes the usual weaning food plan even though it often remains with mashed foods for longer and sometimes is integrated with bottle-fed foods.

A self-feeding program in a child with dysphagia is often postponed until the infant is older and coping with more solid food. In the meantime, the other rehabilitation therapists are working on upper limb control, handgrip of an object, and eye-hand-mouth coordination in play activities, including pretend feeding of doll. Some can be introduced at mealtime, such as assisted holding of the cup during drinking and finger feeding with manual guidance of support at the elbow and/or the hand-to-mouth movement itself.

In the child with feeding difficulties, where assisted feeding is prolonged through the weaning months and beyond, the challenges for the SLT will be to facilitate the child and caregiver in the transition to spoon-feeding and drinking from a cup or beaker instead of a bottle. Using a spoon requires voluntary opening of the mouth as the spoon approaches, the lingual protrusion with flattening of the tongue on the floor of the mouth, and mandibular stability.

Practical Suggestions for Promoting Assisted Spoon-Feeding

- Choose a spoon with the suitable characteristics:
  - *Suitable material: Metal is a good heat conductor and is perceived at a temperature similar to the food; plastic will not give this perception.*
  - *Appropriate size: The spoon should not be larger than the child's mouth.*
- Use and share oral control facilitations as needed (see Sect. 10.5).
- Choose the best approach of the spoon to the mouth:
  - *Lateral approach technique: The placing of the spoon lengthwise from the side under the child's lower lip* (Fig. 10.1), *through a rocking movement carried out by the adult, facilitates the contact between the food in the spoon and the upper lip, creating stability of the central part of the lips and promoting the active emptying of the spoon* (Winstock 2019).
  - *Frontal approach technique: Here, the spoon is introduced directly from the front into the mouth* (Fig. 10.2), *which should actively manage the bolus. It is advised to not passively empty the contents of the spoon into the mouth through the upper gingival arch.*

Fig. 10.1 Proposing the spoon with a lateral approach

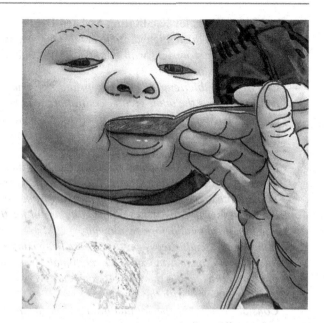

Fig. 10.2 Proposing the spoon with a frontal approach

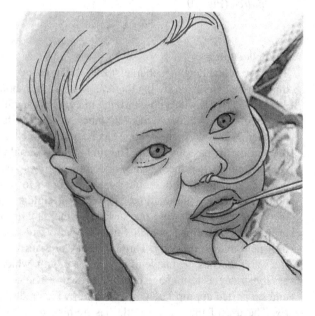

Using a tumbler requires effective lip sealing and anterior thrust protrusion of the tongue. This way of drinking should be proposed early in the weaning phase (gradually reducing and eliminating the use of sucking from a bottle) because it is a more mature, age-appropriate skill, which supports the acquisition of food feeding. The caregiver will need to be supported in this very positive developmental stage and in eliciting an active response of the child.

Practical Suggestions for Facilitating Assisted Drinking from a Tumbler/Cup

- *Position the child in an aligned, stable, and safe posture. The head and the trunk need to be straight upright with the head in the midline and the chin pointed toward the sternum (Fig. 10.3).*
  - *Choose a tumbler/cup of an appropriate size and material. A transparent material allows the adult greater control of the motor aspects; soft materials can facilitate biting to be deformed; obviously, a glass cup or tumbler must be made of very thick glass even though it is not recommended in the self-drinking learning phase to prevent accidents.*
  - *Place the edge of the tumbler resting between the child's lips to facilitate active lip sealing, adding manual facilitation if necessary.*
  - *To facilitate the learning process of drinking from a tumbler, the liquid can be thickened (syrup consistency), especially useful for the phase of holding the liquid in the mouth before swallowing.*
  - *If the head extends excessively, a recessed cup can be useful (Fig. 10.4a, b).*
  - *Integrate oro-motor and general relational, sensory, and postural facilitations into the feeding therapy sessions and everyday mealtimes, sharing the useful maneuvers with the caregivers.*
  - *Consider the use of special facilitating tools, as the Keller bottle, for certain children (Fig. 10.5).*

The Keller Bottle

The speech and language therapist Zita Keller proposed to use a plastic bottle that can be assembled by the therapist. This bottle should have a cap at least 3 cm in diameter, with a hole through its center. A small tube is inserted inside the hole (small-caliber irrigation tubes or suction tubes with a diameter between 12 and 16 French gauge can be used), which adhere completely to it, preventing the passage of air. The rubber straw should be resistant to occlusion by biting (therefore, the use of common straws available on the market is not recommended) and should be long enough to reach the bottom of the bottle. By placing the small tube between the child's lips and facilitating contact between the lips and the surface of the cap, an increase in lip tone is immediately obtained, which causes an active response of the lip control, indispensable for drinking. Through gentle pressure on the walls of the bottle, the water reaches the inside of the child's mouth, which can activate the necessary strategies to manage the right pressure. The head is always positioned and supported appropriately in extension, which reduces the risk of *ab ingestis*. The use of the Keller bottle has nothing to do with the suction action involved in the intake of liquids with a straw but uses the external pressure that is applied by the person holding the bottle.

Fig. 10.3 Postural
alignment with upright
head and trunk (Figure
adapted from Pre-Feeding
Skills (p. 139–139), by
Suzanne Even Morris,
Marsha Dunn Klein 1987,
Austin, TX:
PRO-ED. Copyright 1987
by PRO-ED, Inc. Adapted
with permission)

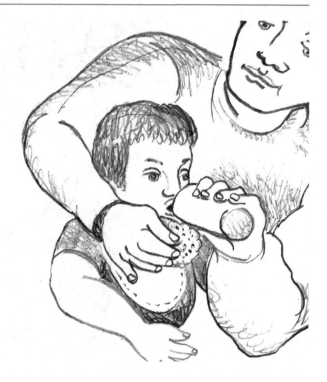

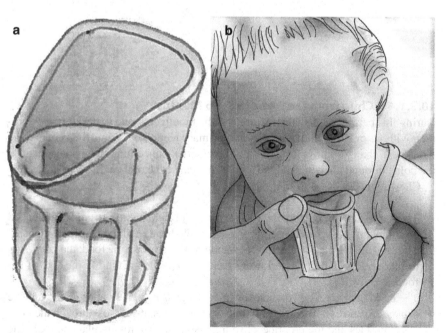

Fig. 10.4 (a, b) Recessed cup used to facilitate drinking

Fig. 10.5 The Keller
bottle

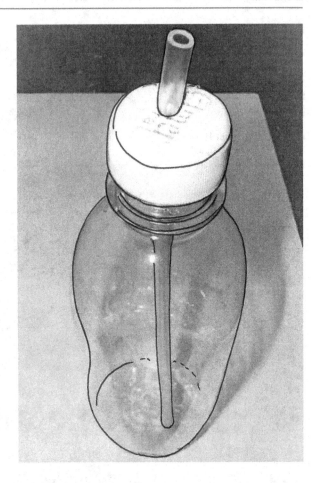

10.3.1.4   Child from the Age of 18–36 Months

During this period, the facial structure and the mouth continue to develop, and children without impairment have full set of primary teeth by the time they are 3 years old. These changes allow for new skills to emerge, concerning the management of the bolus through chewing and the ability to cleanse the oral cavity.

Chewing is divided into four phases:

1. The approach phase: How the food is brought to the mouth, strongly influenced by sociocultural habits involving the use of the hands and the choice of utensils.
2. The grasping phase: As the lips open and prepare to grasp the food, the jaw needs to increase its stability as it lowers and calibrates its opening to the size of the food in arrival.
3. The incision phase: Food particles are mixed together and are stabilized through the *orbicularis* muscle. The lowering of the jaw activates this muscle through the *masseter* muscles and the proprioceptive impulse to the neuromuscular spindles. The impulse is conducted through the section of the trigeminal nucleus, which regulates the order of the muscle contractions and the subsequent elevation of the jaw.

4. The shredding phase: Food comes into contact with the chewing surface of molars and premolars and is shredded through the active and coordinated actions of the tongue and the *buccinator* muscles and the opening and closing movements of the mandible. It finds its evolutionary roots in the bite reflex: a reflex present at birth up to about 4–6 months; it ends its reflex nature with the control of contact from the eroding teeth. Vertical mandibular movements precede lateral ones.

   Some children with CP do not manage to chew using both types of movement.

   As said before, the priority of feeding in all children, and especially infants, children, and adolescents with CP, is an adequate nutrition that guarantees first and foremost sufficient physical maturation (growth rate, body weight, and height). Therefore, all feeding decisions involving changes in food somministration (quality and quantity) must be decided by the child's neonatologist and/or pediatrician and the parents.

Practical Suggestions to Facilitate Chewing

 – *As before, position the child in an aligned, stable, and safe posture. The head and the trunk need to be straight upright with the head in the midline and the chin pointed toward the sternum.*
 – *Evaluate the child's functional capacity and food tolerance: assess when it is appropriate to offer the infant chewable food. When the first upper and lower incisors are organized in occlusal contacts, the proprioceptive information is transmitted to the central nervous system, allowing the coordination of chewing movements.*
 – *Gradually introduce new food proposals (without any force), consulting the caregiver and assessing the child's abilities and their likes and dislikes.*
 – *Try to propose new feeding activities through mealtime models shared with family members and other children. Promote learning through creating interest and curiosity to discover and imitate.*
 – *Propose assisted and independent finger feeding when appropriate* (Fig. 10.6).

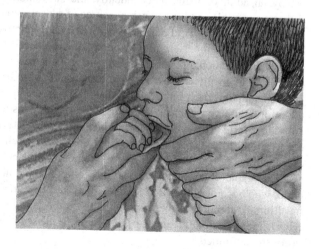

Fig. 10.6 Finger-feeding proposal

- Stimulate the twisting and curling movements of the tongue with touch and rubbing along its edge with food of different tastes and consistencies and play with
  small objects (e.g., using a toothbrush and watching the movements together in
  a mirror).
- Facilitate chewing by placing the food directly on the chewing surface.

10.3.1.5   Child from the Age of 3–6 Years

Rehabilitation therapy for dysphagia and feeding disorders in CP by a specialized
SLT needs to start very early with babies, still of a young age, preferably in the
NICU, and continue through infancy. The therapist intervenes as a member of the
rehabilitation team to treat and resolve the feeding difficulties of the young baby
through therapy sessions and counseling and support to family members and caregivers in the home environment. By the age of 3–4 years, the potential for basic
feeding skills in the CP child should have matured. At this point, the SLT's intervention usually continues for severe cases of CP and becomes focused on good nutrition, the maintenance of the acquired feeding skills, mealtime enjoyment and
independence as much as possible, and food safety.

Food safety and risk reduction are based on attention to different aspects:

1. The use of the most suitable and safest posture during food and drink
   consumption
2. Careful assessment of changes in the consistencies of food
3. The consideration of the suspension of oral feeding in preference for enteral
   feeding to guarantee a good nutritional intake
4. Measures to ensure protection of the child from aspiration of food

10.4   The Care of the Mealtime Environment

It is important to keep in mind that, during mealtimes for the child with CP who is
fed by an adult or feeds independently, the surrounding environment is full of
numerous variables and is a constant source of sensory information which, through
feedback and feedforward mechanisms, will create adaptive responses. The child's
brain receives the inputs coming from the environment and integrates taste, smell,
sight, hearing, touch, position, gravity, and movement, in an automatic physiological process that solicits these adaptive responses (Ayres 2005).

It is within this daily environment that the adult (therapist and caregiver) acquires
the information necessary to understand the facilitations that will be useful for the
individual child. This knowledge will be enriched by careful listening and constant
observation of the verbal and nonverbal messages the child communicates, whatever their age or stage of development (Ramella and Panella 2011).

A favorable environment creates the conditions for active participation of the
child, who becomes curious, attentive, interested, and an active protagonist in their
mealtimes. Attention to the environment is important when the newborn is in the
NICU, breastfeeding/feeding at home, and in all social settings where food and
drink are consumed.

10.4.1 Vestibular Information

The vestibular receptors give information regarding the position of the head in space, the movement in progress, and its speed and direction. In children with CP, who often present with delayed or permanently impaired head control, it is essential that caregivers pay particular attention to the position and stability of the child's head in space, in order to avoid any unwanted tonic reactions and postural compensations. Comfort needs to be considered as well, remembering also that unpredictable situations can easily upset these sensitive children, leading to a tense state of alert, associated with an increase in muscle tone.

10.4.2 Proprioceptive Information

The proprioceptive inputs are important because they facilitate the child to carry out functional and selective movements. They influence activities such as chewing, drinking, and swallowing. This information arrives from the tendons and joints and, above all, from the muscles, and therefore their state of tension, relaxation, and elongation. Excessive, poor, and fluctuating muscle tone influences the execution of the sequence of movements involved in feeding and drinking, making these functions difficult and, in some cases, even impossible and potentially dangerous.

Practical Suggestions for Mealtimes

- *Try to organize the mealtime environment around the child predicting the variables of what can happen, thus allowing them to find adaptive responses.*
- *Check the child's motor and postural state before feeding and improve as necessary.*
- *During mealtime, facilitate the motor initiative of the child and wait for their active response.*
- *Provide precise sensory inputs to the epithelial and intrabuccal areas to facilitate the child's self-awareness and improve oral functioning.*

10.4.3 Tactile Information

Touch is the first sense to develop in the fetus. During gestation, there is progressive development of tactile receptors around the face and mouth area, and the peculiarity of the highly sensitive facial and oral areas remains throughout life. When feeding, tactile inputs come from both the whole body and the specific perioral and endoral contact with the food and the utensils used (i.e., teat, fingers, spoon, fork, cup).

Practical Suggestions

- *Provide clear, "easy to perceive," and precise tactile stimuli.*
- *Pay attention to the supporting surfaces (postural systems, clothing, bibs, etc.).*
- *Choose adequate utensils to feed the child and/or to facilitate self-feeding (teats, spoons, forks, cups/tumblers).*

10.4.4 Visual Information

Visual inputs provide the child with a whole series of information about their surroundings. Through central and peripheral vision, they can recognize people, objects, and situations and understand distances, directions, and the types of movement necessary to reach the objects they desire (vertical, horizontal, diagonal, circular). For further information, see Chap. 14.

Practical Suggestions
- *Prepare the child for the approach of the utensil toward and into their mouth, anticipating with simple words what is about to happen; avoid that utensils appear unexpectedly.*
- *Propose food types separately so each can be appreciated and learned with their own taste and aroma; avoid foods mixed together, where they lose their specific characteristics, making the food become monotonous and uninteresting.*
- *Remember that the colors in the environment influence the mood and relaxation of the people sharing it (soft hues potentially induce calm; bold hues can trigger greater reactivity).*

Note
- Check for postural-kinetic difficulties, such as continual head movements, which do not allow eye fixation and the prediction of what is going on in the environment (e.g., the approaching of the fork with food to the mouth).

10.4.5 Auditory Information

During mealtimes, appropriate auditory facilitations can quickly attract the child's attention; anticipate what will happen, support concentration, and encourage them to actively participate in the actions involved. However, unorganized sound input from the environment has the risk of diverting the child's attention from the tasks of feeding.

Note
- Loud, sudden, intermittent sounds attract attention more quickly.
- Familiar and repetitive sounds tend to be ignored or can take on a reassuring connotation.
- Remember that distractions from the task reduce the opportunities for the child to learn from the experience and adapt to the actions involved.

10.4.6 Taste and Olfactory Information

Through specialized epithelial cells, the tongue provides information regarding the chemical composition of the food particles with which it comes into contact, whereas the nose provides information on the particles which are suspended in the air and produce odors and aromas. In situations of feeding difficulties and/or dysphagia, specific and facilitated gustatory and olfactory learning experiences are often postponed because the priority of the guided feeding intervention is first directed to satisfying the child's nutritional needs (Lipchock et al. 2011).

Practical Suggestions
- *Propose foods that are different in appearance, taste, and texture, respecting the timing of neurodevelopmental phases.*
- *Gradually propose all the various types of taste experiences: sweet, bitter, sour, and salty.*
- *Vary the liquid-semisolid-solid properties of foods, including the characteristics of viscosity and denseness.*
- *Propose various olfactory experiences.*

10.5 Positioning the Child with CP

Appropriate positioning is a basis for the success of all motor learning experiences. It involves the whole body and the posture modified continually to allow movements and activities to occur according to the functional goal of the performance.

Moving one part of the body makes it necessary to stabilize the others. A child with CP in an uncomfortable position will have difficulty carrying out functional tasks, whereas a safe and comfortable position facilitates the child in achieving their potential in the best way. This is also valid for the functions of feeding and drinking. "If you cannot sit/be sat, you cannot do" (Winstock 2019).

The posture of the adults caring for these children is equally important: an adult in discomfort or pain due to their posture is at risk not only of transmitting these feelings to the child, but the discomfort can also reduce their attention to the child's communication and to the goals to be achieved.

For example, while feeding of a child with dyskinesia, the unexpected, sudden, and disorderly movements on the part of the adult could compromise the positive effects of the postural assistance being offered by the caregiver.

Components of Appropriate Positioning for Feeding
The following postural care for feeding is recommended:

1. Alignment of the head, trunk, and upper and lower limbs on the midline
2. Proximal head and trunk stability, which allows for better oral control
3. Control of stiffness and containment of disturbing synergies
4. Close attention to comfort in all parts of the body, checking for any possible painful input or excessive pressure

5. In case of insufficient uprighting of the head and trunk, provision of the necessary support to the postural alignment that reduces the risk of possible gastroesophageal reflux
6. Protection from any risk of aspiration by appropriate positioning of the head, never in hyperextension
7. Positioning of the child and the caregiver in such a way that their eyes are at the same level (Winstock 2019)
8. Integration of adjustments and postural-motor facilitations that promote the active participation of the child and self-feeding as far as possible

10.5.1 Child Held in the Arms of the Caregiver

The adult's body often offers the best postural containment for the small infant with CP, because it naturally adapts to the baby's movements and needs of support. When they hold their baby, the parents themselves spontaneously provide that very special affective, physical, and sensory well-being. This excellence carries over into and facilitates breast- and bottle-feeding. In the case of feeding difficulties, holding the child in the adult's arms is often the best "postural container" during the initial weaning phase.

As already described, children with CP often show poor postures and/or excessive and uncontrollable synergies. The posture with extensor synergy, as often seen in bilateral spastic cerebral palsy (BSCP), includes, together with the rigid extension of the head, shoulder girdle and lower limbs, an open mouth, fisted hands, and an extended trunk with forced inspiration, sometimes in an arching backward opisthotonos position. During feeding this child can react with an exaggerated extension of the head, trunk, and all limbs (Fig. 10.7).

On the contrary, the child with prevalent flexor synergy has shoulders and arms flexed forward, semi-open hands, and a predominantly flexed head with poor mouth

Fig. 10.7 Child with extensor synergy

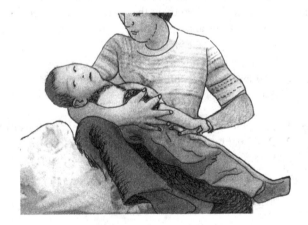

Fig. 10.8 Child with flexor synergy

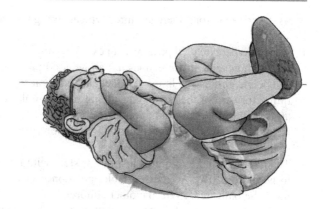

control. The more severe child usually has a poor motor initiative, which does not allow them to change their position or adapt to their surroundings. During feeding time this child should be able to maintain an upright posture of the head and trunk to facilitate swallowing (Fig. 10.8).

10.5.2 Child in Sitting

An optimal sitting position is fundamental for the stability of the head, trunk, and pelvic girdle and the consequent facilitation of the swallowing action, a function that is comprised even more in children with CP when they are in an inappropriate posture, whereas the same child, within a proper sitting system, is more stable and has better use of the upper limbs and so is available for new initiatives and active participation in their feeding activities, such as taking finger food and holding the spoon.

If the child has difficulty maintaining the upright position of the trunk due to hypotonia or incomplete trunk control, they need to be seated with the back of the chair tilted slightly backward. Care needs to take with this inclined positioning during mealtime to avoid the risk of the *ab ingestis* when the food at the back of the mouth falls by gravity and is inhaled into the lungs.

For feeding, the child needs to experience the advantages offered by an organized, upright, and stable position, without hyperextension, with their head and trunk well aligned in the midline. All these features facilitate an efficient and safe swallowing mechanism.

The most common position for mealtimes in small children with CP is sitting in a high chair. The choice of a high chair, commercially available or custom-built, should respond to the characteristics of providing good support, stability, and safety as described above. The base of the chair on the floor needs to be very wide to guarantee stability and that it cannot topple over, whereas the width, height, and depth measurements of the seating area need to correspond to the individual size of the child's body, adding reduction liners, cushions, and rolls as necessary. Most of the time, a normal or recessed table is placed in front of the chair.

As described before, there are three typical sitting postures in children with CP:

1. A rigid hyperextended posture with excessive tonic recruitment:
   The high general stiffness does not allow good postural control of the shoulder and pelvic girdles and limbs. An adequate postural adjustment requires a slightly tilting forward of the pelvis, uprighting of the trunk, feet on support, and forearms on the table providing good eye contact.
2. A "floppy," hypotonic posture with poor tonic recruitment, with poor core stability:
   The hypotonic child requires a sitting system with many supports to help them to be more active. A recessed table, positioned at the height of their armpits, might be indicated, as for the other children.
3. An instable, hypermobile posture with continual fluctuations of tone:
   The chair for positioning of this child with dyskinesia should offer comfort and stability and allow a reasonable amount of movement (avoiding containment that forces the child to stay still).

Note
- In some children it can be indicated to incline the back of the chair slightly backward.

10.6   Oro-motor Facilitation Maneuvers

10.6.1 Oro-motor Facilitation in Preterm Infant

The inability to efficiently suckle for nutritional purposes is often encountered in preterm newborns, due to their particular immaturity for what concerns head control and stabilization of the mandible, indispensable prerequisites for oral movements. The tongue can present fragmentary peristaltic movements, unfinalized lingual movements, contraction movements, muscle hypertonus of the base tongue, retraction of the tongue in the direction of the pharynx, and absence of cupping. Poor lip seal and incoordination of mandibular movements can also be found (Hwang et al. 2010).

Oro-motor facilitations are based on the principle that stability of a proximal part of the body improves the functional activity of a distal part (Bobath and Bobath 1975). Therefore, as necessary, the caregiver should stabilize the child's cheeks and jaw during feeding to facilitate fine and coordinated movements of the tongue (distal action) (Morris and Klein 1987).

10.6.1.1   Facilitations of the Nutritive Sucking in the Preterm and Term Baby
There are two useful maneuvers that improve the efficiency of nutritive sucking in babies who need assistance: the *mandibular support* technique and the *cheek support* technique. They can be used separately or simultaneously, as necessary.

- **Manual support to the mandible** during suckling improves the efficiency of nutritive sucking by reducing the effort involved in the movement of the jaw when the infant compresses the teat and by stabilizing and facilitating oro-motor control.

Practical Suggestion

– *During sucking, the caregiver places the tip of their little finger of the hand holding the bottle under the baby's chin and uses it to stabilize the jaw (Fig. 10.9)*

- **Manual support to the cheeks** facilitates the lip seal and improves sucking, particularly during the negative pressure phase of suction, from either the breast or the teat. The tactile stimulation also helps the baby maintain a quiet alert state.

Practical Suggestion

– *The caregiver uses the ring finger of the hand holding the bottle to slightly compress the baby's cheek while the thumb of their other hand supporting the baby's head compresses the opposite cheek* (Fig. 10.10).

Fig. 10.9 The mandibular support technique

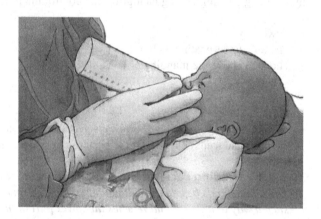

Fig. 10.10 The cheek support technique

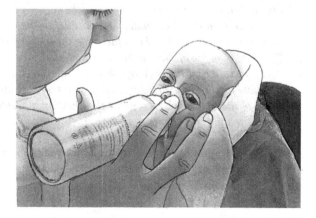

10.6.2 Oro-motor Facilitations in Children with CP

Difficulties in children with CP that can limit feeding and drinking skills include the problem of a continual open mouth and an ineffective lip seal, both due to insufficient tone recruitment. Then, there is the difficulty in regulating the movements of the mandible, which leads to an excessive opening of the mouth and limitation in tongue and lip control. In addition, there is the problem of aligning the posture of the head, neck, and trunk, so it is essential that the caregiver organizes good postural support (alignment and stability) at mealtimes because this will improve the movements of the lips and tongue.

The caregiver can provide direct oro-motor facilitations with two supporting maneuvers:

1. From the side position
2. From the front position

The choice of the maneuvers is based on the postural stability necessary for optimal feeding the child, using handgrips that control the following key points:

- Lower lip
- The area underneath the chin
- The area above the mandibular bone

Note
- As said above, for feeding it is always necessary to take care of the alignment of the head and trunk, elongating the posterior cervical region.

10.6.2.1 Feeding Facilitations with Maneuver from the Side

1. *The adult stands beside the child and places one arm behind the child's head in such a way that their hand reaches the lower part of the child's face.*
2. *Maintaining the appropriate position of the child's head (chin toward the sternum and elongation of cervical region), the caregiver positions their index finger transversely on the chin, under and parallel to the lower lip, so that the finger stabilizes the lower lip and can facilitate the opening of the mouth.*
3. *The middle finger of the caregiver is then placed crosswise under the jaw over the central area of the* mylohyoideus *muscle sheet, the floor of the oral cavity. This hold facilitates the closing of the mouth and the upward and forward movements of the mandible, as well as the chewing movements of the jaw independently from the splanchnocranium (Fig. 10.11).*

An expert is able to feel the forward and backward movements of the child's tongue with their fingers and facilitate those specific movements by exerting pressure on the area under the chin:

Fig. 10.11 Maneuver from the side

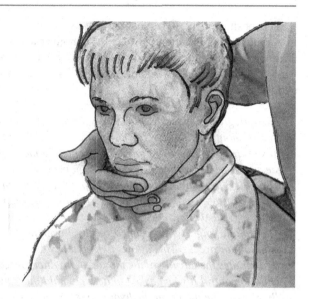

– *The tongue can be felt clearly by slightly flexing the middle finger within the space between the two mandibular arches.*
– *Pressure in the direction of front to back can facilitate the backward movements of the tongue, while the opposite pressure from the back of the mouth to the front facilitates its forward movement.*
– *Very careful intermittent pressure in the area of the hyoid bone can accompany and facilitate the swallowing action (taking extreme care not to stimulate the vomiting reflex!).*
– *As possible, involve the child directly by asking them to actively reduce and control the protrusion of the tongue.*
– *To reduce the stiffness of the cheek muscles and maintain the alignment of the mandible (preventing possible deviations), the thumb of the caregiver can be placed on the child's cheek, following approximately the direction of the* masseter *muscle fibers. This contact will also stabilize the facilitator's hand, but care must be taken not to exert pressure on the cheek because it could lead to biting. The hand should not be too close to the child's eyes, which can be annoying and a distraction. If the assistance offered by this thumb is not necessary, it can be kept away from the child's face, taking care not to block their vision.*

10.6.2.2   Feeding Facilitations with Maneuver from the Front

In this case, the caregiver is positioned in front of the child, which has the advantage of being a better observation point of the child's face and their oral cavity. However, this postural setting must not provoke hyperextension of the child's head, which would increase the risk of aspiration.

This frontal approach for manual feeding guidance is particularly indicated in children who have active and reliable head control or where their postural system provides sufficient head alignment and stability.

This position also offers pleasant face-to-face contact and facilitates the circular in-and-out communication between the caregiver and the child. Depending on the different contexts, the adult can sit on a stool with adjustable height or find other ways to facilitate good eye contact, which does not provoke hyperextension of the child's head.

1. *The caregiver's thumb is placed on the* mentalis *muscle, perpendicular to the lips, without touching the lower lip. It is used to help the child open their mouth, to stabilize the lower lip, and to facilitate the movement of the chin toward the sternum and elongation of cervical region.*
2. *The index finger of the same hand is placed on the child's cheek, along the jaw, mainly to stabilize the hand. Be careful not to exert pressure, so as not to evoke the bite* (Fig. 10.12).
3. *The middle finger is positioned on the lower part of the jaw between the two mandibular arches. This allows to feel and influence the stiffness of the muscles; it facilitates the closure of the mouth and reduces lingual protrusion, helping the child to control it when asked to actively hold the tongue well within the mouth. By placing the finger on the hyoid bone, the act of swallowing can be perceived and even evoked, but it is important to be careful not to stimulate a pharyngeal reflex* (Fig. 10.13).

Note
- It is important for the child to experience a trial run of these facilitation actions in neutral and calm situations, before actually using them during feeding and drinking, because they may not tolerate these manual grips throughout the meal. The caregiver needs to remain alert for any signs of discomfort in the child, which could force them not only to stop the maneuver but also to interrupt feeding.

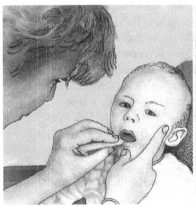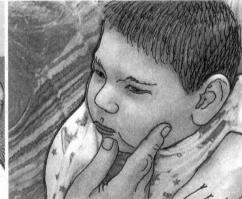

Figs. 10.12 and 10.13 Frontal maneuvers

• As always, these facilitations should be reduced as the child's feeding skills improve, remembering the concept that unnecessary help reduces learning and the development of functional independence.

10.7 Oral Hygiene

Adding to their other responsibilities, the parents of children with CP often need to oversee their youngsters' special diets, administer their medications, and, in all cases, carefully manage their oral hygiene. The latter can be a problem because these children often have difficulties opening their mouths and in keeping them open.

The oral health of children and young people is an integral part of general health and well-being. Good oral hygiene goes hand in hand with good nutrition and a diet that includes a balanced intake of nutritional cariogenic foods. Regular dental checkups are advised, and nowadays there are dentists specialized in managing children with CP.

Careful oral hygiene and regular cleansing of the mouth are aimed at the removal of plaque and the prevention of mouth infections. In children with CP, it keeps the mucous membranes intact and moist and can help normalize abnormal responses to buccal stimuli. In the case of posterior drooling at the back of the oral cavity, a clean mouth also contributes to the reduction of airway infections, because it decreases the bacterial load of the oral secretions (Dougherty 2009; Grzić et al. 2011; Maiya et al. 2015).

Practical Suggestions for Oral Hygiene
• Oral hygiene is an intimate activity to be carried out in a quiet and distraction-free environment:
  – *The child can be prepared for their oral hygiene procedure beforehand, through play situations of "cleaning the teeth" of a doll or teddy bear, showing the child the utensils and how they are used. The caregiver can give a practical demonstration of teeth cleaning on themselves as well.*
  – *The adult caregiver assisting oral hygiene should proceed slowly, remembering to ask for the child's permission and help them to be collaborative and participate actively.*
  – *Care should be given to posture: the child should be comfortable, aligned in the midline with the head slightly tilted toward the sternum.*
  – *It is important to use a soft-bristled or electric toothbrush. A commercial toothbrush can be used if the child has only a normal level of discomfort from the toothbrush. Otherwise, and in the case of children with severe impairment, it is suggested to use the adult's index finger with moistened gauze wrapped around it.*
  – *If using toothpaste, water, and a plaque detector mouthwash, they should not be ingested or, even worse, sucked.*
  – *Before introducing the utensils into the child's mouth, remind the youngster of what will happen, and help them follow the hygiene routine throughout the*

procedure; different sensory channels can be used as facilitations (touch, sight, smell, noise, etc.).

– *If the child shows any discomfort or gets tired during the procedure, respect their tolerance and fatigue, and give them some pauses and rest breaks.*
– *Begin by first introducing the smooth side of the head of the toothbrush into the child's mouth from the side. The bristle side first could cause a withdrawal reaction. So, the second step is then to gently rotate the toothbrush so that the bristles are in contact with the teeth and gums.*
– *Place the bristles perpendicular to the tooth, and then move the head of the toothbrush in the direction from gum to tooth. Clean the outside, inside, and top of the molars; use a steady and predictable rhythmic pattern.*
– *If the child cannot spit, do not use toothpaste or mouthwash but a solution of water and baking soda.*
– *Clean the inner surface of the cheeks and possibly the palate, particularly if the child has an ogival palate and consequently accumulates food.*
– *To facilitate rinsing, keep the child adequately positioned with the chin pointing to the sternum. Introduce a small amount of water into the mouth using a recessed tumbler or the Keller bottle. Then, quickly tilt the tumbler forward and downward to facilitate the liquid to come out by gravity with a manual guidance to the oral area.*
– *Dry the area around the mouth by dabbing, avoiding any annoying friction and rubbing.*

References

Arvedson J (2008) Assessment of pediatric dysphagia and feeding disorders: clinical and instrumental approaches. Dev Disabil Res Rev 14(2):118–127. https://doi.org/10.1002/ddrr.17

Arvedson JA, Brodsky L, Lefton-Grief MA (2020) Pediatric swallowing and feeding. In: Assessment and management, 3rd edn. Plural Publ.

Ayres AJ (2005) Sensory integration and the child. Western Psychological Services Publ.

Baley J, Committee on Fetus and Newborn (2015) Skin-to-skin care for term and preterm infants in the neonatal ICU. Pediatrics 136(3):596–599. https://doi.org/10.1542/peds.2015-2335

Bobath B, Bobath K (1975) Motor development in the different types of cerebral palsy. The Whitefriars Press Ltd, London

Brazelton TB, Nugent JK (2011) Neonatal behavioral assessment scale. In: Clinics in developmental medicine, No. 190, 4th edn. Mac Keith Press, London

da Costa SP, van der Schans CP (2008) The reliability of the Neonatal Oral-Motor Assessment Scale. Acta Paediatr 97(1):21–26. https://doi.org/10.1111/j.1651-2227.2007.00577.x

Dougherty NJ (2009) A review of cerebral palsy for the oral health professional. Dent Clin N Am 53(2):329–338. https://doi.org/10.1016/j.cden.2008.12.001

Ericson J, Palmér L (2019) Mothers of preterm infants' experiences of breastfeeding support in the first 12 months after birth: a qualitative study. Birth 46(1):129–136. https://doi.org/10.1111/birt.12383

Frakking TT, Chang AB, O'Grady KF, David M, Walker-Smith K, Weir KA (2016) The use of cervical auscultation to predict oropharyngeal aspiration in children: a randomized controlled trial. Dysphagia 31(6):738–748. https://doi.org/10.1007/s00455-016-9727-5

Fujinaga CI, de Moraes SA, Zamberlan-Amorim NE, Castral TC, de Almeida e Silva A, Scochi CG (2013) Clinical validation of the preterm oral feeding readiness assessment scale. Rev Lat Am Enfermagem 21 Spec No:140-5. English, Portuguese. https://doi.org/10.1590/s0104-11692013000700018

Galván GM, Mendoza SAG (2020) Video fluoroscopic alterations in the mechanics of swallowing in patients with cerebral palsy. Rev Mex Med Fis Rehabil 32(1–2):6–10. https://doi.org/10.35366/98513

Ghomi H, Yadegari F, Soleimani F, Lessen Knoll B, Mhdi Noroozi M, Mazouri A (2019) The effects of premature infant oral motor intervention (PIOMI) on oral feeding of preterm infants: a randomized clinical trial. Int J Pediatr Otorhinolaryngol 120:202–209. https://doi.org/10.1016/j.ijporl.2019.02.005

Grosso E, Cerchiari A, Panella M (2011) Chapter 12: Il percorso diagnostico-terapeutico nella pedofagia. In: Schindler O, Ruoppolo G, Schindler A (eds) Deglutologia, 2nd edn. Omega Publ.

Grzić R, Bakarcić D, Prpić I, Jokić NI, Sasso A, Kovac Z, Lajnert V (2011) Dental health and dental care in children with cerebral palsy. Coll Antropol 35(3):761–764

Hilditch C, Howes A, Dempster N, Keir A (2019) What evidence-based strategies have been shown to improve breastfeeding rates in preterm infants? J Paediatr Child Health 55(8):907–914. https://doi.org/10.1111/jpc.14551

Hwang YS, Lin CH, Coster WJ, Bigsby R, Vergara E (2010) Effectiveness of cheek and jaw support to improve feeding performance of preterm infants. Am J Occup Ther 64:886–894. https://doi.org/10.5014/ajot.2010.09031

Jensen D, Wallace S, Kelsay P (1994) LATCH: a breastfeeding charting system and documentation tool. J Obstet Gynecol Neonatal Nurs 23(1):27–32. https://doi.org/10.1111/j.1552-6909.1994.tb01847.x

Joffe N, Webster F, Shenker N (2019) Support for breastfeeding is an environmental imperative. BMJ 367:l5646. https://doi.org/10.1136/bmj.l5646

Leal-Martínez F, Franco D, Peña-Ruiz A, Castro-Silva F, Escudero-Espinosa AA, Rolón-Lacarrier OG, López-Alarcón M, De León X, Linares-Eslava M, Ibarra A (2020) Effect of a nutritional support system (diet and supplements) for improving gross motor function in cerebral palsy: an exploratory randomized controlled clinical trial. Foods 9(10):1449. https://doi.org/10.3390/foods9101449

Lessen Knoll BS (2012) Premature Infant Oral Motor Intervention (PIOMI) translating interventional research into interdisciplinary practice. In: 15th National Academy of Neonatal Nurses: Mother Baby Conference, Chicago, USA

Lipchock SV, Reed DR, Mennella JA (2011) The gustatory and olfactory systems during infancy: implications for development of feeding behaviors in the high-risk neonate. Clin Perinatol 38(4):627–641. https://doi.org/10.1016/j.clp.2011.08.008

Maastrup R, Rom AL, Walloee S, Sandfeld HB, Kronborg H (2021) Improved exclusive breastfeeding rates in preterm infants after a neonatal nurse training program focusing on six breastfeeding-supportive clinical practices. PLoS One 16(2):e0245273. https://doi.org/10.1371/journal.pone.0245273

Maiya A, Shetty YR, Rai K, Padmanabhan V, Hegde AM (2015) Use of different oral hygiene strategies in children with cerebral palsy: a comparative study. J Int Soc Prev Community Dent 5(5):389–393. https://doi.org/10.4103/2231-0762.165925

Majoli M, Artuso I, Serveli S, Panella M, Calevo MG, Ramenghi A (2021a) A key developmental step for preterm babies: achievement of full oral feeding. J Matern Fetal Neonatal Med. 2021 Feb.;34(4):519-525, https://doi.org/10.1080/14767058.2019.1610733

Majoli M, De Angelis LC, Panella M et al. (2021b) Parent-Administered Oral Stimulation in Preterm Infants: a Randomized, Controlled, Open-Label Pilot Study. Am. J of Perinatology 2021 Jun., https://doi.org/10.1055/s-0041-1731452

McClure V (2017) Infant Massage: a handbook for loving parents, 4th edn. Bantam Pub.

McFadden A, Gavine A, Renfrew MJ, Wade A, Buchanan P, Taylor JL, Veitch E, Rennie AM, Crowther SA, Neiman S, MacGillivray S (2017) Support for healthy breastfeeding mothers with healthy term babies. Cochrane Database Syst Rev 2(2):CD001141. https://doi.org/10.1002/14651858.CD001141

Molinaro A, Fedrizzi E, Calza S, Pagliano E, Jessica G, Fazzi E, GIPCI Study Group (2017) Family-centred care for children and young people with cerebral palsy: results from an Italian multicenter observational study. Child Care Health Dev 2017(43):463–625. https://doi.org/10.1111/cch.12449

Morris SE, Klein MD (1987) Pre-feeding skills. Therapy Skills Builders

Nyqvist KH, Rubertsson C, Ewald U, Sjödén PO (1996) Development of the Preterm Infant Breastfeeding Behavior Scale (PIBBS): a study of nurse-mother agreement. J Hum Lact 12(3):207–219. https://doi.org/10.1177/089033449601200318

Parkes J, Hill N, Platt MJ, Donnelly C (2010) Oromotor dysfunction and communication impairments in children with cerebral palsy: a register study. Dev Med Child Neurol 52:1113–1119. https://doi.org/10.1111/j.1469-8749.2010.03765.x

Ramella B, Panella M (2011) Pedofagia: quale il ruolo del caregiver? In: Raimondo S, Accornero A, RossettoT (eds) Logopedia e Disfagia. Carrocci Faber ed.

Rempel G (2015) The importance of good nutrition in children with cerebral palsy. Phys Med Rehabil Clin N Am 26(1):39–56. https://doi.org/10.1016/j.pmr.2014.09.001

Ross ES, Philbin MK (2011) Supporting oral feeding in fragile infants: an evidence-based method for quality bottle-feedings of preterm, ill, and fragile infants. J Perinat Neonatal Nurs 25(4):349–57; quiz 358–359. https://doi.org/10.1097/JPN.0b013e318234ac7a

Schindler O, Ruoppolo G, Schindler A (2011) Deglutologia, 2nd edn. Omega Publ., Torino

Sellers D, Mandy A, Pennington L, Hankins M, Morris C (2014) Development and reliability of a system to classify the eating and drinking ability of people with cerebral palsy. Dev Med Child Neurol 56:245–251. https://doi.org/10.1111/dmcn.12352

Sellers D, Pennington L, Bryant L, Benfer K, Weir K, Morris C (2019) Mini-EDACS: Eating and Drinking Ability Classification System for young children with cerebral palsy. In: Ann. Meeting Europ. Acad. of Childhood Disability (EACD), 31st EACD Conf., 23–25 May 2019, Paris

Setaro AM, Fedrizzi E (2016) Paralisi Cerebrale Infantile- Cosa i genitori vogliono sapere. Fondazione Mariani, Milano, p 80

Sitton M, Arvedson J, Visotcky A, Braun N, Kerschner J, Tarima S, Brown D (2011) Fiberoptic endoscopic evaluation of swallowing in children: feeding outcomes related to diagnostic groups and endoscopic findings. Int J Pediatr Otorhinolaryngol. 2011 Aug;75(8):1024-31, https://doi.org/10.1016/j.ijporl.2011.05.010

Van Hulst K (2019) Oral Motor Performance in children with neurodevelopmental disabilities—about dysphagia and drooling. ISBN: 978-90-9032176-9, ProefschriftMaken.nl

WHO (World Health Organization (2007) The International Classification of Functioning, Disability and Health; children and youth version (ICF CY), Geneva, World Health Organization

Winstock A (2019) Eating and drinking difficulties in children. Routledge Publ., USA

The Child with Cerebral Palsy and Visual Impairment

Viviana Baiardi and Tiziana Battistin

The dominant role of vision in human development has been recognized in Western culture since the age of the Greek philosophers.

Vision is the most complex among sensory and perceptual systems: its distinctive feature stems from the capability of transforming physical light stimuli, which reach the retina, into meaningful perception, which terminates in stable mental representations of a three-dimensional world. Even if recent neuroimaging studies on individuals with blindness have shown a supramodal functional cortical organization, with the overlapping of perceptive and affective areas in them and sighted individuals (Pietrini et al. 2004; Bedny et al. 2009; Klinge et al. 2010; Ricciardi et al. 2014), it is still clear that vision is the only sense which has both an analytical and synthetic perceptive interaction with the external environment. Vision has characteristics of perceptive continuity and immediate synthesis of numerous input peculiarities, such as shape, size, colour, and contrast (Fazzi et al. 2010a). Fraiberg (1977) gave vision the principal role of coordinating all other perceptual sensory systems and of driving interaction with the external world, it being the "synthesizer of experience" and the central agency of sensorimotor adaptation.

Vision usually precedes action: Prechtl et al. (2001) showed how the absence of sight has an effect on motor development even before birth. The discovery of mirror neurons (Di Pellegrino et al. 1992; Umiltà et al. 2001) confirmed the role of vision in guiding the neuropsychomotor development of the child through imitation of motivating gestures, postures, and movement. Vision is the driving force of a secure bond between the parent and the baby because, according to the theory of infant

V. Baiardi (✉)
Fondazione Robert Hollman, Cannero Riviera (VB), Italy
e-mail: v.baiardi@fondazioneroberthollman.it

T. Battistin
Fondazione Robert Hollman, Padova, Italy
e-mail: T.battistin@fondazioneroberthollman.it

© The Author(s), under exclusive license to Springer Nature Switzerland AG 2022
P. Giannoni, L. Zerbino (eds.), *Cerebral Palsy*,
https://doi.org/10.1007/978-3-030-85619-9_11

intersubjectivity (Trevarthen and Aitken 2001), the innate aptitude of newborns to relational life evokes, in the caregivers, behaviours which promote interaction, mostly driven by the eyes.

Therefore, the visual system, which develops in early life, assumes the guiding role in the structuring of all other neuropsychic functions and in the neurodevelopment of the whole child (Table 11.1), including emotional and affective growth, motor abilities, learning, and social communication (Purpura and Tinelli 2020).

Literature shows that 20–30% of the cerebral cortex in humans is devoted to visual processing (Orban et al. 2004) and that 80% of the information, coming from the external environment, reaches in the brain through visual pathways (Haupt and Huber 2008). The visual pathways are already developed at birth, but their maturing is a long process, which is strongly influenced by experience-dependent plasticity, especially in the first years of life, in the critical periods (Berry and Nedivi 2016; Consorti et al. 2019). The early years of the children's lives (Tierney and Nelson 3rd. 2009) are especially fundamental in their development since they represent a continuous path of curiosity, exploration, discovery, interaction, and learning. The daily interaction with the surrounding environment, starting with faces/people and then objects/situations, becomes, beginning with the separation of self, gradually internalized by the children over a period of time (Stern 1985). This allows the development of their internal world and their expertise. In this way, children acquire relational, motor, cognitive and affective skills, which are constantly sustained by vision.

Fraiberg's studies showed, 50 years ago, that visual impairment (VI), especially if early-onset/congenital, affects all developmental areas and functions, such as attachment, the sleep-wake cycle, learning, gross and fine motor ability, communicative skill, and cognitive ability. Her studies have been confirmed over the years by other authors in the respective specialties (Prechtl et al. 2001; Sonksen and Dale 2002; Hallemans et al. 2011; Braddick and Atkinson 2013; Bathelt et al. 2019).

Visual impairment is defined by the World Health Organization (WHO 2019a) in six categories, according to residual visual acuity, and it is classified in the International Statistical Classification of Diseases and Related Health Problems

Table 11.1 Neurodevelopmental processes in which vision has a key role

- Attachment
- Differentiation between self and the external environment
- Development of the concept of an object permanence
- Interaction with and recognition and comprehension of the environment (objects, people, situations)
- Comprehension of both details and context
- Social communication
- Learning through observation and imitation
- Guidance in motor development
- Spatial orientation and exploration
- Locomotion and mobility
- Anticipation, protection, and feedback
- Reading/writing

10th Revision (ICD-10) in the H54 section, with the new ICD-11 revision coming into effect from 2022 (WHO 2019b). Visual impairment is essentially a decrease in visual functions and abilities, which has a profound impact on the child's daily life and development and which cannot be affected merely by the use of corrective aids such as glasses (WHO 2019c).

According to the experience of the Robert Hollman Foundation (RHF,[1]Vaglio et al. 2018), a private non-profit Dutch institution that has been working on the support and development of children with visual impairment since 1979, in addition to visual acuity, the visual field also has a very important function in determining low vision, because its reduction significantly affects the child's visual functionality both in orientation and mobility and in the visual analysis-synthesis processes. This parameter is taken into account, as binocular perimetrical residual, in the Italian classification of VI, but this measurement in percentage terms is very difficult to assess in children with cerebral palsy and can often present a real challenge. It is, therefore, preferable to use a test called "behavioural visual field screening test (BEFIE)", which uses degree measurements and which was developed by Porro, specifically for neurologically impaired children (Porro et al. 1998; Koenraads et al. 2015).

Visual impairment is mainly classified in two categories, according to the anatomical origin or site involved (Sonksen and Dale 2002):

1. *Cerebral visual impairment (CVI):* here neurological impairment involves the visual retrochiasmatic system (optic tracts, geniculate bodies, optic radiations, and visual cortex) and/or the visual associative areas and pathways. Usually, children with CVI have a pre-existing neurological/neurodevelopmental disease, such as cerebral palsy (CP).

   Children with CVI can be classified into three groups:
   (a) Those with profound visual impairment
   (b) Those with impaired but functionally useful vision and often associated cognitive and/or motor impairments
   (c) Those with impaired but functionally useful vision, mostly near their academic level, the high-functioning CVI (Philip and Dutton 2014)
2. *Ocular impairment:* here the visual impairment consists of disorders of the eye, retina or optic nerves, giving rise to prechiasmatic pathologies. These pathologies may be confined only to the eye/s provoking low vision, or they may also be part of complex plurimalformative/genetic syndromes, thus belonging to a rare disease category.

The aetiology of VI is different in its two categories and is shown in Table 11.2.

The main causes of visual impairment vary from country to country, and they depend on socio-economic development and the availability of primary health and eye care services (WHO 2019c). In low-income countries, cataracts are still the leading cause of VI (WHO 2020), but there is also a shift to a scenario more

---

[1] Robert Hollman Foundation, (IT), http://www.fondazioneroberthollman.it/home-english.html

Table 11.2 Causes of VI

Cerebral visual impairment (Lueck et al. 2019)	Ocular impairment
Hypoxic-ischemic encephalopathy	Retinopathies
Periventricular leukomalacia	Opticopathies
Traumatic brain injury	Anterior segment abnormalities
Infections of the central nervous system (i.e. encephalitis, meningitis)	Ocular malformations
Occipital epilepsy	Strabismus
Metabolic disorders (i.e. mitochondrial diseases)	Refractive errors
Chromosomal anomalies	Infectious diseases

Table 11.3 CVI: visual characteristics and behaviours (Vaglio et al. 2018)

Visual characteristics	Visual behaviours
Lacking visual orienting to the stimuli	Fluctuation of visual performances
Unstable/brief fixation	Visual inattention
Hyperfixation	Stimulus avoidance
Oculomotor dyspraxia	Preference for pattern and coloured, moving stimuli
Difficult saccades	Dilated visual perception (time to adapt to the environment)
Visual field defects	Reduced visual perception in situations of crowding
Strabismus may be present	Facilitated visual perception with environmental stability
Refraction deficits may be present	Difficulty in environmental exploration

resembling the one present in high-income countries (Solebo et al. 2017) where the lesions of the higher visual pathways, such as CVI, are the main cause (Pereins and Ortibus 2016; Philip and Dutton 2014; Chokron and Dutton 2016).

Prematurity, especially in very low-birth-weight (VLBW) or extremely low-birth-weight (ELBW) children, is also a risk factor for visual impairment (Siatkowski et al. 2013), for CVI (Geldof et al. 2015), and also for CP (Marret et al. 2013; Hafström et al. 2018). These premature children undergo disorders of the posterior visual pathways, like CVI and the retinopathy of preterm (ROP), which is an ocular impairment described later in the paragraph regarding the pathologies.

A significant percentage of children with cerebral palsy (34–43%) present also a VI (Surman et al. 2009; Philip et al. 2020), which worsens the disability; about 10% of children with CP have severe VI or functional blindness (Novak et al. 2012).

The main visual difficulties, in children with CP and VI, are due to brain injury and belong to the umbrella term of CVI (Philip and Dutton 2014; Philip et al. 2020); it is present in children with CP in a percentage, which can vary from 16 to 80% (Alimovic 2012).

CVI is characterized by a range of visual disorders, including ophthalmological, oculomotor, and perceptual abnormalities. Its peculiarity is the difficulty in the processing of visual input, which results in a visuo-cognitive pathology (Vaglio et al. 2018; Lueck et al. 2019; Pereins and Ortibus 2016) (Table 11.3).

In literature, a complete neuro-ophthalmological profile for each of the four forms of CP (Rosenbaum et al. 2007) has not yet been defined: Himmelmann et al.

(2006) showed how severe VI is, especially when present in the spastic bilateral and the dyskinetic forms of CP; Jan et al. (2001) showed dyskinetic eye movements in children with the dyskinetic form of CP; Pavone et al. (2017) showed nystagmus and oculomotor apraxia in ataxic children; Saunders et al. (2010) showed a higher number of refractive errors in non-spastic forms compared to spastic ones.

Fazzi et al. (2010b, 2012) showed that each form of spastic CP has a typical neuro-ophthalmological profile:

- Children with bilateral spastic CP (BSCP)/tetraparesis show the most severe reduction, or even absence, in visual acuity and major impairment in the basic oculomotor functions (such as smooth pursuit and saccades) and ocular abnormalities (such as refractive errors and altered fundus oculi).
- Children with BSCP/diplegia show mostly strabismus, refractive errors, dysmetric saccades, visual field deficit, a usually mild or moderate reduction of visual acuity, and oculomotor impairments (dyspraxic pursuit).
- Children with unilateral spastic CP show higher visual acuity, impaired visual field, and neglect (whose association can be sometimes misunderstood as hemianopia); they also show strabismus and refractive errors but less oculomotor involvement.

The "take-home message" is that, whatever the form and its clinical signs, every child is unique. Therefore, for a therapist, whose aim is to design tailor-made rehabilitative care, it is essential not only to take into account clinical classifications but also to keep in mind that a different sign may always be present. It is possible, for example, to meet a child with a BSCP/tetraparesis whose visual acuity is not so severe or a child with ataxia who has blindness.

The addition of visual impairment, and particularly blindness, in children with CP, compromises further all developmental areas, including those already negatively influenced by neurological damage. For this reason, in these particular children with CP and VI, there are important risk factors for their future neuropsychic development, even if there are individual potentials and the opportunity to favour cerebral plasticity through dedicated experiences. It is therefore important to promote the postnatal development of the visual system, especially in the critical periods of the maximum reorganization of the central nervous system.

Early intervention is strategic for the future development and the quality of life of these little children. The empirical experience of decades of work at the RHF confirms that early attention to the specific needs of both parents, caregivers, and children promotes a fuller overall development of the child (Lanners et al. 1999; Mercuriali et al. 2016). The main aims of the Robert Hollman Foundation are:

- To offer early attention to the family affective-relational system
- To create "nurturing care" to support and promote the development of the child with visual impairment
- To support the child's parents, who are an integral part and recipients of the intervention, from the moment of acceptance and understanding of the clinical diagnosis to the nurturing care of their child

Table 11.4 Specific factors arising from sensory deprivation

– **Loss of eye contact**: it is difficult, especially with children with congenital blindness or severe visual impairment, to understand their signals, because they mimic less. Eye contact allows mirroring and tuning to happen, so its loss can provoke a feeling of rejection in the adult
– **Difficulty in sending effective communicative signals and eliciting a response**: the visual impairment deeply affects communication, requiring the intervention of the other senses, such as hearing and touch
– **Difficulty in interacting with the environment**: the sensory deprivation requires the children to interact with their surroundings through the other senses (hearing, touch, sense of smell, taste)

This means giving the family their own tailored-made space and time, listening to them and becoming aware of and sharing their specific needs, understanding the strengths and the weaknesses of their child, and offering concrete help regarding all the aspects of the child's life (daily rhythms such as sleep, awakening, playing, feeding, postural hygiene, holding and handling, bonding, sensory and neuromotor aspects). This attention affects the neuronal plasticity of the brain (Purpura and Tinelli 2020), a fact which has been also scientifically proven in the child's overall development (Hadders-Algra 2014; Dale et al. 2019).

There are some specific factors, linked to the child's visual deprivation, which should be considered because they represent an important element of disorientation in the affective relationship between parents and their child, and they can hinder the future child's development (Table 11.4). Parents need therefore to be accompanied in the relationship with their child, discovering together other ways of mutual, equally meaningful interaction (Lanners and Salvo, 2000).

The different paths, designed and developed at the RHF over the years, begin with an assessment, which usually completes the clinical diagnosis and helps the therapists propose specific rehabilitative "tailor-made" care. It is important to start every care path by listening carefully to parents' observations of the visual behaviour of their child in the family environment, as being parents, they are the best experts (Brazelton and Sparrow 2007). Table 11.5 reports some of the questions the therapist asks the parents in the first meeting with the child and its family.

The RHF protocol for assessing visual functions and visual functionality integrates with the medical assessment, which includes neuro-ophthalmological and electrophysiological examinations.

The basic visual functions to observe in a rehabilitative context are the following:

- *Perception*: the brain's ability to process and interpret the information received by the eyes, beginning with the ability to detect light
- *Localization*: the ability to find the location of a visual target in the surrounding space
- *Fixation*: the ability to maintain the visual gaze on a steady visual target
- *Smooth pursuit*: the ability to move the eyes to follow the trajectory of a slow-moving visual target

Table 11.5 Questions to parents

- Can you describe your child's everyday routine?
- What in particular amuses your child?
- What does your child prefer doing?
- Is there anything your child does not like at all?
- What do you notice at home in your child's visual behaviour (gaze/eventual asymmetries or difficulties in eye movements)?
- Does your child have any particular way of looking at people/objects?
- Does your child turn their head to a visual target?
- Does your child habitually look to the left or right or both?
- Does your child hold their head in a preferred position?
- Does your child have a preferred posture?
- Have you noticed any difference in your child's visual response between a natural environment with normal light and the dark when switching on a light source?
- Does your child smile when presented with a toy?
- Does your child have a favourite toy?
- What are the characteristics of your child's favourite toy (colour, shape, texture)?
- Does your child try to reach for or grasp the object or both?
- Does your child do this predominantly with the same hand?
- Does your child look at the object when reaching for or grasping it?

- *Saccades*: simultaneous and rapid eye movements which change abruptly the point of foveal fixation
- *Visual comparison*: the ability to detect and compare two or more visual targets presented simultaneously

These functions can be evaluated in an orthoptic/oculistic/neuro-ophthalmological assessment. To assess them, there are tests for visual acuity, contrast sensitivity, colour vision, visual field, ocular motility, and stereopsis. This assessment aims at clinical diagnosis (because of the loss of function) and to test the residual function and the "functional vision", contributing in this way to taking care of the child.

11.1 Assessment of Visual Functions

Below are some of the tests used by the RHF rehabilitative team to measure these visual functions. These tests are those considered most suitable for children with CP and VI and are based on years of experience with children with visual impairment:

- *Teller Acuity Cards* (Preston et al. 1987; Huurneman and Boonstra 2016): this is a test which gives a quantitative measurement of the grating acuity, and it is suitable for children with CP and VI. It is easy to use because it does not require any verbal response and it tests the visual behaviour of the child when looking at grating spatial frequency cards with decreasing widths. The child's acuity is determined by the smallest grating that is detected by the child. It is important to keep in mind that this is a resolution acuity test, due to a sensory-motor response to a threshold stimulus of known size at a known testing distance. It gives you therefore an approximation of the real visual acuity.

- *Lea Hyvärinen (LH) recognition acuity test* (Hyvärinen et al. 2014): this is a recognition acuity test, which means that the children can verbally identify (or point to) the smallest target of known size at a known testing distance. This test is used in situations in which the children can recognize forms, even if they are not able to name them yet. There are four symbols to be recognized at a distance of 3 m, but with children with visual impairment it is possible to move closer and then to mathematically convert the results. This test, even if usually presented when a child is 18–24 months old, is usable with children with visual impairment usually after 3 years of age.
- *Tumbling E charts*: this recognition test is more difficult for the child than the LH test, because it requires also the presence of good spatial orientation skills, so it is not used so often in children with CP and VI.
- *Video screen visual acuity optotype with linear progression*: this test is used in children over 6 years old who can distinguish and recognize letters on a standard chart at a known distance.
- *Hiding Heidi Hyvärinen test*: this test allows the measurement of contrast sensitivity. It is very suitable for children with CP and VI because it evaluates the preferential looking cards/"palettes" with the social face stimulus (similar to Fantz face: see Fantz 1961) with decreasing contrast. With older children with mild visual impairment, it is also possible to try the Tumbling E contrast charts or the Octotype contrast chart.
- *Montessori test rack division*: this is a test, which allows the assessment of colour vision through the association of equal colours. For colour vision, there is also the Ishihara plates test (Ishihara 1972), but with children with both CP and VI, the Montessori test is preferable.
- *Lang stereotest* (Lang 1983): this test allows the assessment of the presence or absence of stereopsis. It is a simple card where children should recognize four hidden images, but it is not always applicable to children with CP and VI.
- *Behavioral Visual Field (BEFIE) screening test* (Koenraads et al. 2015): this test measures the peripheral visual field extension in degrees, by observing an individual's response to a stimulus on a graded arc that is moved from the periphery to the centre of the visual field along different meridians.

In Table 11.6 (below), some important observations on the visual functionality by therapists on children with CP and VI are reported, beginning with an observation of the child's spontaneous behaviour in a normally lit environment and then moving to neurovisual functional observation in an adapted environment, if necessary (e.g. darkened with a light source as a visual target). In the observation of visual functionality visuoperceptive aspects, environmental visual exploration and hand-eye coordination are considered.

In children with CP and CVI, it is particularly important to assess hand-eye coordination and manual praxis (Table 11.7).

Table 11.6 Observation of the visual functionality

General
– How does the child enter the therapy room (in parent's arms/in a stroller)?
– Can the child differentiate between the parent and the therapist?
– Is the child awake/restless/sleepy?
– Is there any form of communication (verbal/non-verbal)?
– Which behavioural characteristics are present (attention, motivation, curiosity, liveliness, discomfort, crying, indifference)?
– Are timeout signals present?
– Which postures are utilized? Is there a preferred one?
– Does the child make postural transitions? Does the child make any kind of autonomous movement within the environment?
– Is there any postural misalignment?
– Has the child an environmental intolerance?
– Has the child a preferred sense?
– Has the child a spontaneous use of vision, hearing, and touch?
Specific
– Does the child need environmental aids to help with the surroundings?
– Does the child react to light sources/black and white patterns/coloured objects?
– Does the child complain about light (i.e. dazzle)?
– Does the child adopt unusual postures of the body or the head?
– Does the child smile at an unfamiliar face or object?
– Does the child direct arm movement towards the face/object?
– Does the child show non-verbal response to the visual target?
– Is there a functional use of vision?
– Does the child move in the surrounding space?
– Does the child explore the environment? How and at what distance? Does the child navigate without help?
– Are there any particular repetitive visual behaviours (light-gazing, eye-pressing, eye-poking, eye-rubbing, flickering)?

Lanners and Goergen (2001); Battistin et al. (2005)

Table 11.7 Hand-eye coordination and manual praxis

Hand-eye coordination and manual praxis
– Orientation towards the object
– Reaching for the object
– Adaptation to the form and orientation of the hand after the contact with the object
– Preadaptation and orientation of the hand to the object's form
– Evaluation errors of the distance of the object to reach (dysmetrias)
– Grasping of the object (radial palmar, radial digital, inferior pincer or superior pincer)

Recently, a Visual Function Classification System (VFCS) for children with CP was developed and validated (Baranello et al. 2020) in order to classify how children with CP use visual abilities in daily life, as previously done with Motor, Manual, Communication, Eating and Drinking abilities. A CVI range was also developed by Roman Lantzy (2018) to evaluate how much the visual and behavioral characteristics associated with CVI interfere with the functional vision of the child, affecting it.

11.2   Cerebral Visual Impairment and Cerebral Palsy

What does it mean in practice to relate to children with CP and CVI? The therapist should be aware in advance of the characteristics of the children with CP and CVI in order not to have difficulties both in the relationship with them and how to plan the treatment.

The characteristics which can be present are:

- *No eye contact and no smile*: a baby or child with motor and visual impairment very often does not have eye contact and does not smile at all; therefore, it is important to start to relate through other senses, especially hearing (e.g. the tone, the rhythm, and the use of words and sounds of the therapist's voice) and touch (e.g. soft touch and caresses, cuddling, playing with the child's hands and feet) and also through body language while an adult is holding the child. A gentle touch and baby massage can help.
- *On-off gaze*: a toddler/child with CP and CVI, even if the visual acuity is not so low, very often does not gaze at people, and this is a factor that is independent of the degree of relationship and affection. Toddlers/children with CP and CVI do not look the therapist in the eyes because of their visual disorder. These children usually give a very quick glance to the therapist, and then they turn their head aside, i.e. the on-off gaze, as it is known.
- In this case, it is important to create a relationship with them through the other senses, playing with sounds and by using adequate handling and playful touch (Provenzi et al. 2020).
- *Oculomotor dyspraxia*: the children with CP and CVI usually present oculomotor disorganization, which can be in different degrees of severity and which causes dyspraxic ocular movements, characterized by:
  - Difficulty in fixation, which is usually very brief and unstable
  - Possible hyperfixation
  - Difficulty in smooth pursuit because there is no fluidity of eye movements, being instead sudden and discontinuous

This means that the children are not able to move their eyes voluntarily and smoothly towards an object or a person. This oculomotor dyspraxia affects the relationship between the child and the therapist because of the problem of sharing the gaze due to the difficulty of fixation; at the same time, it affects the visual strategies used in scanning and exploring the environment, creating a misperception in the visuoperceptual processing and consequently an impairment in the representation processes, which allows the brain to build the images of the living environment. Subsequently, all the visual learning processes are affected by this impairment. This means that it will be important to work on basic visual functions with motivating proposals, integrating them into the neuromotor approach. A subsequent step, where possible, will be the work on scanning and exploring visual strategies.

- *No hand-eye coordination*: children with CVI and CP adopt the same behaviour in reaching for an object, in which they first take a quick look at the object and then reach for it with their head turned away from the object.
- *Fluctuation of attention*: another important visual behaviour, which characterizes the children with CP and CVI, is the fluctuation of their attention and consequently of their visual performance. Inattention is typical in these children; therefore, it is not surprising that visual behaviour is not constant during the treatment, as it can frequently vary and is often linked to the difficulty of the task required of them. It is much easier to get a visual and also motor response if the proposal is part of play activity and within a familiar context and if the proposal is presented intermittently. These children very often do not perform well at all during the eye examinations, while on the contrary, they give their best at home.
- *Crowding effect*: this is another factor to consider because it affects visual perception, creating and increasing visual perceptual confusion: this is important to know when arranging the setting, which should be simple and functional.
- *Light-gazing*: it is another visual behaviour that is characteristic of these children: this means staring at the light sources in the ceiling. It is important to avoid this behaviour, which could increase and become repetitive and could "close" and isolate the children. In this case, it is necessary to distract them and motivate them in a different direction.
- *Preference for colours*: a child with CP and CVI shows a preference for saturated colour patterns compared to black-white, which is usually used with children with visual impairment. It is the experience of the RHF team that the child prefers black-yellow, red-yellow, or yellow-blue much more than black-white toys.
- *Preference for fluorescent multisensory toys*: sometimes, it is possible to capture the child's gaze with very simple fluorescent, home-made toys, such as rounded lids covered with glittering adhesive paper.
- *Preference for moving objects*: very often due to the integrity of the peripheral vision. Motion may be useful as a stimulus to glimpse the target, even by the children themselves, who move as a stimulation to "see better".
- *Distance*: it is an important factor to be considered; a child with CP and CVI will need the targets to be presented at a very close distance, like the near-sighted child. This means that the nearer the target is, the better it is seen, and all the background disappears reducing perceptive confusion.

Note

- Repetition of the experience is also very important because it allows a better consolidation and internalization of the visual information, helping perception and representative cognitive processes. In children with visual impairment, response times are more dilated than in children with no visual impairment; therefore, it is important to wait a long time, especially if the condition is severe. This increased latency may be due to the difficulty in information processing.
- A multisensory approach with visual facilitating characteristics is important, since it usually allows a better response time in these children and it is used also to trigger motor initiative.

11.3   Facilitation in the Treatment Planning and Practical Suggestions

An early rehabilitative intervention, guided by professionals such as therapists, supports and promotes learning and behavioural strategies in the child with CP and VI.

It is important to always maintain good integration between the child's postural control, posturo-kinetic skills, visual abilities, and abnormal visual behaviours.

Different aims of the therapist:

- *For the child (autonomy and life quality)*
  - Maximization of visual potential
  - Integration of visual potential with other senses and with other developmental areas (motor, affective, relational, and cognitive)
  - Adaptation of environment to all daily life situations
- *For the parents/caregivers (child management)*
  - Provision of tips to promote and support the use of the child's visual potential (e.g. design of an individualized play corner and introduction of environmental visual facilitations linked to specific moments of daily life)
  - Evaluation together with parents/caregivers of the most functional posture and the handling of the child
  - Evaluation of the selected environment (lighting, ecological/structured environment, distances between the child and the visual targets)
- *For the treatment planning*
  - Promotion of the child's initiative in all aspects
  - Assessment of the selected posture
  - Assessment of the selected environment
  - Maintenance of the functional use of the visual residue in the child with visual impairment
  - Perceptual sensory integration through multisensory proposals
  - Development of the representative process (construction of mental images), improving praxis (hand functional use), enhancing motor imagery (exploration of the environment through tactile-motor-acoustic experiences)
  - Selection of the proposed target, for example, contrasted o lighting objects
  - Selection of the most visually facilitating background

The concept of facilitation is fundamental when dealing with children with CP and VI: this means adopting some external modifications of their environment to improve the children's quality of life, to support their residual visual and motor potentialities, to prevent any possible regressions, and to take into account their needs.

The main suggested facilitations are:

11.3.1 Environmental Facilitations

It is necessary to create a contained and appropriate environment, considering also adequate lighting.

Sight can provide, at the same time, a series of environmental characteristics, such as colour, form, and dimension, which are important for the child's attainment of knowledge. For this reason, it is opportune to use high contrasts and/or structured panels in the play corner to support and reassure the children because of their visual difficulties. It is important to give a spatial and temporal boundary to the proposals to reassure the children at a perceptual level and to offer greater predictability and adaptation. Particularly with children with CP, it is fundamental to offer breaks, the right rhythm, and dynamism to the activities while at the same time respecting the children's response times and needs.

Note

- It is important not to create visual perceptual crowding but rather to create and offer a visually contained space, not too big, starting from the child's first perceptive area and slowly enlarge it.
- It is essential to keep in mind the child's visual acuity to define the longest distance that the child can potentially reach; at a rehabilitative level, it is mandatory to maintain the distance at which the child perceives, localizes, and is able to reach the object. According to the concept of "affordance", it is important that the child can easily grasp the object, according to their abilities (Gibson and Walker 1984; Ellis and Tucker 2000).
- It is crucial to maintain the difference between the visual target and the background in terms of sensitivity and chromatic contrast (if the background has a structured pattern, it is fundamental that the object has plain chromatic characteristics and vice versa)

Setting the appropriate light is fundamental before starting the treatment. In visual rehabilitation, there are three different kinds of light, depending on:

- Natural environment with normal light
- Semi-darkened environment
- Darkened environment

The first moment of spontaneous observation of the visual function should always be in a natural environment with normal light, to observe the spontaneous use of the visual function of the child in daily life. In this case, the environment should be as neutral as possible.

According to the child's responses, some environmental changes may be necessary, i.e. an increase/decrease in light, in line with a different postural support of the child.

The degree of environmental light affects considerably the child's attention:

- The bright or lit object represents the easiest visual target to perceive, after direct or filtered light.
- In the semi-darkened or darkened environment, the child can concentrate more on the object of the activity.

Note
- It is important to integrate the visual information with other senses because "seeing" only the light is of little interest and not motivating; moreover, it affects the visual abilities less; it is important to localize but more so to touch, to explore, and to know what can be visually perceived.
- The darkened environment is a "rehabilitative environment"; therefore, it should be used sparingly in everyday life;
- It is important to use the "rehabilitative cues" not as "exercises with the light".
- The reduction of light is not always effective with these children.

11.3.2 Targets and Their Characteristics

The therapist should always consider the most appropriate toys or targets to use, taking into consideration their dimensions and distance from the child. Furthermore, the therapist should evaluate and vary as necessary the multisensory characteristics of the proposed toys.

Multisensoriality is the main characteristic of the target, always bearing in mind the aim of helping the child.

The multisensorial object allows the perception not only of visual features, such as colours and high chromatic contrast, but also of tactile, auditory, and smelling inputs.

It is important to assess and carefully support the child's visual and behavioural response regarding the different sensory inputs:

- Sound can help to localize people/objects, but the environmental sounds and noises should be considered so as not to create confusion.
- Tactile input helps the perception of the object in the environment.

Note
- In case of low visual residue and poor neuromotor abilities, the sensory proposal is enlarged, keeping stable modulation of the incoming sense not to involve too many senses.

11.3.3 Postural Setting

The therapist should verify the most suitable posture for the child previously evaluated, also proposing, if necessary, various personalized aids.

It is possible to begin with the initial supine posture and then transfer the child to the side and/or sitting positions, with or without assistance.

Temporary aids (baby's chair, high chair, or postural systems) can be used and adapted according to the rehabilitative goals, helping them to be reached. In children with CP and VI, it is advised to prepare the child for a possible change of the environment or of the situation (room, stroller or postural aids, light, noises).

The purpose of a proper posture is:

- To encourage the aligned posture, trying to contain reflexes and massive pathological synergies
- To enhance the use of the visual sense
- To allow visuomotor integration

Below is a list of postures suggested for treatment:

11.3.3.1 Supine

This posture is used in the treatment of children, also at an early age, who still do not have good antigravity control and for those with a very severe motor case history such as BSCP.

The main aims of the treatment are:

- To use as much as possible the visual residue in a posture which allows the child to have better head-trunk axial control
- To promote and facilitate basic visual functions

Suggestion
- Position the child in supine, in a play-corner with environmental perceptual facilitation and personalized targets (Fig. 11.1) The aims of these kinds of environment and position are:
  - Support and facilitate the child in achieving the median line, even with the guidance of an adult, if necessary.
  - Enhance the oculomotor coordination.

Fig. 11.1 Child in the supine position in a play corner

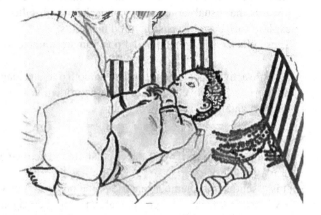

- Introduce multisensory proposals (e.g. with vertical splints, toy activity centre, etc.) which activate and support the child's visual potential.
- Allow a better eye contact or gaze and favour a relational communication through face-to-face playing.
- Facilitate basic visual functions.
- Support the head of the child with a proper pillow, to facilitate head control in the midline.

Note
- It is important to be sure that the child avoids light-gazing and avoids hyperextension patterns, which can cause deviations of the eyes upwards.
- It is fundamental to avoid the eliciting of an asymmetric tonic neck reflex, which can induce a deviation of the gaze, in addition to misalignment.
- The therapist should bear in mind that some children, hospitalized for a long time, may show a strong perceptual intolerance in the supine position.
- It is essential to foster the activity of the child, according to their potential.

11.3.3.2 Prone
This posture is particularly indicated for children with BSCP because it engages them in responding to gravity and counteracts their pathological attitude. Nevertheless, this posture allows more postural stability, but not good gaze control, and therefore the caregiver should give verbal guidance to sustain the child's motivation.

The main aims of the treatment are:

- Use as far as possible the visual residue in the position that allows the activation of the posterior muscle chain, the cervical area included, and could enhance the activation of the visual function.
- Promotion and facilitation of visual functions, particularly visual scanning and smooth pursuit.

Suggestion
- Lie the child down on a wedge, in a confined setting with visual environmental aids (Fig. 11.2), and promote the orientation, the localization, and the gaze towards the visual target, integrating them with other senses, e.g. the touch to explore surfaces/objects/structured materials.
  These kinds of environment and position are suitable to:

- Propose activities of exploration and smooth pursuit along the horizontal trajectory
- Support and improve the oculomotor coordination
- Support and improve visual contact

Note
- It is important to verify that the child started to actively reach and maintain antigravity stability.
- It is essential to remember that the prone position is challenging for a child with a VI, because it involves considerable postural engagement, such as being supported by arms, and therefore might have little interest in the anterior space.

Fig. 11.2 Child in prone
position in play corner
with guidance

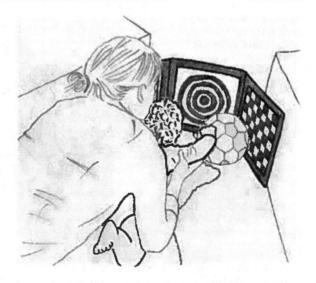

11.3.3.3   Rolling to Side

Before proposing this transition, it is necessary to check the availability of the two girdles, scapular and pelvic, enabling the child to move independently, as necessary for rolling.

The main aims of the treatment are:

– Foster the use of the visual sense in a position that facilitates the arm's movement of the free side for reaching the proposed targets.
– Guide the child through attracting a visual target during the transition from the supine position to the side one.
– Favour the visual and gestural approach on the median line.

Suggestion

• Start with the child supine in an adapted play-corner with visual facilitation; propose the visual catching of an object approaching with slow movement, from the centre to the periphery assisting the movement from supine to the side. This can be proposed to both sides (Fig. 11.3).

In this way, the child can hold the moving object and is guided by the therapist's hand to do the complete passage, allowing the maintenance of visual control for the whole motor sequence.

These kinds of environment and posture are suitable for:

– Improving hand-eye coordination
– Allowing the use of objects or materials which perceptually hold the child, offering in this way a greater perceptual continuity
– Using facilitations, such as aids and the support (pillows, wedges, small rollers)
– Allowing the visual exploration of the anterior and the top space
– Fostering face-to-face play
– Inserting a light source oriented towards the target, depending on the child's visual residue

Fig. 11.3 Child pivoting to the side with multisensorial target and light behind

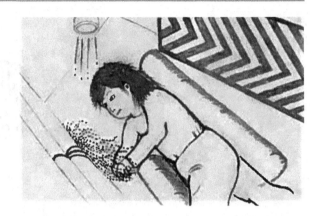

Note

It is essential to:

- Take care of how to propose targets and to avoid hyperextension and consequently the loss of the proper positioning
- Minimize the handling and foster the child's motivation to move actively
- Control the child's alignment when holding a toy moved slowly in front of the child's eyes

11.3.3.4 Semi-chair Sitting

The semi-seated posture is a halfway position between the supine and the sitting one. This position is very significant in children who still do not have good head-trunk axial control, or when such a control cannot be achieved. Moreover, it is a posture that helps to lower muscle stiffness and facilitates the alignment of the child.

The main aims of the treatment are to:

- Facilitate the use of the visual sense in a posture that does not require important muscular activity
- Motivate the child with an interesting visual target proposed in the peripersonal space

Suggestion

- Position the child in a nest, which surrounds and creates a peripersonal circular space offering perceptual and proprioceptive inputs.

  For example, visual and multisensory targets can be proposed, to be glimpsed first by the child's eyes, to then touch the body, or be moved into the middle-low space in such a way that the child can reach for, grasp, and explore them with hands. Wedges and ring-shaped or "U"-shaped pillows can help to maintain a proper alignment (Fig. 11.4)

  These kinds of environment and posture are suitable for:

- Facilitating the achievement and maintenance of the median line
- Facilitating eye and "face-to-face" contacts
- Facilitating the insertion of multisensory proposals, with simple structured materials, or splints with mobile toys with visually attractive characteristics.

Fig. 11.4 Child sitting in
U-shaped pillow with
target in front of their eyes

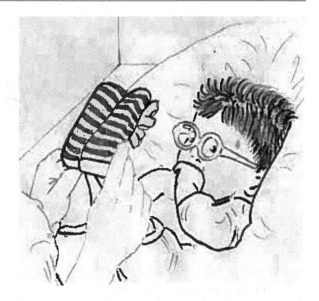

Note

It is important to:

- Ensure a proper position of the head to facilitate easy breathing and swallowing
- Avoid light-gazing

11.3.3.5   Sitting

With the child with CP, there are different ways of reaching and maintaining the sitting position. In this section, a situation which is adapted to a child who has good head-trunk axial control and who can maintain the sitting position autonomously, without achieving it independently, is described.

The main aims are to:

- Allow the child to have new experiences in a different antigravity position, which also requires an organization of the visual and vestibular functions
- Favour the positioning with feet on the foot support because of the tactile and proprioceptive information received
- Foster the child's interpersonal relationships with the environment, because of its enhancement on the cognitive level

Suggestion

- Depending on axial control, the child can be positioned in long sitting or on a small bench, inside a soft corner surrounded by stable visuoperceptive boundaries to support perceptual and proprioceptive continuity.

  It is also possible to add a small table in front, assisting the child to sense an environmental boundary and also to facilitate arms and upper trunk motor initiative. For example, visual and multisensory proposals, showed in front of or on the sides of the child, can foster the reaching and grasping movements (Fig. 11.5). These kinds of environment and posture are suitable for:

Fig. 11.5 Two multisensorial patterns placed at the side of a sitting child

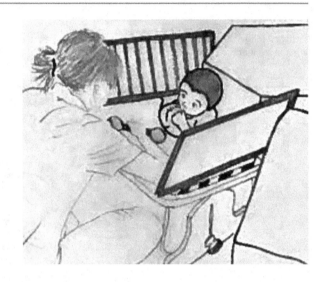

- Improving hand-eye coordination
- Proposing the sitting position during daily life to foster the child's autonomies (e.g. self-feeding, playing), introducing some visual facilitation to attract attention
- Introducing playing activities with some cognitive meaning, to enhance hand-eye coordination and mono-/bimanual activities
- Organizing the exploration of the environment to foster visual scanning, smooth pursuit, and saccades

Note
- During all these proposals, it is fundamental that the child maintains the upright position, particularly when rotating.

11.3.3.6   Sitting with the Therapist's Guidance

The therapist's guidance is necessary when the child with CP does not yet have good trunk control. The therapist's body works as a mediator and facilitator to let the child feel a stable position and to guide the child's hands in the haptic exploration of the environment and objects, according to the child's specific motor and visuo-cognitive needs.

When the child needs some guidance and help to maintain axial control, the therapist can sit behind the child. Instead, in other situations, the therapist sits in front of the toddler/child to increase attention and participation.

Sometimes, a mirror can be used to improve the child's visual control and increase motivation, but its use is not always recommended and should be carefully evaluated because in children with CVI it can often cause a crowding effect.

Suggestion

- In a soft contained and controlled environmental setting, the child is positioned in long sitting between the therapist's legs or sitting on a roll with feet on the floor and the therapist behind him. If the child shows some tactile resistance, the therapist can propose some perceptual aids, such as a medium-large sized toy, with interesting perceptual characteristics placed in front of the child or in the peripersonal space, so that it can become both an interesting visual target and a mediator of the guided movement.

These kinds of environment and posture are considered for children with low visual residue, because it is a useful situation that offers more meaningful and less fragmentary perceptual information through a more global proposal when using an object which can be multisensorial, such as visuo-auditory or visuo-tactile.

11.3.3.7   Sitting on Chair

With the growth of the child, the positioning system becomes fundamental for the child as well as a micro-environment which becomes a very important postural alternative in daily life and at specific times such as moments of structured playing or mealtimes. Moreover, the positioning system becomes essential in clinical cases with considerable reduction or absence of postural control.

The main aim of the treatment are to:

- Support the visual function in a facilitating posture, frequently used during the day by the child, where there is low motor engagement. Also in this situation, the affective relationships are encouraged and therefore the motivation and the "face-to-face" playing.

Suggestion

- The child is seated in a positioning system with a small cut-out table in the front, which facilitates the sighting of an object and the reaching for/grasping it. A perceptive structured or a C-shaped panel gives multisensorial information so that the child can be more aware of the anterior space and more interested in exploring a wider range of environments (Fig. 11.6). Visual proposals may be introduced in front or next to the child within a short distance, using, for example, a toy activity centre, tactile trays, or small mats with Velcro and small wooden boards, to create a more attractive perceptual screen.

These kinds of environment and posture are suitable for:

- Improving the child's basic visual functions being well postured but, at the same time, without the need for motor control
- Helping the child to communicate, even through aids (e.g. voca, sensors, communication board, etc.) if necessary

Fig. 11.6 Child in the
chair set with a
multisensorial target in the
anterior space

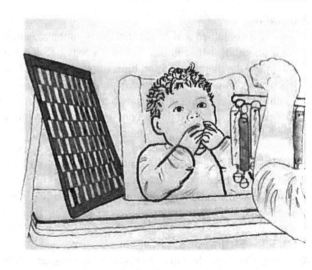

Importance of a Bookstand or Inclined Surface
From a rehabilitative point of view, as previously stated, it is very important
to propose a perceptual screen in front of the child. An inclined surface or a
bookstand can be used to allow better motor reaching or grasping of the object
and to improve visual perception, localization, and fixation of the proposed
target. It is possible to propose multisensory, coloured tridimensional toys and
enhance trials of hand-eye coordination in the anterior space, sustaining at the
same time the child's motivation and visuomotor integration. If necessary, the
therapist guides the child proposing multisensory objects and materials to
improve the child's experience of the environment and surrounding objects.

11.3.3.8   Standing with Aids

Before proposing the standing position, a good assessment should be carried out,
evaluating if the child can maintain the position independently or with some aid,
such as a standing frame equipped with all its options.

The main aim of the treatment is to:

– Favour the visual function in a different position, which relates child, people, and
environment differently and support visual potential

Suggestion
• The child is positioned in a customised standing system, always inside a confined
environment. It is possible to place some multisensory toys on the table of the
standing frame, as interesting visual targets which guide sight and motion in the
peri-personal space (Fig. 11.7). It is moreover possible, depending on the child's
visual residue, to insert a light source oriented towards the target.

Fig. 11.7 A child plays on a standing frame

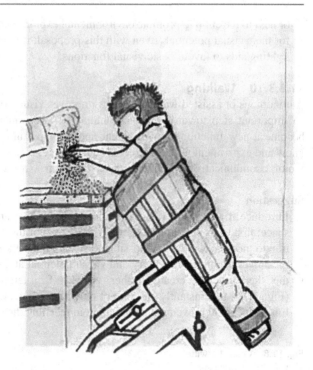

These kinds of environment and posture are suitable for:

- Promoting the reaching of an object with better visual control
- Challenging the child in an antigravity posture, which can improve visual potential

11.3.3.9 Standing

The standing position without aids is possible in children with milder forms of CP, such as the unilateral or mild bilateral spastic forms. The therapist's aim is, as always, to offer the child experiences such as to be able to use and increase visual potential.

The main aim of the treatment is to:

- Foster the visual function in this antigravity position to promote environmental exploration and locomotion, with all the novelties that they entail

Suggestion

- Allow the child to experiment with and experience the standing position, initially with some support, such as leaning with the shoulders against a wall-corner, maintaining the environmental facilitations with stable visuoperceptual boundaries. In this situation, it is possible to propose some multisensory toys in front of or next to the child to promote environmental exploration at an adequate distance for their visual potential. Even with this proposal, it is possible to include some lighting aids to favour basic visual functions.

11.3.3.10 Walking

Autonomous or assisted walking always improves visuomotor integration, and it is an important step towards personal autonomy. Every postural improvement can become a new functional environment and an opportunity for these children, to know and experiment with themselves and to express their skills and visual, neuro-motor, communicative, emotional, and relational resources.

Suggestion

- Introduce the first experiences of locomotion inside an initially not too large space; first trials should be extremely attractive for the child to increase motivation to move forwards. It is possible to sustain the walking initiative with verbal incentives to improve auditory and visual potential at the same time. Moreover, the therapist can create further visually facilitating environmental paths (Fig. 11.8), to constantly sustain not only visual potential but also, at the same time, functional movement culminating in reaching the target.

Fig. 11.8 A corridor with visually facilitation path

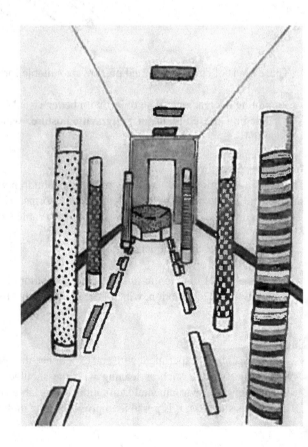

Note

- It is important to remember that the initial environment does not have to be not too large but characterized by spatial reference points, such as a small play corner with coloured furniture or a well-defined corridor with clear and obvious signs.

11.4 The Child with Blindness

Up to now, the problems of children with CP and VI have been focused on those with a visual residue to support and strengthen. However, there is also the possibility of meeting children with CP and total blindness.

The main aims of the treatment in children with blindness are to:

- Support the bonding and the relationship between child and parents through other senses from the first months in which they experience shared sounds, smells and touch
- Enhance the discovery of space, starting with the anterior proximal space and then gradually increasing the range of distance and direction
- Favour developmental stages through anticipatory and physical hand guidance by both parents and therapist
- Encourage neuromotor acquisition and environmental exploration using tactile and auditory stimuli

11.5 Specific Rehabilitative Tools

In this paragraph, the use of some rehabilitative tools is described, specifically those which are mainly used in the daily work of the RHF. Beyond these, in recent years many computerized and technological tools have been developed, such as interactive mats and applications for tablets and computers, and many research projects are still ongoing. These devices are particularly suitable for school children (see Chap. 14).

11.5.1 Light Box

Light box is a box with a bright surface inside which allows the presence of homogeneous light. On this surface, it is possible to use objects which become bright to facilitate the child in seeing them. There are two versions of this box: a larger one with a dimmer to calibrate the light intensity and a smaller one with only the on/off options. There are also some specific materials, which differ according to the child's developmental stage: under 18 months, the 18–36 months age range, and over 36 months (Fig. 11.9).

Fig. 11.9 A child plays
with light box

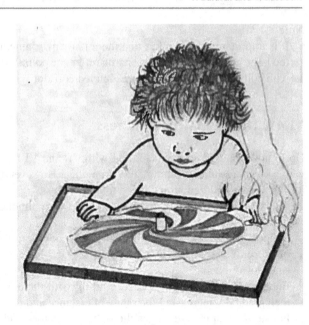

This tool is very suitable for the following children:

– Those who are visually impaired, to stimulate their visual residue and attention
– Those with peripheral eye damage or with a reduced visual field

There are many ways of and reasons for using this tool, among which are:

– For assessing light perception, switching the light on/off, and observing the way
  the child reacts
– By changing the intensity of the light, dimming, and using sheets with different
  opacity to compare the different reactions of the child
– By comparing different colourings to understand which is best perceived by
  the child
– By comparing different patterns (e.g. striped or chequered)
– By presenting the first faces (e.g. stylized faces in black and white)
– For favouring not only the first basic visual functions, such as fixation and pur-
  suit, but also manipulation, grasping, and hiding of transparent tridimen-
  sional objects
– For promoting the first visuo-cognitive tasks, such as selecting, associating, con-
  structing, inserting, forming a line, and categorizing
– For introducing the first activities of drawing and the prerequisites of writing

11.5.2 Multisensory Search Set

A multisensory search set is intended as a small environment of sensory exploration, which could be a wooden or cardboard structure with some holes in it, which

Fig. 11.10 Child at play with a multisensory search set

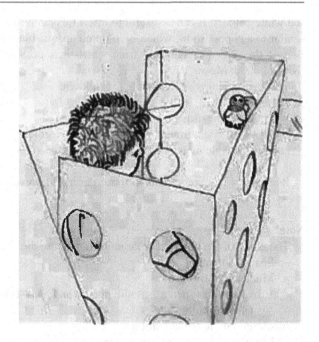

are horizontally and vertically aligned at a minimum distance of 5 cms from each other, which is the distance useful in evoking a saccade (Fig. 11.10) (Signorini et al. 2016).

This tool is very suitable for use with the following children:

- Those who are visually impaired to stimulate the visual residue and attention
- Those with oculomotor dyspraxia
- Those with peripheral eye damage or with a reduced visual field

It also helps the child to acquire the cognitive concept of an object's permanence.

This tool is used is to make objects which appear and disappear from holes, resulting in the child's search for them in different points of the space and to evoke saccades. It is also possible to enrich the cardboard structure, making it more attractive by drawing different shapes and change contexts to improve the child's ability to categorize. In this way, the child, observing what is happening and listening to a fairy tale, is encouraged to direct the gaze in different directions and to reach for and grasp the objects nearby.

For some children, it is possible and fundamental to propose a multisensory object and therefore the possibility of touching the object they are looking for and following.

11.5.3 Black Light

It is an ultraviolet lamp with cold light, known also as the lamp of Wood; this lamp increases the fluorescence and brightness of toys with particular colours such as fluo and white colours. It can be useful to insert this lamp in a box to create something similar to a puppet show, which is coloured opaque black inside to avoid the diffusion of the screened light and from which it is possible to make things appear (Kitchel 2000; Meeus 1994).

This instrument is very suitable for children:

- With visual impairment, who present dazzle.
- With visual impairment with inattention; colours, particularly fluorescent colours, activate more some cortical brain areas (Good et al. 1994).

Its ways of use are similar to those described previously for the multisensory search set.

Note
- The effect of the fluorescent target is to increase the child's:
  - Span of attention
  - Moments of fixation
  - Visual abilities such as smooth pursuit and hand-eye coordination
  - Visual exploration
- It is important to pay attention to:
  - Limiting the exposure times, (max. 15 min); the ultraviolet light, if directed and for a long time exposure, can favour the formation of cataracts or retinal degeneration.
  - Putting the light source behind the child or screening, in such a way it is not directed on the child's eyes.
  - Using protective glasses with aphakic or albino children or those with coloboma.
  - Using the instrument in a moderate and not exclusive way.
  - Turning on the black light in natural light of the room and gradually lowering it.

11.5.4 Snoezelen

The word Snoezelen derives from the fusion of two Dutch words "snuffelen" (to smell) and "doezelen" (to relax) (Hotz et al. 2006). This approach was born in the Netherlands in the 1970s, and it considers the stimulation of the five senses to help the child relax and sustain the multisensory proposals in a non-demanding context. In all multisensory approaches, the stimulations are produced by devices appropriately chosen by the therapist, depending on the characteristics of the single child. This allows the use of the multisensory target also by a caregiver.

Multiple proposals are possible, among them are the following:

- Relaxing the child on a mat or in a rocking chair or hammock, thereby activating the vestibular system
- Playing with intermittent or moving lights to trigger the visual sense
- Using natural scents to favour the olfactory sense

- Experimenting with vibrations to integrate a more perceptive sense
- Activating and listening to rhythmic, melodic sounds, which recall nature to reinforce the auditory sense.

11.6 Pathologies and Comorbidity

Some conditions, with important visual components and associated with CP, are described below.

11.6.1 Retinopathy of the Premature Child

Several children with CP were born prematurely (Vincer et al. 2006), and the main visual pathology is the retinopathy of prematurity (ROP).

In literature, ROP appeared in 1942 (Fagerholm and Vesti 2017), described as an abnormality in the process of the formation of the blood vessels, which nourish the retina and which grow from the posterior to the anterior part of the eye. This development ends after the birth term.

The developmental periods of retinopathy are classified according to the localization, the extent, and the stage (ICCRP 2005).

The extension or stadiation defines the severity of the pathology:

Stage 1: An ischemic area, delimited by a light/pale stripe, is highlighted.
Stage 2: There is no vascular proliferation.
Stage 3: Classified as light, moderate, severe.
Stage 3-PLUS: It is necessary a surgical treatment.
Stage 4: Partial retinal detachment.
Stage 5: Total retinal detachment.

The degree of ROP severity affecting a child is the key element to consider in the planning of a visual rehabilitation programme (Lanners et al. 2005).

In recent years, the clinical pictures of the disease changed considerably because ROP practically disappeared over the 28th week of gestational age (GA), and the classical pictures became unusual. ROP is confirmed before the 26th week, with deeply different ophthalmoscopical pictures and its clinical course still in evolution. The ICCRP felt the need to describe the typical form of ELBW children, called aggressive posterior ROP (ICCRP 2005; Drenser et al. 2010). It is an extremely aggressive form which appeared from 2000 onwards, simultaneously to the increased survival of newborns with ELBW (less than 700 gr.) and GA at birth less than 26 weeks (Sanghi et al. 2014).

11.6.2 Congenital Oculomotor Apraxia, Type Cogan

This is another pathology which has comorbidity with CP and VI, which was described for the first time in 1952 (Wente et al. 2016) and which is very specific because there is an inability to make voluntary gaze movements. The child, intentionally, is not able to shift the gaze with a consequent inability in environmental and object exploration and difficulty in the adaptive and recognition functions.

Some distinctive characteristics are present:

- Hyperfixation
- Spasms in fixation
- Compensatory movements of the head
- Palpebral blinks of a compensatory nature
- Compensatory slowing down of the movements of the body and of the head to explore the environment more
- Inability to effect saccades

Oculomotor apraxia is also a clinical sign, which characterizes many motor and ophthalmological pathologies, including CP. It is often associated with ataxia; in fact, there is the ataxia with oculomotor apraxia 1 (AOA1), which is a neurological disease belonging to recessive autosomical cerebellar ataxias.

Oculomotion defects can be found in children with CP, who show apraxia or dyspraxia that indicates a total or partial disorganization of the oculomotor movements (Wente et al. 2016).

11.6.3 Joubert Syndrome

Joubert syndrome is another pathology, which is sometimes associated with CP; it is caused by brain malformations, particularly in the cerebellum vermis (Romani et al. 2013; Parisi 2019).

Joubert syndrome is a recessive autosomical disease characterized by episodic hyperpnea, abnormal ocular movements, ataxia, psychomotor retardation, and hypoplasia of the cerebellar vermis (molar tooth sign-MTS). It can also present retinal dystrophy (Wang et al. 2018) and renal abnormalities, with the possible following characteristics:

- Oculomotor apraxia from birth which impedes pursuit eye movements.
- Horizontal or rotatory nystagmus or chaotic eye movements.
- Oculo-digital signs, which can indicate almost blindness. These signs are common in childhood and tend to vanish during adolescence. The oculo-digital signs consist of three different behaviours:
  1. Pressure of the eyeball with the hand's palm ("eye-pressing")
  2. Pressure of the eyeball with the tip of the index finger introduced with strength near the side limits of the eye socket of the eyeball up to the medial shift of the eyeball ("eye-poking")
  3. Rubbing of the eyeball ("eye-rubbing")

In the Joubert syndrome, precise diagnosis and care are fundamental, to prevent complications and to be able to carry out multiple rehabilitative strategies (oculomotor rehabilitation, physiotherapy ...), thereby greatly improving the quality of life of the individual. The physiotherapy should aim to improve postural control and functioning. It is important to remember that sometimes the delay in motor development and communication may be secondary to the visual impairment; therefore, a rehabilitative neurophthalmological approach is important, particularly in the child with oculomotor apraxia.

It is therefore fundamental to support a multidisciplinary approach among all professionals who work in the rehabilitation field.

References

Alimovic S (2012) Visual impairments in children with cerebral palsy. Hrvatska Revija Za Rehabilitacijska Istrazivanja 48(1):96–103

Baranello G, Signorini S, Tinelli F, Guzzetta A, Pagliano E, Rossi A, Foscan M, Tramacere I, Romeo DMM, Ricci D (2020) Visual Function Classification System for children with cerebral palsy: development and validation. Dev. Med. Child Neurology, 62:104–110. https://doi.org/10.1111/dmcn.14270

Bathelt J, de Haan M, Dale NJ (2019) Adaptive behaviour and quality of life in school-age children with congenital visual disorders and different levels of visual impairment. Res Dev Disabil 85:154–162. https://doi.org/10.1016/j.ridd.2018.12.003

Battistin T, Lanners J, Vinciati M, Pinello L, Caldironi P (2005) Visual assessment in multidisabled children. ICS Elsevier 1282C:21–25. https://doi.org/10.1016/j.ics.2005.04.033

Bedny M, Pascual-Leone A, Saxe RR (2009) Growing up blind does not change the neural bases of Theory of Mind. Proc Natl Acad Sci U S A 106(27):11312–11317. https://doi.org/10.1073/pnas.0900010106

Berry KP, Nedivi E (2016) Experience-dependent structural plasticity in the visual system. Annu Rev Vis Sci 2:17–35. https://doi.org/10.1146/annurev-vision-111815-114638

Braddick O, Atkinson J (2013) Visual control of manual actions: brain mechanisms in typical development and developmental disorders. Dev Med Child Neurol 55(Suppl 4):13–18. https://doi.org/10.1111/dmcn.12300

Brazelton TB, Sparrow J (2007) The Touchpoints TM model of development. Brazelton Touchpoints Center, pp 1–10. https://www.touchpoints.org

Chokron S, Dutton GN (2016) Impact of Cerebral Visual Impairments on motor skills: implications for developmental coordination disorders. Front Psychol 7:1471. https://doi.org/10.3389/fpsyg.2016.01471

Consorti A, Sansevero G, Torelli C, Berardi N Sale A (2019) From basic visual science to neurodevelopmental disorders: the voyage of environmental enrichment-like stimulation. Neural Plast ID 5653180, 1–9. https://doi.org/10.1155/2019/5653180

Dale NJ, Sakkalou E, O'Reilly MA et al (2019) Home-based early intervention in infants and young children with visual impairment using the Developmental Journal: longitudinal cohort study. Dev Med Child Neurol 61(6):697–709. https://doi.org/10.1111/dmcn.14081

Di Pellegrino G, Fadiga L, Fogassi L, Gallese V, Rizzolatti G (1992) Understanding motor events: a neurophysiological study. Exp Brain Res 91:176–180. https://doi.org/10.1007/BF00230027

Drenser KA, Trese MT, Capone A (2010) Aggressive posterior retinopathy of prematurity. Retina 30(4 Suppl):S37–S40. https://doi.org/10.1097/IAE.0b013e3181cb6151

Ellis R, Tucker M (2000) Micro-affordance: the potentiation of components of action by seen objects. Br J Psychol 91:451–471. https://doi.org/10.1348/000712600161934

Fagerholm R, Vesti E (2017) Retinopathy of prematurity—from recognition of risk factors to treatment recommendations. Duodecim 133(4):337–344. PMID: 29205980

Fantz RL (1961) The origin of form perception. Sci Am 204:66–72. https://doi.org/10.1038/scientificamerican0561-66

Fazzi E, Signorini SG, Lanners J (2010a) The effect of impaired vision on development. In: Dutton GN, Bax M (eds) Visual Impairment in children due to damage to the brain. MacKeith Press, London, pp 162–173

Fazzi E, Signorini SG, Bianchi PE (2010b) Visual impairment in cerebral palsy. In: Dutton GN, Bax M (eds) Visual impairment in children due to damage to the brain. MacKeith Press, London, pp 194–204

Fazzi E, Signorini SG, LA Piana R et al (2012) Neuro-ophthalmological disorders in cerebral palsy: ophthalmological, oculomotor, and visual aspects. Dev Med Child Neurol 54(8):730–736. https://doi.org/10.1111/j.1469-8749.2012.04324.x

Fraiberg S (1977) Insights for the blind: comparative studies of blind and sighted infants. Plenum Press, New York

Geldof CJ, van Wassenaer-Leemhuis AG, Dik M, Kok JH, Oosterlaan J (2015) A functional approach to cerebral visual impairments in very preterm/very-low-birth-weight children. Pediatr Res 78(2):190–197. https://doi.org/10.1038/pr.2015.83

Gibson EJ, Walker AS (1984) Development of knowledge of visual-tactual affordances of substance. Child Dev 55(2):453–460. https://doi.org/10.2307/1129956

Good W, Jan J, DeSa L, Barkovich J, Groenveld M, Hoyt C (1994) Cortical visual impairment in children. Surv Ophthalmol 38:351–364. https://doi.org/10.1016/0039-6257(94)90073-6

Hadders-Algra M (2014) Early diagnosis and early intervention in cerebral palsy. Front Neurol 5:185. https://doi.org/10.3389/fneur.2014.00185

Hafström M, Källén K, Serenius F et al (2018) Cerebral palsy in extremely preterm infants. Pediatrics 141(1):e20171433. https://doi.org/10.1542/peds.2017-1433

Hallemans A, Ortibus E, Truijen S, Meire F (2011) Development of independent locomotion in children with a severe visual impairment. Res Dev Disabil 32:2069–2074. https://doi.org/10.1016/j.ridd.2011.08.017

Haupt C, Huber AB (2008) How axons see their way—axonal guidance in the visual system. Front Biosci 13:3136–3149. https://doi.org/10.2741/2915

Himmelmann K, Beckung E, Hagberg G, Uvebrant P (2006) Gross and fine motor function and accompanying impairments in cerebral palsy. Dev Med Child Neurol 48:417–423. https://doi.org/10.1017/S0012162206000922

Hotz GA, Castelblanco A, Lara IM, Weiss AD, Duncan R, Kuluz JW (2006) Snoezelen: a controlled multi-sensory stimulation therapy for children recovering from severe brain injury. Brain Inj 20:879–888. https://doi.org/10.1080/02699050600832635

Huurneman B, Boonstra FN (2016) Assessment of near visual acuity in 0-13 year olds with normal and low vision: a systematic review. BMC Ophthalmol [Internet] 16(1):1–15. https://doi.org/10.1186/s12886-016-0386-y

Hyvärinen L, Walthes R, Jacob N, Chaplin KN, Leonhardt M (2014) Current understanding of what infants see. Curr Ophthalmol Rep 2(4):142–149. https://doi.org/10.1007/s40135-014-0056-2

ICCRP (International Committee for the Classification of Retinopathy of Prematurity) (2005) The international classification of retinopathy of prematurity revisited. Arch Ophthalmol 123(7):991–999. https://doi.org/10.1001/archopht.123.7.991

Ishihara S (1972) The series of plates designed as tests for colour-blindness. Kanehara Shuppan Co. Ltd, Tokyo

Jan J, Lyons C, Heaven R, Matsuba C (2001) Visual impairment due to a dyskinetic eye movement disorder in children with dyskinetic cerebral palsy. Dev Med Child Neurol 43(2):108–112. https://doi.org/10.1017/S0012162201000184

Kitchel E (2000) The effects of blue light on ocular health. J Vis Impair Blindness 94(6):399–403. https://doi.org/10.1177/0145482.X0009400606

Klinge C, Röder B, Büchel C (2010) Increased amygdala activation to emotional auditory stimuli in the blind. Brain 133:1729–1736. https://doi.org/10.1093/brain/awq102

Koenraads Y, Braun KP, van der Linden DC, Imhof SM, Porro GL (2015) Perimetry in young and neurologically impaired children: the Behavioral Visual Field (BEFIE) Screening Test revisited. JAMA Ophthalmol 133(3):319–325. https://doi.org/10.1001/jamaophthalmol.2014.5257

Lang J (1983) A new stereotest. J Pediatr Ophthalmol Strabismus 20(2):72–74

Lanners J, Salvo R (2000) Un bambino da incontrare. Fondazione Robert Hollman

Lanners J, Goergen E (2001) Functional evaluation and rehabilitation of severely visually impaired children (0-4 years). Vis Impair Res 3(1):1–5. https://doi.org/10.1076/vimr.3.1.1.4416

Lanners J, Piccioni A, Fea F, Goergen E (1999) Early intervention for children with cerebral visual impairment: preliminary results. J Intellect Disabil Res 43(Part 1):1–12. https://doi.org/10.1046/j.1365-2788.1999.43120106.x

Lanners J, Battistin T, Del Negro E, Segnacasi S, Caldironi P (2005) Early rehabilitation in ROP children. Int Congr Ser 1282(1):191–195. https://doi.org/10.1016/j.ics.2005.05.095

Lueck AH, Dutton GN, Ophth FRC, Chokron S (2019) Profiling children with Cerebral Visual Impairment using multiple methods of assessment to aid in differential diagnosis. Semin Pediatr Neurol 31:5–14. Elsevier Inc. https://doi.org/10.1016/j.spen.2019.05.003

Marret S, Marchand-Martin L, Picaud JC et al (2013) Brain injury in very preterm children and neurosensory and cognitive disabilities during childhood: the EPIPAGE cohort study. PLoS One 8(5):e62683. https://doi.org/10.1371/journal.pone.0062683

Meeus L (1994) Stimulation of the visual possibilities in the Dark Room by means of black light and other light sources. Series Studies in Health Technology and Informatics, vol 11, Low vision: 320–322. https://doi.org/10.3233/978-1-60750-855-7-320

Mercuriali E, Battistin T, Schoch V, Di Maggio I, Suppiej A (2016) L'importanza del counseling precoce alla famiglia: L'esperienza presso la Fondazione Robert Hollman. Il counselling in Italia. Funzioni, criticità, prospettive e applicazioni, Ed. Cleup, pp 501–516

Novak I, Hines M, Goldsmith S, Barclay R (2012) Clinical prognostic messages from a systematic review on cerebral palsy. Pediatrics 130:e1285. https://doi.org/10.1542/peds.2012-0924

Orban GA, Van Essen D, Vanduffel W (2004) Comparative mapping of higher visual areas in monkeys and humans. Trends Cogn Sci 8(7):315–324. https://doi.org/10.1016/j.tics.2004.05.009

Parisi MA (2019) The molecular genetics of Joubert syndrome and related ciliopathies: the challenges of genetic and phenotypic heterogeneity. Transl Sci Rare Dis 4(1–2):25–49. https://doi.org/10.3233/TRD-190041

Pavone P et al (2017) Ataxia in children: early recognition and clinical evaluation. Ital J Pediatr 43:6. https://doi.org/10.1186/s13052-016-0325-9

Pereins G, Ortibus E (2016) Concept and overview of cerebral visual impairment: a clinical perspective. In: Visual impairment and Neurodevelopmental disorders: from diagnosis to rehabilitation. John Libbey Eurotext, pp 71–84

Philip SS, Dutton GN (2014) Identifying and characterising cerebral visual impairment in children: a review. Clin Exp Optom 97:196–208. https://doi.org/10.1111/cxo.12155

Philip SS, Guzzetta A, Chorna O, Gole G, Boyd RN (2020) Relationship between brain structure and Cerebral Visual Impairment in children with Cerebral Palsy: a systematic review. Res Dev Disabil 99, 1–16, 103580. https://doi.org/10.1016/j.ridd.2020.103580

Pietrini P, Furey ML, Ricciardi E et al (2004) Beyond sensory images: object-based representation in the human ventral pathway. Proc Natl Acad Sci U S A 101(15):5658–5663. https://doi.org/10.1073/pnas.0400707101

Porro G, Dekker EM, Van Nieuwenhuizen O et al (1998) Visual behaviours of neurologically impaired children with cerebral visual impairment: an ethological study. Br J Ophthalmol 82(11):1231–1235. https://doi.org/10.1136/bjo.82.11.1231

Prechtl HF, Cioni G, Einspieler C, Bos AF, Ferrari F (2001) Role of vision on early motor development: lessons from the blind. Dev Med Child Neurol 43(3):198–201. https://doi.org/10.1111/j.1469-8749.2001.tb00187.x

Preston KL, McDonald M, Sebris SL, Dobson V, Teller DY (1987) Validation of the acuity card procedure for assessment of infants with ocular disorders. Ophthalmology [Internet] 94(6):644–653. https://doi.org/10.1016/S0161-6420(87)33398-6

Provenzi L, Rosa E, Visintin E, Mascheroni E, Guida E, Cavallini A, Montirosso R (2020) Understanding the role and function of maternal touch in children with neurodevelopmental disabilities. Infant Behav Dev 58:101420. https://doi.org/10.1016/j.infbeh.2020.101420

Purpura G, Tinelli F (2020) The development of vision between nature and nurture: clinical implications from visual neuroscience. Childs Nerv Syst 36:911–917. https://doi.org/10.1007/s00381-020-04554-1

Ricciardi E, Bonino D, Pellegrini S, Pietrini P (2014) Mind the blind brain to understand the sighted one! Is there a supramodal cortical functional architecture? Neurosci Biobehav Rev 41:64–77. https://doi.org/10.1016/j.neubiorev.2013.10.006

Roman-Lantzy C (2018) Cortical visual impairment: an approach to assessment and intervention, 2nd edn. AFB Press, New York

Romani M, Micalizzi A, Valente EM (2013) Joubert Syndrome: congenital cerebellar ataxia with the molar tooth. Lancet Neurol 12(9):894–905. https://doi.org/10.1016/S1474-4422(13)70136-4

Rosenbaum P, Paneth N, Leviton A, et al. (2007) A report: the definition and classification of cerebral palsy. April 2006. Dev Med Child Neurol Suppl 109:8–14. Erratum in: Dev Med Child Neurol (2007) 49(6):480. https://doi.org/10.1111/j.1469-8749.2007.00001.x

Sanghi G, Dogra MR, Katoch D, Gupta A (2014) Aggressive posterior retinopathy of prematurity in infants ≥1500 g birth weight. Indian J Ophthalmol 62(2):254–257. https://doi.org/10.4103/0301-4738.128639

Saunders KJ, Little JA, Mc Clelland J, Jackson AJ (2010) Profile of refractive errors in cerebral palsy: impact of severity of motor impairment (GMFCS) and CP subtype on refractive outcome. Invest Ophthalmol Vis Sci 51(6):2885–2890. https://doi.org/10.1167/iovs.09-4670

Siatkowski RM, Good WV, Summers CG, Quinn GE, Tung B (2013) Clinical characteristics of children with severe visual impairment but favorable retinal structural outcomes from the Early Treatment for Retinopathy of Prematurity (ETROP) study. J AAPOS 17(2):129–134. https://doi.org/10.1016/j.jaapos.2012.10.022

Signorini SG, Fedeli C, Luparia A et al (2016) A multidisciplinary and multidimensional approach to visual function in childhood: from neurovisual disorders to strategies of intervention for promoting neuropsychomotor development. In: Fazzi E, Bianchi PE (eds) Visual impairment and neurodevelopmental disorders—from diagnosis to rehabilitation. John Libbey Eurotext, London-Paris, pp 155–170

Solebo AL, Teoh L, Rahi J (2017) Epidemiology of blindness in children. Arch Dis Child 102(9):853–857. https://doi.org/10.1136/archdischild-2016-310532

Sonksen PM, Dale N (2002) Visual impairment in infancy: impact on neurodevelopmental and neurobiological processes. Dev Med Child Neurol 44:782–791. https://doi.org/10.1111/j.1469-8749.2002.tb00287.x

Stern DN (1985) The interpersonal world of the infant. Basic Books, New York

Surman G, Hemming K, Platt MJ, Parkes J, Green A, Hutton J, Kurinczuk JJ (2009) Children with cerebral palsy: severity and trends over time. Paediatr Perinat Epidemiol 23(6):513–521. https://doi.org/10.1111/j.1365-3016.2009.01060.x

Tierney AL, Nelson CA 3rd. (2009) Brain development and the role of experience in the early years. Zero Three 30(2):9–13

Trevarthen C, Aitken KJ (2001) Infant intersubjectivity: research, theory, and clinical applications. J Child Psychol Psychiatry 42(1):3–48. https://doi.org/10.1017/S0021963001006552

Umiltà MA, Kohler E, Gallese V, Fogassi L, Fadiga L, Keysers C, Rizzolatti G (2001) I know what you are doing: a neurophysiological study. Neuron 31(1):155–165. https://doi.org/10.1016/S0896-6273(01)00337-3

Vaglio S, Battistin T, Lanners J, Lodigiani S, Panizzolo L, Segnacasi S, Zaccheo D, Schoch V (2018) Caratteristiche e comportamenti visivi nei bambini ipovedenti con danno neurologico associato. Oftalmol Soc 3:29–36

Vincer MJ, Allen AC, Joseph KS, Stinson DA, Scott H, Wood E (2006) Increasing prevalence of cerebral palsy among very preterm infants: a population-based study. Pediatrics 118(6):e1621–e1626. https://doi.org/10.1542/peds.2006-1522

Wang SF, Kowal TJ, Ning K, Koo EB, Wu AY, Mahajan VB, Sun Y (2018) Review of ocular manifestations of Joubert Syndrome. Genes (Basel) 9(12):605. https://doi.org/10.3390/genes9120605

Wente S, Schröder S, Buckard J, Büttel HM, von Deimling F, Diener W, Häussler M, Hübschle S et al (2016) Nosological delineation of congenital ocular motor apraxia type Cogan: an observational study. Orphanet J Rare Dis 11(1):104. https://doi.org/10.1186/s13023-016-0486-z

WHO (2019a) World Health Organization. International Statistical Classification of Diseases and Related Health Problem. 10th Revision, https://icd.who.int/browse10/2019/en#/H53-H54

WHO (2019b) World Health Organization. International Statistical Classification of Diseases and Related Health Problem. 11th Revision https://icd.who.int/browse11/l-m/en

WHO (2019c) World report on vision. https://www.who.int/publications/i/item/world-report-on-vision

WHO (2020) Blindness and vision impairment prevention. https://www.who.int/blindness/causes/priority/en/index1.html

Augmentative and Alternative Communication in Severe Motor Impairment

12

Gabriella Veruggio and Monica Panella

"The silence of speechlessness is never golden. We all need to communicate and connect with each other – not just in one way, but in as many ways as possible. It is a basic human need, a basic human right. And more than this, it is a basic human power..." (Williams 2000).

From birth and all through the first years of life, communication plays a fundamental role in the child's development. Effective communication is essential for personal maturation, social participation, personal care, education and work. It is also an essential component for patient safety in healthcare and the defence of rights in the legal context (ASHA 2004).

The National Joint Committee for the Communication Needs of Persons with Severe Disability (NJC) defines communication as *"every act through which a person provides or receives information from another person about needs, wants, perceptions, knowledge, or emotional states"* (NJC, USA 1992, 2016).

A good communicator masters the complex interaction between oromotor articulation, linguistic and auditory skills (Kent 2004; Smith and Goffman 2004; Nip et al. 2011). Communication, as defined by Schindler (1990), is an exchange of messages between two or more people, through one or more communication channels (pragmatic, analogic and digital) with the use of arbitrarily chosen signs.

"People cannot act as main players in their lives if they are unable to communicate effectively with others, to make decisions and make recognized and understood choices" (Light and Gulens 2000).

G. Veruggio (✉)
AAC Service of Benedetta d'Intino Centre, Milan, Italy

M. Panella
Rehabilitation Department, Degli Infermi Hospital, Ponderano (Biella), Italy
e-mail: panella.monica@aslbi.piemonte.it

© The Author(s), under exclusive license to Springer Nature Switzerland AG 2022
P. Giannoni, L. Zerbino (eds.), *Cerebral Palsy*,
https://doi.org/10.1007/978-3-030-85619-9_12

12.1 Communication Disorders in Severe Motor Impairment

Communication disorders in children with severe motor disabilities are present in a wide range of cases that varies from 30% (Pellegrino 2002) to 80% (Odding et al. 2006). They are characterized by heterogeneity in type and severity of dysfunction, depending on the extent and location of the neurological lesion, on environmental experiences and on how soon the intervention is started. Whereas, in situations of severe pathologies, attention is often focused on the clinical and medical complexities of the child and communication needs tend to be postponed.

When children have temporary or permanent difficulties in using speech, they encounter many challenges, because they are unable to communicate their basic needs, desires, knowledge and emotions to their family members, peers and teachers and to the wider community. When motor disabilities are present, there are communication disorders on several levels, related to speech and language and often both. These will limit the child's general development, participation and autonomy.

12.1.1 Speech Disorders

Verbal production requires the cortical motor control of the speech subsystems and difficulty at any level compromises the communicative act with varying levels of severity. Articulation motor control (speech) requires involvement and coordination between peripheral and central structures, including four anatomical and physiological subsystems: respiratory, laryngeal, velopharyngeal and orofacial (Netsell 1986). The brain regions involved in articulatory motor control are organized into two distinct but interconnected networks that relate to planning and motor articulatory execution (Riecker et al. 2005).

In severe motor impairments, dysarthria is the most common speech disorder resulting from neural lesions that compromise the sensory processes needed for motor articulatory programming and planning (Darley et al. 1975; Netsell 2001). Strength, speed, timing, pitch, tone and accuracy are affected.

Depending on the location and extent of neurological damage, the symptoms that may occur in the dysarthric child range from difficulties in controlling saliva and feeding skills (swallowing and chewing), difficulty in pneumo-phonic coordination and difficulty in articulating speech. They can reach a gravity of complete anarthria. These dysfunctions affect breathing, phonation, resonance, articulation and prosody as well as respiratory, larynx, velopharyngeal and orofacial control (Arvedson and Brodsky 2002). Structural anomalies can also interfere with verbal production, such as severe malocclusions (Darley et al. 1975; Yogi et al. 2018). During the assessment phase, it is essential to evaluate all the speech subsystems and the interactions between them (McNeil 2008; Lowit and Kent 2010; Swigert 2010; Duffy 2013).

The other speech disorder observed in children with severe motor impairment is verbal dyspraxia, a neurological language disorder in which the accuracy and the consistency of speech subsystem movements are altered in the absence of neuromuscular deficits. The verbal dyspraxia core deficit relates to space-time planning and/or programming, involving inconsistent errors, articulatory transitions and prosody alteration (ASHA 2007). Often, dysarthria and verbal dyspraxia can coexist.

There are specific speech assessment scales, such as the Viking Speech Scale (Pennington et al. 2010) which uses four levels to classify the children's voice production intelligibility and the Hustad-Gorton-Lee (Hustad et al. 2010) classification, concerning speech and language impairment.

12.1.2 Language Disorders

Linguistic competence was defined by Chomsky (1965) as the language knowledge and the human faculty of communication. This competence can be grammatical (the set of knowledge about the language unit organization) and pragmatic. Language, understood as the mental act underlying the communicative one, involves the cognitive-linguistic domain. It represents the ability to perceive and interpret sensory input, conceptual categories and executive functions (Hayden 2004) and includes five components: pragmatic, semantics, syntax, morphology and phonology (Paul and Norbury 2012).

The children who use AAC often have disorders or delay in all these areas. Therefore strategies that are specifically aimed at language development need to be an integral part of every communication intervention.

12.2 Augmentative and Alternative Communication (AAC)

AAC was officially initiated in 1983 in Toronto, together with the creation of the International Society of Augmentative Alternative Communication (ISAAC). However, as a field of study and intervention, AAC's history has its roots in the past (Zangari et al. 1994).

"AAC refers to an area comprised of research, clinical practice and education. AAC involves actions to study and to compensate for when necessary, temporary or permanent communication impairments, activity limitations, and participation restriction of persons with severe disorders of speech-language production and/or comprehension, including spoken and written modes of communication" (ASHA 2004; Beukelman and Light 2020).

The term "augmentative" indicates that AAC's techniques, methods and tools are primarily aimed not at replacing existing communication means but at increasing natural communication through the enhancement of the natural communication modes (vocal, mimic-gestural, visual, etc.). The term "alternative" means that the AAC uses, when necessary, special means and communication tools that may include special techniques and strategies as well as tools such as graphic symbols, writing, gestures, communication devices, etc.

Evidence in the literature and emerging from clinical experience underlines how the use of AAC approach is extremely effective in children with severe motor impairment and complex communication needs (CCN). AAC can be used both to promote expressive communication and to support language comprehension, which are essential for development. Although its most obvious role is to provide severely motor-challenged children with an augmented and/or alternative communication means, the AAC can also be used to increase speech and existing vocalizations and to improve the intelligibility of the message (Romski and Sevcik 1988). Where possible, AAC enhances speech development, as it increases the interaction opportunities and language skills and provides language models both through the communication partner's modelling and through the speech-generating devices (Millar et al. 2006).

The AAC scope is to support communication development, providing a communication means as independent as possible and maximizing the skills and participation opportunities of individuals with CCN. This CCN term indicates complex communication needs that concern not only the need to communicate with others but also the means, forms and tools necessary to satisfy it.

Over the years, AAC field has progressively addressed the many changes and development in interpersonal and social communication modalities and means. In the 1980s, the AAC focus was primarily on maximizing the communication of individuals with communication difficulties within face-to-face interactions, whereas now there is increased recognition that communication needs to extend well beyond these face-to-face interactions. Nowadays, for example, there is major use of written and remote communication at school and the workplace for personal expression, Internet access, social media, cell phones, texting, blogging, e-commerce, etc. (Light and McNaughton 2014). These changes in everyday custom have resulted in increased communication demands that need to be addressed through AAC intervention, in order to guarantee that all individuals with CCN develop the necessary knowledge, judgment and skills to facilitate their communicative competencies (see Sect. 12.4: "Become a good communication partner").

The characteristics of people receiving AAC services are changing continually in terms of age, types of disabilities, environments and living conditions. Children and adolescents with severe cerebral palsy (CP) make up one etiological group in which AAC interventions are or should be implemented almost routinely (Mirenda and Mathy-Laikko 1989).

12.3 General Intervention Guidelines

In children with severe motor impairment, communication disorders can be predictable and are often described as an associated disorder. AAC interventions should be initiated as early as possible integrated into the overall rehabilitation project. The child with CCN and their family need access to AAC interventions starting from the first months of the child's life. This support will be aimed at promoting the baby's communication and language skills, as well as their relational and cognitive development (Romski et al. 2015).

As with all rehabilitation interventions, AAC needs a wide-ranging multidisciplinary team so that a "communication culture" can be shared, not only among the different rehabilitation professionals (Blackstone 2010) but also with others that are involved with the child and the family for different reasons (e.g. paediatrician, nurses, educators and caregivers).

Over the course of life, people with CCN obviously change in their clinical evolution, partners and daily environments, usually requiring long-term AAC interventions. In children with CP it is essential to continue intervention throughout schooling and beyond. The general communication system (GCS) of the children with severe motor impairment needs to be designed and constantly adapted to the interpersonal communication and participation needs, considering their various life contexts, such as home, school, day care or residential living centre and leisure environments.

Assistive technology (AT) plays a key role in enabling access to communication devices, computers, mobile technologies and social media and more generally in fostering communication and participation in the community.

The ultimate aim of AAC interventions is to improve the active participation of individuals with CCN in daily and social life, following the indications of the International Classification of Functioning, Disability and Health (ICF) (WHO 2001, 2007; Raghavendra et al. 2007), and to increase their level of participation in social life, allowing them to become protagonists of their own lives (Hill and Romich 2006; Brady et al. 2016).

For all these reasons, AAC projects are highly personalized and based on the individual person, their communication partners and their living environments. They should be implemented by an AAC team.

12.3.1 Assessment of Communication Disorders

All AAC interventions need to be based on appropriate assessments.

Because of the wide variety of motor disabilities in children with CP, the assessment requires the expertise of a team of professionals, comprised of AAC experts (including technicians trained in AAC and Assistive Technology) and other rehabilitation professionals (neurologists, occupational therapists, speech therapists, physiotherapists, orthopedics specialists). In addition, the child's family members and, if possible, the child/adolescent themselves, along with caregivers, educators, teachers and other significant people in the child's life, should be involved. It is necessary to determine the appropriate general level communication system (GCS) for each individual child, which responds not only to current communication needs but also considers those of the future.

The AAC assessment relies on the participation model (Beukelman and Mirenda 1988), which provides a dynamic and systematic evaluation process, leading to the implementation of functional interventions, based on the individual communication needs. In this model, it is also considered the participation needs of nondisabled peers of the same age, in the various situations and activities of daily life, co-using the AAC system.

Access barriers can contribute to limiting the child's participation, and therefore it is important to carry out a detailed analysis of the individual's resources, rather than of their deficits, to identify the real opportunities to improve their communication (Schlosser and Lee 2000).

- Opportunity barriers refer to restrictions on participation not directly related to the individual person with CCN but to environmental factors. They may relate to the policies and operational practices existing in the individual's living environments and also to the skills and abilities of their partners, attitudes and beliefs.
- Access barriers refer to the limits in abilities and resources of the individual person with CCN and can relate to their motor, perceptual, cognitive, linguistic and learning impairments. Comprehension problems can be relatively more difficult to assess and they may depend on various factors. At the same time they are crucial in setting up any AAC intervention (Romski et al. 1997). The access barriers' assessment is conducted using the typical clinical tools and, for the specific aspect of communication, also the dynamic assessment (DA) (Snell 2002).

In AAC, communication assessment relies on observation and on DA, during which interactive strategies are used (Iacono et al. 1998). The observer proposes play activities which provide opportunities to evaluate the child's communication intentions and competences.

The child's spontaneous means of expressing themself are also assessed together with their receptive abilities, degree of intentionality, the communicative functions in use (e.g. attention-getting, choice-making, object or action request, etc.) and the ability to modify strategies used to repair communication breakdowns.

An early intervention program will be set up based on the DA data, the results of which will contribute to a more accurate communication assessment (circular evaluation and intervention process) during communicative exchanges in different life contexts and with different partners.

Many other assessment tools can be used in various environments, starting from easier communicators, such as the Communication Matrix (Rowland 2004), the Interactive Checklist for Augmentative Communication (INCH) (Bolton and Dashiell 1991), the SETT Model (Zabala 1993) and Triple C (Bloomberg et al. 2009).

12.3.1.1 Assessing Communication and Participation Opportunities

The therapist can use many different strategies and tools to assess the real opportunities for communication and participation existing in the child's life: direct observations in everyday environments, videos, interviews and the compilation of specific forms (Beukelman and Light 2020). The aim is to identify the discrepancies in different contexts and activities, between peer communication behaviours and participation patterns, compared to those of the children using AAC.

AAC intervention may also aim at rethinking or building real and personalized opportunities for communication and participation at home, school, rehabilitation services, day care centre, pool and leisure settings. Moreover, it is important to identify all the necessary environmental adaptations in play and for access to daily routines (Musselwhite 1986).

Finally, it is essential to identify the child's communication partners and enhance their communication modalities and interaction patterns. This is because, according to the Participation ICF Model, these "partners" can become facilitators and implementors of AAC intervention or, on the contrary, a potential source of a barrier to communication (Blackstone and Hunt Berg 2003).

12.3.1.2 Alternative Access Assessment

The term "access" refers here to how a person with CCN can use an AAC system that could be unaided or aided. Unaided systems are intended as those modalities of linguistic expression, like speech and deictic gestures, which do not involve external objects while aided systems do use physical objects. These can be low technological devices like a simple pen and paper, a communication board or a book containing photographs and/or symbols or devices considered high technology such as a speech-generating device (SGD) with voice output.

In children with communication disorders and severe motor impairment, the AAC team should make an early assessment of the feasible access methods (alternative access) to AAC systems (Goossens' and Crain 1992; Silverman 1995; Higginbotham et al. 2007; Curry and Robinson 2010).

During the first evaluation, the therapist should immediately identify an access method to be used during the assessment itself (e.g. can the child communicate *yes* and *no*?) and the kind of AAC systems suitable for the child in the short and possibly long term.

Children with CP can also have visual and auditory impairments, sensory-perceptual disorders, cognitive impairments, postural control and positioning problems, especially in sitting. It is, therefore, essential that the occupational therapist or physiotherapist makes an initial assessment of the child's positioning (York and Weimann 1991; Costigan and Light 2011). If the child is not adequately positioned and supported in the seated position, their real communication abilities can be greatly underestimated (Fig. 12.1).

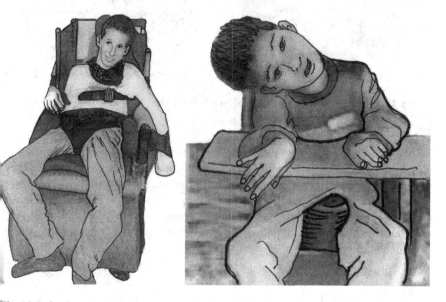

Fig. 12.1 Inadequate positioning compromises face-to-face interactions and AAC systems access

The seated posture assessment and positioning optimization are the starting conditions for the initial AAC assessment and for the identification of a more functional method of accessing the AAC, both unaided and aided. However, in the later stages of intervention, it will be necessary to evaluate the communication access possibilities in the different postures used during the day, because the child with CCN should be able to communicate at all times.

Communicating Throughout All the Day
Depending on the different postures used by the child, it will often be necessary to identify different AAC access methods. For example, when the child is well-positioned in their wheelchair, they might be able to use an index finger to point to a symbol on their communication board inserted in the lap tray. On the contrary, when lying in bed, the child might be unable to use their upper limbs in the same way and so here they need to use eye pointing.

Different types of communication support may be needed, depending on the postural and mobility aids used during the day. For example, a communication board can be placed on a mobility aid (Fig. 12.2).

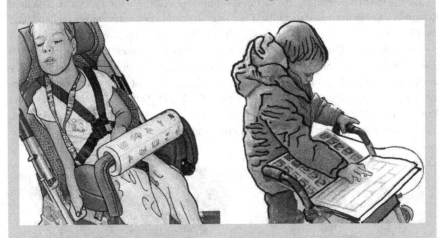

Fig. 12.2 Communication boards placed on a mobility aid

After the initial evaluation phase, the occupational and/or physical therapist will have to implement the positioning system most suitable for the child's needs. They will need to identify not only an adequate sitting aid but also the possible use of other components of the positioning system, e.g. supports to the pelvis, trunk, lower and upper limbs and often head (York and Weimann 1991) (Fig. 12.3), and also the most suitable lap tray desk type (transparent, opaque, padded or unpadded, with or without a border, etc.).

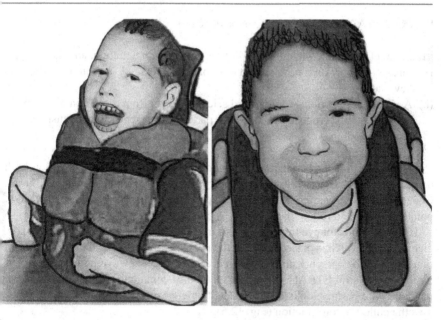

Fig. 12.3 Head supports and anchoring systems to facilitate access to AAC systems

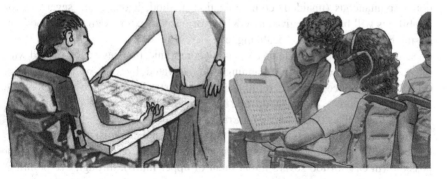

Fig. 12.4 The constant inclusion of AAC systems on the lap tray promotes communication initiative and allows greater autonomy

The constant presence of a lap tray is often a key condition for allowing children with severe CP to access to an AAC system (Fig. 12.4). It not only provides the child with a more appropriate postural alignment and greater stability, but it also acts as an essential support for assembling the communication devices (e.g. communication board, SGDs, environmental control systems, etc.). In this way the child can independently access his communication device, without depending on the availability of another person, for example, as when their teacher has to get the communication board stored in the backpack attached to the wheelchair.

Access to AAC-aided systems can be done either by

(a) A direct selection, when a child directly points to an item (e.g. an object, a picture, a symbol) on a communication board or presses a key on a SGD or the keyboard
(b) A scanning selection, when a child selects an item from those that are verbally and/or visually proposed to him by a partner or presented on the display of a scanning aid

Direct selection can be made with fingers or through eye pointing on a low-tech device (e.g. ETRAN) or a high-tech device (e.g. Eye Tracking device, iMotions, Copenhagen, NL) or even with pointers applied to the head (e.g. headstick, light pointers) or more rarely to the foot or to the mouth.

ETRAN stands for eye transfer and is a transparent panel with letters, symbols or pictures on it, which is placed between the person with CCN and their communication partner. The person with CCN selects sequentially—by eye pointing—the letters or symbols on ETRAN, using this method to communicate the desired word/message. The partner looks at the selected letters, receives the message and then asks the child for confirmation (Fig. 12.5).

In the scanning selection, the child selects an item among those proposed by a partner, communicating their choice—i.e. giving an Ok—through their more functional spontaneous (unaided) communication method. People with severe motor disabilities will be able to give an "OK" in various ways, for example, by nodding, raising their eyes upwards, vocalizing, etc.

Scanning can also be made on a scanning communication device, organized with linear, circular, row/column, scanning and activated by one or two switches (Fig. 12.6). It is necessary to carefully select the most suitable switches based on the functional resources of the child and also decide how to place and mount the switches themselves (Goossens' and Crain 1992).

During the initial access assessment, the occupational therapist evaluates first the child's ability to make a direct selection with his fingers or hand or, if that is not possible (in case of too severe impairment of upper limbs), through eye pointing.

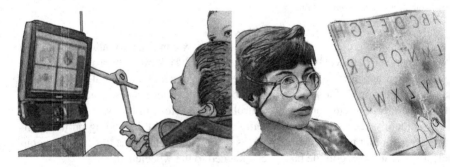

Fig. 12.5 Direct selection trough eye pointing (ETRAN use) and eye tracking device

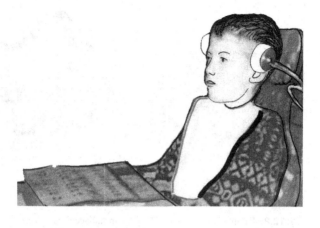

Fig. 12.6 Scanning selection via switches activated by head movements

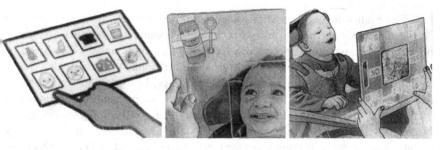

Fig. 12.7 Various types of communication supports for initial access assessment

The child can use various types of preset communication supports, for example, a simple choice board or an ETRAN device (Fig. 12.7) or even a simple VOCA (voice output communication aids) operated by big size switches, as BIGmack[1] (Fig. 12.8).

When direct selection is not possible in any way, the therapist uses visual/auditory scanning, proposing interesting choices for the child, for example, "do you want to play with the doll, with the washing machine, with the oven"? or "do you want a coke, a juice, or water"?

In the later stages of the intervention, the AAC team identifies a long-term alternative access technique and delves into the factors that may influence its use.

Another important aspect to assess is that relating to visual and visual-perceptual problems, which is essential to define both the characteristics of the AAC system and the visual environmental adaptations required by alternative access. Colour, background, size and distribution/organization of the identified set of symbols are fundamental characteristics to take into consideration when proposing a communication tool (Utley 2002).

---

[1] AbleNet, Inc., Roseville, MN (USA), https://www.ablenetinc.com/

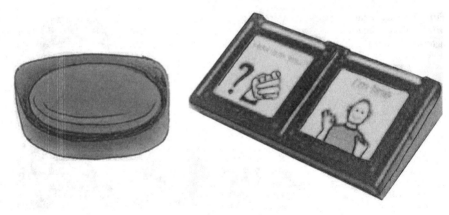

Fig. 12.8 BIGmack and other VOCA for initial access assessment

When evaluating children with severe motor disabilities, the AAC team may decide that the child needs more than a single communication device, such as mixed-mode communication systems, for example, a multimodal GCS, based on both the use of natural spontaneous means and aided communication tools.

Different techniques, strategies and AAC tools may be used in different contexts and with different partners, depending on the real communication functions and participation opportunities. For example, a child can use natural communication means with their family but a communication board to communicate at school. They can communicate with classmates or the teacher using a tablet or an ETRAN or follow the school activities using a computer with scanning software or a headstick equipped with a brush when painting.

However, it is important to periodically reassess the child's potential to update and optimize the functional access to AAC systems, for example, to improve the upper limb use for a direct selection or a head movement to activate a switch.

12.3.1.3 Language Assessment

Language assessment for AAC should include an evaluation of the individual's single-word vocabulary capabilities as well as their common language structures (i.e. morphemes, syntax).

In recent years, several AAC researchers have noted the importance of assessing morphosyntactic and grammatical knowledge, since those who have not mastered skills in these areas are likely to have difficulty conveying ideas, fulfilling academic requirements, etc. (Blockberger and Johnston 2003).

Speech therapists can use standardized instruments (Beukelman and Light 2020), but some adaptations could be necessary when assessing children with severe motor impairment. Often the speech therapist relies on a functional evaluation both to support the relationship with the family and the cognitive and linguistic development of the child (ASHA 2004).

12.4   Strategies to Enhance Communication

In severe CP child, AAC intervention is aimed at evolving, where possible, their communication from pre-intentional forms to intentional non-symbolic forms and later to the most evolved forms of symbolic expression.

As Light (1989) first proposed, communicative competences rest on the integration of knowledge, judgment and skills, in four interrelated domains: linguistic, operational, social and strategic. These competencies also depend on psychosocial factors (motivation, attitude, confidence and resilience) as well as environmental barriers and supports (Light and McNaughton 2014).

- Linguistic domain refers to skills in the native language spoken and written in the home and in the broader social community
- Operational domain is to produce unaided symbols, operates aided AAC systems/apps accurately and efficiently (e.g. plan and produce required coded body movements, such as looking upwards to say "yes") and other social media and mainstream communication tools
- Social domain is to develop appropriate sociolinguistic skills (e.g. fulfil turns in interaction, as request for information) and socio-relation skills (e.g. be responsive to partners)
- Strategic domain is the use of compensatory strategies to bypass limitations in the linguistic domain (e.g. ask the partner to provide choice to overcome vocabulary limitation), in the operational domain (e.g. ask the partner to predict how the message is spelled to reduce fatigue and enhance the rate of communication) or in the social domain (e.g. utilize social media)

The intervention project also has to support and train the different communication partners that the child will meet in their life (Blackstone and Hunt Berg 2003; Pepper and Weitzman 2004). It is also important to create a communicative environment that optimizes the child's communication development.

Becoming a Good Communication Partner

It is essential, for children with CCN, to have communication partners who can interact and relate effectively with them, recognizing their communication means and promoting their communication initiative. Some essential communication partner competences are as follows:

- **Observe and respond**
  Communication is more than just words! A good partner observes and recognizes all the child communicative signals through facial expression, body language, vocalization, etc., to understand their communicative func-

tions (e.g. understand how the child expresses acceptance or rejection) and to respond to all the child's communicative attempts.

- **Wait—give time—take turns**
  During a conversation, a competent partner (a) waits, (b) gives the child their turn and (c) gives the child the time to start the communicative exchange to express interests and feelings, to answer questions using their unaided and aided communication means and to share the control of the conversation and not only just responding to the partner's questions.

- **Create communication opportunities**
  It is essential to create real communication opportunities, starting from daily routines during feeding and bath time, outdoor walks and play, to enhance all communicative functions to support the child's self-determination (e.g. to make choices and requests, share information and considerations, etc.).

- **Add language and experiences appropriate to the child's level of development**
  During the daily routines, which allow for shared interaction a competent partner describes what is happening with simple sentences using words, gestures, facial expressions, voice tone, etc. They give the child the words they need to understand add information and experiences and expand what the child is doing and communicating. They also model the messages used during the communication exchange on the child's aided AAC system.

12.4.1 Early Communication Intervention

Early communication intervention needs to be implemented as early as possible (Cress and Marvin 2003; Beukelman and Light 2020), and it is aimed at the beginning communicator, their partners and the environment. The purpose is to support comprehension, increase the use of the most functional natural communication modes and enhance and support communicative intentionality, together with the development of the first basic communication skills such as attention-getting, accepting and rejecting. Later it creates the basis for symbolic communication, within the real communication and participation opportunities identified in daily life.

The child's first communicators primarily use non-symbolic communication means such as vocalizations, facial expressions, body language, etc. These behaviours may be unintentional or intentional.

12.4.1.1 Partner Awareness Training

Early intervention focuses mainly on improving the partner's communication ability to recognize and perceive, i.e. give meaning, to the child's behaviours. These behaviours can be vocalizations and actions, often not yet intentional and frequently atypical, nuanced, subtle and conditioned by the pathology, responding contingently to such signals (Kent Walsh and McNaughton 2005).

All the child's partners should give and share the same communication meaning, recognizing the child's signals, e.g. their way of expressing acceptance/rejection by facial expressions or by limbs movements, and eventually using specific tools, e.g. communication passports, communication dictionary, etc. (Siegel and Wetherby 2000; Millar and Aitken 2003; Bloomberg et al. 2004; Beukelman and Light 2020).

12.4.1.2 Create Participation and Communication Opportunities: Daily Routines and Play

AAC intervention aims at creating opportunities to influence the behaviours of the first communicator and their partner and more generally the child's everyday environments, using *unaided* and *aided* communication means. Early intervention is therefore the only real prerequisite for undertaking an AAC intervention (Mirenda et al. 1990).

Opportunities for participation and communication are built into daily routines, shared between children with CCN and their natural caregivers, during shared attention situations. They will need to be interesting for the child, taking into account their functional and developmental profile but also their chronological age (Butterworth and Cochran 1980).

The primary communicative opportunities occur in the play context and therefore the caregiver should select toys and activities with interaction goals to foster the child's communication skill development (Beukelman and Light 2020). The child with severe CP needs to discover that their behaviour affects the human/non-human environment, e.g. when activating a reactive toy or using a VOCA. This is one of the first steps toward communicative intentionality (Siegel and Cress 2002).

Toys Selection, Communication and Participation
- The caregivers need to select toys and activities with interaction goals. Some types of toys (e.g. balls, puppets, toy vehicles, bubble, blocks, etc.) can promote interactions more than others (e.g. paper and crayons, play dough, puzzles, etc.).
- To foster attention and participation of children with motor impairment and CCN, it is important to select toys that are easy to hold, carry and manipulate as well as being safe and attractive. Play, toys, activities and books may be adapted and modified (Musselwhite 1986; Goossens" 1989; Goossens' et al. 1992).
- Children with severe disabilities prefer to play with reactive toys that produce sound, movements and lights, and therefore it is often necessary to fit these toys with a personalized switch (Fig. 12.9). However, it should always be kept in mind that playing with a battery-operated toy serves as the means to an end (i.e. participation) not as an end itself!

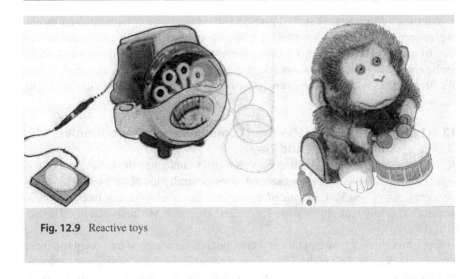

Fig. 12.9 Reactive toys

12.4.1.3 Early Access Intervention

To allow participation and communication of the child with severe impairment, it is often essential to early identify an alternative access mode (see paragraph on Alternative access assessment). The therapist needs to promote improvement in the use of unaided communication resources (e.g. eye pointing for choice-making) and/or the physical access to aided communication means (e.g. a symbol on a communication board with arm/hand control for selection). The seated posture assessment and positioning are starting conditions that identify the more functional mode/modes of accessing the AAC (Giannoni and Zerbino 2000; Costigan and Light 2011).

12.4.1.4 Building Early Communication Skills

Once the AAC team has created participation and communication opportunities, the group can begin to plan a multimodal approach to encouraging the development of the basic communication skills and then introducing the child, when possible, to symbolic communication.

> **Building Early Communication Skills**
> **Attention getting**
> The child mainly uses signals to get attention, such as laughing, crying, moving limbs, vocalizing, or making eye contact, to initiate social interactions with other people. Communication partners should respond to any intentional behaviour of the child so that the youngster can repeatedly experience the communicative results of their efforts (Smeybe 1990). For example, a caregiver may respond to behaviour such as tapping on a lap tray as an indicator of a desire for attention (Baumgart et al. 1990). Once an acceptable attention-seeking behaviour has been established and then used intentionally, caregivers can filter and respond to only the most socially acceptable ones. Simple technology can also be used to increase the importance of attention-seeking

behaviour, e.g. a call buzzer equipped with a switch or a VOCA with a single message: "Come here, please", etc. (Beukelman and Light 2020).

Accepting and Rejecting

Acceptance signals are those used to communicate that whatever is currently happening is tolerable or enjoyable, while the rejection signals are used to communicate the opposite. Accept and reject signals may be overt and obvious, such as smiling, laughing, frowning, etc., or maybe very subtle, such as averted eye gaze, increased body tension, increase rate of respiration, or sudden passivity.

As with attention-getting signals, the caregiver initially responds to and complies with any socially and culturally tolerated communicative behaviour of the child to strengthen their behaviour over time. Once the child uses these signals intentionally, caregivers begin to limit their responses to the most desirable, socially tolerated and functional behaviours only (Beukelman and Light 2020). Sometimes, in children with severe motor impairment, some accepting/rejecting signal can be even non-functional, especially in the long term, for example, when the child protrudes their tongue as an accepting signal.

12.4.1.5 Early Communication (EC) and General Rehabilitation Project

During the first years of the child's life, it is important that all the rehabilitation team shares a common "communication culture", also considering the collaborative participation of the child's family, that determines the successful communication outcome (Blackstone 2010).

Paediatricians and other medical and rehabilitation professionals, who often have the first chance to identify children with CCN, should promptly refer them to programs that support access to AAC and functional communication, integrating EC goals into their rehabilitation interventions.

Furthermore, it is now widely recognized as essential to provide quality communication access to young people with chronic communication disabilities. Rehabilitation specialists can play a key role in preparing these young people by teaching them to express their future health needs to use social services and to self-advocate with healthcare specialists (McNaughton et al. 2010).

12.4.1.6 Intervention General Guidelines for Symbolic Communication and Communication Competence Development

The AAC intervention aims at enhancing symbolic communication development, evaluating emerging skills and estimating if and to what extent the child can integrate the use of any aided systems for further linguistic and communicative development.

The introduction of the first symbolic modalities is based on the modelling process during which the partner while interacting with the child introduces and points to the corresponding symbol (tangible symbol, photo, picture, graphic symbol) to the keywords and progressively models, expands and reframes subsequent child's productions (Romski and Sevcik 1988; Goossens" 1989).

This initiates a process of shared meanings co-construction within the daily routines, play and other everyday activities of the child, where the partner and child with CCN will begin to agree and to conventionalize the modalities to express them, whether they are vocal, gestural, or with the use of visual symbols. At this early stage, the intervention addressed at communication partners is essential. This intervention by the AAC team is aimed at teaching the modelling process to the partner and, more generally, at the use of an appropriate language to support understanding (Sevcik and Romski 1997, 2002). Furthermore, it aims at improving strategies to support expressive communication, not limiting it to the expression of desires and needs but by expanding communication functions to other components such as comments, requests for information, narrations, etc. (Light et al. 2002).

Introducing the first AAC-aided modalities, the team should identify the most appropriate aided system, concerning the present capabilities, i.e. access modes and techniques, cognitive, sensory, linguistic skills, etc. (Beukelman and Light 2020):

(a) Symbol type, e.g. tangible symbols, photos and more suitable symbols system/ set such as Mayer-Johnson PCS,[2] Widgit,[3] Bliss,[4] etc.
(b) Communication support type, e.g. communication board, ETRAN type, first VOCAs, etc.
(c) Functional organizational layout, e.g. on a semantic/syntactic or pragmatic basis, etc.

For children with motor disabilities using the wheelchair, it is necessary to identify adequate low- and/or high-tech aids mounting systems and adaptations (e.g. lap tray use) that allow constant and autonomous access to the aided systems themselves (see also Chap. 13).

After the initial symbolic communication introduction phase, the AAC team intervention will then be aimed, where possible, at encouraging further development of symbolic communication in the various contexts of life and the acquisition of even wider communication competences. It will also be important to ensure that the vocabulary, which will be implemented over time, is not limited to the request for objects and actions but allows the child to express feelings, actions, emotions and more evolved communication functions (Light et al. 2002; Beukelman and Light 2020).

In recent years, the need for differentiated interventions aimed at communication and receptive and expressive language development has been reiterated both by analysing and intervening in the most general contexts of language learning (Light

---

[2] Crick Software Ltd., Northampton (UK), https://www.cricksoft.com

[3] Widgit Software, Cubbington (UK), https://www.widgit.com

[4] Blissymbol Communication, Oxford (UK), http://www.blissymbols.co.uk

1997) and through evaluations and subsequent specific interventions on language skills, in particular on morphosyntactic ones (Soto and Zangari 2009).

Special attention should be paid to the acquisition, where possible, of literacy skills. Lindsay (1989) thus expresses the importance of this acquisition: *"Teaching literacy skills is the thing – among those we can do for people who rely on the AAC – that most confers autonomy and power"*.

Starting from appropriate assessments and identifying any specific difficulties, a team approach to literacy is needed that involves the drafting of a specific intervention plan by speech therapists, with appropriate literacy intervention knowledge in children using AAC. The involvement of teachers and the share of the most appropriate teaching methods are fundamental, taking into account the principles of Universal Design for Learning (Rose 2000; Moore 2007) and the implementation of times specifically dedicated to literacy learning. Access to literacy activities can also be facilitated by the assistive technology use that allows children and young people with severe motor disabilities to participate in academic learning.

AAC intervention is an ongoing, longitudinal intervention. Throughout life, the individuals with CCN's communication needs and abilities can change with age to clinical picture evolution (skills acquisition or lost) and also to the partners and context changes (school, home, rehabilitation environments, day care centre, etc.). The AAC team has to continue to identify and implement appropriate strategies and tools for face-to-face, written and remote communication over time (Light and McNaughton 2014). Moreover, it should ensure the continuity of intervention, and his adaptation to the communication and participation need evolution, continuously supporting and involving the life communication partners and living contexts (high schools, universities, day care and residential centre, leisure, independent living, etc.) and the person with CCN himself (Lund and Light 2007).

References

Arvedson JC, Brodsky L (2002) Pediatric swallowing and feeding: assessment and management. Singular Thomson Learning, Albany

ASHA (2004) American speech-language-hearing association—special interest division 12: augmentative and alternative communication—roles and responsibility of speech-language pathologist with respect to Augmentative and Alternative Communication. Technical Report—ASHA Supplement, vol 24

ASHA (2007) American speech-language-hearing association—ad hoc committee on childhood apraxia of speech—childhood apraxia of speech. https://www.asha.org/policy/tr2007-00278/

Baumgart D, Johnson J, Helmstetter E (1990) Augmentative and Alternative Communication systems for persons with moderate and severe disabilities. Paul H. Brookes Publishing Co., Baltimore

Beukelman DR, Light JC (2020) Augmentative and Alternative Communication; supporting children and adults with complex communication needs, 5th edn. Paul H. Brookes Publishing Co., Baltimore

Beukelman DR, Mirenda P (1988) Communication options for persons who cannot speak: assessment and evaluation. In: Coston CA (ed), Proceedings of the National Planners Conference on Assistive Device Service Delivery, Association for the Advanced of Rehabilitation Technology, Washington, DC, pp 151–165

Blackstone S (2010) Communication access for children: the role of augmentative and alternative communication technologies and strategies in pediatric rehabilitation. J Pediatr Rehabil Med 3(2010):247–250. https://doi.org/10.3233/PRM-2010-0145

Blackstone S, Hunt Berg M (2003) Social networks: a communication inventory for individuals with complex communication needs and their communication partners. Augmentative Communication Inc., Monterey

Blockberger S, Johnston J (2003) Grammatical morphology acquisition by children with complex communication needs. Augment Altern Commun 2003(19):207–221. https://doi.org/10.1080/07434610310001598233

Bloomberg K, Johnson H, West D (2004) InterAACtion: strategies for intentional and unintentional communicators, Communication Resource Centre, SCOPE. http://www.scopevic.org.au

Bloomberg K, West D, Johnson H, Iacono T (2009) The triple C: checklist of communication competence—revised. Victoria, Australia, Scope Communication Resource Centre

Bolton S, Dashiell S (1991) Interaction checklist for augmentative communication—revised ed. PRO-ED, Austin

Brady NC, Bruce S, Goldman A, Erickson K, Mineo B, Ogletree BT, Paul D, Romski M, Sevcik R, Siegel E, Schoonover J, Snell M, Sylvester L, Wilkinson K (2016) Communication services and supports for individuals with severe disabilities: guidance for assessment and intervention. Am J Intellect Dev Disabil 2016:121,121–121,138. https://doi.org/10.1352/1944-7558-121.2.121

Butterworth G, Cochran E (1980) Towards a mechanism of joint visual attention in human infancy. Int J Behav Dev 1980(3):253–272. https://doi.org/10.1177/016502548000300303

Chomsky N (1965) Aspects of the theory of syntax. M.I.T. Press, Cambridge

Costigan FA, Light J (2011) Functional seating for school-age children with cerebral palsy: an evidence-based tutorial. Lang Speech Hear Serv Sch 2011:42. https://doi.org/10.1044/0161-1461(2010/10-0001)

Cress CJ, Marvin C (2003) Common questions about AAC services in early intervention. Augment Altern Commun 19(4):254–272. https://doi.org/10.1080/07434610310001598242

Curry SK, Robinson NB (2010) Assistive technology for young children. Paul Brookes Publishing

Darley FL, Aronson AE, Brown JR (1975) Motor speech disorders. Saunders, Philadelphia

Duffy JR (2013) Motor speech disorders: substrates, differential diagnosis, and management, 3rd edn. Elsevier Mosby, St. Louis

Giannoni P, Zerbino L (2000) Fuori schema. Chap. 9. Springer, pp 273–286

Goossens' C (1989) Aided communication intervention before assessment; a case study of a child. Augment Altern Commun 1989(5):14–26. https://doi.org/10.1080/07434618912331274926

Goossens' C, Crain S (1992) Utilizing switch interfaces with children who are severely physically challenged. Pro-Ed Inc.

Goossens' C, Crain S, Elder P (1992) Engineering the preschool environment for interactive symbolic communication. Southeast Augmentative Communication Conference Publications

Hayden DA (2004) PROMPT: a tactually grounded treatment approach to speech production disorders. In: Stockman I (ed) Movement and action in learning and development: clinical implications for pervasive developmental disorders. Elsevier, San Diego, pp 255–297

Higginbotham DJ, Shane H, Russel S, Caves K (2007) Access to AAC: present, past and future. Augment Altern Commun 2007(23):243–257. https://doi.org/10.1080/07434610701571058

Hill KJ, Romich BA (2006) AAC evidence-based clinical practice: a model for success. http://www.aacinstitute.org/Resources/Press/EBPpaper/EBPpaper.html

Hustad KC, Gorton K, Lee J (2010) Classification of speech and language profiles in 4-year-old children with cerebral palsy: a prospective preliminary study. J Speech Lang Hear Res 2010(53):1496–1513. https://doi.org/10.1044/1092-4388(2010/09-0176)

Iacono T, Carter M, Hook J (1998) Identification of intentional communication in students with severe and multiple disabilities. Augment Altern Commun 1998(14):102–114. https://doi.org/10.1080/07434619812331278246

Kent RD (2004) Models of speech motor control: implications from recent developments in neurophysiological and neurobehavioral science. In: Maassen B, Kent R, Peters H, Van Lieshout

P, Wouther H (eds) Speech motor control in normal and disordered speech. Oxford University Press, pp 3–28

Kent Walsh JE, McNaughton D (2005) Communication Partner Instruction in AAC: present practices and future directions. Augment Altern Commun 2005(21):195–204. https://doi.org/10.1080/07434610400006646

Light J (1989) Toward a definition of communicative competence for individuals using Augmentative and Alternative Communication systems. Augment Altern Commun 1989(5):137–144. https://doi.org/10.1080/07434618912331275126

Light J (1997) "Let's go star fishing": reflections on the context of language learning for children who use aided AAC. Augment Altern Commun 1997(13):158–171. https://doi.org/10.1080/07434619712331277978

Light J, Gulens M (2000) Rebuilding communicative competence and self-determination. In: Beukelman, Yorkston, Reichle (eds) Augmentative and Alternative Communication for adults with acquired neurological disorders. Paul H. Brookes, Baltimore, pp 137–179

Light J, McNaughton D (2014) Communicative competence for individuals who require Augmentative and Alternative Communication: a new definition for a new era? Augment Altern Commun 30:1–18. https://doi.org/10.3109/07434618.2014.885080

Light J, Parsons AR, Drager K (2002) "There's more to life than cookies": developing interactions for social closeness with beginning communicators who use AAC. In: Reichle, Beukelman (eds) Light. Exemplary practice for beginning communicators: implications for AAC. Paul Brookes Publishing

Lindsay P (1989) Literacy and the disabled: an unfilled promise or the impossible dream? Presentation at the Pacific Conference on Technology in Education and Rehabilitation. Vancouver, Canada

Lowit A, Kent R (2010) Assessment of motor speech disorders. Plural Publishing, San Diego

Lund S, Light S (2007) Long-term outcome for individual who use augmentative and alternative communication: part III. Contributing factors. Augment Altern Commun 2007(23):323–335. https://doi.org/10.1080/02656730701189123

McNaughton D, Balandin S et al (2010) Health transitions for youth with complex communication needs: the importance of health literacy and communication strategies. J Pediatr Rehabil Med 2010(3):311–318. https://doi.org/10.3233/PRM-2010-0143

McNeil M (2008) Clinical management of sensorimotor speech disorders. Thieme, New York

Millar S, Aitken S (2003) Personal communication passports: guidelines for good practice. Call Centre ed.

Millar DC, Light JC, Schlosser RW (2006) The impact of Augmentative and Alternative Communication intervention on the speech production of individuals with developmental disabilities. Journal of Speech. Lang Hear Res 2006(49):248–264. https://doi.org/10.1044/1092-4388(2006/021)

Mirenda P, Mathy-Laikko P (1989) Augmentative and Alternative Communication applications for persons with severe congenital communication disorders: an introduction. Augment Altern Commun 1989(5):3–13. https://doi.org/10.1080/07434618912331274916

Mirenda P, Iacono T, William R (1990) Communication options for persons with severe and profound disabilities: state of art and future directions. J Assoc Pers Sev Handicaps 15:3–21. https://doi.org/10.1177/154079699001500102

Moore SL, (2007) David H. Rose, Anne Meyer, Teaching Every Student in the Digital Age: Universal Design for Learning, *Education Tech Research Dev 55, 521–525 (2007)*, https://doi.org/10.1007/s11423-007-9056-3 (2007).

Musselwhite C (1986) Adaptive play for special needs children. College Hill, San Diego

National Joint Committee for the Communication Needs of Persons with Severe Disability (USA) (1992) Communication Bill of Rights—guidelines for meeting the communication needs of persons with severe disabilities. Asha 34(Suppl 7):2–3

National Joint Committee for the Communication Needs of Persons with Severe Disability (USA) (2016) Communication Bill of Rights (revised) in Brady et al. (2016) Communication services and supports for individual with severe disabilities. Am J Intellect Dev Disabil 121:121–138. https://doi.org/10.1352/1944-7558-121.2.121

Netsell R (1986) A neurobiologic view of speech production and the dysarthrias. College-Hill Press, San Diego

Netsell R (2001) Speech aeromechanics and the dysarthrias: implications for children with traumatic brain injury. J Head Trauma Rehabil 2001(16):415–425. https://doi.org/10.1097/00001199-200110000-00002

Nip ISB, Green JR, Marx DB (2011) The co-emergence of cognition, language and speech motor control in early development: a longitudinal correlation study. J Commun Disord 2011(44):149–160. https://doi.org/10.1016/j.jcomdis.2010.08.002

Odding E, Roebroeck ME, Stam HJ (2006) The epidemiology of cerebral palsy: incidence, impairments and risk factors. Disabil Rehabil 2006(28):183–191. https://doi.org/10.1080/09638280500158422

Paul R and Norbury F (2012) Language Disorders from Infancy through Adolescence, Listening, Speaking, Reading, Writing, and Communicating, 4th Edition, C.V.Mosby Co. Publ.

Pellegrino L (2002) Cerebral palsy. In: Bastshaw ML (ed) Children with disabilities, 5th edn. Paul H Brookes, Baltimore, pp 443–466

Pennington L, Miller N, Robson S, Steen N (2010) Intensive speech and language therapy for older children with cerebral palsy: a systems approach. Dev Med Child Neurol 2010(52):337–344. https://doi.org/10.1111/j.1469-8749.2009.03366.x

Pepper J, Weitzman E (2004) It takes two to talk. A practical guide for parents of children with language delay. The Hanen Program

Raghavendra P, Bornman J, Granlund ME, Björck-Ändersson E (2007) The World Health Organization's International Classification of Functioning, Disability and Health: implications for clinical and research practice in the field of Augmentative and Alternative Communication. Augment Altern Commun 2007(23):349–361. https://doi.org/10.1080/07434610701650928

Riecker A, Mathiak K, Wildgruber D, Erb M, Hertrich I, Grodd W, Ackermann H (2005) fMRI reveals two distinct cerebral networks subserving speech motor control. Neurology 2005(64):700–706. https://doi.org/10.1212/01.WNL.0000152156.90779.89

Romski M, Sevcik R (1988) Augmentative communication system acquisition and use: a model for teaching and assessing progress. NSSLHA J 1988(16):61–74

Romski M, Sevcik R, Adamson L (1997) Framework for studying how children with developmental disabilities develop language through augmented means. Augment Altern Commun 1997(13):172–178. https://doi.org/10.1080/07434619712331277988

Romski M, Sevcik R, Barton-Hulsey A, Whitmore AS (2015) Early intervention and AAC: what a difference 30 years makes. Augment Altern Commun 31(3):181–202. https://doi.org/10.3109/07434618.2015.1064163

Rose D, Universal Design for Learning, J of Special Ed Tech, March 1, 2000, https://doi.org/10.1177/016264340001500208 (2000).

Rowland C (2004) Communication matrix. Oregon Health and Science University, Portland

Schindler O (1990) Morbidity, epidemiology and systems analysis in phoniatrics: introduction, literature, updating. Folia Phoniatr Logop 1990(43):320–326. https://doi.org/10.1159/000266089

Schlosser R, Lee O (2000) Promoting generalization and maintenance in augmentative and alternative communication: a meta-analysis of 20 years of effectiveness research. Augment Altern Commun 2000(16):208–227. https://doi.org/10.1080/07434610012331279074

Sevcik R, Romski M (1997) Comprehension and language acquisition: evidence from youth with severe cognitive disabilities. In: Adamson, Romsky (eds) Communication and language acquisition: discoveries from atypical development. Paul Brookes Publishing

Sevcik R, Romski M (2002) The role of language comprehension in establishing early augmented conversations. In Reichle, Beukelman, Light (eds) Exemplary Practice for Beginning Communicators: implications for AAC—Paul Brookes Publishing

Siegel E, Cress J (2002) Overview of the emergence of early AAC behaviors: progression from communicative to symbolic skills. In: Reichle, Beukelman, Light (eds) Exemplary Practice for Begininng Communicators: implications for AAC. Paul Brookes Publishing, pp 25–57

Siegel E, Wetherby A (2000) Non symbolic communication. In: Snell ME, Brown F (eds) Instruction of students with severe disabilities, 5th edn. Merrill/Prentice-Hall, Upper Saddle River, pp 409–451

Silverman F (1995) Communication for the speechless, 3rd edn. Needham Heighs, MA, Allyn and Bacon

Smeybe H (1990) A theoretical basis for early communication intervention. Paper presented at the fifth biennial conference of the ISAAC, Stockholm

Smith A, Goffman L (2004) Interaction of motor and language factors in the development of speech production. In: Maassen B, Kent R, Peters H, Van Lieshout P, Wouther H (eds) Speech motor control in normal and disordered speech. Oxford University Press, pp 225–252

Snell M (2002) Using dynamic assessment with learners who communicate non symbolically. Augment Altern Commun 2002:18,163–18,172. https://doi.org/10.108 0/07434610212331281251

Soto G, Zangari C (2009) Practically speaking: language, literacy and academic development of students with AAC needs. Paul Brookes Publishing

Swigert NB (2010) The source for dysarthria, 2nd edn. Pro-Ed., Austin

Utley BL (2002) Visual assessment consideration for the design of AAC systems. In: Reichle, Beukelman, Light (eds) Exemplary practice for beginning communicators: implications for AAC—Paul Brookes Publishing

Williams B (2000) More than exception to the rule. In: Fried-Oken, Bersani (eds) Speaking up and spelling it out: personal essays on augmentative and alternative communication. Paul H. Brookes Publishing Co., Baltimore

World Health Organization (WHO) (2001) The international classification of functioning, disability and health (ICF). World Health Organization, Geneva

World Health Organization (WHO) (2007) The international classification of functioning, disability and health; children and youth version (ICF CY). World Health Organization, Geneva

Yogi H, Alves LAC, Guedes R, Ciamponi AL (2018) Determinant factors of malocclusion in children and adolescents with cerebral palsy. Am J Orthod Dentofac Orthop 154(3):405–411. https://doi.org/10.1016/j.ajodo.2017.11.042

York J, Weimann G (1991) Accommodate severe physical disabilities. In: Reichle, York, Sigafoos (eds) Implementing augmentative and alternative communication: strategies for learners with severe disabilities. Paul H. Brookes Publishing Co., Baltimore

Zabala J (1993) The SETT framework. Closing the Gap 2005(23):6

Zangari C, Lloyd LL, Vicker B (1994) Augmentative and Alternative Communication: an historic perspective. Augment Altern Commun 1994(10):27–59. https://doi.org/10.108 0/07434619412331276740

Rehabilitation Technologies for Sensory-Motor-Cognitive Impairments

13

Psiche Giannoni

Rehabilitation technology (RT) is an umbrella term that includes a great number and a large variety of applications of modern technologies and technological systems designed to address the physical and/or psychological needs of people with disability, by providing practical tools and devices that may be used by a child/adolescent/adult as well as their caregivers/assistants/therapists. The technological systems usually combine hardware (sensors, actuators, monitors, processors of biological signals, generators of stimuli of various types) and software, frequently nicknamed as 'apps', running on smartphones, laptop or desktop personal computers with or without functional connections to local or global networks.

The purpose of the technological aids is to improve selected functions of the person with an impairment, decrease the level of handicap in specific areas, evaluate critical aspects of sensory-motor-cognitive deficits, train the person for the recovery of at least partially normal levels of sensory-motor abilities and facilitate social interaction in terms of mobility, education, recreation and the possibility of employment.

The novelty of many RT systems makes them intrinsically attractive for persons with impairment, their relatives and sometimes the clinicians and rehabilitators themselves, somehow hiding the pros and cons of the practical introduction of these aids in a realistic and rational treatment plan. This is the case, for example, of robotic systems that are typically associated with Star Wars or WALL-E characters with human-like or pet-like features. Real robots are mostly used for industrial applications in manufacturing, have no anthropomorphic or biomorphic appearance and do not interact with humans during their work cycle. Different from industrial robots, service robots carry out several functions that imply interactions with human users or partners, with applications in medicine, entertainment, etc. However, this is

P. Giannoni (✉)
DIBRIS, University of Genoa, Genoa, Italy

still a minor sector that requires massive technological innovations both in terms of hardware (the robot's *body*) and software (the robot's *mind*) before achieving a functional level comparable, for example, to that of a therapist. At present, the field is characterized mostly by research prototypes, and the market can offer devices at the level of more or less sophisticated technological toys.

However, further progress is expected in this field in the near future, which will motivate the new entry of technology into the numerous and multifaceted aspects of disability, highlighting the urgency of team work between professionals who previously did not have occasions and/or motivations to interact with each other. Bioengineers and rehabilitators, despite their different backgrounds and professional experiences, should improve the communication channels to combine the rigor and objectivity of scientific work on one side with a holistic 'human' sensitivity on the other, always for the benefit of the person with impairment.

RT is usually subdivided according to three main application areas:

1. *Assistive*: to help the person with impairment to compensate or overcome specific handicaps without training or evaluation functions
2. *Assessment*: to evaluate quantitatively the impairment level of the person in specific sensory-motor-cognitive functions in comparison with accepted standards
3. *Training*: to train the person with impairment to improve or recover their sensory-motor capabilities

However, the three categories above are not mutually exclusive. For example, good training RT systems must include assessment functions to adapt the training to the general needs and changing the performance of any specific person in treatment.

Of course, these considerations are equally true of the interaction with the person with impairment by a 'human' therapist, who must *assess* the given person to formulate a personalized *treatment protocol*, carrying it out in an *adaptive way*, and complement/enrich the decided protocol with the appropriate *assistive aids* if necessary, possibly including RT systems in a rational manner.

13.1   Assistive Technology

The World Health Organization (WHO 2015), always attentive to the International Classification of Functioning, Disability and Health (ICF), strongly supports the application of assistive technology (AT) as a facilitator for the inclusion and participation of people with disabilities, so that they can maintain or improve their functioning and well-being. According to the WHO, the range of applications is not only restricted to prostheses and aids, but it also includes the implementation of software and hardware aids to facilitate mobility and improve sensory experience and communication. The WHO is also supporting the Global Cooperation on Assistive Technology (GATE) program (2016) aimed in particular to help children with disabilities to achieve sustainable development. Unfortunately, nowadays AT is still not readily accessible and applicable in countries with scarce clinical resources and funding (Bustamante Valles et al. 2016; Johnson et al. 2017).

AT is intended to provide devices capable to perform physical tasks for the person with impairment, immersed in a context of daily life activities, that the person is unable to carry out by themself and thus would require the intervention of an assistant/caregiver. AT plays the role of a cybernetic interface that allows the person to use their severely limited motor capabilities for controlling an operational device or robot, capable of carrying out a functional task. For example, if the task is to allow a person to drink a glass of water, the robot should be able to identify an empty glass in the environment, grasp and bring it to an appropriate position near the person. Thereafter, it is possible to envisage two technical solutions of very different levels of complexity: in the simpler one, the robot would fetch a straw and insert it in the glass, allowing the user to drink by himself; in the more complex solution, the robot should be able to appropriately tilt the glass and carefully approach the user's mouth, monitoring the whole operation. The choice depends on the user's needs, and, in any case, this is not a kind of technology that one can buy off the shelf and then learn how to use it by reading a complex user's manual, as a smartphone of the last generation. These kinds of devices should be carefully adapted and personalized to the single user to be functionally useful: again, this requirement calls for a close three-way collaboration between the therapist, who should have a clear understanding of the user's needs, and the technician/engineer, who knows the limits and the constraints of the proposed device and the user himself.

The fields of application of AT for people with cerebral palsy (CP) are multiple and growing because the available technologies are constantly improving, allowing better adaptation to the specific user's needs, taking into account the general level of impairment, the specific sensory-motor-cognitive deficits and the age of the subject. Roughly, these fields concern:

– Activities of daily life
– Environmental control
– Communication
– Mobility
– Social participation

13.1.1 Robots as Assistive Devices

Robotic devices, often shaped like one or two mechanical arms, can be used in several contexts. They can be mounted in a fixed location, e.g. a desk, or on an electric wheelchair, thus combining mobility and activities of daily life (ADLs). The users of these devices, either children or adults, are persons with severe disability as a consequence of greatly impaired voluntary control of movements in terms of force, range of motion and/or smoothness. The goal of a careful and smart application of this technology is to help such persons to gain more independence during eating, drinking, washing, shaving, teeth cleaning or controlling environmental devices in a 'smart home'. Two examples of robot assistive devices are the Jaco[1] 'arm'

---

[1] NuMotion, Brentwood (USA), https://www.numotion.com

(Campeau-Lecours et al. 2016) and Handy 1 (Topping 2000) that can offer a glass to a person or even help a girl with cosmetics. They are usually mounted on a wheelchair (e.g. Manus Wheelchair Robot: Driessen et al. 2001), to provide functions like writing on a keyboard when the child is attending school.

13.1.2 Brain-Computer Interfaces and Body-Machine Interfaces

An important module of many AT systems, whatever their specific function, is the use of an appropriate control interface to offer the possibility for the seriously disabled to manage the chosen AT system for performing important tasks while exploiting in the best possible way the few residual movements available. There are several technical solutions available, which can be more or less sophisticated, more or less invasive, more or less effective in the end but always needing careful adaptation and personalization to the user's need. Two large classes of interfaces of this kind are brain-computer interfaces (BCIs) or body-machine interfaces (BMIs).

Different types of BCI are supposed to detect the intention of the user to perform an action or induce the robot to perform it with their assistance (i.e. motor imagery) by processing brain activity in a non-invasive or invasive manner: with some hype, these systems are described by saying that they allow the person with disability to control the robot with their 'thoughts'. In any case, the former proposal is based on processing electroencephalographic activity (EEG) by using standard electrodes attached to the skull (McFarland and Wolpaw 2011; Daly et al. 2013; Zhang et al. 2019). Invasive solutions, in contrast, require insertion of electrodes in the brain, a technology somehow similar to the one used for deep brain stimulation of Parkinson patients. For example, invasive BCI systems like BrainGate Neural Interface (Nuyujukian et al. 2018) uses ECoG (electrocorticography), based on intra-skull electrodes placed on the dura and the activation by the user of motor imagery. What is gained by the invasive technology is essentially speed, which allows a quasi-real-time use of the AT system: in the non-invasive case, unfortunately, long delays in detecting motor imagery and controlling the robot deteriorate the performance of the robot as well the motivation of the user.

Different from BCIs, BMIs do not use motor imagery but directly attempt to extract as much information as possible from the reduced motility of impaired users. Typically, these AT systems are based on motion sensors applied to parts of the body, e.g. the shoulder, head or eyes, that the person is somehow able to control voluntarily, although such movements may not be directly functional for the action that they are required to control. The rationale of the BMI approach is to translate such controlled movements into the motion parameters of the assistive device, e.g. an electric wheelchair (Casadio et al. 2012; Lee et al. 2016; Abdollahi et al. 2017). It is important to note that, although this technology is not invasive, it requires a rather complex training for the user, who should learn to modulate and coordinate their reduced voluntarily controlled gestures in a reliable way in order to transmit their intention to the AT system. Thus, to be used efficiently, BMI controlled devices require double training and adaptation: the user should adapt to the device and the device should adapt to the user, with the help of a technician or technically oriented therapist. In comparison with non-invasive BCIs, the non-invasive BMI is potentially more effective in terms of speed, although a minimal set of motor abilities are required. For example, in the case of severe tetraplegic persons, invasive or non-invasive BMI is probably the only technology that would work.

Also, to support the impaired person in ADLs, BCIs or BMIs have been used for educational and/or entertainment applications by integrating them in video games and more generally in more serious games. Finally, it is worth mentioning that the BCI non-invasive technology can also be used, by appropriate processing of the EEG signals, for detecting emotional states and/or the attentional level of the user.

13.1.3 Writing Aids

For very severely impaired people who are unable to use simple, low-technology writing aids, like orthoses for handwriting, adapted/enlarged keyboards for typewriting, or for using personal computers (see Chap. 12 for further details), an almost ready-made technology is based on the measurement of eye movements or more generally gaze control, in such a way to implement eye pointer computer interfaces (Breuninger et al. 2011; Borgestig et al. 2016; Caceres and Rios 2018; Wachner et al. 2018), integrated with a virtual keyboard visualized on a video screen. In even more severe cases in which gaze control by the impaired person is not reliable, possibly as a consequence of the attentive stress implied by this unnatural control action, the selection of characters on the virtual keyboard can be implemented by a single-switch scanning mechanism, where the interface with the user intention consists of a single on-off command or switch delivered by means of a BCI, sucking/blowing detector, etc. For example, EyeMobile Plus[2] is an example of a device with gaze-enabled communication and computer access with many options.

13.1.4 Reading Aids

For persons with blindness or reduced vision capabilities, there are different technologies for accessing visual information, either text or images. For people with partial vision problems but who need more than magnifying glasses, there are electronic video magnifiers, which can provide continuous magnification and high contrast images. Regarding the access to written texts, there are audio text readers that scan and recognize printed documents and transform them into spoken language: they can be used either by people with blindness or reduced vision who find reading tiring. On the other hand, while audio text readers relieve the user of actions related to actively managing the written material, including choosing the rhythm, stopping and going back on the text, they may also induce a kind of passive attitude, like listening to a radio program which may be good for entertainment but not for

TobiiDynavox, Danderyd (S), https://us.tobiidynavox.com

education or professional activities. Another technical approach that requires the full participation of the user with blindness and allows access to both text and images is exemplified, for example, by the Optacon device (Linvill and Bliss 1966), which is an electromechanical device that consists of two parts: a scanner (a very small camera), which the user actively runs over the material to be read/visualized, and a finger pad, which translates the visual pixels detected by the camera into corresponding vibratory pixels felt on the finger tip of the user. There is no recognition by the machine, but the user should learn to interpret and recognize the vibratory patterns by himself. Finally, for Braille readers, there are several Braille devices that provide access to computers, tablets or smartphones, intended to allow the user to be independent and flexible in the home and work environment.

13.1.5 Mobility Aids

For people with a mild level of impairment regarding locomotion, there are robotized versions of the standard rollator walkers, namely walking assistance robots, that actively improve stability and can also avoid obstacles, for example, PAMM (Spenko et al. 2006) or Guido walker (Rentschler et al. 2008). For people who cannot walk, there are a large number of electric wheelchairs with a variety of electronic interfaces for adapting the control of the chair (direction, speed, brake) to the residual capabilities of the user. There are also mobility systems, conceived in particular for paraplegic users, that combine the mobility function with robotic support to the user, for standing up from a chair or bed, as well as sitting down: an example is the Tek Robotic Mobilization Device.[3]

An alternative to different types of electric/electronic wheelchairs is provided by robotized exoskeletons applied over the legs with suitable straps. The main function of such systems is to keep the users upright by providing the necessary antigravity activation of the motors, namely unloading the legs of a given percentage of the body weight; the control unit is also supposed to generate activation patterns of the motors that approximately emulate the stepping patterns of normal gait. Since the activation patterns of the exoskeleton are generated only in an approximate manner, the overall stability is the responsibility of the user themself, who typically holds balancing sticks while aided by the exoskeleton to generate functional stepping movements. Among the most currently used exoskeletons are ReWalk,[4] Phoenix Exoskeleton[5] and EksoNR.[6] Although exoskeletons were originally conceived for people with spinal cord injuries, characterized by a severe strength deficit of the leg muscles, there are recent studies that also address children with CP, to facilitate the achievement of physiological gait patterns while challenging the balance control system (Andrade et al. 2019; Eguren et al. 2019; Lerner et al. 2019). In most cases,

---

[3] Matia Robotics, Salt Lake City (USA), https://matiarobotics.com

[4] ReWalk Robotics, Marlborough (USA), https://rewalk.com

[5] suitX Co., Emeryville (USA), https://www.suitx.com

[6] Ekso Bionics, Richmond (USA), https://eksobionics.com

however, the exoskeletons are applied to the children only as a facilitator during a training session, e.g. during treadmill walking (see Sect. 13.3.2).

13.1.6 Domotics

Nowadays, everyday life is normally facilitated by numerous gadgets and devices that help a person in their home environment. With regard to communication or writing, technology has significantly contributed to the creation of smart homes, equipped to allow a person with impairment to easily access them and use the various accessories according to their needs, and so gain a little more independence. The person can take advantage of operating many electrical devices simply by using remote sensors or connecting these devices via an internal network that is also connected to the Internet and operate them even with a smartphone or a voice command (Harper 2006; Ghazal and Khatib 2015; Varriale et al. 2020). Wästlund et al. (2015) have also tested a system that allows the user to move functionally and safely in their home environment with a gaze-driven powered wheelchair and with navigation support.

These automation systems, called assistive domotics, have become a viable option for those who would rather stay in their homes than move to assisted living facilities. Services for automatic light controls, automated doors and locks, home safety and security, automated appliances, medicine dispensing devices, automated reminder systems, etc. are presently offered by some providers, such as smartofficesandsmarthomes.com, abilitynet.org.uk, atwiki.assistivetech.net, gettecla.com, iot.ilifesmart.com, unipi.technology, etc. Moreover, the new IoT[7] technology will probably increase the networking capability of the smart home and the integration of large-scale services.

13.1.7 Socially Assistive Robots

In the context of the large, variegated and scattered area of assistive technologies, the caregivers *par excellence* are undoubtedly a group of service robots known as socially assistive robots (SARs) that are supposed to replace the user in most activities of daily life (Pieskä et al. 2012; Mettler et al. 2017; Wirtz et al. 2018). Very often these robots have a captivating, semi-humanoid look, to convey a sense of empathy and have a good emotional impact on the user, as the Cognitive Service Robot Cosero[8] (Behnke et al. 2016) or Care-O-bot II[9] (Graf et al. 2004). In many cases, these robots are provided with the technology of spoken language production and recognition, a technology imported from consumer electronics that has nothing

---

[7] Internet of Things, https://www.softwaretestinghelp.com/iot-devices
[8] NimbRo, Bonn (D), http://www.nimbro.net/robots.html
[9] Fraunhofer IPA, Stuttgart (D), https://www.care-o-bot.de

to do with a disability but has the main purpose of simple and fun interaction with the user, by creating the illusion of understanding.

A popular social robot is Pepper,[10] a quasi-humanoid robot designed with the ability to observe some aspects of facial expressions and therefore capable to interact with the user as though capable of reading emotions and behaving accordingly. It is sometimes possible to meet Peppers in unexpected locations somewhere, such as on a luxury cruise ship, trained to behave as a perfect receptionist, able to identify visitors, through the facial recognition technology and, if appropriate, meet them with a welcome drink. For a disabled user, Pepper can be programmed to carry out more specific, functional services, like a helpful and attentive caregiver as well as a gym trainer (Lotfi et al. 2017).

Some care robots were designed to play the role of affective partners, like a kind of nanny to look after children or the elderly; affective robots can have a humanoid look like the NAO[11] robot or a pet look like the furry-covered seal Paro.[12] In particular, Paro is equipped with tactile sensors and touch-sensitive whiskers, capable to induce an effective response to the patting behaviour of the user by silently moving the tail, opening/closing the eyes or producing a kind of purring response. Children with autistic spectrum disorders seem to be benefited from this kind of human-robot interaction, probably because it is predictable and reliable; in contrast, in elderly users, this interaction may induce a sense of anxiety for fear of breaking a complex toy (Sharkey and Sharkey 2011; Huijnen et al. 2016; Alcorn et al. 2019), although such affective gadgets were given to them to attenuate their sense of solitude in the first place. In any case, the whole rationale and the related ethical issues regarding the use of these robots are largely debated, questioning if they only give an illusion of a deep and healthy human relationship (Coeckelbergh et al. 2015; Wachsmuth 2018).

There is also another aspect related to technology involving people with disability in their social and recreational moments. It concerns all those gadgets and software programs that require some technical adaptation to allow people with impairment to manage games to be played alone or in the company of their peers with impairment or not. Video games are also offered for educational purposes, but in the same way that it is not entirely possible to distinguish between assessment and rehabilitation situations, it is difficult to make the same distinction also for video games that could be assistive and therapeutic at the same time. For this reason, they will be considered here in the rehabilitation section.

13.2 Assessment Technology

According to the dictionary, *assessment is the act of judging or deciding the amount, value, quality or importance of something.* Here, the 'something' is the level of impairment of a person in one of the many facets of perception, motor control and

---

[10] SoftBank Robotics, Tokyo (JP), https://www.softbank.jp/en/robot

[11] SoftBank Robotics, Tokyo (JP), https://www.softbankrobotics.com/emea/en/nao

[12] Intelligent System Co., Kyoto (JP), https://intsys.co.jp/english; http://www.parorobots.com

cognition, in comparison with a population of controls, for diagnostic and prognostic purposes. As implicit in the dictionary entry, assessment implies quantitative and qualitative evaluations: in the former case, technology may compete with human healthcare professionals with some competitive edge caused by a large spectrum of sensors and measuring devices. In the latter case, well-trained and experienced rehabilitation professionals have a significant advantage over expert software package of the last generation, even if based on artificial intelligence (AI). Indeed, the problem is that AI lacks common sense reasoning, based on intuition and experience in the field that will remain a specific human feature in the foreseeable future particularly in the medical and healthcare field. Nevertheless, professionals need to take on the challenge of accepting and understanding the quantitative aspects of assessment that are provided by modern technology, taking into account continuous improvement.

Technological advancement of the last decades has contributed greatly to scientific knowledge. From its beginning, it was possible to understand more about movement and human behaviour, obtaining much more precise and reliable data to study than the results of an exclusively human and subjective investigation.

Over time, the study of human movement has gone from simple subjective observation to the photographic eye of Eadweard Muybridge and then to the use of electronic equipment capable of providing precise data (Gilliaux et al. 2015; Laut et al. 2016). The undoubted objectivity and precision of the data provided by a computer-aided assessment is extremely positive compared to the subjective data obtained from the use of clinical scales, even though a rehabilitator must continue to consider and compile (see also Chap. 1 Sect. 1.3.2). Where and when possible, it is very advantageous for the professional to collect these data, reflect on them and give meaning to the results. On this basis, they can customize a client-centred rehabilitation plan. Nevertheless, a 'human' approach to the evaluation of a person should never be overlooked. In any case, the quantitative measurement-based evaluations provided by assessment technologies are typically used in comparison and as a complement of qualitative clinical scales.

An Indian Story

In his book 'One more ride on the Merry-Go-Round' (2004, engl. version 2016), Tiziano Terzani, an Italian reporter from war areas and writer, explains very well how a scientific and detached approach to a health problem is extremely positive and efficient, but it also has the risk of losing sight of the person as a whole.

He has described an ancient Indian story, in which five blind men have to touch and describe an elephant. The first man touches its legs and describes the animal as a temple with columns, the second touches its trunk and says it is like a snake, the third describes its abdomen like a mountain, the fourth feels its ears like fans and the last thinks the tail like a whip.

All these descriptions have some truth, but none of them describe what the elephant really is. The same can happen if, taking into account only objective limited aspects, the practitioner forgets to put them together with the personality and needs of the individual person in care.

Considering the field of rehabilitation, technology assessment is basically applied to evaluate deficits of motor coordination and motor control, in the context of any specific pathological syndrome. The number and types of measurement systems and biomedical signal processing units are extremely large and diversified, as well as steadily growing with general technology innovations, and thus its detailed analysis is beyond the scope of this handbook. The general message for the therapists is that they should neither accept these tools in an acritical manner nor ignore the opportunity of exploiting these tools for improving their practice and enriching their experience on the field. A rule of thumb is to look with a critical eye at the daily activity with children, where treatment should always be the consequence of clinical reasoning driven by an articulated diagnostic/prognostic assessment, and answering the following question: is my qualitative assessment enough or can it be improved by quantitative technology-based evaluations? Below, a short exemplary list of instrumental assessment methods is outlined, mentioning the ones that are entering into clinical practice:

- General kinematic movement analysis
- Gait analysis
- Free spontaneous movements
- Other applications of motion capture
- Proprioceptive acuity
- Balance
- Haptic perception
- Stiffness and spasticity

13.2.1 General Kinematic Movement Analysis

Kinematics of body movements describes the spatio-temporal patterns of joint rotations, including joint angles, rotational velocities and accelerations, as well as the corresponding spatio-temporal patterns of the movements of the end-effectors (hands and feet). Kinematics describes the movement, namely, what happens to each joint but does not tell us why. In other words, it does not consider the forces that cause the movement, which is the role instead of kinetic analysis.

Kinematic analysis is employed in many contexts, for many purposes and in combination with other types of measurement systems. Pure kinematic analysis can be used, for example, for the evaluation of free spontaneous movements in newborns (see specific entry later on), for the evaluation of the degree of coordination/accuracy/jerkiness of reaching movements in subjects with different forms of apraxia in comparison with control subjects, who are known to generate smooth and accurate reaching movements characterize by a bell-shaped speed profile (Morasso 1981). Moreover, kinematic analysis is combined with other techniques in clinical gait analysis labs (see specific entry later on).

Different types of technologies are available for carrying out kinematic analysis and can be subdivided into two major categories:

- Systems based on markers
- Systems that do not use markers, i.e. markerless systems

Another subdivision is related to the type of sensing technology:

- Optical, based on cameras, either sensitive to visual light or infrared light
- Inertial, based on the accelerometer or more generally IMU sensors (inertial measurement units)
- Magnetic, based on a source of electromagnetic field and small magnetic sensors as targets of a 3D digitizing function

The choice among the different motion capture technologies depends on the requirement of the applications, for example, the spatial resolution, the rate of sampling, the number of markers or body segments that need to be measured, how invasive the system is, concerning the range of motion of the user, the operating volume, etc.

Markers in motion capture systems are small objects firmly attached to different parts of the body, for example in correspondence of the joints.

They can be passive, i.e. small light-reflecting spheres, or active, i.e. LEDs capable of emitting their light.

For example, in the case of the Vicon Vantage[13] system or the Smart DX[14] system of BTS, the markers (typically used in large numbers) are small reflective discs illuminated by infrared sources coaxial with a number of infrared cameras (typically 12) aimed at the volume of analysis.

In the case of the Polhemus Fastrak magnetic 3D digitizer,[15] the markers are small, rounded antennas: a rather small number are compatible with this technology but, different from the Vicon or BTS optical systems that suffer from a visibility problem (the markers may be hidden from the field of view of a camera), the magnetic markers are always sensitive inside the operational volume.

There are also hybrid optical motion capture systems as Miqus Hybrid[16] that combine within the same camera both marker-based or markerless detection and tracking.

The motion capture systems with active markers are mostly optical, as Simi Aktisys,[17] using small infrared light-emitting diodes that are quickly flashed one after the other, to simplify the real-time identification of the spot detected by each camera, with the result of achieving a higher frequency rate of motion capture.

---

[3] Vicon Motion Systems Ltd., Oxford (UK), https://www.vicon.com

[4] BTS Bioengineering, Garbagnate Mil. (IT), https://www.btsbioengineering.com

[5] Polhemus, Colchester (USA), https://polhemus.com

[6] Qualisys, Göteborg (S), https://www.qualisys.com

[7] Biosense Medical, UK, https://biosensemedical.com

Non-optical markerless systems typically are based on inertial sensors, as the Motion Capture Suit[18] with 19 inertial sensors and the MTi[19] inertial sensor modules.

13.2.2 Gait Analysis

Clinical gait analysis labs are typically operated for orthopaedic or neurological users, to be evaluated in comparison with control populations within specific experimental protocols (Cappozzo 1984; Benedetti et al. 1998; Perry and Burnfield 1992; Armand et al. 2016). Gait analysis is not focused on a single type of measurement but requires the integration of different types of evaluations that require different devices to be carefully synchronized:

(a) *Kinematic analysis*. It can be performed with one of the systems described above, although most clinical labs are equipped with infrared cameras with passive markers and floor mounted force platforms, with standardized dimensions of the lab to compare the measured patterns to the established control base. The output is spatial movements of the body including joint angles, displacements, velocities and accelerations.

(b) *Kinetic analysis*. By measuring the ground reaction force of the walking subject, with force platforms embedded in the walkway and integrating it with the synchronized kinematic analysis above, it is possible to evaluate the time course of the internal and external forces involved in the execution and control of the observed locomotion movement.

(c) *Plantar pressure*. By using pressure sensors embedded in the walkway or pedobarographic systems, it is possible to evaluate the distribution of pressure and path of pressure progression during a step and the contact and pressure exerted by the foot on the ground are also recorded.

(d) *Temporal parameters*. Typical temporal parameters that are extracted from the measurements above and that are relevant from the clinical point of view are the following ones: cadence (steps/min), speed (m/s), stride and step length (m) and stride and step time (s).

(e) *Electromyography* (EMG). The kinematic/kinetic analysis above is frequently associated with the analysis of the activation of the leg muscles involved in gait by means of electromyography. Routinely, large surface muscle groups can be measured with surface electrodes such as *rectus femoris, hamstrings, gastrocnemius* and *tibialis anterior*. Deeper muscles can be measured with fine wire, such as the *tibialis posterior*.

(f) *Energy expenditure*. This kind of measurement is important for evaluating the efficiency of the gait patterns used by an impaired subject in comparison with controls: it is usually carried out by measuring oxygen consumption by means of some kind of portable respirometer.

---

[18] Rokoko, Copenhagen (DK), https://www.rokoko.com

[19] Xsens, Hong Kong (HKSAR), https://www.xsens.com

Three-dimensional instrumented gait analysis (3DGA) collects kinematic data regarding the spatio-temporal values of the gait cycle that are important to evaluate regarding development and impairment in children. It is important to remember that the evaluated values must be referred to the typical parameters of the child's gait in its various stages of development, and the markers are positioned according to a conventional gait model. There are many such models, the most used being the Plug-In Gait model (PiG) (Armand et al. 2016), the calibrated anatomical system technique (CAST) (Cappozzo et al. 1996) and the human body model (HBM). Nevertheless, a recent study conducted by Flux et al. (2020) concludes that all the three models are equivalent since the significant elements between them are minimal.

Russell et al. (2011) used a VICON system and applied markers both to able-bodied and diplegic children with CP according to the LifeMod model, to highlight the differences of the angular momentum at the joints during their gait. The result of the study was significantly increased internal work, in terms of expenditure of energy, in these children. The importance of EMG analysis in motor-impaired children is related to the detailed characterization of the activity of the main muscles related to gait, reporting data about their activation timing, co-contraction periods and even muscle spasticity, giving fundamental hints to understand the deviated gait patterns used by the assessed children with CP.

Gait analysis is also a valid assessment tool for the planning of lower limb surgery and the verification of the effective post-surgical functional acquisitions of the child (Lee et al. 1992; Lofterød et al. 2007; Brunner et al 2008; Ferrari et al. 2015) and for integrating clinical assessments with gait analysis, in the process of treatment decision-making (Franki et al. 2014; Ferrarin et al. 2015; Õunpuu et al. 2015; Rethlefsen et al. 2017; Wren et al. 2020).

The development of strategies by toddlers in the first months after the onset of their independent walking is a frequent subject of analysis, as reported by many scientific studies that used force platforms (Ledebt et al. 1995; Ledebt and Bril 2000; Roncesvalles et al. 2000; Ivanenko et al. 2004, 2007; Looper and Chandler 2013).

Although most gait analysis studies are based on optical motion capture, there have been clinical studies based on markerless inertial sensors, motivated by their low cost and preparation simplicity. For example, inertial sensors were applied at the wrist of unilateral spastic CP children to highlight the increased asymmetry of the less-able arm during different walking speeds (Wolff et al. 2020) or to evaluate clinical spasticity (van den Noort et al. 2009). Bisi and Stagni (2015) used them to analyse the different strategies of walking in toddlers, with the motivation that the child can wear this kind of sensors also outside a laboratory environment and for a long time, and they need no calibration.

13.2.3 Analysis of Free Spontaneous Movements

While gait analysis requires a standardized environment and measurement protocol for evaluating the spatio-temporal features of a single representative step to be repeated periodically during undisturbed planar gait, spontaneous free movements have been investigated in depth in infants because many studies, initiated by Prechtl (Prechtl 1990, 1997; Einspieler et al. 2012, 2016) have demonstrated that their intrinsic features are indicative from the diagnostic and prognostic point of view of newborns at risk of pathology. Unfortunately, the critical features are somehow qualitative and difficult to identify in a well-defined manner. In practice, the protocol suggested by Prechtl consisted of video recording the newborn in their cot with a traditional video camera and entrusting the video sequence to specifically trained evaluators to detect the presence/absence of the critical features. This is a time-consuming procedure, limited by fatigue and inter-rater reliability. As a consequence, there have been many studies attempting to adapt motion capture technologies to this specific problem that implies specific implementation constraints, before becoming viable for daily clinical practice, in particular in the case of preterm babies.

On the other hand, wearable sensors may be based on inertial measurements, for example with the use of accelerometers (Ohgi et al. 2008; Cliff et al. 2009; Heinze et al. 2010; Gravem et al. 2011) or magnetic measurements (Karch et al. 2008, 2010; Philippi et al. 2014) to measure the manual coordination in infants. In both cases, the sensors must be firmly connected to the appropriate body part by a strap or other means; they can be wireless or use wires for transmission of signals and power.

It is easy to realize how both technologies are rather invasive, particularly if applied on newborns or infants and require accurate positioning on the body to obtain a sufficient degree of precision. With the aim of overcoming this aspect of invasiveness, Airaksinen et al. (2020) carried out a study on the spontaneous movements of the newborn—but extendable to subjects of all ages—designing a 'smart jumpsuit' with sensors consisting of an accelerometer and gyroscope, attached at the level of the shoulder and hip joints of the child.

Motion capture systems based on markers have been used for many studies on the motor development of very young infants or aiming to detect newborns at risk for developing spasticity (Meinecke et al. 2006; Kanemaru and Watanabe 2012; Kanemaru et al. 2014).

As understandable, in the studies above the presence of markers or sensors attached to the body of the infant is invasive, in particular for preterm newborns. Thus, there have been several approaches to the computerized analysis of spontaneous movements in fully ecological conditions, i.e. without markers or other attachments to the body. For example, several studies used the Microsoft Kinect Sensor[20] (Ilg et al. 2012; Chang et al. 2013; Luna-Oliva et al. 2013; Marcroft et al. 2015; Olsen et al. 2018; Hesse et al. 2018).

Another possibility is markerless motion capture, based on the quantitative analysis of video sequences, recorded with a single semi-professional camera and processed with software packages specifically designed for the spontaneous movements of the newborns: MIMAS (Marker-less Infant Movement Analysis System: Osawa

---

[20] Microsoft Corp., Redmond (USA), https://www.microsoft.com

et al. 2008; Tsuji et al. 2020; Tacchino et al. 2021; Doi et al. 2021), GMT (General Movement Toolbox: Adde et al. 2009, 2010), AVIM (Orlandi et al. 2015).

In particular, different from GMT and AVIM software packages, which operate with grey level images, MIMAS uses a preliminary adaptive binarization stage, which minimizes the variability due to illumination conditions and thus increases its applicability in a common clinical setting. Moreover, there is no need for manual identification by a human operator of the features of interest as required by other systems, e.g. AVIM. Furthermore, MIMAS evaluation uses a large number of indices that can be used to identify potential infants at risk in a very early stage of development.

13.2.4 Other Applications of Motion Capture in Children

The pneumotachograph or spirometer is a device that measures airflow quantitatively by detecting the flow of respiratory fluids and comparing it to the pressure drop against a small resistive field. These devices, which are used to measure breathing potential and pulmonary ventilation, are not always usable by subjects with impairment because they are somehow invasive and require the subject's collaboration. Aliverti and Pedotti (2003) developed a non-invasive optoelectronic system of motion capture called optoelectronic plethysmography, which was derived from the same technology used for gait analysis (i.e. the BTS optical system). It consists of the application of reflective markers on the chest wall to record the 3D movements of the chest during respiration. In particular, this system can be very useful to measure the lung volume in newborns and children (Dellaca et al. 2010), or in neuromuscular disorders (Bonato et al. 2011).

A pure optical system, without markers, was used by Eishima (1991), who applied a video camera and fiberscope to the feeding bottles of newborns on the fifth day after birth and accurately recorded their sucking patterns and adaptability to a changing environment. Along the same line, another possibility of motion capture is to study quantitatively, with older children, the characteristics of jaw movements during their chewing (Nip et al. 2018).

13.2.5 Proprioceptive Acuity

Proprioceptive acuity is a specific indicator of perceptual efficiency, namely, the ability to sense joint position, movement and force of muscle contraction and to discriminate movements of limb segments individually and relative to each other. This is an integrated perceptual function that employs many sensory channels (through the muscle spindles, the joint receptors and the skin) with a fundamental cognitive component related to what is known as body image (Paillard 1980; Schwoebel and Coslett 2005; Pitron et al. 2018). A good level of proprioceptive acuity is fundamental for carrying out skilled activities of daily life, particularly with regard to the proprioceptive acuity of the upper limbs. As a consequence, the deterioration of this perceptual ability, due to cerebral palsy or other neuromotor impairments, negatively affects all these abilities (Goble et al. 2005, 2009; Pickett and Konczak 2009; Wang et al. 2009; Li et al. 2015), and thus its evaluation is important for planning the treatment of a child with impairment.

Unfortunately, since this is a multimodal perception, its qualitative estimate, using clinical scales, is not very sensitive and thus is not very useful from the clinical point of view. Instead, advanced technology can help researchers particularly to investigate the different aspects of proprioceptive functioning, using different techniques to measure the joint position sense with or without the passive motion threshold detection and the active motion amplitude discrimination (Han et al. 2016).

Scientific literature reports that passive motion detection and the joint position sense have been measured both with custom-built devices or with more sophisticated ones.

Advanced technological systems use manipulanda to measure the proprioceptive acuity of the upper limb joints or of the wrist (Masia et al. 2008, 2009; Iandolo et al. 2015; Cappello et al. 2015; Holst-Wolf et al. 2016; Tseng et al. 2017; Kuczynski et al. 2017; Marini et al. 2017a, b), or of the ankle (Willems et al. 2002; Yasuda et al. 2014).

Since proprioceptive acuity is the prerequisite to perform precisely coordinated movements, it is interesting to consider studies that, using inertial or magnetic measurement systems, focus on the 3D orientation of body segments and joint angles, e.g. at the wrist level, to evaluate the finger movements during handwriting (Fujisawa and Okajima 2015; Li et al. 2019).

On the other hand, custom-built devices have been used to measure rotation around the axis of a semi-goniometer and record the orientation angles in normal and subjects with CP (Wingert et al. 2009; de Andrade et al. 2020). Low-cost devices, like Microsoft Kinect 2, have been used with children with CP (Chin et al. 2017) as well as the compact measuring system to investigate the correlation between joint position and kinesthetic sense and ideogram handwriting legibility in children with physiological development (Hong et al. 2016).

Using custom devices, Hoseini et al. (2015) applied psychometric adaptive staircase procedures to measure hand proprioception with a simple tablet-style apparatus and a tactile marker applied at index fingers. Subjects were asked to position their finger according to what saw on a screen, or to match the movement/position in two opposite joints relative to each other, and to discriminate the passive movement direction of one finger.

The ability to detect passive motion at one or more joints is different from the detection of a joint position; however, the two skills are still closely related. Indeed, the Nottingham Sensory Assessment clinical scale (Lincoln et al. 1998) considers these two evaluations in the same section.

As discussed above, proprioception is usually related to the articulations of the body, one at a time or in combination. Another proprioceptive estimate, which is essential for balance and requires even greater integration of multimodal information, is the evaluation of the position of the centre of pressure (CoP) during bipedal standing. This evaluation requires integrating the touch sensors under the feet with proprioceptive sensors of both legs to relate the CoP position to the base of support, information that is essential for balance control.

Proprioceptive acuity for active motion, i.e. movement amplitude discrimination, can be assessed accurately only through instrumented technologies. In the case of single or multijoint reaching movements, it is possible to measure the reaching accuracy; in the case of a person standing or sitting on a force platform, it is possible to measure the shifting accuracy of the CoP, visualized on a screen monitor.

A major problem in setting this assessment in children with CP could be the presence of muscle weakness and/or a severe level of stiffness. In fact, most scientific studies measure proprioceptive acuity on healthy adults or those with disability (Waddington and Rogers 1999; Han et al. 2015; Pellegrino et al. 2017; Gurari et al. 2019; Cai et al. 2020).

13.2.6 Balance

Avoiding the tendency to fall determined by gravity, in normal control subjects is under-evaluated as a kind of reflex, with little coordination and no cognitive involvement. However, this is completely wrong, and there are reasons to believe that maintaining equilibrium against gravity is a kind of generalized skill, applied in a wide range of situations, from daily life activities to challenging sports gestures (Morasso 2020). In particular, Shumway-Cook and Woollacott (2016) clarify that the successful performance of many ADLs requires that the subject is capable of mastering different balance skills:

(a) Steady-state balance when maintaining a steady position
(b) Dynamic steady-state balance, e.g. while walking
(c) Proactive balance as anticipation of a predictive disturbance
(d) Reactive balance in response to an unexpected disturbance

These types of balance are highly interlinked, but they can be assessed in detail both with clinical scales and, even more precisely, with force platforms, which measure different aspects of the ground reaction forces generated by a person standing on or moving across them.

Early clinical studies based on the application of a computerized force platform date back to 1976 when it was used for gait analysis at the Boston Children's Hospital. After that, force platforms have been used also to register different postural responses and to describe in detail the body sway of subjects facing different kinds of perturbation.

Nowadays, there are different types of force platforms with different complexity, precision and cost. In the case of gait analysis labs, the adopted platforms are the more complex ones, namely, multi-axis platforms that simultaneously measures three force components and three-moment components about the three coordinate axes (x, y and z) for a total of six output components (e.g. the AccuGait platform by AMTI[21], the multicomponent force plate Type 9281EA by Kistler[22] and the 4060-XX model series of platforms by Bertec[23]). With the six components of this kind of platforms, it is possible to evaluate the instantaneous position of the CoP, which corresponds to the point of application of the ground reaction force and the three components of this force vector: the vertical component, i.e. the body weight ± the body mass multiplied by the vertical acceleration of the centre of mass of the body (CoM) and the two horizontal components (in the anterior-posterior and the medio-lateral directions) that play a role in evaluating the risk of slipping during gait or when recovering balance after a perturbation. It is important to note that the CoP does not coincide with the projection of the CoM on the support base, although they are related according to a dynamic model (Baratto et al. 2002).

In the case of posturographic analysis for the measurement of body sway during quiet upright standing, it is possible to use simpler and less costly force platforms that only provide the position of the CoP, combined for the two feet, or, for some clinical application, it may be useful to decompose the composite CoP of the standing body in the CoPs of the two feet, utilizing two coupled platforms located closely side to side. In the same class of devices, low-cost force platforms are often considered, originally developed for the consumer electronic market of videogame, like the Wii Balance Board[24] (WBB) that trade-off cost with measurement precision.

Another technology is based on plantar pressure maps, i.e. distributed arrays of pressure sensors that provide an image of the distribution of pressure between the feet and the support base. Different types of pressure maps are produced, for example, by Tekscan.[25] This kind of information is not available from a force plate, which can only provide information on the overall ground reaction force and its point of application, namely the CoP.

As regards steady-state balance, namely balance in quiet upright standing on a rigid surface, many studies present dynamic models of the elements of instability and control mechanisms of upright posture (Peterka 2002; Baratto et al. 2002; Winter et al. 2003; Casadio et al. 2005). It has been investigated also the postural control in standing in children with CP, with open or closed eyes (Rose et al. 2002; Donker et al. 2008) and recently also on a large number of healthy children/adolescents (Ludwig et al. 2020).

The situation par excellence for studying dynamic balance is walking, which, as described above, is investigated using motion capture devices and a series of force platforms (Assaiante et al. 2005). Nevertheless, the analysis of gait does not saturate to the issue of dynamic balance: other postural transfers are worth

---

[21] AMTI, Watertown (USA), https://amti.biz

[22] Kistler, Winterthur (CH), www.kistler.com

[23] Bertec, Columbus (USA), www.bertec.com

[24] Nintendo, Redmond (USA), www.nintendo.com

[25] Tekscan, South Boston (USA), www.tekscan.com

considering, as sit-to-stand or back-to-sit. These are very common transitions in the daily life of normal but rather difficult for children with CP to perform properly. Several studies have investigated the quality of postural control in children with CP, highlighting the different performances with open or closed eyes (Park et al. 2003; dos Santos et al. 2011). El Shemy (2018) even reported better results when training children with CP to walk on a treadmill with their eyes closed than with eyes open.

Pavão et al. (2015) have also analysed the steady-balance characteristics during a static upright position versus a dynamic one, highlighting the need to better prepare the first to move efficiently during more demanding functional tasks.

However, most of the investigations are aimed at analysing data concerning both the proactive and reactive balance. Proactive balance is a feedforward strategy, which involves the activation of the balance system in anticipation of a perturbing force, either internal (self-generated) or external. For example, picking up an object from the floor and putting it on a table implies a disturbance to the performing subject's own stability that can be predicted and thus anticipated proactively. Preparing to catch an incoming ball is another example that, again, can be predicted and anticipated. These gestures are called anticipatory postural adjustments (APA), which rely on feedforward control and depend to large extent on the previous sensory-motor experience of the subject, on their ability to use visual information and on a process of sensorimotor learning that involves both motor cognition and motor control (Massion 1992).

In a reactive balance response, the subject is not aware of the upcoming situation, and therefore, there is not any APA. Most laboratory studies investigate reactive and unplanned balance reactions causing a sudden and unexpected movement of the force plate on which the subjects are standing, as opposed to a predicted adaptive situation, where the platform does not move but the environment and the task change.

Many studies are milestones for the understanding of the proactive/reactive balance on healthy subjects (Nashner 1982; Horak and Nashner 1986; Horak et al. 1990; Aruin 2002, 2016) and many other report data about the behaviour of the elderly or people with sensory disorders (Lin et al. 2004; Aruin 2015; McGeehan et al. 2017). Moreover, several investigations have also been made on the balance of children with CP when they are standing or walking, also compared with the behaviour of children with physiological development (Woollacott and Shumway-Cook 2005; Girolami et al. 2011; Sobera et al. 2011; Akbarfahimi et al. 2012; Shiratori et al. 2016; Mills et al. 2018).

More information about physical activity, and therefore indirectly about anti-gravity performance of a subject, can also be obtained using simpler tools than platforms, such as accelerometers and inclinometers, with sensors attached to some parts of the body, according to the aim of the data collection. Inclinometers, which are tilting sensors, are often used to process data during the STS (Sit to Stand) sequence and vice versa (Lanningham-Foster et al. 2005; Vähä-Ypyä et al. 2018; Valkenet and Veenhof 2019; Darwish et al. 2019).

13.2.7 Haptic Perception

Gibson (1966) wrote about haptic perception as 'the sensibility of the individual to the world adjacent to his body by use of his body', identifying it not only as the process allowing the recognition of an object by touch but also a combination of somatosensory perception through the skin and proprioception. As described in Chap. 6, haptic perception consists of the active exploration, mainly not only through the hand but also with different parts of the body, e.g. a foot. In every case, it involves the integration of purposive control, proprioceptive information and tactile information. Vision can help but is not essential. For example, the ability to select an orange in a basket instead of an apple or a banana, in the absence of vision, implies using haptic perception. The failing to carry out the task by a subject with impairment may be due to a deficit in one or other function above or a combination of both. Consequently, this is a perceptual channel difficult to assess quantitatively.

Technology can help to propose assistive programs for the assessment and improvement of the upper limb functioning, including haptic perception. In the case of children with impairment, where constant motivation will be needed to have their commitment to the active participation required, it is understandable that a game-like environment is preferred (Frascarelli et al. 2006; Ríos-Rincón et al. 2016). For this reason, most of the activities proposed for the upper limb assessment and training in children with CP are mainly based on virtual reality or serious games, as described further on.

Focusing particularly on assessment, it is possible to program robotic devices, according to different strategies of physical interaction with the user, that may implement a combined assessment/treatment purpose. However, in this case, there are no off-the-shelf devices that can be used without careful adaption to the type and severity of the impairment and the age and other specific characteristics of the user.

Two different types of robotic devices can be distinguished, according to how they are connected to the user:

- End-point connection: In the case of upper limb systems, the hand of the robot is connected to the hand of the user, for example, through a handle. The earliest example is the MIT Manus, now out of production, or the Kinarm[26] end-point system. Through this connection, the robot can help or resist the action of the user and, at the same time, measure the force transmitted in one sense or the other and the corresponding motion. In the case of the lower limb applications, such as a walking aid, the point of contact is the foot, an example being G-EO[27].
- Exoskeleton connection: In this case, the robot motion mirrors the motion of the body segment of the user to which it is connected, exchanging forces through

---

[26] BKIN Technologies Ltd., Kingston (CDN), https://kinarm.com
[27] Reha Technology AG, Olten (CH), https://www.rehatechnology.com

multiple points. An example for the upper limb is Armeo,[28] the bimanual Kinarm exoskeleton, ReoGo,[29] the Wristbot[30] or 'Braccio di Ferro' of the Genoa University (Casadio et al. 2006). In the case of the lower limb, an example is Lokomat by Hocoma.

There are infinite interaction strategies that can be implemented in the robot software for both assessment or treatment, according to the specific goal, for a given subject with impairment. At the same time, this infinite number of possibilities is also the 'palette' available to the hand and the mind of the therapist when attempting to evaluate and address the specific needs of the person with an impairment in the best way possible.

Typical interaction strategies that are frequently made available for the kind of robotic manipulators mentioned above can be summarized as follows:

(a) *Active mode*: the person is fully active and receives no assistance by the robot, even when interacting with it; in this case, the robot simply measures the motion of the user.

(b) *Passive mode*: the robot passively moves part of the body of the user, imposing trajectory and speed profile, whatever the muscle activation of the user. Passive mobilization is ineffective for (re)learning by recruiting neural plasticity because of 'slacking', i.e. the general psychological phenomenon for which, if one is helped too much by the trainer when learning a gesture, the person will simply give up and not participate (Wolbrecht et al. 2008). However, passive mobilization may help to preserve the thixotropic properties of muscles and ligaments by compensating for the effects of immobilization of paretic limbs.

(c) *Resistive mode*: the robot interferes with the movements of the user, opposing in some way their active control. In this manner, it is possible to simulate the action of an elastic (spring-like) load, generating resistive forces proportional to the distance of the hand from a given equilibrium point. Along the same line, the resistive force can be delivered by the robot to be proportional to the speed of the motion generated by the user in the opposite direction, thus simulating the action of a viscous load. The resistance may also be delivered as a disturbing element, for example a force proportional to speed but oriented sideways (to the left or the right) concerning the direction intended by the user, such as the approximately straight line of normal reaching movements. The reason for this disturbance is to challenge the user when learning (or relearning, after a stroke) to coordinate the movement in the most economic way (Shadmehr and Mussa-Ivaldi 1994).

(d) *Assistive mode*: the robot implements an impedance-based assistance paradigm that corresponds to a mild spring-like force generated by the robot in such a way as to attract the user's hand from its current position to the ideal one for the

---

[28] Hocoma, Volketswil (CH), https://www.hocoma.com

[29] Motorika USA Inc., Mount Laurel (USA), http://motorika.com

[30] Italian Institute of Technology, Genova (IT), www.iit.it

function. The intensity of this assistance should be modulated carefully, according to the 'assist-as-needed' principle that does help the user but challenges them to avoid the 'slacking phenomenon' mentioned above (Wolbrecht et al. 2008; Casadio et al. 2009; Elsaeh et al. 2017). A more challenging variation of this paradigm is to use an 'error enhancing' force that tends to slightly increase the deviation of the trajectory produced by the user instead of decreasing it. In a specific study (Abdollahi et al. 2014), it was demonstrated that the error enhancing strategy is more effective than the error reducing strategy, in inducing learning based on neural plasticity, provided that the impairment level of the user is not too high.

However, this field of clinical research is still a work in progress, particularly in the case of child users, and, indeed, most publications are related to adult subjects. In most cases, the robotic equipment in use has been designed for both evaluation and training.

For example, we may consider the ReHapticKnob[31] (Metzger et al. 2014), an end-effector-based hand rehabilitation robot with sensing and actuation capabilities, for therapy for grasping and forearm rotation tasks, and capable of providing precise and objective measurements of interaction dynamics and performance. Such information can be used to drive assist-as-needed control strategies or to complement clinical assessments by reconstructing the scores from robot data. In-Motion2,[32] a commercial version of MIT-MANUS, has been used extensively, particularly by subjects with impairment managed by the USA Veterans Administration, but there have also been several studies involving hemiplegic children (Fasoli et al. 2008). Another device also tailored for children is the AMADEO Hand Robot System,[33] which can move the fingers of the child with passive or assistive modalities (Sale et al. 2012; Bishop et al. 2017), or WristBot (Marini et al. 2014, 2015, 2017a, b) for the evaluation and training of distal upper limb movements.

13.2.8 Stiffness and Spasticity

Haptic perception and stiffness evaluation are related and, in a sense, represent the same physiological phenomenon in a dual, complementary way, i.e. they are the two faces of the same coin. In the case of haptic perception of a subject, the therapist (or the haptic robot, acting as a robotic therapist) is trying to evaluate extent to which the assessed subject is capable of integrating exploratory movements, proprioceptive and tactile information for successfully carrying out specific ADLs. Stiffness evaluation focuses on the level of coactivation of antagonist muscles chosen by a subject when executing a given action. A given posture or a given trajectory, for example, a reaching trajectory, can be executed with infinite coactivation levels. The

---

[31] Eidgenössische Technische Hochschule Zürich, Zürich (CH), https://relab.ethz.ch

[32] Interactive Motion Technologies, Inc., Watertown (USA), http://www.interactive-motion.com

[33] Tyromotion GmbH, Graz (A), https://tyromotion.com

higher the coactivation, the higher the rigidity of the posture or the movement. This is the consequence of muscles having non-linear elastic properties, namely, their stiffness increases with the activation level. It is quite clear that high activation levels require higher energetic costs for the same movement, and thus the reduction of coactivation is one of the basic requirements in motor learning, a concept that is quite clear in sports training and should also be better emphasized in the treatment of motor impairments.

For evaluating stiffness, it is necessary to apply a quick, small perturbation to a given posture or movement and measure the resisting force in amplitude and direction: the higher the resisting force, the higher the stiffness. This is an evaluation that clearly can be performed by a human professional only in highly qualitative terms, while it perfectly fits the capability of end-point haptic robots. This technique was developed about three decades ago (Flash and Mussa-Ivaldi 1990; Tsuji et al. 1995), with experiments on normal, adult subjects, focusing on the spatial characteristics of stiffness, namely, its dependence on the direction of the perturbation that is usually expressed graphically by stiffness ellipses.

More recently, this kind of technology was applied to children with CP (Vaz et al. 2006), using a hand-held dynamometer associated with EMG recording, or to adult stroke patients (Piovesan et al. 2013), monitoring the evolution of stiffness amplitude during robot treatment according to an 'assist-as-needed protocol'. It was found that stiffness decreased while voluntary control was slowly recovered.

It should be clarified that although stiffness and spasticity correspond to modifications of the mechanical response of muscles to perturbations, as a consequence, the underlying physiology, together with the measurement protocols, is quite different. The modulation of stiffness is under voluntary control through the increase/decrease of the coactivation level of antagonist muscles. Excessive stiffness involves hypertonus of the involved muscles, and this hypertonus can be decreased by training. The measurement protocol has been defined decades ago and remains the same nowadays.

Spasticity is completely different issue. It certainly is not under voluntary control and is probably determined by an exaggerated tonic stretch reflex. Despite the clear phenomenology of the clinical condition, it is an impairment that is poorly defined and poorly assessed (Malhotra et al. 2009). Spasticity has been defined in many ways over the years. The following definition by Lance (1980) is the most accepted, although it is more descriptive than operational: 'Spasticity is a motor disorder characterized by an increase in the tonic-stretch reflexes due to hyper-excitability tensions, resulting from the hyper-excitability of the stretch reflex, as a component of the upper motor neuron syndrome'. Among the numerous clinical scales focused on spasticity and related pathological conditions, even the most popular ones, based on manual tests of resistance to stretch, namely the modified Ashworth scale (MAS) and modified Tardieu scale (MTS), have been reported to have poor reliability and validity (Abolhasani et al. 2012). Moreover, both scales are examiner-dependent and time-consuming and have scarce sensitivity to progressive improvements during treatment, a sensitivity that is crucial for rational, assessment-driven rehabilitation.

The alternative to clinical scales is the use of electromechanical or robotic systems, to provide precisely controlled stretches, integrated with the concurrent analysis of the short and long-latency components of the stretch reflex (Thilmann et al. 1991). Different studies have involved adult subjects (Pisano et al. 2000; Mirbagheri et al. 2000; Formica et al. 2012; Seth et al. 2015; Popovic-Maneski et al. 2018) and a smaller number of children with CP (Boiteau et al. 1995; Germanotta et al. 2017). However, this matter remains a work in progress and no specific approach has emerged as a de facto standard.

13.3 Training Technology

Training technology to a large extent is based on robotics, with the more or less explicit goal of programming the robot in such a way as to imitate a physiotherapist, thus somehow behaving as a robot-therapist. In this framework, it should be considered that many persons, even if not very fond of science fiction, know the three laws of robotics devised by Isaac Asimov in his novel 'I, Robot' (1950), the first of which—the fundamental one—declares that 'a robot may not injure a human being or, through inaction, allow a human being to come to harm'. Certainly, this should not be a major problem for the application of robotics in rehabilitation, as it is assumed that the design of a rehabilitation device will benefit the person and not be harmful. Nonetheless, as suggested by Iosa et al. (2016), a new version of Asimov's three laws could be written looking at neuro-robotics and taking into consideration not only the ethical aspects of safety but also the usefulness of a robotic machine towards the real needs of a person, its actual role in a rehabilitation program and its contribution to the other professionals working in the rehabilitation field (Wolbrecht et al. 2008; Morasso et al. 2009; Gassert and Dietz 2018). However, it is fair to say that the goal of an effective robot-therapist is still far away as in general is the whole issue of human-robot symbiosis (Sandini et al. 2018). Symbiosis means full, bidirectional interaction and cooperation (consistent with Asimov's laws), and the robot-therapist should have a three-way symbiotic relationship: with a subject with impairment and a human therapist, acting as a partner and as a trainer. From the technological point of view, this requires massive technological innovation in perceptual, motor and cognitive capabilities. According to realistic evaluations from roboticists, at least a decade will be necessary to reach this level. In the meantime, haptic manipulators with adaptive interaction capabilities are what is offered by the state of the art of technology. Largely due to great expectations as technology began to be applied more systematically in the clinical environment, robots are often referred to as therapeutic devices that might work in the place of rehabilitation professionals. As can be easily deduced from the topics and problems addressed in the chapters of this book, client-centred therapeutic planning, well focused on the real needs of the individual, is much more complex and demanding of solutions than only with the use of a device, even if it is very sophisticated. Nevertheless, advanced technology can be of great help where a lengthy repetition of actions is required, with the application of more reliable and measurable parameters. On this basis, it is more correct to refer to the robots currently available in the market and in research labs not as therapeutic but as training devices.

Many interesting publications discuss the role of current robots for a better practice, highlighting their positive contribution for training and as reliable tools for repeated measurements (Krebs and Hogan 2006; Finley et al. 2009; Lins et al. 2019). On the other hand, Kager et al. (2019) observe that, beyond a training threshold, the impaired subject can be overwhelmed and their performance saturated. This brings the clinicians' and engineers' attention back to the need for careful multidisciplinary work planning. The effective final goal should be to enhance functional training, by providing additional training to conventional therapy in a controlled way.

13.3.1 Types of Assistance Provided by Rehabilitation Robots

Going back in time, an ancient ancestor of rehabilitative robots can be found in a 'movement-care' apparatus designed in 1910 by Büdingen, to exercise gait movements in people with heart disease. Later on, rehabilitation devices were always designed according to a passive motion paradigm, which is simpler to implement, and it was only around the 1990s that the first machines were designed providing for an active, bidirectional interface with a subject (Krebs et al. 1998).

This distinction between devices providing passive motion assistance and others supporting active movement (namely, haptic robots) is very important, not because one is always better than the other but because they have different aims and implement a different interaction with the subject. This has already been discussed in the previous Sect. 13.2.7, underlining the distinction between active/passive/resistive/ assistive modes of interaction and the fundamental concepts of 'slacking effect' (to be avoided) and 'assist as needed' (to be optimized). Such distinctions and concepts should be clear in the therapist's mind in order to choose the device best suited to the needs of the user and consequently to optimize and supervise the adopted protocol. Sometimes, a phase of passive mobilization is indeed necessary to support the maintenance or delay the modification of the intrinsic properties of soft tissues, with all the beneficial positive effects in benefit of severely impaired persons for those with severe impairment (see Chap. 7). However, in most situations, the main goal of rehabilitation is to make the person reach an optimal level of function, exploiting neural plasticity even through intense and demanding training sessions.

Current evidence suggests that the number of repetitions of action during a training session, with or without the use of robots, is very important (with due attention as suggested by Krager et al., as mentioned previously) to favour tissue releasing or muscle strengthening and, in particular, to enhance learning, as the repetition of an interesting task can improve motivation, stimulate cognition and facilitate CNS plasticity (Kwakkel et al. 1999; Langhorne et al. 2011; Wandell et al. 2014).

Lang et al. (2009) underline the great difference in the number of actions performed by a person during a robot training session compared with those of a traditional therapy session. However, despite this obvious consideration, during treatment the therapist is supposed to modulate the level of difficulty of the proposed exercise, considered as a full problem-solving task, not a mere assisted movement, keeping the difficulty level just beyond the ability limit of the subject, to challenge and motivate them, without inducing frustration. This requires that the therapist can 'resonate' with the physical-mental needs of the subject, what was referred to before as a 'symbiotic relationship'. This typical human capability, unavailable in the existing robotic machines, explains the rationale of the quantity/quality trade-off of the treatment that supports the integration of robot training with human treatment.

Many robotic machines currently in use are capable of compliant, haptic inter-action, are provided with on-board sensors and can adapt their interaction param-eters in real time to the level of the subject's performance. These features allow to differentiate haptic robots from other electromechanical machines, a distinc-tion that in a rehabilitation environment is often not well focused. For example, there is difference between a traditional treadmill, the parameters of which are set by the therapist but remain fixed thereafter and a Lokomat[34] that can apply an assist-as-needed protocol to the gait of the subject. That does not mean that the treadmill or other non-compliant gait trainers should be eliminated in rehabilita-tion. Indeed, sizeable scientific literature reports that, if electromechanical train-ers are used in children with CP, and applied in appropriate situations and in a rational way, there are positive results regarding improvements in endurance, muscle strength, functional balance and walking ability in general (Richards et al. 1997; Cherng et al. 2007; Meyer-Heim et al. 2009; Smania et al. 2011; Grecco et al. 2013; Wu et al. 2017).

In any case, before proposing the use of a robotic device, it is essential to under-stand its peculiarities, for what purpose it was designed, and what kind of assistance each device can provide. As clarified by Meyer-Heim and van Hedel (2013), differ-ent devices provide a different level of support, requiring the child to be more or less active according to their structure, low-level control software and higher-level task management. The greater the assistance level, the less active the child is motivated to be, and vice versa. For example, this is the case, in the large amount of assistance given by Bi-Manu-Track[35] compared to Armeo®Spring,[36] which does not provide any assistive force. This is because it is a motorless exoskeleton and provides strong support to the arm against gravity through a clever set of springs. We may also quote the YouGrabber System[37] that can deliver virtual reality-based therapy exploiting video game technology appropriate for more able and active children. In general, it is crucial to focus on the great need of linking technological applications with tar-geted therapeutic aims, in such a way as to differentiate different types of advanced devices, depending on their proposal of active or passive exercises and which kind of assistance they provide, as considered above when describing assessment robot-ics (Maciejasz et al. 2014; Falzarano et al. 2019).

---

[34] Hocoma, Volketswil (CH), https://www.hocoma.com
[35] Reha-Stim Medtec AG, Schlieren (CH), https://reha-stim.com
[36] Hocoma, Volketswil (CH), https://www.hocoma.com
[37] Rehab Management, Sidney (AUS), https://rehabpub.com

13.3.2 Robot Training of the Lower Limbs

Wearable robotic exoskeletons have been mentioned previously, such as ReWalk,[38] Phoenix Exoskeleton[39] and EksoNR[40], which were specifically designed for people with spinal cord injuries, who have severe leg muscle strength deficit, rather than motor control deficit. Thus, such devices fundamentally carry out an assistive function. However, the assistive function assured by a suitably adapted exoskeleton may also be useful to subjects with neuromotor problems who require specific gait sessions, to help them acquire adequate neuromotor control of locomotion and consolidate the therapeutic project during ADLs outside the clinic, at home and in the workplace.

In general, this consideration clarifies the fact that assistive, assessment and training technologies can be combined creatively by a therapist supported by a clear understanding of the user's need and their potential for improvement and recovery.

Conventional physiotherapy of subjects with motor difficulties, e.g. stroke patients, focuses on the practice of preparatory gait activities, proposing transfers at all antigravity levels. Innovation to improve walking speed and increase the number of steps trained during a therapy session was the adoption of the treadmill with partial body weight support (Dodd and Foley 2007; Willoughby et al. 2009). However, by itself, this technology is only one-way, without any feedback between the machine and the trained subject, thus sacrificing the quality of interactive assistance to the number of trained movements. This has been the motivation for the development of robotic-assisted gait training (RAGT), supposed to include at least some element of adaptation to the user's need, so bypassing these limiting factors. Robotic gait machines move the legs of the user through specified patterns, and this function can be implemented either by an exoskeleton or an end-point system.

The exoskeletons for RAGT embrace the lower limbs, supporting the body weight in the vertical position and engaging the subject in an active simulation of gait training (Digiacomo et al. 2019; Jin et al. 2020; Kawasaki et al. 2020). There are many examples of such devices, e.g. the Lokomat (Colombo et al. 2000), the LOPES (Veneman et al. 2007), the AutoAmbulator[41] (Healthsouth Corporation 2004) and the Sarà (MPD Costruzioni Meccaniche 2010). However, the Lokomat system is the one that has been used most extensively so far, mainly for adult stroke subjects, although also a paediatric model of this robot has been developed, for children at least 5 years old (Meyer-Heim et al. 2007; van Hedel et al. 2016; Wallard et al. 2017, 2018). Recently, a FreeD module has been added to this robotic orthosis, guiding lateral translation and transverse rotation of the pelvis, an important function not present in previous models (Aurich-Schuler et al. 2019).

Nevertheless, despite the positive results of RAGT, less positive assessments should also be considered. An interesting study on motor learning strategies in

---

[38] ReWalk Robotics Inc., Marlborough (USA), https://rewalk.com
[39] suitX Co., Emeryville (USA), https://www.suitx.com
[40] Ekso Bionics, Richmond (USA), https://eksobionics.com
[41] Encompass Health, Birmingham (USA), http://www.encompasshealth.com

gait-based interventions (Ryan et al. 2020) reported how therapists can be limited by a reduced range of task options using these gait-robot systems with children, compared with more simply and immediate task-oriented activities, and consequently underlies how training is the main function of robots. Moreover, there are still some doubts between the rehabilitation professionals on how these RAGT devices really mimic the natural gait with its typical organization and spatio-temporal parameters, while agreeing about the positive effects of robot training, particularly regarding an increase of muscle strength and endurance (Swank et al. 2019). A general evaluation is also provided by a Cochrane review by Mehrholz et al. in 2017.

Moreover, regarding the end-point RAGT devices, different systems have been developed, like the GangTrainer GT I and II[42] (Hesse and Uhlenbrock 2000), the HapticWalker (Schmidt 2004), the LokoHelp[43] (Freivogel et al. 2008), the 6 Degrees of Freedom Gait Robot (Yoon et al. 2010) and the G-EO systems (Hesse et al. 2010). In particular, the Haptic Walker and the G-EO systems comprise two programmable foot platforms on which the user stands on and the robot control unit enables movements in three degrees of freedom (DOF) of each foot in the sagittal plane, requiring the person to actively adapt to the movements proposed by the trainer. Such devices have been used mostly for adolescent or adult subjects (Schmidt 2004; Esquenazi et al. 2017; De Luca et al. 2018), but at present, a semi-mobile CPWalker[44] is also proposed for the training of children with CP (Bayón et al. 2018).

As to treadmill training in with impairment, there is a general acceptance of the potential benefits of careful training if therapists are fully involved in providing guidance to the child. Nowadays, there is a new generation of advanced treadmill protocols that integrates the traditional body weight-supported treadmill training (BWSTT) with RAGT, which means the child is asked to move on a treadmill eventually with the assistance of a robotic gait training device. To give a sensation of real movement in the environment, which otherwise would remain limited within the confines of the device and therefore be lacking the creation of that optical flow typical of a targeted movement, these advanced treadmills create a virtual environment through the application of a monitor in front of the subject, to simulate their forward-going (Booth et al. 2018). This is the case for example with the ReoAmbulator.[45]

Of course, the application of all these promising technologies for the improvement of the impaired child raises many expectations, but, at the moment, there is only weak evidence regarding the use of RAGT for children with CP or other people with impairment, and the rehabilitator should always monitor individual progress closely with appropriate outcome measures (Lefmann et al. 2017; Veerbeek et al. 2017; Beretta et al. 2020; Petrarca et al. 2021).

---

[42] Reha-Stim Medtec AG, Schlieren (CH), https://reha-stim.com

[43] Woodway, Waukesha (USA), https://www.woodway.com

[44] C P Walker & Son, Beeston (UK), https://www.cpwalker.co.uk

[45] Motorika USA Inc., Mount Laurel (USA), http://motorika.com

13.3.3 Robot Training of the Upper Limbs

Both types of designs, namely exoskeletons and end-point manipulators, are being used for rehabilitation training of the upper limbs of persons with motor impairment. Regarding the former type, the most used system is Armeo®Spring, which is a non-motorized passive skeleton designed in such a way as to compensate for the weight of the arm. Considering also the size of the system and the difficulty of adapting exoskeletons in general to the body of a child, the number of studies involving children with CP is rather limited (Keller and Van Hedel 2017; El-Shamy 2018; Cimolin et al. 2019), and they are focused on the effect of weight-supported training of the upper extremity in learning a goal-directed movement. Another example concerning a research prototype is the IOTA device, i.e. a 2 DOFs exoskeleton to train thumb movements in 7–12 year children (Aubin et al. 2013).

However, to be effective, a robot trainer should be designed in such a way as to integrate both assessing and training capabilities in its structure and function in order to provide a flexible and adaptive interaction with the user, as is sketched in Fig. 13.1. From this point of view, the end-point or end-effector design is better because it allows to measure the exchange of force and energy flow between the robot and the user and the haptic modification of the interacting patterns. In contrast, this is hardly possible with exoskeletons that best operate at two extremes of the interaction modalities: as rigid mobilization machines, at one extreme, or as pure weight-support systems with no mobilization assistance, at the other.

Fig. 13.1 Scheme of haptic interaction for robot training

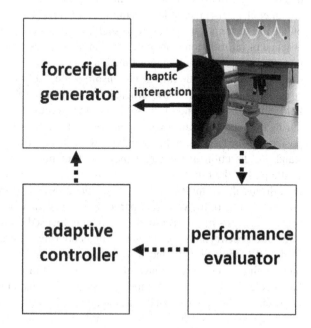

Unfortunately, in this case, the literature on the application of end-point robot training to children is rather scarce, in comparison with the literature that reports studies related to adults (Fasoli et al. 2008; Mazzoleni et al. 2013; Marini et al. 2014, 2015, 2017a, b).

Some preliminary studies exploit the potentialities of haptic interaction and only in a superficial manner, considering the rather unsatisfactory appreciation of robotic training of the upper limb after stroke portrayed by a recent Cochrane review (Mehrholz et al. 2018).

Devices with this kind of haptic adaptation to the user's performance match in some way the action of the physical therapist, who interacts with the assisted subject through carefully modulated forces and movements with the double goal of evaluating the crucial elements of the subject's pathology and assisting them in to improving the voluntary control of their goal-oriented actions. Undoubtedly, the robot has an advantage over the human therapist because it has access to precise quantitative measurements of the interaction, while the human therapist can only rely on their subjective qualitative perceptions. However, the current haptic robots have important technological limitations. For example, they cannot provide real three-dimensional interaction and have even greater limitations in enriching the physical interaction with a motivational, empathic involvement.

Given the importance of proprioception for motor control, research was more and more focused on the issue of 'proprioceptive training', as the hidden side of the training process after neural damage (Schabrun and Hillier 2009; Aman et al. 2014). Several clinical approaches claim to constitute a form of training that improves proprioception and aids motor recovery, but there is no universal agreement in what this training actually constitutes. It may help to consider the following definition of Aman et al. (2014) that at least is quite clear: 'Proprioceptive training [...] focuses on the use of somatosensory signals such as proprioceptive or tactile afferents in the absence of information from other modalities such as vision. Its ultimate goal is to improve or restore sensorimotor function'.

In particular, this definition has inspired the study of robot training of stroke subjects (Casadio et al. 2009), where a reaching task was assisted by minimal force field, attracting the hand of the subject to the target in two experimental conditions during training: (a) subject with open eyes and therefore with visual feedback of the position of the target and their hand; (b) with no vision and the subject could understand the direction of the target they were attempting to reach only through the gentle pull of the robot, i.e. their proprioceptive information. Results demonstrated that, during the training, the level of haptic assistance decreased dramatically and the smoothness of the voluntary part of the movements increased. Moreover, a subsequent analysis of the recorded experiments focused on the analysis of the haptic interaction between the robot and the subject during the training sessions (Piovesan et al. 2013) showed that hand stiffness decreased during training. This is in agreement with the desirable features of motor learning in general, and visual feedback had a deleterious effect on compliance, suggesting that eliminating vision, the soft assistance of the haptic robot had a beneficial effect on the proprioceptive awareness of the subject. Moreover, similar results of a combined motor/proprioceptive training were demonstrated in a similar set of experiments where the reaching task was substituted by a tracking task, in which the subjects were assisted to follow a moving target, marking out a figure of eight (Vergaro et al. 2010).

13.4   Virtual Reality

Virtual reality (VR) is a technology that generalizes the well-known technique of biofeedback. In biofeedback systems, a biological signal of a subject is measured, and the measured variable is presented to the subject in an explicit form, typically visual, acoustic, tactile or in a combination of the three channels. The task assigned to the subject may be of different types, e.g. maintaining it stable in face of disturbances, reaching a target value, tracking a moving target, etc. In the case of VR, biofeedback is integrated with the virtual representation (typically visual) of an environment where the task is defined and the performance of the subject is evaluated and fed back to the subject themselves. Usually, VR systems are subdivided into two classes: full-immersion vs. normal VR implementation. In the former case, the technology has the purpose to induce the subject to feel the perception of being physically present in a non-physical world. The perception is created by surrounding the user with multimodal stimuli (images, sound or other stimuli) that provide a realistic impression of a totally virtual environment, where the real actions of the user interact with the virtual objects of the virtual world, intended as a simulated experience that can be akin or different from the real world.

Despite the impressive effects of immersive VR systems, we believe that they are not appropriate for subjects with sensorimotor impairment because the realistic but physically false interaction is likely to induce confusion and overstimulation. The training process of these subjects requires focusing their attention on what is relevant for their treatment, rather than overstimulating them for entertainment and false fun.

In the non-immersive VR, the user is not isolated from the physical surroundings when interacting with the virtual environment. In these situations, participants could be involved for entertainment, e.g. video games, or educational purposes, including rehabilitation training. In fact, in most of the implementations, at least those carried out for young people with motor impairments, the proposed solutions are a combination of the two aspects, basically to foster motivation of child/adolescent for training (Bonnechère 2018).

To give a more therapeutic look to the use of VR, it is now common to refer to video games for rehabilitation training as 'serious games' (SG). During the last few decades, youngsters have become very able to engage themselves in compelling video games, using commercial game controllers operated through a mouse or keyboard. After the early experiments, the idea of using these games for therapeutic purposes have taken over, adapting the game consoles with new controller interfaces that can also be managed by people with impairment.

This rehabilitation approach is frequently appreciated by users because the aspect of entertainment and little competition is very welcome, but the motivation to participate decreases drastically when the main purpose of the games adapted to specific rehabilitation exercises increases the challenge and lowers enjoyment (Lopes et al. 2018). Furthermore, at present, there is a lack of standardized protocols and robust outcome measurements for an acceptable validation of SGs, although there is marginal evidence of a positive contribution of this therapy as a complementary activity to more conventional rehabilitation treatments (Turolla et al. 2013; Tarakci et al. 2016; Levac et al. 2018; Mills et al. 2019; Avcil et al. 2020).

Bonnechère (2018) refers that most of the devices used for studies on children with CP are designed with specially developed solutions, based on the specific needs of the children (Velasco et al. 2017). In addition to these custom-built devices, the commercial WBB, the PlayStation[46] and the Kinect Xbox[47] are the most—but not the only—consoles used in a rehabilitation environment. In particular, WBB is thought to be a good tool for balance assessment and force measurement (Clark et al. 2010; Bartlett et al. 2014) but is intended also as a platform on which to perform Wii-Fit games. However, there are contrasting evaluations about the therapeutic efficacy of the use of these games with children with CP. Some studies are dubious (Gatica-Rojas et al. 2017); others are positive but mostly for children with USCP or mild CP in combination with NDT treatment (Ramstrand and Lygnegård 2012; Tarakci et al. 2016).

Kinect differs from WBB because it is not a force platform but a cost-effective device with a depth camera and software able to detect and track the shape of a body, redesigning it as a simplified stick-like skeleton. For these characteristics, it has often been used to evaluate motor performances in persons with impairment (Van Sint et al. 2015; Summa et al. 2015), as well as to investigate the effects of its interactive Xbox 360 games on children with cerebral palsy, deducing their possible effectiveness as complementary tools to conventional therapy (Luna-Oliva et al. 2013; Zoccolillo et al. 2015; Machado et al. 2017).

YouGrabber is another interactive game system proposed to improve upper limb movements. In addition to a computer and an infrared localization camera, the system uses adjustable data gloves with Bend Sensor.[48] Training requires the execution of different selective finger and arm movements, challenging the subject in stimulating video games, engaging also visual attention and reaction times. There are few studies on the use of YouGrabber in CP, some of which report satisfactory results, but others doubt the effectiveness of the home-use system beyond the entertainment aspect, because of the need for the support of clinical therapists is often necessary (van Hedel et al. 2011; Gerber et al. 2016).

Apart from the rather small number of applications cited above with a clear rehabilitation purpose, the developments in most cases could be classified more as assistive, in the sense of lowering or eliminating the barriers faced by children with impairment for accessing devices and services useful for ADLs.

---

[46] Sony Interactive Entertainment, Tokyo (JP), https://www.playstation.com

[47] Microsoft Corp., Redmond (USA), https://www.microsoft.com

[48] Flexpoint Sensor System Inc., Draper (USA), https://www.flexpoint.com

A consistent area of interest is entertainment, and here the problem is related to the use of the videogames by subjects with impairment. In particular, concerning the interaction of the child with devices requiring upper limb activities, there is the need to evaluate extent to which the child can use standard controllers and interfaces and, if needed, which kind of modification or adaptation is appropriate for every child. There is a vast range of possible modification and just a set of possibilities is presented as follows:

- An updated version of the Xbox One Elite controller, originally designed in such a way to make the use by people with limitations rather difficult, now has buttons, triggers and extra inputs which can all be remapped to different locations and so facilitate access to the games.
- Switch Joy-Con is a single hand adapter for Nintendo's Switch console.
- GEAR[49] is a device allowing gamers with disabilities to play by only using tilting their feet up or down to simulate eight different button combinations.
- Wearing GlassOuse,[50] a pair of glasses that allow the use of computers hands-free. It is possible to control the mouse cursor with head movements and then biting the selected item;
- Jouse3[51] is an all-encompassing controller operated entirely by the head. It only requires a minimal movement, e.g. only of a cheek, the mouth, the tongue or even the wings of the nose.
- Nintendo manufactured a hands-free controller. The person operates it by using their mouth, acting with the tongue on a stick-like structure to control direction while sucking and blowing on a straw to operate on the buttons.
- A bum controller has been designed to allow gamers to use Xbox 360 to control the movement by shifting the person's own weight in certain directions.

For the purpose of independent living, domotics is another important area where it is necessary to enhance the access to available services (see also Sect. 13.1.6). Here, there are even more sophisticated devices, designed to control the environment without physically touching any kind of controller. Leap Motion Controller[52] is an innovative computer sensor device with two cameras and three infrared LEDs, able to capture and track hand and finger motion in VR. It acts as a mouse but requires no hand contact or touching. The software knows six basic gestures: circle, swipe, key tap, screen tap, plus pinching and grabbing. Some studies with children and adolescents with CP (Tarakci et al. 2019) and elderly people with disability (Iosa et al. 2015; Wang et al. 2017; Fernández-González et al. 2019) have reported rather satisfactory results after the training of upper limbs with this device.

---

[49] Samsung, Suwon (ROK), https://www.samsung.com
[50] GlassOuse, Shenzhen (PRC), https://glassouse.com
[51] Compusult, Mount Pearl (CDN), https://www.compusult.com
[52] Ultraleap Inc., San Francisco (USA), https://www.ultraleap.com

13.5 Telerehabilitation

Telerehabilitation is the provision of assessment and rehabilitation services using telecommunication networks, allowing persons to interact remotely with technological interfaces. Telerehabilitation is a work-in-progress field, where there is the opportunity to develop many interesting rehabilitation paradigms according to the cost/benefit ratio. For example, one of the main opportunities is to increase the intensity and the duration of rehabilitation programs.

The first papers reporting the possible benefits of telerehabilitation are dated around the year 2000. Winters (2002) writes: 'The tools of telerehabilitation help minimize the barrier of distance, both of patients to rehabilitative services and of researchers to subject populations'. At first, the fields of application were addressed to assessment and then spread to almost all the rehabilitation sectors, meaning physiotherapy, but also occupational and speech therapy, audiology, and more recently individual or group motor training, using VR or human-like robot trainers.

There are many pros favouring telerehabilitation, but its use is not always easy and intuitive for the end user, so the management of these remote systems often requires the presence of technicians and, in the case of training children, the supervision of parents or caregivers (Syamimi et al. 2014; Ferre et al. 2017; Anton et al. 2018). Good results are recorded mainly for patients following orthopaedic surgery, but higher-quality research is needed, especially with neurological patients (Agostini et al. 2015; Tyagi et al. 2018).

Concerning children with CP, several studies report telerehabilitation experiences aimed at training lower extremities and also at improving upper extremities through VR videogames (Golomb et al. 2010; Reifenberg et al. 2017; Surana et al. 2019). Syamimi et al. (2014) even offered children with CP home-training where the 'coacher' was the humanoid robot NAO (see before), with a training program including not only lower limb functions but also trunk balance, stand-up, sit-down, and other balance abilities.

Tele-rehabilitation is perfectly tailored for the action observation treatment (AOT), which can propose the child activities through a home video and with the remote supervision by a professional. Many studies report a positive result in favour of children with unilateral CP, also in conjunction with CIMT (Simon-Martinez et al. 2020; Molinaro et al. 2020; Beani et al. 2020).

And in AOT, several initiatives are aimed at the treatment of speech and language disorders, also swallowing dysfunctions. Looking back, as far as language problems are concerned, the telephone was the ancient ancestor of telerehabilitation, which today even allows computer video conferencing and face-to-face treatments of many people at the same time.

Regarding the specific assessment of speech and swallowing disorders, there are some reports with positive results of online assessments of both children and adults, albeit with the obvious limitations of the situation (Lalor et al. 2000; Waite et al. 2010; Ward et al. 2012).

Tele-rehabilitation has recently proved to be a very important resource for dealing with problems such as pandemic situations, for example, the one that recently was caused by Covid-19. This fact has made clinicians rethink the possibility of transforming healthcare in various ways, including remote services. Remote support and counselling have proven to be of great advantage for the family of a child with CP on these occasions, as well as the opportunity of a home-training for adults or other persons in chronic conditions (Ben-Pazi et al. 2020; Azhari and Parsa 2020; Middleton et al. 2020).

Summing up, telerehabilitation can be considered useful, and it is important to further develop the technology behind it, but its use requires special attention, at least on two basic points: it should be able to help rehabilitators for the selection of the most appropriate therapies for the individual user, to manage them remotely and to evaluate the results of the therapy. Furthermore, treatment based on remote systems should strongly motivate and empower users to carry out their therapy programs and not abandon them, asking them also to independently evaluate the rehabilitation sessions and the goals achieved.

References

Abdollahi F, Case Lazarro ED, Listenberger M, Kenyon RV, Kovic M, Bogey RA, Hedeker D, Jovanovic BD, Patton JL (2014) Error augmentation enhancing arm recovery in individuals with chronic stroke: a randomized crossover design. Neurorehabil Neural Repair 28(2):120–128. https://doi.org/10.1177/1545968313498649

Abdollahi F, Farshchiansadegh A, Pierella C, Seáñez-González I, Thorp E, Lee M, Ranganathan R, Pederson J, Chen D, Roth E, Casadio M, Mussa-Ivaldi FA (2017) Body-Machine Interface enables people with cervical Spinal Cord Injury to control devices with available body movements: proof of concept. Neurorehabil Neural Repair 31(5):487–493. https://doi.org/10.1177/1545968317693111

Abolhasani H, Ansari NN, Naghdi S, Mansouri SK, Ghotbi N, Hasson S (2012) Comparing the validity of the Modified Gobi Ashworth Scale (MMAS) and the Modified Tardieu Scale (MTS) in the assessment of wrist flexor spasticity in patients with stroke: protocol for a neurophysiological study. BMJ Open 2(6):e001394. https://doi.org/10.1136/bmjopen-2012-001394

Adde L, Helbostad JL, Jensenius AR, Taraldsen G, Støen R (2009) Using computer-based video analysis in the study of fidgety movements. Early Hum Dev 85(9):541–547. https://doi.org/10.1016/j.earlhumdev.2009.05.003

Adde L, Helbostad JL, Jensenius AR, Taraldsen AG, Grunewaldt KH, Støen R (2010) Early prediction of cerebral palsy by computer-based video analysis of general movements: a feasibility study. Dev Med Child Neurol 52:773–778. https://doi.org/10.1111/j.1469-8749.2010.03629.x

Agostini M, Moja L, Banzi R, Pistotti V, Tonin P, Venneri A, Turolla A et al (2015) Telerehabilitation and recovery of motor function: a systematic review and meta-analysis. J Telemed Telecare 21(4):202–213. https://doi.org/10.1177/1357633X15572201

Airaksinen M, Räsänen O, Ilén E, Häyrinen T, Kivi A, Marchi V, Gallen A, Blom S, Varhe A, Kaartinen N, Haataja L, Vanhatalo S (2020) Automatic posture and movement tracking of infants with wearable movement sensors. Sci Rep 10:169. https://doi.org/10.1038/s41598-019-56862-5

Akbarfahimi N, Arslan SA, Hosseini SA, Rassafiani M (2012) The reactive postural control in spastic cerebral palsy children. Iran Rehabil J 10(1):66–74

Alcorn AM, Ainger E, Charisi V, Mantinioti S, Petrović S, Schadenberg BR, Tavassoli T, Pellicano E (2019) Educators' views on using humanoid robots with autistic learners in special education settings in England. Front Robot AI 6:107. https://doi.org/10.3389/frobt.2019.00107

Aliverti A, Pedotti A (2003) Opto-electronic plethysmography. In: Mechanics of breathing. pp 47–59. https://doi.org/10.1007/978-88-470-2916-3_5

Aman JE, Elangovan N, Yeh IL, Konczak J (2014) The effectiveness of proprioceptive training for improving motor function: a systematic review. Front Hum Neurosci 8:1075

Andrade RM, Sapienza S, Bonato P (2019) Development of a "transparent operation mode" for a lower-limb exoskeleton designed for children with cerebral palsy. In: 2019 IEEE 16th international conference on rehabilitation robotics (ICORR), Toronto, Canada, 24–28 June 2019. https://doi.org/10.1109/ICORR.2019.8779432

Anton D, Berges I, Bermúdez J, Goñi A, Illarramendi A (2018) A telerehabilitation system for the selection, evaluation and remote management of therapies. Sensors (Basel) 18(5):1459. https://doi.org/10.3390/s18051459

Armand S, Decoulon G, Bonnefoy-Mazure A (2016) Gait analysis in children with cerebral palsy. EFORT Open Rev 1:448–460. https://doi.org/10.1302/2058-5241.1.000052

Aruin AS (2002) The organization of anticipatory postural adjustments. J Autom Control 12(1). https://doi.org/10.2298/JAC0201031A

Aruin AS (2015) Anticipatory and compensatory postural adjustments in individuals with multiple sclerosis in response to external perturbations. Neurosci Lett 591:182–186. https://doi.org/10.1016/j.neulet.2015.02.050

Aruin AS (2016) Enhancing Anticipatory Postural Adjustments: a novel approach to balance rehabilitation. J Nov Physiother 6(2):e144. https://doi.org/10.4172/2165-7025.1000e144

Assaiante C, Mallau S, Viel S, Jover M, Schmitz C (2005) Development of postural control in healthy children: a functional approach. Neural Plast 12:art.523497. https://doi.org/10.1155/NP.2005.109

Aubin PM, Sallum H, Walsh C, Stirling L, Correia A (2013) A pediatric robotic thumb exoskeleton for at-home rehabilitation: the Isolated Orthosis for Thumb Actuation (IOTA). In: Proceedings IEEE 13th Int Conf on Rehab Robotics (ICORR), Seattle, USA, 24–26 June 2013, pp 1–6. https://doi.org/10.1109/ICORR.2013.6650500

Aurich-Schuler T, Gut A, Labruyère R (2019) The FreeD module for the Lokomat facilitates a physiological movement pattern in healthy people—a proof of concept study. J Neuroeng Rehabil 16(1):26. https://doi.org/10.1186/s12984-019-0496-x

Avcil E, Tarakci D, Arman N, Tarakci E (2020) Upper extremity rehabilitation using video games in cerebral palsy: a randomized clinical trial. Acta Neurol Belg 121(4):1053–1060. https://doi.org/10.1007/s13760-020-01400-8

Azhari A, Parsa A (2020) Covid-19 Outbreak Highlights: importance of home-based rehabilitation in orthopedic surgery. Arch Bone Jt Surg 8(Suppl 1):317–318. https://doi.org/10.22038/abjs.2020.47777.2350

Baratto L, Morasso P, Re C, Spada G (2002) A new look at posturographic analysis in the clinical context: sway-density versus other parameterization techniques. Mot Control 6(3):246–270. https://doi.org/10.1123/mcj.6.3.246

Bartlett HL, Ting LH, Bingham JT (2014) Accuracy of force and center of pressure measures of the Wii Balance Board. Gait Posture 39(1):224–228. https://doi.org/10.1016/j.gaitpost.2013.07.010

Bayón C, Martín-Lorenzo T, Moral-Saiz B, Ramírez O, Pérez-Somarriba A, Lerma-Lara S, Martínez I, Rocon E (2018) A robot-based gait training therapy for pediatric population with cerebral palsy: goal setting, proposal and preliminary clinical implementation. J Neuroeng Rehabil 15:69. https://doi.org/10.1186/s12984-018-0412-9

Beani E, Menici V, Ferrari A, Cioni C, Sgandurra G (2020) Feasibility of a home-based Action Observation Training for children with unilateral cerebral palsy: an explorative study. Front Neurol 11:16. https://doi.org/10.3389/fneur.2020.00016

Behnke S, Schwarz M, Stückler J (2016) Mobile manipulation, tool use and intuitive interaction for cognitive service robot Cosero. Front Robot AI 3. https://doi.org/10.3389/frobt.2016.00058

Benedetti MG, Catani F, Leardini A, Pignotti E, Giannini S (1998) Data management in gait analysis for clinical applications. Clin Biomech 13(3):204–215. https://doi.org/10.1016/S0268-0033(97)00041-7

Ben-Pazi H, Beni-Adani L, Lamdan R (2020) Accelerating telemedicine for cerebral palsy during the COVID-19 pandemic and beyond. Front Neurol. https://doi.org/10.3389/fneur.2020.00746

Beretta E, (2020) Effect of Robot-Assisted Gait Training in a Large Population of Children With Motor Impairment Due to Cerebral Palsy or Acquired Brain Injury, Arch Phys Med Rehabil. 2020 Jan; 101(1):106–112. https://doi.org/10.1016/j.apmr.2019.08.479 (2020).

Bishop L, Gordon AM, Heakyung K (2017) Hand robotic therapy in children with hemiparesis: a pilot study. Am J Phys Med Rehabil 96(1):1–7. https://doi.org/10.1097/PHM.0000000000000537

Bisi MC, Stagni R (2015) Evaluation of toddler different strategies during the first six-months of independent walking: a longitudinal study. Gait Posture 41(2):574–579. https://doi.org/10.1016/j.gaitpost.2014.11.017

Boiteau M, Malouin F, Richards CL (1995) Use of a hand-held dynamometer and a Kin-Coma dynamometer for evaluating spastic hypertonia in children: a reliability study. Phys Ther 75(9):796–802

Bonato S, d'Angelo MG, Gandossini S, Romei M, Colombo D, Turconi AC, Aliverti A, Bresolin N (2011) Optoelectronic Plethysmography for respiratory assessment in muscular Duchenne dystrophy (P03.5). Eur J Paediatr Neurol 15:S43. https://doi.org/10.1016/j.gaitpost.2009.07.102

Bonnechère B (2018) Serious games in physical rehabilitation: from theory to practice. Springer Int. Publ. https://doi.org/10.1007/978-3-319-66122-3

Booth ATC, Buizer AI, Meyns P, Oude Lansink ILB, Steenbrink F, van der Krogt MM (2018) The efficacy of functional gait training in children and young adults with cerebral palsy: a systematic review and meta-analysis. Dev Med Child Neurol 60(9):866–883. https://doi.org/10.1111/dmcn.13708

Borgestig M, Sandqvist J, Parsons R, Falkmer T, Hemmingsson H (2016) Eye gaze performance for children with severe physical impairments using gaze-based assistive technology—a longitudinal study. Assist Technol 28(2):93–102. https://doi.org/10.1080/10400435.2015.1092182

Breuninger J, Lange C, Bengler K (2011) Implementing gaze control for peripheral devices. In: ACM PETMEI'11, Beijing, China, 18–22 Sept, pp 3–7. https://doi.org/10.1145/2029956.2029960

Brunner R, Dreher T, Romkes J, Frigo C (2002) Effects of plantarflexion on pelvis and lower limb kinematics, Gait Posture. 2008 Jul;28(1):150–6, https://doi.org/10.1016/j.gaitpost.2007.11.013 (2008).

Büdingen T (1910) Movement-cure apparatus. Patent United States: Theodor Buedingen 0964898. https://www.freepatentsonline.com/0964898.html

Bustamante Valles K, Montes S, Madrigal MJ, Burciaga A, Martinez ME, Johnson MJ (2016) Technology-assisted stroke rehabilitation in Mexico: a pilot randomized trial comparing traditional therapy to circuit training in a Robot/technology-assisted therapy gym. J Neuroeng Rehabil 13:83. https://doi.org/10.1186/s12984-016-0190-1

Caceres E, Rios S (2018) Evaluation of an eye-pointer for human-computer interaction. Heliyon 4:e00574. https://doi.org/10.1016/j.heliyon.2018.e00574

Cai NM, Dewald JPA, Gurari N (2020) Accuracy of older adults in judging self-generated elbow torques during multi-joint isometric tasks. Sci Rep 10:13011. https://doi.org/10.1038/s41598-020-69470-5

Campeau-Lecours A, Maheu V, Lepage S, Lamontagne H, Latour S, Paquet L, Hardie N (2016) JACO assistive robotic device: empowering people with disabilities through innovative algorithms. Rehabilitation Engineering and Assistive Technology Society of North America (RESNA) Annual Conference, July 2016, Washington DC

Cappello L, Elangovan N, Contu S, Khosravani S, Konczak J, Masia L (2015) Robot-aided assessment of wrist proprioception. Front Hum Neurosci 9:198. https://doi.org/10.3389/fnhum.2015.00198

Cappozzo A (1984) Gait analysis methodology. Hum Mov Sci 3(1–2):27–50. https://doi.org/10.1016/0167-9457(84)90004-6

Cappozzo A, Catani F, Leardini A, Benedetti MG, Della Croce U (1996) Position and orientation in space of bones during movement: experimental artefacts. Clin Biomech (Bristol, Avon) 11(2):90–100. https://doi.org/10.1016/0268-0033(95)00046-1

Casadio M, Morasso PG, Sanguineti V (2005) Direct measurement of ankle stiffness during quiet standing: implications for control modelling and clinical application. Gait Posture 21(4):410–424. https://doi.org/10.1016/j.gaitpost.2004.05.005

Casadio M, Morasso P, Sanguineti V, Arrichiello V (2006) Braccio di Ferro: a new haptic worksta-tion for neuromotor rehabilitation. Technol Health Care 14:123–142. https://doi.org/10.3233/THC-2006-14301

Casadio M, Morasso P, Sanguineti V, Giannoni P (2009) Minimally assistive robot train-ing for proprioception enhancement. Exp Brain Res 194:219–231. https://doi.org/10.1007/s00221-008-1680-6

Casadio M, Ranganathan R, Mussa-Ivaldi FA (2012) The Body-Machine Interface: a new per-spective on an old theme. Mot Behav 44(6):419–433. https://doi.org/10.1080/00222895.2012.700968

Chang YJ, Han WY, Tsai YC (2013) A Kinect-based upper limb rehabilitation system to assist people with cerebral palsy. Res Dev Disabil 34(11):3654–3659. https://doi.org/10.1016/j.ridd.2013.08.021

Cherng RJ, Liu CF, Lau TW, Hong RB (2007) Effect of treadmill training with body weight sup-port on gait and gross motor function in children with spastic cerebral palsy. Am J Phys Med Rehabil 86(7):548–555. https://doi.org/10.1097/PHM.0b013e31806dc302

Chin K, Soles L, Putrino D, Dehbandi B, Nwankwo V, Gordon A, Friel K (2017) Use of marker-less motion capture to evaluate proprioception impairments in children with unilateral spastic cerebral palsy: a feasibility trial. In: Abstracts of 71st Annual Meeting of the AACPDM, vol 59, issue S3, 13–16 Sept, pp 24–25. https://doi.org/10.1111/dmcn.33_13511

Cimolin V, Germiniasi C, Galli M, Condoluci C, Beretta E, Piccinini L (2019) Robot-Assisted Upper Limb Training for Hemiplegic Children with Cerebral Palsy, J of Devel and Physical Disabilities, 31:89–101. https://doi.org/10.1007/s10882-018-9632-y (2019)

Clark RA, Bryant AL, Pua Y, McCrory P, Bennell K, Hunt M (2010) Validity and reliability of the Nintendo Wii Balance Board for assessment of standing balance. Gait Posture 31(3):307–310. https://doi.org/10.1016/j.gaitpost.2009.11.012

Cliff DP, Reilly JJ, Okely AD (2009) Methodological considerations in using accelerometers to assess habitual physical activity in children aged 0 to 5 years. J Sci Med Sport 12:557–567. https://doi.org/10.1016/j.jsams.2008.08.008

Coeckelbergh M, Pop C, Simut R, Peca A, Pintea S, David D, Vanderborght B (2015) A sur-vey of expectations about the role of robots in robot-assisted therapy for children with ASD: ethical acceptability, trust, sociability, appearance and attachment. Sci Eng Ethics. https://doi.org/10.1007/s11948-015-9649-x

Colombo G, Joerg M, Schreier R, Dietz V (2000) Treadmill training of paraplegic patients using a robotic orthosis. J Rehabil Res Dev 37(6):693–700

Daly I, Billinger M, Laparra Hernandez J, Aloise F, Lloria Garcia M, Faller J, Scherer R, Müller-Putz G (2013) On the control of brain-computer interfaces by users with cerebral palsy. Clin Neurophysiol 124(9):1787–1797. https://doi.org/10.1016/j.clinph.2013.02.118

Darwish MH, Ahmed S, Ismail ME, Khalifa HA (2019) Influence of pelvic inclination on sit to stand task in stroke patients. Egypt J Neurol Psychiatr Neurosurg 55:89. https://doi.org/10.1186/s41983-019-0132-5

de Andrade E, Souza Mazuchi F, Mochizuki L, Hamill J, Martins Franciulli P, Bigongiari A, de Almeida Martins IT, Ervilha UF (2020) Joint-Position Sense Accuracy is equally affected by vision among children with and without Cerebral Palsy. J Mot Behav 1–8. https://doi.org/10.1080/00222895.2020.1756732

De Luca A, Vernetti H, Capra C, Pisu I, Cassiano C, Barone L, Gaito F, Danese F, Antonio Checchia G, Lentino C, Giannoni P, Casadio M (2018) Recovery and compensation after robotic assisted gait training in chronic stroke survivors. Disabil Rehabil Assist Technol 9:1–13. https://doi.org/10.1080/17483107.2018.1466926

Dellaca RRL, Ventura MML, Zannin EA, Natile M, Pedotti A, Tagliabue P (2010) Measurement of total and compartmental lung volume changes in newborns by optoelectronic plethysmogra-phy. Pediatr Res 67:11–16. https://doi.org/10.1203/PDR.0b013e3181c0b184

Digiacomo F, Tamburin S, Tebaldi S, Pezzani M, Tagliafierro M, Casale R, Bartolo M (2019) Improvement of motor performance in children with cerebral palsy treated with exoskeleton robotic training: a retrospective explorative analysis. Restor Neurol Neurosci 37(3):239–244. https://doi.org/10.3233/RNN-180897. Erratum in: Restor Neurol Neurosci (2020) 38(2):185

Dodd KJ, Foley S (2007) Partial body-weight-supported treadmill training can improve walking in children with cerebral palsy: a clinical controlled trial. Dev Med Child Neurol 49(2):101–105. https://doi.org/10.1111/j.1469-8749.2007.00101.x

Doi H, Iijima N, Furui A, Soh Z, Shinohara K, Iriguchi M, Shimatani K, Tsuiji T (2021) Markerless Video Analysis of Spontaneous Bodily Movements in 4-Month-Old Infants Predicts Autism-like Behavior in 18-Month-Olds, medRxiv, https://doi.org/10.1101/2021.10.11.21264725 (2021)

Donker SF, Ladebt A, Roerdink M, Savelsbergh GJP, Beek PJ (2008) Children with cerebral palsy exhibit greater and more postural sway than typically developing children. Exp Brain Res 184:363–370. https://doi.org/10.1007/s00221-007-1105-y

dos Santos AN, Pavão SL, Rocha NA (2011) Sit-to-stand movement in children with cerebral palsy: a critical review. Res Dev Disabil 32(6):2243–2252. https://doi.org/10.1016/j.ridd.2011.05.001

Driessen BJ, Evers HG, van Woerden JA (2001) MANUS—a wheelchair-mounted rehabilitation robot. Proc Inst Mech Eng H 215(3):285–290. https://doi.org/10.1243/0954411011535876

Eguren D, Cestari M, Luu TP, Kilicarslan A, Steele A, Contreras-Vidal JL (2019) Design of a customizable, modular pediatric exoskeleton for rehabilitation and mobility. In: 2019 IEEE international conference on systems, man and cybernetics (SMC) Bari, Italy, 6–9 Oct 2019. https://doi.org/10.1109/SMC.2019.8914629

Einspieler C, Marschik PB, Bos AF, Ferrari F, Cioni G, Prechtl HFR (2012) Early markers for cerebral palsy: insights from the assessment of general movements. Future Neurol 7(6):709–717. https://doi.org/10.2217/fnl.12.60

Einspieler C, Bos AF, Libertus ME, Marschik PB (2016) The General Movement assessment helps us to identify preterm infants at risk for cognitive dysfunction. Front Psychol 7:406. https://doi.org/10.3389/fpsyg.2016.00406

El Shemy SA (2018) Effect of treadmill training with eyes open and closed on knee proprioception, functional balance and mobility in children with spastic diplegia. Ann Rehabil Med 42(6):854–862. https://doi.org/10.5535/arm.2018.42.6.854

Elsaeh M, Pudlo P, Djemai M, Bouri M, Thevenon A, Heymann I (2017) The effects of haptic-virtual reality game therapy on brain-motor coordination for children with hemiplegia: a pilot study. In: Proceedings of the IEEE 2017 international conference on virtual rehabilitation (ICVR), Montreal, QC, Canada, 19–22 June 2017, pp 1–6. https://doi.org/10.1109/ICVR.2017.8007472

El-Shamy SM (2018) Efficacy of Armeo® robotic therapy versus conventional therapy on upper limb function in children with hemiplegic cerebral palsy. Am J Phys Med Rehabil 97(3):164–169. https://doi.org/10.1097/PHM.0000000000000852

Eishima K (1991) The analysis of sucking behaviour in newborn infants. Early Hum Dev. 1991 Dec;27(3):163–73. https://doi.org/10.1016/0378-3782(91)90192-6

Esquenazi A, Lee S, Wikoff A, Packel A, Toczylowski T, Feeley J (2017) A comparison of locomotor therapy interventions: Partial-Body Weight-Supported Treadmill, Lokomat and G-EO training in people with traumatic brain injury. PM R 9(9):839–846. https://doi.org/10.1016/j.pmrj.2016.12.010

Falzarano V, Marini F, Morasso P, Zenzeri J (2019) Devices and protocols for upper limb robot-assisted rehabilitation of children with neuromotor disorders. Appl Sci 9(13):2689. https://doi.org/10.3390/app9132689

Fasoli SE, Fragala-Pinkham M, Hughes R, Hogan N, Krebs HI, Stein J (2008) Upper limb robotic therapy for children with hemiplegia. Am J Phys Med Rehabil 87(11):929–936. https://doi.org/10.1097/PHM.0b013e31818a6aa4

Fernández-González P, Carratalá-Tejada M, Monge-Pereira E, Collado-Vázquez S, Sánchez-Herrera Baeza P et al (2019) Leap motion controlled video game-based therapy for upper limb rehabilitation in patients with Parkinson's disease: a feasibility study. J Neuroeng Rehabil 16:133. https://doi.org/10.1186/s12984-019-0593-x

Ferrari A, Brunner R, Faccioli S, Reverberi S, Benedetti MG (2015) Gait analysis contribution to problems identification and surgical planning in CP patients: an agreement study. Eur J Phys Rehabil Med 51(1):39–48

Ferrarin M, Rabuffetti M, Bacchini M, Casiraghi A, Castagna A, Pizzi A, Montesano A (2015) Does gait analysis change clinical decision-making in poststroke patients? Results from a pragmatic prospective observational study. Eur J Phys Rehabil Med 51(2):171–184

Ferre CL, Brandão M, Surana B, Dew AP, Moreau NG, Gordon AM (2017) Caregiver-directed home-based intensive bimanual training in young children with unilateral spastic cerebral palsy: a randomized trial. Dev Med Child Neurol 59(5):497–504. https://doi.org/10.1111/dmcn.13330

Finley MA, Dipietro L, Ohlhoff J, Whitall J, Krebs HI, Bever CT (2009) The effect of repeated measurements using an upper extremity robot on healthy adults. J Appl Biomech 25(2):03–110. https://doi.org/10.1123/jab.25.2.103

Flash T, Mussa-Ivaldi FA (1990) Human arm stiffness characteristics during maintenance of posture. Exp Brain Res 82:315–326

Flux E, van der Krogt MM, Cappa P, Petrarca M, Desloovere K, Harlaar J (2020) The Human Body Model versus conventional gait models for kinematic gait analysis in children with cerebral palsy. Hum Mov Sci 70:102585. https://doi.org/10.1016/j.humov.2020.102585

Formica D, Charles SK, Zollo L, Guglielmelli E, Hogan N, Krebs HI (2012) The passive stiffness of the wrist and forearm. J Neurophysiol 108(4):1158–1166. https://doi.org/10.1152/jn.01014.2011

Franki I, De Cat J, Deschepper E, Molenaers G, Desloovere K, Himpens E, Vanderstraeten G, Van den Broeck C (2014) A clinical decision framework for the identification of main problems and treatment goals for ambulant children with bilateral spastic cerebral palsy. Res Dev Disabil 35(5):1160–1176. https://doi.org/10.1016/j.ridd.2014.01.025

Frascarelli F, Masia L, Di Rosa G, Cappa P, Petrarca M, Castelli E, Krebs H (2006) The impact of robotic rehabilitation in children with acquired or congenital movement disorders. Eur J Phys Rehabil Med 2009(45):135–141

Freivogel S, Mehrholz J, Husak-Sotomayor T, Schmalohr D (2008) Gait training with the newly developed 'LokoHelp'-system is feasible for nonambulatory patients after stroke, spinal cord and brain injury. A feasibility study. Brain Inj 22(7):625–632. https://doi.org/10.1080/02699050801941771

Fujisawa Y, Okajima Y (2015) Characteristics of handwriting of people with cerebellar ataxia: three-dimensional movement analysis of the pen tip, finger and wrist. Phys Ther 95(11):1547–1558. https://doi.org/10.2522/ptj.20140118

Gassert R, Dietz V (2018) Rehabilitation robots for the treatment of sensorimotor deficits: a neurophysiological perspective. J Neuroeng Rehabil 15:46. https://doi.org/10.1186/s12984-018-0383-x

Gatica-Rojas V, Méndez-Rebolledo G, Guzman-Muñoz E, Soto-Poblete A, Cartes-Velásquez R, Elgueta-Cancino E, Cofré Lizama LE (2017) Does Nintendo Wii Balance Board improve standing balance? A randomized controlled trial in children with cerebral palsy. Eur J Phys Rehabil Med 53(4):535–544. https://doi.org/10.23736/S1973-9087.16.04447-6

Gerber CN, Kunz B, van Hedel HJA (2016) Preparing a neuropediatric upper limb exergame rehabilitation system for home-use: a feasibility study. J Neuroeng Rehabil 13:33. https://doi.org/10.1186/s12984-016-0141-x

Germanotta M, Taborri J, Rossi S, Frascarelli F, Palermo E, Cappa P, Castelli E, Petrarca M (2017) Spasticity measurement based on tonic stretch reflex threshold in children with cerebral palsy using the PediAnklebot. Front Hum Neurosci 11:277. https://doi.org/10.3389/fnhum.2017.00277

Ghazal B, Khatib K (2015) Smart home automation system for elderly and handicapped people using XBee. Int J Smart Home 9(4):203–210. https://doi.org/10.14257/ijsh.2015.9.4.21

Gibson JJ (1966) The senses considered as perceptual systems. Houghton Mifflin, Boston

Gilliaux M, Dierckx F, Berghe LV, Lejeune TM, Sapin J, Dehez B, Stoquart G, Detrembleur C (2015) Age effects on upper limb kinematics assessed by the REAplan robot in healthy school-aged children. Ann Biomed Eng 2015(43):1123–1131. https://doi.org/10.1007/s10439-014-1189-z

Girolami GL, Shiratori T, Aruin AS (2011) Anticipatory postural adjustments in children with hemiplegia and diplegia. J Electromyogr Kinesiol 21(6):988–997. https://doi.org/10.1016/j.jelekin.2011.08.013

Goble DJ, Lewis CA, Hurvitz EA, Brown SH (2005) Development of upper limb proprioceptive accuracy in children and adolescents. Hum Mov Sci 24(2):155–170. https://doi.org/10.1016/j.humov.2005.05.004

Goble DJ, Hurvitz EA, Brown SH (2009) Deficits in the ability to use proprioceptive feedback in children with hemiplegic cerebral palsy. Int J Rehabil Res 32(3):267–269. https://doi.org/10.1097/MRR.0b013e32832a62d5

Golomb MR, McDonald BC, Warden SJ, Yonkman J, Saykin AJ, Shirley B et al (2010) In-home Virtual Reality videogame telerehabilitation in adolescents with hemiplegic cerebral palsy. Arch Phys Med Rehabil 91(1):1–8.e1. https://doi.org/10.1016/j.apmr.2009.08.153

Graf B, Hans M, Schraft R (2004) Care-O-bot II—development of a next generation robotic home assistant. Auton Robot 16(2):193–205. https://doi.org/10.1023/B:AURO.0000016865.35796.e9

Gravem D, Singh M, Chen C, Rich J, Vaughan J, Goldberg K, Waffarn F, Chou P, Cooper D, Reinkensmeyer D, Patterson D (2011) Assessment of infant movement with a compact wireless accelerometer system. J Med Devices 6(2):1–7. https://doi.org/10.1115/1.4006129

Grecco LAC, Tomita SM, Christovão TCL, Pasini H (2013) Effect of treadmill gait training on static and functional balance in children with cerebral palsy: randomized controlled clinical trial. Braz J Phys Ther 17(1). https://doi.org/10.1590/S1413-35552012005000066

Gurari N, van der Helm NA, Drogos JM, Dewald JPA (2019) Accuracy of individuals post-hemiparetic stroke in matching torques between arms depends on the arm referenced. Front Neurol 10:921. https://doi.org/10.3389/fneur.2019.00921

Han J, Anson J, Waddington G, Adams R, Liu Y (2015) The role of ankle proprioception for balance control in relation to sports performance and injury. Biomed Res Int 2015:842804. https://doi.org/10.1155/2015/842804

Han J, Waddington G, Adams R, Anson J, Liu Y (2016) Assessing proprioception: a critical review of methods. J Sport Health Sci 5(1):80–90. https://doi.org/10.1016/j.jshs.2014.10.004

Harper R (2006) Inside the smart home. Springer, Berlin

Healthsouth Corporation (2004) Powered gait orthosis and method of utilizing same. US Patent US2004/0143198

Heinze F, Hesels K, Breitbach-Faller N, Schmitz-Rode T, Disselhorst-Klug C (2010) Movement analysis by accelerometry of newborns and infants for the early detection of movement disorders due to infantile cerebral palsy. Med Biol Eng Comput 48(8):765–772. https://doi.org/10.1007/s11517-010-0624-z

Hesse S, Uhlenbrock D (2000) A mechanized gait trainer for restoration of gait. J Rehabil Res Dev 37(6):701–708

Hesse S, Waldner A, Tomelleri C (2010) Innovative gait robot for the repetitive practice of floor walking and stair climbing up and down in stroke patients. J Neuroeng Rehabil 7(30):1–10. https://doi.org/10.1186/1743-0003-7-30

Hesse N, Pujades S, Romero J, Black MJ, Bodensteiner C, Arens M, Hofmann UG, Tacke U, Hadders-Algra M, Weinberger R, Muller-Felber W, Schroeder AS (2018) Learning an Infant Body Model from RGB-D Data for Accurate Full Body Motion Analysis. In: Proceedings Int. Conf. on Medical Image Computing and Computer Assisted Intervention (MICCAI), Sept 2018. https://doi.org/10.1007/978-3-030-00928-1_89

Holst-Wolf JM, Yeh IL, Konczak J (2016) Development of proprioceptive acuity in typically developing children: normative data on forearm position sense. Front Hum Neurosci. https://doi.org/10.3389/fnhum.2016.00436

Hong SY, Jung NH, Kim KM (2016) The correlation between proprioception and handwriting legibility in children. J Phys Ther Sci 28(10):2849–2851. https://doi.org/10.1589/jpts.28.2849

Horak FB, Nashner LM (1986) Central programming of postural movements: adaptation to altered support-surface configurations. J Neurophysiol 55:1369–1381. https://doi.org/10.1152/jn.1986.55.6.1369

Horak FB, Nashner LM, Diener HC (1990) Postural strategies associated with somatosensory and vestibular loss. Exp Brain Res 82(1):167–177. https://doi.org/10.1007/BF00230848

Hoseini N, Sexton BM, Kurtz K, Liu Y, Block HJ (2015) Adaptive staircase measurement of hand proprioception. PLoS One. https://doi.org/10.1371/journal.pone.0135757

Huijnen CAGJ, Lexis MAS, Jansens R, de Witte LP (2016) Mapping robots to therapy and educational objectives for children with autism spectrum disorder. J Autism Dev Disord 46(6):2100–2114. https://doi.org/10.1007/s10803-016-2740-6

Iandolo R, Squeri V, De Santis D, Giannoni P, Morasso P, Casadio M (2015) Proprioceptive bimanual test in intrinsic and extrinsic coordinates. Front Hum Neurosci. https://doi.org/10.3389/fnhum.2015.00072

Ilg W, Schatton C, Schicks J, Giese MA, Schöls L, Synofzik M (2012) Video game-based coordinative training improves ataxia in children with degenerative ataxia. Neurology 79(20):2056–2060. https://doi.org/10.1212/WNL.0b013e3182749e67

Iosa M, Morone G, Fusco A, Castagnoli M, Fusco FR, Pratesi L, Paolucci S (2015) Leap motion controlled videogame-based therapy for rehabilitation of elderly patients with subacute stroke: a feasibility pilot study. Top Stroke Rehabil 22(4):306–316. https://doi.org/10.1179/1074935714Z.0000000036

Iosa M, Morone G, Cherubini A, Paolucci S (2016) The Three Laws of neurorobotics: a review on what neurorehabilitation robots should do for patients and clinicians. J Med Biol Eng 36:1–11. https://doi.org/10.1007/s40846-016-0115-2

Ivanenko YP, Dominici N, Cappellini G, Dan B, Cheron G, Lacquaniti F (2004) Development of pendulum mechanism and kinematic coordination from the first unsupported steps in toddlers. J Exp Biol 207(Pt 21):3797–3810. https://doi.org/10.1242/jeb.01214

Ivanenko YP, Dominici N, Lacquaniti F (2007) Development of independent walking in toddlers. Exerc Sport Sci Rev 35(2):67–73. https://doi.org/10.1249/jes.0b013e31803eafa8

Jin LH, Yang S, Choi JY, Sohn MK (2020) The effect of Robot-Assisted Gait Training on locomotor function and functional capability for daily activities in children with cerebral palsy: a single-blinded, randomized cross-over trial. Brain Sci 2020(10):801. https://doi.org/10.3390/brainsci10110801

Johnson MJ, Rai R, Barathi S, Mendonca R, Bustamante-Valles K (2017) Affordable stroke therapy in high-, low- and middle-income countries: from Theradrive to Rehab CARES, a compact robot gym. J Rehabil Assist Technol Eng 4:1–12. https://doi.org/10.1177/2055668317708732

Kager S, Hussain A, Budhota A, Dailey WD, Hughes CML, Deshmukh VA, Kuah CWK, Yin Ng C, Yam LHL, Xiang L, Ang MH Jr, Chua KSG, Campolo D (2019) Work with me, not for me: relationship between robotic assistance and performance in subacute and chronic stroke patients. J Rehabil Assist Technol Eng 6:1–9. https://doi.org/10.1177/2055668319881583

Kanemaru N, Watanabe H (2012) Increasing selectivity of interlimb coordination during spontaneous movements in 2- to 4-month-old infants. Exp Brain Res 218:49–61. https://doi.org/10.1007/s00221-012-3001-3

Kanemaru N, Watanabe H, Kihara H, Nakano H, Nakamura T, Nakano J (2014) Jerky spontaneous movements at term age in preterm infants who later developed cerebral palsy. Early Hum Dev 90(8):387–392. https://doi.org/10.1016/j.earlhumdev.2014.05.004

Karch D, Kim KS, Wochner K, Pietz J, Dickhaus H, Philippi H (2008) Quantification of the segmental kinematics of spontaneous infant movements. J Biomech 41(13):2860–2867. https://doi.org/10.1016/j.jbiomech.2008.06.033

Karch D, Wochner K, Kim K, Philippi H, Hadders-Algra M, Pietz J, Dickhaus H (2010) Quantitative score for the evaluation of kinematic recordings in neuropediatric diagnostics. Methods Inf Med 49(05):526–530. https://doi.org/10.3414/ME09-02-0034

Kawasaki S, Ohata K, Yoshida T, Yokoyama A, Yamada S (2020) Gait improvements by assisting hip movements with the robot in children with cerebral palsy: a pilot randomized controlled trial. J Neuroeng Rehabil 17(1):87. https://doi.org/10.1186/s12984-020-00712-3

Keller JW, Van Hedel HJ (2017) Weight-supported training of the upper extremity in children with cerebral palsy: a motor learning study. J Neuroeng Rehabil 2017(14):87. https://doi.org/10.1186/s12984-017-0293-3

Krebs HI, Hogan N (2006) Therapeutic robotics: a technology push. Proc IEEE Inst Electr Electron Eng 94(9):1727–1738. https://doi.org/10.1109/JPROC.2006.880721

Krebs HI, Hogan N, Aisen ML, Volpe BT (1998) Robot-aided neurorehabilitation. IEEE Trans Rehabil Eng 6(1):75–87. https://doi.org/10.1109/86.662623

Kuczynski AM, Semrau JA, Kirton A, Dukelow SP (2017) Kinesthetic deficits after perinatal stroke: robotic measurement in hemiparetic children. J Neuroeng Rehabil 14:13. https://doi.org/10.1186/s12984-017-0221-6

Kwakkel G, Wagenaar RC, Twisk JW, Lankhorst GJ, Koetsier JC (1999) Intensity of leg and arm training after primary middle-cerebral-artery stroke: a randomised trial. Lancet 354(9174):191–196. https://doi.org/10.1016/S0140-6736(98)09477-X

Lalor E, Brown M, Cranfield E (2000) Telemedicine: its role in speech and language management for rural and remote patients. ACQ Speech Pathol Aust 2:54–55

Lance JW (1980) Symposium synopsis. In: Feldman RG, Young RR, Koella KP (eds) Spasticity: disorder of motor control. Year Book, Chicago, pp 17–24

Lang CE, Macdonald JR, Reisman DS et al (2009) Observation of amounts of movement practice provided during stroke rehabilitation. Arch Phys Med Rehabil 90(10):1692–1698. https://doi.org/10.1016/j.apmr.2009.04.005

Langhorne P, Bernhardt J, Kwakkel G (2011) Stroke rehabilitation. Lancet 377(9778):1693–1702. https://doi.org/10.1016/S0140-6736(11)60325-5

Lanningham-Foster LM, Jensen TB, McCrady SK, Nysse LJ, Foster RC, Levine JA (2005) Laboratory measurement of posture allocation and physical activity in children. Med Sci Sports Exerc 37(10):1800–1805. https://doi.org/10.1249/01.mss.0000175050.03506.bf

Laut J, Porfiri M, Raghavan P (2016) The present and future of robotic technology in rehabilitation. Curr Phys Med Rehabil Rep 4:312–319. https://doi.org/10.1007/s40141-016-0139-0

Ledebt A, Bril B (2000) Acquisition of upper body stability during walking in toddlers. Dev Psychobiol 36:311–324. https://doi.org/10.1002/(SICI)1098-2302(200005)36:4<311::AID-DEV6>3.0.CO;2-V

Ledebt A, Bril B, Wiener-Vacher S (1995) Trunk and head stabilization during the first months of independent walking. Neuroreport 6:1737–1740. https://doi.org/10.1097/00001756-199509000-00008

Lee EH, Goh JCH, Bose K (1992) Value of gait analysis in the assessment of surgery in cerebral palsy. Arch Phys Med Rehabil 73(7):642–646

Lee MH, Ranganathan R, Kagerer F, Mukherjee R (2016) Body-machine interface for control of a screen cursor for a child with congenital absence of upper and lower limbs: a case report. J Neuroeng Rehabil 13:34. https://doi.org/10.1186/s12984-016-0139-4

Lefmann S, Russo R, Hillier S (2017) The effectiveness of robotic-assisted gait training for paediatric gait disorders: systematic review. J Neuroeng Rehabil 14:1. https://doi.org/10.1186/s12984-016-0214-x

Lerner ZF, Harvey TA, Lawson JL (2019) A battery-powered ankle exoskeleton improves gait mechanics in a feasibility study of individuals with cerebral palsy. Ann Biomed Eng 47(6):1345–1356. https://doi.org/10.1007/s10439-019-02237-w

Levac D, McCormick A, Levin MF, Brien M, Mills R, Miller E, Sveistrup H (2018) Active video gaming for children with cerebral palsy: does a clinic-based Virtual Reality component offer an additive benefit? A pilot study. Phys Occup Ther Pediatr 38(1):74–87. https://doi.org/10.1080/01942638.2017.1287810

Li KY, Su WJ, Fu HW, Pickett KA (2015) Kinesthetic deficit in children with developmental coordination disorder. Res Dev Disabil 38:125–133. https://doi.org/10.1016/j.ridd.2014.12.013

Li L, Li SW, Li YX (2019) Wrist joint proprioceptive acuity assessment using inertial and magnetic measurement systems. Int J Distrib Sensor Netw 15(4). https://doi.org/10.1177/1550147719845548

Lin SI, Woollacott M, Jensen JL (2004) Postural response in older adults with different levels of functional balance capacity. Aging Clin Exp Res 16(5):369–374. https://doi.org/10.1007/BF03324566

Lincoln NB, Jackson JM, Adams SA (1998) Reliability and revision of the Nottingham Sensory Assessment for stroke patients. Physiotherapy 84(8):358–365. https://doi.org/10.1016/S0031-9406(05)61454-X

Lins AA, de Oliveira JM, Rodrigues JJPC, de Albuquerque VHC (2019) Robot-assisted therapy for rehabilitation of children with cerebral palsy—a complementary and alternative approach. Comput Hum Behav 100:152–167. https://doi.org/10.1016/j.chb.2018.05.012

Linvill JG, Bliss JC (1966) A direct translation reading aid for the blind. Proc IEEE 54(1):40–45

Lofterød B, Terjesen T, Skaaret I, Huse AB, Jahnsen R (2007) Preoperative gait analysis has a substantial effect on orthopedic decision making in children with cerebral palsy: comparison between clinical evaluation and gait analysis in 60 patients. Acta Orthop 78(1):74–80. https://doi.org/10.1080/17453670610013448

Looper J, Chandler LS (2013) How do toddlers increase their gait velocity? Gait Posture 37(4):631–633. https://doi.org/10.1016/j.gaitpost.2012.09.009

Lopes S, Magalhães P, Pereira A, Martins J, Magalhães C, Chaleta E, Rosário P (2018) Games used with serious purposes: a systematic review of interventions in patients with cerebral palsy. Front Psychol 9:1712. https://doi.org/10.3389/fpsyg.2018.01712

Lotfi A, Langensiepen C, Yahaya SW (2017) Socially Assistive Robotics: robot exercise trainer for older adults. Technologies 2018(6):32. https://doi.org/10.3390/technologies6010032

Ludwig O, Kelm J, Hammes A, Schmitt E, Fröhlich M (2020) Neuromuscular performance of balance and posture control in childhood and adolescence. Heliyon 6(7):e04541. https://doi.org/10.1016/j.heliyon.2020.e04541

Luna-Oliva L, Ortiz-Gutierrez RM, Cano-de la Cuerda R (2013) Kinect Xbox 360 as a therapeutic modality for children with cerebral palsy in a school environment: a preliminary study. Neurorehabilitation 33(4):513–521. https://doi.org/10.3233/NRE-131001

Machado FRC, Pereira Antunes P, De Moura Souza J, Cardoso Dos Santos A, Centenaro Levandowski D, De Oliveira AA (2017) Motor improvement using motion sensing game devices for cerebral palsy rehabilitation. J Mot Behav 49(3):273–280. https://doi.org/10.1080/00222895.2016.1191422

Maciejasz P, Eschweiler J, Gerlach-Hahn K, Jansen-Troy A, Leonhardt S (2014) A survey on robotic devices for upper limb rehabilitation. J Neuroeng Rehabil 11:3. https://doi.org/10.1186/1743-0003-11-3

Malhotra S, Pandyan AD, Day CR, Jones PW, Hermens H (2009) Spasticity, an impairment that is poorly defined and poorly measured. Clin Rehabil 23(7):651–658. https://doi.org/10.1177/0269215508101747

Marcroft C, Khan A, Embleton ND, Trenell M, Plötz T (2015) Movement recognition technology as a method of assessing spontaneous general movements in high risk infants. Front Neurol. https://doi.org/10.3389/fneur.2014.00284

Marini F, Cappello L, Squeri V, Morasso P, Moretti P, Riva A, Doglio L, Masia L (2014) Online modulation of assistance in robot aided wrist rehabilitation a pilot study on a subject affected by dystonia. In: Proceedings of the 2014 IEEE Haptics Symposium (HAPTICS), Houston, TX, USA, 23–26 Feb 2014, pp 153–158. https://doi.org/10.1109/HAPTICS.2014.6775448

Marini F, Squeri V, Cappello L, Morasso P, Riva A, Doglio L, Masia L (2015) Adaptive wrist robot training in pediatric rehabilitation. In: Proceedings of the 2015 IEEE International Conference on Rehabilitation Robotics (ICORR), Singapore, Singapore, 11–14 Aug 2015, pp 175–180. https://doi.org/10.1109/ICORR.2015.7281195

Marini F, Hughes CML, Squeri V, Doglio L, Moretti P, Morasso P, Masia L (2017a) Robotic wrist training after stroke: adaptive modulation of assistance in pediatric rehabilitation. Robot Auton Syst 91:169–178. https://doi.org/10.1016/j.robot.2017.01.006

Marini F, Squeri V, Morasso P, Campus C, Konczak J, Masia L (2017b) Robot-aided developmental assessment of wrist proprioception in children. J Neuroeng Rehabil 14:3. https://doi.org/10.1186/s12984-016-0215-9

Masia L, Casadio M, Morasso P, Pozzo T, Sandini G (2008) Using a wrist robot for evaluating how human operators learn to perform pointing movements to a rotating frame of reference. In: Proceed IEEE BioRob., 19–22 Oct 2008, Scottsdale, AZ, USA

Masia L, Casadio M, Giannoni P, Sandini G, Morasso P (2009) Performance adaptive training control strategy for recovering wrist movements in stroke patients: a preliminary, feasibility study. J Neuroeng Rehabil 6(44):1–11. https://doi.org/10.1186/1743-0003-6-44

Massion J (1992) Movement, posture and equilibrium: interaction and coordination. Prog Neurobiol 38:35–56

Mazzoleni S, Sale P, Franceschini M, Bigazzi S, Carrozza MC, Dario P, Posteraro F (2013) Effects of proximal and distal robot-assisted upper limb rehabilitation on chronic stroke recovery. Neurorehabilitation 33:33–39. https://doi.org/10.3233/NRE-130925

McFarland DJ, Wolpaw JR (2011) Brain-Computer Interfaces for communication and control. Commun ACM 54(5):60–66. https://doi.org/10.1145/1941487.1941506

McGeehan MA, Woollacott MH, Dalton BH (2017) Vestibular control of standing balance is enhanced with increased cognitive load. Exp Brain Res 235:1031–1040. https://doi.org/10.1007/s00221-016-4858-3

Mehrholz J, Thomas S, Werner C, Kugler J, Pohl, M, Elsner B (2017) Electromechanical-assisted training for walking after stroke. Cochrane Library 5(CD006185). https://doi.org/10.1002/14651858.CD006185.pub4

Mehrholz J, Pohl M, Platz T, Kugler J, Elsner B (2018) Electromechanical and robot-assisted arm training for improving activities of daily living, arm function and arm muscle strength after stroke. Cochrane Library 9(CD006876). https://doi.org/10.1002/14651858.CD006876.pub5

Meinecke L, Breitbach-Faller N, Bartz C, Damen R, Rau G, Disselhorst-Klug C (2006) Movement analysis in the early detection of newborns at risk for developing spasticity due to infantile cerebral palsy. Hum Mov Sci 25(2):125–144. https://doi.org/10.1016/j.humov.2005.09.012

Mettler T, Sprenger M, Winter R (2017) Service robots in hospitals: new perspectives on niche evolution and technology affordances. Eur J Inf Syst 26(5):451–468. https://doi.org/10.1057/s41303-017-0046-1

Metzger J, Lambercy O, Chapuis D, Gassert R (2014) Design and characterization of the ReHapticKnob, a robot for assessment and therapy of hand function. Journal of NeuroEngineering and Rehabilitation 11:154. https://doi.org/10.1109/IROS16071.2011

Meyer-Heim A, van Hedel HJ (2013) Robot-assisted and computer-enhanced therapies for children with cerebral palsy: current state and clinical implementation. Semin Pediatr Neurol 20(2):139–145. https://doi.org/10.1016/j.spen.2013.06.006

Meyer-Heim A, Borggraefe I, Ammann-Reiffer C, Berweck S, Sennhauser FH, Colombo G, Knecht B, Heinen F (2007) Feasibility of robotic-assisted locomotor training in children with central gait impairment. Dev Med Child Neurol 49(12):900–906. https://doi.org/10.1111/j.1469-8749.2007.00900.x

Meyer-Heim A, Ammann-Reiffer C, Schmartz A, Schäfer J, Sennhauser FH, Heinen F, Knecht B, Dabrowski E, Borggraefe I (2009) Improvement of walking abilities after robotic-assisted locomotion training in children with cerebral palsy. Arch Dis Child 94(8):615–620. https://doi.org/10.1136/adc.2008.145458

Middleton A, Simpson KN, Bettger JP, Bowden MG (2020) COVID-19 pandemic and beyond: considerations and costs of telehealth exercise programs for older adults with functional impairments living at home—lessons learned from a pilot case study. Phys Ther 100(8):1278–1288. https://doi.org/10.1093/ptj/pzaa089

Mills R, Levac D, Sveistrup H (2018) Kinematics and postural muscular activity during continuous oscillating platform movement in children and adolescents with cerebral palsy. Gait Posture 66:13–20. https://doi.org/10.1016/j.gaitpost.2018.08.002

Mills R, Levac D, Sveistrup H (2019) The effects of a 5-day Virtual-Reality Based Exercise Program on kinematics and postural muscle activity in youth with Cerebral Palsy. Phys Occup Ther Pediatr 39(4):388–403. https://doi.org/10.1080/01942638.2018.1505801

Mirbagheri MM, Barbeau H, Kearney RE (2000) Intrinsic and reflex contributions to human ankle stiffness: variation with activation level and position. Exp Brain Res 135(4):423–436. https://doi.org/10.1007/s002210000534

Molinaro A, Micheletti S, Pagani F, Garofalo G, Galli J, Rossi A, Fazzi E, Buccino G (2020) Action Observation Treatment in a tele-rehabilitation setting: a pilot study in children with cerebral palsy. Disabil Rehabil. https://doi.org/10.1080/09638288.2020.1793009

Morasso P (1981) Spatial control of arm movements. Exp Brain Res 42:223–227. https://doi.org/10.1007/BF00236911

Morasso P (2020) Centre of pressure versus centre of mass stabilization strategies: the tightrope balancing case. R Soc Open Sci 7:200111. https://doi.org/10.1098/rsos.200111

Morasso P, Casadio M, Giannoni P, Masia L, Sanguineti V, Squeri V, Vergaro E (2009) Desirable features of a "humanoid" robot-therapist. Conf Proc IEEE Eng Med Biol Soc 2009:2418–2421. https://doi.org/10.1109/IEMBS.2009.5334954

MPD Costruzioni Meccaniche (2010) Robot motor rehabilitation device, World Patent WO 2010/105773

Nashner LM (1982) Adaptation of human movement to altered environments. Trends Neurosci 5(10):358–361. https://doi.org/10.1016/0166-2236(82)90204-1

Nip ISB, Wilson EM, Kearney L (2018) Spatial characteristics of jaw movements during chewing in children with cerebral palsy: a pilot study. Dysphagia 33(1):33–40. https://doi.org/10.1007/s00455-017-9830-2

Nuyujukian P, Albites Sanabria J, Saab J, Pandarinath C, Jarosiewicz B, Blabe CH et al (2018) Cortical control of a tablet computer by people with paralysis. PLoS One 13(11):e0204566

Ohgi S, Morita S, Loo KK, Mizuike C (2008) Time series analysis of spontaneous upper-extremity movements of premature infants with brain injuries. Phys Ther 88(9):1022–1033. https://doi.org/10.2522/ptj.20070171

Olsen J, Marschik P, Spittle A (2018) Do fidgety general movements predict cerebral palsy and cognitive outcome in clinical follow-up of very preterm infants? Acta Paediatr 107:361–362. https://doi.org/10.1111/apa.14126

Orlandi S, Guzzetta A, Bandini A, Belmonti V, Barbagallo SD, Tealdi G, Mazzotti S, Scattoni ML, Manfredi C (2015) AVIM—a contactless system for infant data acquisition and analysis: software architecture and first results. Biomed Signal Process Control 20:85–99

Osawa Y, Shima K, Bu N, Tsuji T, Tsuji T, Ishii I, Matsuda H, Orito K, Ikeda T, Noda S (2008) A motion-based system to evaluate infant movements using real-time video analysis. In: Lim CT, Goh JCH, (eds) Proceedings ICBME 2008, Springer, pp 2043–2047. https://doi.org/10.1007/978-3-540-92841-6_509

Õunpuu S, Gorton G, Bagley A, Sison-Williamson M, Hassani S, Johnson B, Oeffinger D (2015) Variation in kinematic and spatiotemporal gait parameters by Gross Motor Function Classification System level in children and adolescents with cerebral palsy. Dev Med Child Neurol 2015(57):955–962. https://doi.org/10.1111/dmcn.12766

Paillard J (1980) Le corps situé et le corps identifié. Une approche psychophysiologique de la notion de schéma corporel. Rev Méd Suisse Romande 100:129–141

Park ES, Park CI, Lee HJ, Kim DY, Lee DS, Cho SR (2003) The characteristics of sit-to-stand transfer in young children with spastic cerebral palsy based on kinematic and kinetic data. Gait Posture 17(1):43–49. https://doi.org/10.1016/s0966-6362(02)00055-3

Pavão SL, Santos AN, Oliveira AB, Rocha NA (2015) Postural control during sit-to-stand movement and its relationship with upright position in children with hemiplegic spastic cerebral palsy and in typically developing children. Braz J Phys Ther 19(1):18–25. https://doi.org/10.1590/bjpt-rbf.2014.0069

Pellegrino L, Giannoni P, Marinelli L, Casadio M (2017) Effects of continuous visual feedback during sitting balance training in chronic stroke survivors. J Neuroeng Rehabil 14(1):107. https://doi.org/10.1186/s12984-017-0316-0

Perry J, Burnfield JM (1992) Gait analysis: normal and pathological function. SLACK Inc., Thorofare. ISBN 978-1-55642-766-4

Peterka RJ (2002) Sensorimotor integration in human postural control. J Neurophysiol 88:1097–1118. https://doi.org/10.1152/jn.00605.2001

Petrarca M, Frascarelli F, Carniel S, Colazza A, Minosse S, Tavarnese E, Castelli E (2021) Robotic-assisted locomotor treadmill therapy does not change gait pattern in children with cerebral palsy, Int J Rehab Res. 2021 Mar 1;44(1):69–76. https://doi.org/10.1097/MRR.0000000000000451 (2021)

Philippi H, Karch D, Kang KS, Wochner K, Pietz J, Dickhaus H, Hadders-Algra M (2014) Computer based analysis of general movements reveals stereotypies predicting cerebral palsy. Dev Med Child Neurol 56(10):960–967. https://doi.org/10.1111/dmcn.12477

Pickett K, Konczak J (2009) Measuring kinaesthetic sensitivity in typically developing children. Dev Med Child Neurol 2009(51):711–716. https://doi.org/10.1111/j.1469-8749.2008.03229.x

Pieskä S, Luimula M, Jauhiainen J, Spiz V (2012) Social Service Robots in public and private environments. In: Proceedings of the 11th WSEAS International Conference on Instrumentation, Measurement, Circuits and Systems, Rovaniemi, Finland, 18–20 Apr 2012, World Scientific and Engineering Academy and Society (WSEAS): Stevens Point, WI, USA, pp 190–195

Piovesan D, Morasso P, Giannoni P, Casadio M (2013) Arm stiffness during assisted movement after stroke: the influence of visual feedback and training. IEEE Trans Neural Syst Rehabil Eng 21(3):454–465. https://doi.org/10.1109/TNSRE.2012.2226915

Pisano F, Miscio G, Del Conte C, Pianca D, Candeloro E, Colombo R (2000) Quantitative measures of spasticity in post-stroke patients. Clin Neurophysiol 111(6):1015–1022. https://doi.org/10.1016/s1388-2457(00)00289-3

Pitron V, Alsmith A, de Vignemont F (2018) How do the body schema and the body image interact? Conscious Cogn 65:352–358. https://doi.org/10.1016/j.concog.2018.08.007

Popovic-Maneski L, Aleksic A, Metani A, Bergeron V, Cobeljic R, Popovic DB (2018) Assessment of spasticity by a pendulum test in SCI patients who exercise FES cycling or receive only conventional therapy. IEEE Trans Neural Syst Rehabil Eng 26(1):181–187. https://doi.org/10.1109/TNSRE.2017.2771466

Prechtl HFR (1990) Qualitative changes of spontaneous movements in fetus and preterm infant are a marker of neurological dysfunction. Early Hum Dev 23(3):151–158. https://doi.org/10.1016/0378-3782(90)90011-7

Prechtl HFR (1997) State of the art of a new functional assessment of the young nervous system. An early predictor of cerebral palsy. Early Hum Dev 50(1):1–11. https://doi.org/10.1016/S0378-3782(97)00088-1

Ramstrand N, Lyngegård F (2012) Can balance in children with cerebral palsy improve through use of an activity promoting computer game? Technol Health Care 20(6):501–510. https://doi.org/10.3233/THC-2012-0696

Reifenberg G, Gabrosek G, Tanner K, Harpster K (2017) Feasibility of pediatric game-based neurorehabilitation using telehealth technologies: a case report. Am J Occup Ther 71(3):7103190040p1. https://doi.org/10.5014/ajot.2017.024976

Rentschler AJ, Simpson R, Cooper RA, Boninger ML (2008) Clinical evaluation of Guido robotic walker. J Rehabil Res Dev 45(9):1281–1293. https://doi.org/10.1682/JRRD.2007.10.0160

Rethlefsen SA, Blumstein G, Kay RM, Dorey F, Wren TAL (2017) Prevalence of specific gait abnormalities in children with cerebral palsy revisited: influence of age, prior surgery and Gross Motor Function Classification System level. Dev Med Child Neurol 59(1):79–88. https://doi.org/10.1111/dmcn.13205

Richards CL, Malouin F, Dumas F, Marcoux S, Lepage C, Menier C (1997) Early and intensive treadmill locomotor training for young children with cerebral palsy: a feasibility study. Pediatr Phys Ther 158–165

Ríos-Rincón AM, Adams K, Magill-Evans J, Cook A (2016) Playfulness in children with limited motor abilities when using a robot. Phys Occup Ther Pediatr 2016(36):232–246. https://doi.org/10.3109/01942638.2015.1076559

Roncesvalles N, Woollacott M, Jensen JL (2000) The development of compensatory stepping skills in children. J Mot Behav 32(1):100–111. https://doi.org/10.1080/00222890009601363

Rose J, Wolff DR, Jones VK, Bloch DA, Oehlert JW, Gamble JG (2002) Postural balance in children with cerebral palsy. Dev Med Child Neurol 44:58–63. https://doi.org/10.1017/S0012162201001669

Russell S, Bennett B, Sheth P, Abel M (2011) The gait of children with and without cerebral palsy: work, energy and angular momentum. J Appl Biomech 27(2):99–107. https://doi.org/10.1123/jab.27.2.99

Ryan JL, Wright FV, Levac DE (2020) Exploring physiotherapists' use of motor learning strategies in gait-based interventions for children with cerebral palsy. Phys Occup Ther Pediatr 40(1):79–92. https://doi.org/10.1080/01942638.2019.1622623

Sale P, Lombardi V, Franceschini M (2012) Hand robotics rehabilitation: feasibility and preliminary results of a robotic treatment in patients with hemiparesis. Stroke Res Treat 2012(5):82093. https://doi.org/10.1155/2012/820931

Sandini G, Mohan V, Sciutti A, Morasso P (2018) Social cognition for human-robot symbiosis—challenges and building blocks. Front Neurorobot. https://doi.org/10.3389/fnbot.2018.00034

Schabrun SM, Hillier S (2009) Evidence for the retraining of sensation after stroke: a systematic review. Clin Rehabil 23:27–39. https://doi.org/10.1177/0269215508098897

Schmidt H (2004) Haptic Walker—a novel haptic device for walking simulation. In: Proc. of EuroHaptics, 2004, Munich, Germany, 5–7 June 2004

Schwoebel J, Coslett HB (2005) Evidence for multiple, distinct representations of the human body. J Cogn Neurosci 17(4):543–553. https://doi.org/10.1162/0898929053467587

Seth N, Johnson D, Taylor GW, Allen OB, Abdullah HA (2015) Robotic pilot study for analysing spasticity: clinical data versus healthy controls. J Neuroeng Rehabil 12:109. https://doi.org/10.1186/s12984-015-0103-8

Shadmehr R, Mussa-Ivaldi FA (1994) Adaptive representation of dynamics during learning of a motor task. J Neurosci 14(5):3208–3224. https://doi.org/10.1523/JNEUROSCI.14-05-03208

Sharkey A, Sharkey N (2011) Children, the elderly, and interactive robots. IEEE Robot Autom Mag 18:32–38. https://doi.org/10.1109/MRA.2010.940151

Shiratori T, Girolami GL, Aruin AS (2016) Anticipatory postural adjustments associated with a loading perturbation in children with hemiplegic and diplegic cerebral palsy. Exp Brain Res 234(10):2967–2978. https://doi.org/10.1007/s00221-016-4699-0

Shumway-Cook A, Woollacott MH (2016) Motor control. Translating research into clinical practice, 5th edn. Lippincott Williams & Wilkins, Baltimore

Simon-Martinez C, Mailleux L, Hoskens J, Ortibus E, Jaspers E, Wenderoth N, Sgandurra G, Cioni G, Molenaers G, Klingels K, Feys H (2020) Randomized controlled trial combining constraint-induced movement therapy and action-observation training in unilateral cerebral palsy: clinical effects and influencing factors of treatment response. Ther Adv Neurol Disord 13:1756286419898065. https://doi.org/10.1177/1756286419898065

Smania N, Bonetti P, Gandolfi M, Cosentino A (2011) Improved gait after repetitive locomotor training in children with cerebral palsy. Am J Phys Med Rehabil 90(2):137–149. https://doi.org/10.1097/PHM.0b013e318201741e

Sobera M, Siedlecka B, Syczewska M (2011) Posture control development in children aged 2-7 years old, based on the changes of repeatability of the stability indices. Neurosci Lett 491(1):13–17. https://doi.org/10.1016/j.neulet.2010.12.061

Spenko M, Yu H, Dubowsky S (2006) Robotic personal aids for mobility and monitoring for the elderly. IEEE Trans Neural Syst Rehabil Eng 14(3):344–351. https://doi.org/10.1109/TNSRE.2006.881534

Summa S, Pierella C, Giannoni P, Sciacchitano A, Iacovelli S, Farshchiansadegh A, Mussa-Ivaldi FA, Casadio M (2015) A body-machine interface for training selective pelvis movements in stroke survivors: a pilot study. Conf Proc IEEE Eng Med Biol Soc 2015:4663–4666. https://doi.org/10.1109/EMBC.2015.7319434

Surana BK, Ferre CL, Dew AP, Brandao M, Gordon AM, Noelle G, Moreau NG (2019) Effectiveness of Lower-Extremity Functional Training (LIFT) in young children with Unilateral Spastic Cerebral Palsy: a randomized controlled trial. Neurorehabil Neural Repair 33(10):862–872. https://doi.org/10.1177/1545968319868719

Swank C, Wang-Price S, Gao F, Almutairi S (2019) Walking with a robotic exoskeleton does not mimic natural gait: a within-subjects study. JMIR Rehabil Assist Technol 6(1):e11023. https://doi.org/10.2196/11023

Syamimi S, Norjasween AM, Hanafiah Y, Salina M, Fazah AH, Farhana WY (2014) Telerehabilitation in robotic assistive therapy for children with developmental disabilities. In: 2014 IEEE Region 10 Symposium. https://doi.org/10.1109/TENCONSpring.2014.6863060

Tacchino C, Impagliazzo M, Maggi E, Bertamino M, Blanchi I, Campone F, Durand P, Fato M, Giannoni P, Iandolo R, Izzo M, Morasso P, Moretti P, Ramenghi L, Shima K, Shimatani K, Tsuji T, Uccella S, Zanardi N, Casadio M (2021) Quantitative video analysis of spontaneous movements of the newborns: a tool of quantitative video analysis of preterm babies. Comput Methods Prog Biomed 199:105838. https://doi.org/10.1016/j.cmpb.2020.105838

Tarakci D, Huseyinsinoglu BE, Tarakci E, Ozdincler AR (2016) Effects of Nintendo Wii-Fit ® video games on balance in children with mild cerebral palsy. Pediatr Int 58(10):1042–1050. https://doi.org/10.1111/ped.12942

Tarakci E, Arman N, Tarakci D, Kasapcopur O (2019) Leap Motion Controller-based training for upper extremity rehabilitation in children and adolescents with physical disabilities: a randomized controlled trial. J Hand Ther 33(2):220–228.e1. https://doi.org/10.1016/j.jht.2019.03.012

Thilmann AF, Schwarz M, Töpper R, Fellows SJ, Noth J (1991) Different mechanisms underlie the long-latency stretch reflex response of active human muscle at different joints. J Physiol 444(1):631–643. https://doi.org/10.1113/jphysiol.1991.sp018898

Topping M (2000) An overview of the development of Handy 1, a rehabilitation robot to assist the severely disabled. Artif Life Robot 4:188–192. https://doi.org/10.1007/BF02481173

Tseng YT, Tsai CL, Chen FC, Konczak J (2017) Position sense dysfunction affects proximal and distal arm joints in children with developmental coordination disorder. J Mot Behav 51(1):49–58. https://doi.org/10.1080/00222895.2017.1415200

Tsuji T, Morasso P, Goto K, Ito K (1995) Human hand impedance characteristics during maintained posture in multi-joint arm movements. Biol Cybern 72:475–485

Tsuji T, Nakashima S, Hayashi H, Soh Z, Furui A, Shibanoki T, Shima K, Shimatani K (2020) Markerless measurement and evaluation of general movements in infants. Sci Rep 10:1422. https://doi.org/10.1038/s41598-020-57580-z

Turolla A, Dam M, Ventura L, Tonin P, Agostini M, Zucconi C, Kiper P, Cagnin A, Piron L (2013) Virtual reality for the rehabilitation of the upper limb motor function after stroke: a prospective controlled trial. J Neuroeng Rehabil 10:85. https://doi.org/10.1186/1743-0003-10-85

Tyagi S, Lim DSY, Ho WHH, Koh YQ, Cai V, Koh GCK, Legido-Quigley H (2018) Acceptance of tele-rehabilitation by stroke patients: perceived barriers and facilitators. Arch Phys Med Rehabil 99(12):2472–2477.e2. https://doi.org/10.1016/j.apmr.2018.04.033

Vähä-Ypyä H, Husu P, Suni J, Vasankari T, Sievänen H (2018) Reliable recognition of lying, sitting, and standing with a hip-worn accelerometer. Scand J Med Sci Sports 28:1092–1102. https://doi.org/10.1111/sms.13017

Valkenet K, Veenhof C (2019) Validity of three accelerometers to investigate lying, sitting, standing and walking. PLoS One 14(5):e0217545. https://doi.org/10.1371/journal.pone.0217545

van den Noort JC, Scholtes VA, Harlaar J (2009) Evaluation of clinical spasticity assessment in cerebral palsy using inertial sensors. Gait Posture 30(2):138–143. https://doi.org/10.1016/j.gaitpost.2009.05.011

van Hedel HJA, Wick K, Meyer-Heim A, Eng K (2011) Improving dexterity in children with cerebral palsy. Preliminary results of a randomized trial evaluating a glove based VR-system. In: International Conference on Virtual Rehabilitation, 2011, Rehab Week Zurich, ETH Zurich Science City, Switzerland

van Hedel HJ, Meyer-Heim A, Rüsch-Bohtz C (2016) Robot-assisted gait training might be beneficial for more severely affected children with cerebral palsy. Dev Neurorehabil 19(6):410–415. https://doi.org/10.3109/17518423.2015.1017661

Van Sint Jan S, Bonnechère B, Moureau D, Brassine E, Sholukha V, Moiseev F (2015) Novel solution for performing regular objective functional assessments for follow-up of neuro-muscular disorders. Physiotherapy 101(S1):e1577–e1578. https://doi.org/10.1016/j.physio.2015.03.1581

Varriale L, Briganti P, Mele S (2020) Disability and home automation: insights and challenges within organizational settings. In: Lazazzara A, Ricciardi F, Za S (eds) Exploring digital ecosystems. Lecture notes in Information Systems and Organisation, vol 33. Springer, Cham. https://doi.org/10.1007/978-3-030-23665-6_5

Vaz DV, Cotta Mancini M, Fonseca ST, Vieira DS, de Melo Pertence AE (2006) Muscle stiffness and strength and their relation to hand function in children with hemiplegic cerebral palsy. Dev Med Child Neurol 48(9):728–733. https://doi.org/10.1017/S0012162206001563

Veerbeek JM, Langbroek-Amersfoort AC, van Wegen EEH, Meskers CGM, Kwakkel G (2017) Effects of robot-assisted therapy for the upper limb after stroke. Neurorehabil Neural Repair 31(2):107–121. https://doi.org/10.1177/1545968316666957

Velasco MA, Muzzioli L, Morelli D, Otero A, Iosa M, Cincotti F, Rocon E (2017) Evaluation of cervical posture improvement of children with cerebral palsy after physical therapy based on head movements and serious games. Biomed Eng Online 16(Suppl 1):74. https://doi.org/10.1186/s12938-017-0364-5

Veneman J, Kruidhof R, Hekman E, Ekkelenkamp R, Van Asseldonk E, van der Kooij H (2007) Design and evaluation of the LOPES exoskeleton robot for interactive gait rehabilitation. IEEE Trans Neural Syst Rehabil Eng 15(3):379–386. https://doi.org/10.1109/TNSRE.2007.903919. ISSN 1534-4320

Vergaro E, Casadio M, Squeri V, Giannoni P, Morasso P, Sanguineti V (2010) Self-adaptive robot-training of stroke patients for continuous tracking movements. J Neuroeng Rehabil 7:13. https://doi.org/10.1186/1743-0003-7-13

Wachner A, Edinger J, Becker C (2018) Towards gaze-based mobile device interaction for the disabled. In: 3rd IEEE Workshop on Pervasive Health Technologies, Athens, Greece, 19–23 Mar, pp 397–402. https://doi.org/10.1109/PERCOMW.2018.8480159

Wachsmuth I (2018) Robots Like Me: challenges and ethical issues in aged care. Front Psychol 9:432. https://doi.org/10.3389/fpsyg.2018.00432

Waddington G, Rogers A (1999) Discrimination of active plantarflexion and inversion movements after ankle injury. Aust J Physiother 45(1):7–13. https://doi.org/10.1016/s0004-9514(14)60335-4

Waite MC, Theodoros DG, Russell TG, Cahill LM (2010) Internet-based telehealth assessment of language using the CELF-4. Lang Speech Hear Serv Sch 41(4):445–458. https://doi.org/10.1044/0161-1461(2009/08-0131)

Wallard L, Dietrich G, Kerlirzin Y, Bredin J (2017) Robotic-assisted gait training improves walking abilities in diplegic children with cerebral palsy. Eur J Paediatr Neurol 21(3):557–564. https://doi.org/10.1016/j.ejpn.2017.01.012

Wallard L, Dietrich G, Kerlirzin Y, Bredin J (2018) Effect of robotic-assisted gait rehabilitation on dynamic equilibrium control in the gait of children with cerebral palsy. Gait Posture 60:55–60. https://doi.org/10.1016/j.gaitpost.2017.11.007

Wandell KJ, Birkenmeier RL, Moore JL, Hornby TG, Lang CE (2014) Feasibility of high-repetition, task-specific training for individuals with upper-extremity paresis. Am J Occup Ther 68(4):444–453. https://doi.org/10.5014/ajot.2014.011619

Wang TN, Tseng MH, Wilson BN, Hu FC (2009) Functional performance of children with developmental coordination disorder at home and at school. Dev Med Child Neurol 51(10):817–825. https://doi.org/10.1111/j.1469-8749.2009.03271.x

Wang ZR, Wang P, Xing L, Mei LP, Zhao J, Zhang T (2017) Leap Motion-based virtual reality training for improving motor functional recovery of upper limbs and neural reorganization in subacute stroke patients. Neural Regen Res 12(11):1823–1831. https://doi.org/10.4103/1673-5374.219043

Ward EC, Sharma S, Clare Burns C, Theodoros D, Russell T (2012) Managing patient factors in the assessment of swallowing via telerehabilitation. Int J Telemed Appl 2012:132719. https://doi.org/10.1155/2012/132719

Wästlund E, Sponseller K, Pettersson O, Bared A (2015) Evaluating gaze-driven power wheelchair with navigation support for persons with disabilities. J Rehabil Res Dev 52(7):815–826. https://doi.org/10.1682/JRRD.2014.10.0228

Willems T, Witvrouw E, Verstuyft J, Vaes P, De Clercq D (2002) Proprioception and muscle strength in subjects with a history of ankle sprains and chronic instability. J Athl Train 37:487–493

Willoughby KL, Dodd KJ, Shields N (2009) A systematic review of the effectiveness of treadmill training for children with cerebral palsy. Disabil Rehabil 31(24):1971–1979. https://doi.org/10.3109/09638280902874204

Wingert JR, Burton H, Sinclair RJ, Brunstrom JE, Damiano DL (2009) Joint-position sense and kinesthesia in cerebral palsy. Arch Phys Med Rehabil 90(3):447–453. https://doi.org/10.1016/j.apmr.2008.08.217

Winter DA, Patla AE, Ishac M, Gage WH (2003) Motor mechanisms of balance during quiet standing. J Electromyogr Kinesiol 13(1):49–56. https://doi.org/10.1016/s1050-6411(02)00085-8

Winters JM (2002) Telerehabilitation research: emerging opportunities. Annu Rev Biomed Eng 4:287–320. https://doi.org/10.1146/annurev.bioeng.4.112801.121923

Wirtz J, Patterson P, Kunz W, Gruber T, Lu VN, Paluch S, Martins A (2018) Brave new world: service robots in the frontline. J Serv Manag 29(5):907–931. https://doi.org/10.1108/JOSM-04-2018-0119

Wolbrecht ET, Chan V, Reinkensmeyer D, Bobrow JE (2008) Optimizing compliant, model-based robotic assistance to promote neurorehabilitation. IEEE Transactions on Neural Systems and Rehabilitation Engineering 16(3):286–297. https://doi.org/10.1109/TNSRE.2008.918389

Wolff A, Sama A, Lenhoff M, Daluiski A (2020) The use of wearable inertial sensors effectively quantify arm asymmetry during gait in children with unilateral spastic cerebral palsy. J Hand Ther 19:S0894-1130(20)30074-0. https://doi.org/10.1016/j.jht.2020.03.026

Woollacott MH, Shumway-Cook A (2005) Postural dysfunction during standing and walking in children with cerebral palsy: what are the underlying problems and what new therapies might improve balance? Neural Plast 12(2-3):211–9; discussion 263–272. https://doi.org/10.1155/NP.2005.211

World Health Organization (2015) WHO global disability action plan 2014–2021. World Health Organization, Geneva

World Health Organization Global Cooperation on Assistive Technology (GATE) (2016). http://www.who.int/phi/implementation/assistive_technology/phi_gate/en/. Accessed 11 Aug 2016

Wren TAL, Tucker CA, Rethlefsen SA, Gorton GE, Õunpuu S (2020) Clinical efficacy of instrumented gait analysis: systematic review 2020 update. Gait Posture 80:274–279. https://doi.org/10.1016/j.gaitpost.2020.05.031

Wu M, Kim J, Gaebler-Spira DJ, Schmit BD, Arora P (2017) Robotic resistance treadmill training improves locomotor function in children with cerebral palsy: a randomized controlled pilot study. Arch Phys Med Rehabil 98(11):2126–2133. https://doi.org/10.1016/j.apmr.2017.04.022

Yasuda K, Sato Y, Iimura N, Iwata H (2014) Allocation of attentional resources toward a secondary cognitive task leads to compromised ankle proprioceptive performance in healthy young adults. Rehabil Res Pract 2014:7. https://doi.org/10.1155/2014/170304

Yoon J, Novandy B, Yoon C, Park K (2010) A 6-DOF Gait Rehabilitation Robot with upper and lower-limb connections that allows walking velocity updates on various terrains. IEEE Trans Mechatron 15(2):201–215. https://doi.org/10.1109/TMECH.2010.2040834

Zhang J, Jadavji Z, Zewdie E, Kirton A (2019) Evaluating if children can use simple brain computer interfaces. Front Hum Neurosci. https://doi.org/10.3389/fnhum.2019.00024

Zoccolillo L, Morelli D, Cincotti F, Muzzioli L, Gobbetti T, Paolucci S, Iosa M (2015) Video-game based therapy performed by children with cerebral palsy: a cross-over randomized controlled trial and a cross-sectional quantitative measure of physical activity. Eur J Phys Rehabil Med 51(6):669–676

Printed in the United States
by Baker & Taylor Publisher Services